Obstetric and Gynaecological Ultrasound

For Elsevier

Senior Content Strategist: Rita Demetriou-Swanwick
Content Development Specialist: Nicola Lally
Project Manager: Umarani Natarajan
Designer/Design Direction: Miles Hitchen
Illustration Manager: Lesley Fraser
Illustrator: Antbits and Hardlines

Obstetric and Gynaecological Ultrasound

How, Why and When

Fourth Edition

Trish Chudleigh PhD, DMU
Specialist Sonographer for Education & Training,
The Rosie Hospital,
Cambridge University Hospitals NHS Foundation Trust,
Cambridge, UK

Alison Smith MSc, DMU
Tutor Sonographer,
Women's Health & Fetal Medicine,
Guy's & St Thomas' NHS Foundation Trust,
London, UK

Sonia Cumming RGN, RM, PGCert
Midwife Sonographer,
The Rosie Hospital,
Cambridge University Hospitals NHS Foundation Trust,
Cambridge, UK

ELSEVIER
Edinburgh • London • New York • Oxford • Philadelphia • St Louis • Sydney • Toronto 2017

ELSEVIER

© 2017 Elsevier Ltd. All rights reserved.

First edition 1986
Second edition 1992
Third edition 2004

ISBN 978-0-7020-3170-0

Notices

Knowledge and best practice in this field are constantly changing. As new research and experience broaden our understanding, changes in research methods, professional practices, or medical treatment may become necessary.

Practitioners and researchers must always rely on their own experience and knowledge in evaluating and using any information, methods, compounds, or experiments described herein. In using such information or methods they should be mindful of their own safety and the safety of others, including parties for whom they have a professional responsibility.

With respect to any drug or pharmaceutical products identified, readers are advised to check the most current information provided (i) on procedures featured or (ii) by the manufacturer of each product to be administered, to verify the recommended dose or formula, the method and duration of administration, and contraindications. It is the responsibility of practitioners, relying on their own experience and knowledge of their patients, to make diagnoses, to determine dosages and the best treatment for each individual patient, and to take all appropriate safety precautions.

To the fullest extent of the law, neither the Publisher nor the authors, contributors, or editors, assume any liability for any injury and/or damage to persons or property as a matter of products liability, negligence or otherwise, or from any use or operation of any methods, products, instructions, or ideas contained in the material herein.

ELSEVIER your source for books, journals and multimedia in the health sciences

www.elsevierhealth.com

Working together to grow libraries in developing countries

www.elsevier.com • www.bookaid.org

The publisher's policy is to use paper manufactured from sustainable forests

Printed in India

Last digit is the print number: 10 9

Dedication

To Ben

Contents

Contributor

Tony Evans BSc, MSc, PhD, CEng, BC, Sci, FIPEM
Senior Lecturer in Medical Physics,
University of Leeds, Leeds, UK

Foreword

To be invited to write a foreword is an honour, and to be asked to write one for this particular book is a privilege.

The authors are very experienced and knowledgeable clinical sonographers and this has enabled them to understand what information is required in a text such as this. This text is perfect for all students of obstetric and gynaecological ultrasound and should also be a standard bench textbook in every ultrasound department. Experienced sonographers will benefit from consulting this text when specific queries arise, and it will also bring them up to date with current best ultrasound practice.

The authors have used their specific experiences to include areas such as professional issues, reporting and medico legal aspects of ultrasound practice, but this advanced knowledge has not made them forget the very basic aspects such as preparing to scan, that are so important to all new students of ultrasound.

The style, content and information contained in this book make it very important, and it is viewed by many as the most influential text on obstetric and gynaecological ultrasound in the United Kingdom and much farther afield.

I congratulate the authors on this latest edition, which provides sonographers with up to date and best obstetric and gynaecological ultrasound practice.

Jean Wilson DCR(R), DMU, BEd, PGD(Man)
Senior Lecturer
MSc Programme Leader
School of Medicine
University of Leeds

Preface

We are delighted to introduce the fourth edition of this text, which, as in previous editions, combines best practice with practical advice. The principal aims of this edition are essentially unchanged from previous editions. It is designed as a teaching guide for students learning to scan and as a scanning companion for those with more clinical expertise and ultrasound experience.

Ultrasound students traditionally undertake a programme of training which typically incorporates both obstetric and gynaecological ultrasound. Many qualified practitioners perform both obstetric and gynaecological examinations in their routine practice. As there is also an overlap between the two specialities in clinical practice, we have chosen to expand this new text to include four chapters on scanning the nonpregnant pelvis.

We recognize that the ultrasound trainee is faced with the challenges of understanding and appreciating the similarities of and differences in using the transabdominal and transvaginal approaches to scanning. Practical and relevant advice accompanies each section to guide the student in how to obtain the correct sections when using both types of probe.

Since publication of the third edition, significant changes have taken place in how routine obstetric screening programmes are delivered. For those ultrasound practitioners involved in first trimester screening, the remit is ever evolving. Understanding the purpose of the examination, the techniques involved and the interpretation and implications of the results is required. In this edition we have therefore devoted a chapter to dating and screening for chromosomal abnormalities to reflect these advancements in first trimester ultrasound examinations.

The introduction of the national fetal anomaly screening programme has impacted on all departments involved in fetal anomaly screening in England. As ultrasound technologies evolve, the ability to image fetal anatomy in greater detail increases. Subsequently there is a need for the ultrasound practitioner to identify, appreciate and differentiate between what is normal, what is not normal and what is abnormal. We have chosen therefore to discuss both the normal and abnormal ultrasound appearances for each of the body areas together rather than describe them in different chapters. This is because we feel this more closely reflects true clinical practice.

It is very important to understand how imaging and Doppler work, and therefore we are indebted to Dr Tony Evans for explaining the principles of ultrasound, Doppler ultrasound and instrumentation with such clarity.

We hope this text will be a useful aide for those learning to scan and also for those experienced practitioners who are responsible for performing and/or teaching students in their own departments.

Trish Chudleigh, Alison Smith, Sonia Cumming
April 2016

Acknowledgements

Jillian Brown, Dr Ali Al Chami Angela Clough, Elizabeth Daly Jones, Dr Osama Naji, Sharon Watty, Jo Wolfenden, Dr Rob Yates, the administration team and all the sonographers and midwife sonographers from the Rosie Ultrasound Department without whose input and support this book could not have been written and illustrated.

The principles of ultrasound, Doppler ultrasound and instrumentation

Tony Evans

This chapter addresses the physical principles of ultrasound which need to be understood in order to be able to perform ultrasound examinations properly and safely.

The aims of this chapter are to:

- explain the basic principles of how ultrasound and Doppler ultrasound work
- explain the factors that affect the quality of the images obtained
- discuss the issues surrounding the safety of ultrasound.

2D ULTRASOUND

Ultrasound is simply very high frequency (high pitch) sound. Human ears can detect sound with frequencies lying between 20 Hz and 20 kHz. Middle C in music has a frequency of about 500 Hz and each octave represents a doubling of that frequency. Although some animals such as bats and dolphins can generate and receive sounds at frequencies higher than 20 kHz, this is normally taken to be the limit of sound. Mechanical vibrations at frequencies above 20 kHz are defined as ultrasound.

Medical imaging uses frequencies that are much higher than 20 kHz; the range normally used is 3–15 MHz. These frequencies do not occur in nature, and it is only within the last 60 years that the technology has existed to both generate and detect this type of ultrasound wave in a practical way.

WAVE PROPERTIES

In order to describe a wave, it is not sufficient to say that it has a certain frequency; we must also specify the type of wave and the medium through which it is travelling. Ultrasound waves are longitudinal, compression waves. The material through which they travel experiences cyclical variations in pressure. In other words, within each small region

MATERIAL	SPEED OF SOUND (m s⁻¹)
Air	330
Water	1480
Steel	5000
Blood	1575
Fat	1459
Muscle	1580
Cortical bone	3500

Table 1.1 Speed of sound in various materials

FREQUENCY (MHz)	WAVELENGTH (mm)
3	0.51
5	0.31
7	0.22
10	0.15

Table 1.2 Values for the wavelength (mm) of ultrasound waves in soft tissue for different frequencies, assuming a sound speed of 1540 m s⁻¹

there is a succession of compressions or squeezing followed shortly afterwards by rarefactions or stretching. The molecules within any material are attracted to each other by binding forces that hold the material together. These same forces are responsible for passing on the pressure variations. It is as though the molecules were joined by springs such that a stretch and release at one end would create a disturbance that travelled across the material to the other side. If the springs are stiff, i.e. require a lot of force to create a small change in length, then the disturbance will travel quickly. Softer or more compressible materials will require more time to respond fully and hence the disturbance or wave will travel slowly. Some examples of sound wave speeds in different materials are given in Table 1.1.

It is readily seen from Table 1.1 that the stiffer materials are associated with the higher sound speeds. It is also noteworthy that the speed of sound in most soft tissues is similar and close to that of water, which is perhaps not surprising in view of their high water content. It turns out that this is critical in the design of ultrasound scanning systems as we see in the next section. In fact, all ultrasound scanners are set up on the assumption that the speed of sound in all tissues is 1540 m s⁻¹. We can see that this is not strictly true but is nevertheless a reasonable approximation.

Having chosen to generate a wave at a particular frequency f, in a particular material with a speed of sound c, the wavelength λ (lambda) is automatically determined. Their relationship is simple:

$$c = f\lambda$$

If we rearrange the above expression, we see that $\lambda = c/f$ and we can calculate the wavelength for an ultrasound wave in soft tissue, assuming a 1540 m s⁻¹ speed of sound (Table 1.2).

Note that the wavelength is always a fraction of a millimetre and that it gets shorter as the frequency rises. This will have an important influence on the quality of the ultrasound images.

THE PULSE-ECHO PRINCIPLE

The principle underlying the formation of ultrasound images is the same as that of underwater sonar (**so**und **na**vigation and **r**anging) used by submarines and fishing boats. It relies on the generation of a short burst of sound and the detection of echoes from reflectors in front of it. The same principle applies when we hear our voices reflected from, say, walls or in tunnels.

If we consider the case in Fig. 1.1, the person P can detect the presence of the wall but can also work out the distance D to the wall by measuring the time it takes for the burst of sound to travel to the wall and back, provided certain assumptions are made. These include the following:

- sound travels in straight lines
- the speed of sound is the same in all materials through which it is travelling and is known
- all echoes received are generated at the interface between the wall and the surrounding medium.

We can then perform the following substitutions:

- sound becomes ultrasound
- the 'person' becomes a device (a transducer) which can send and receive the ultrasound

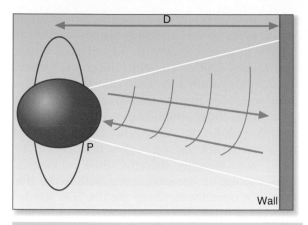

Fig 1.1 • Pulse-echo principle.

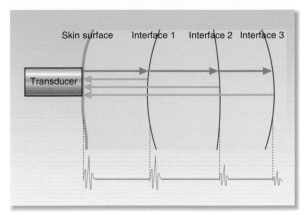

Fig 1.3 • Pulse-echo principle with multiple reflectors.

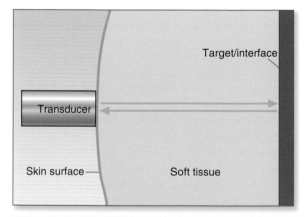

Fig 1.2 • Pulse-echo principle in tissue.

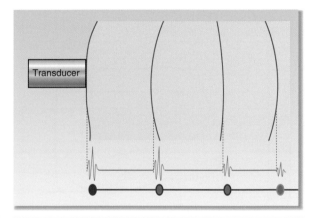

Fig 1.4 • Spot brightness related to echo amplitude.

- the air becomes soft tissue
- the wall becomes a target or interface within the soft tissue.

This creates the situation shown in Fig. 1.2 where echoes are received from a structure inside the body but where the pulse-echo principle still applies and the above assumptions are still made.

If there are two or more targets or interfaces behind each other, we can expect to receive echoes from each, although the echoes from the more distant targets will arrive later. In this way, we can build up a kind of one-dimensional map of the positions of reflectors lying along the direction of the sound beam (Fig. 1.3).

2D SCANNING

The one-dimensional view of Fig. 1.3 is known as the A-scan. It is difficult to interpret anatomically without detailed prior knowledge or assumptions and is of limited clinical value. To produce a more useful two-dimensional (2D) scan, it is necessary to obtain a series of A-scans and assemble them in a convenient format. This is done either by moving the transducer using a suitable mechanical device or else having more than one transducer. The latter option is preferred in modern scanners and the 'transducer' which is held by the operator in fact contains a row or array of many transducers (typically 100–200). In this way a series of A-scans can be obtained in a closely packed regular format. For the purposes of display, the amplitude (height) of each echo is represented by the brightness of a spot at that position. Fig. 1.4 illustrates how the echo amplitudes from the previous section can be turned into spot brightnesses.

This display mode in which the x and y directions relate to real distances in tissue and the greyscale is used to represent echo strength is known as the B-scan (Fig. 1.5).

TIME GAIN COMPENSATION

The echoes shown in Fig. 1.3 show a steady decline in amplitude with increasing depth. This occurs for two reasons. First, each successive reflection removes some energy from the pulse, leaving less for the generation of later echoes. Second, tissue absorbs ultrasound strongly and so there is a steady loss of energy simply because the ultrasound pulse is travelling through tissue. This is generally considered to be a nuisance and therefore attempts are made to correct for it. The amount of amplification or gain given to the incoming signals is made to increase simultaneously with the arrival of echoes from greater depths. The machine control that is used for this is called the time gain compensation (TGC) control and it is fitted to virtually all machines

Of course, the assumption that all echoes should be made equal is not really valid. We will see later that some structures, e.g. organ boundaries, are much more strongly reflective than others, e.g. small regions of inhomogeneity within the placenta. The operator needs to use the TGC control with care if misleading images are not to be produced. Providing excessive TGC can turn the normally echo-poor region within a fluid-filled cyst into one that seems to have many small echoes, thereby resembling a tumour. Also, if excessive TGC is used close to the surface, the receiving circuits can be saturated. This can have the effect of causing a blurring of the fine detail and a loss of information. Fig. 1.6 shows the same anatomical sections of an ovarian cyst with both correct and incorrect TGC settings (see also Chapter 2).

The layout of the TGC controls varies from one machine to another. One of the most popular options is a set of slider knobs. Normally each knob in the slider set controls the gain for a specific depth. It is the task of the operator to set each level for each patient, and often it is necessary to adjust the TGC during a clinical examination when moving from one anatomical region to another.

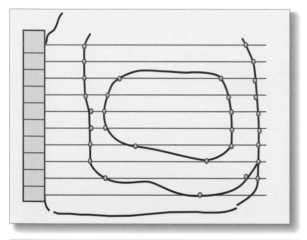

Fig 1.5 • Principle of B-scanning using a linear array.

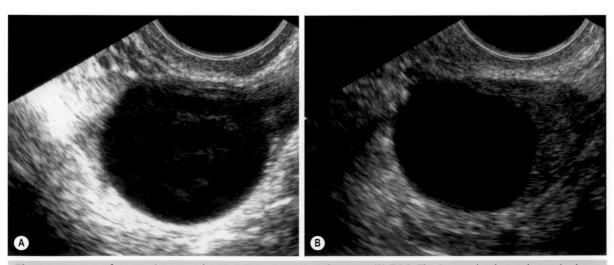

Fig 1.6 • Images of an ovarian cyst showing incorrect (A) and correct (B) TGC. The internal echoes shown in A are artefactual owing to the incorrect TGC settings.

GENERATION, DETECTION AND DIFFRACTION

The device that both generates the ultrasound and detects the returning echoes is the transducer. Transducers are made from materials that exhibit a property known as piezoelectricity. Piezoelectric behaviour is found in many naturally occurring materials including quartz but medical transducers are made from a synthetic ceramic material, lead zirconate titanate. This is fired in a kiln just as any other ceramic and can therefore be moulded into almost any shape. In order to establish an electrical connection, thin layers of silver are evaporated onto the surface to form electrodes. This creates a device which will expand and contract when a voltage is applied to it but will also create a voltage when subject to a small pressure such as a returning echo might exert. Obviously the voltages generated while receiving echoes are normally much smaller than those applied to create the ultrasound wave in the first instance. This process is illustrated in Fig. 1.7.

Diffraction is a process that occurs when a wave encounters an obstacle which has dimensions which are comparable to its wavelength. In this case, the transducer itself can be seen as such an obstacle. The diffraction process has a strong influence on the shape of the beam that is generated by ultrasound transducers, and in some respects this is unexpected. In Fig.1.5 the 2D image is shown as being assembled from a series of parallel scan lines. The implied assumption made is that each individual scan line or beam is very 'thin' and neither convergent nor divergent. It might be assumed that a thin beam would best be produced by a narrow source in the same way as a beam of light from a small torch would be narrower than that from a larger one. However, for diffractive sources this is not true. Fig. 1.8A shows a simplified version of the beam shape from three transducers of different sizes. In all three cases two different regions can be seen. The first region, closer to the source, roughly approximates to the ideal parallel beam concept. This is known as the near field. At some point, this pattern changes into a shape that is divergent and appears to have come from a point at the centre of the source. This region is called the far field. In Fig. 1.8A most of the beam is in the near field. Fig. 1.8B shows a much smaller source from where it can be seen that the divergent far field dominates. Fig. 1.8C shows an intermediate source. The distance at which the near field pattern changes to the far field pattern clearly depends upon the source diameter. In fact, it turns out that for a circular source, the distance d at which this transition takes place is given by

$$d = a^2/\lambda$$

where a is the radius of the source and λ is the wavelength. Therefore we have a conflict. If we want a narrow beam, we would normally select a small diameter source, but this will also result in a beam that will diverge readily. If we want a beam that is reluctant to diverge, then this requires a

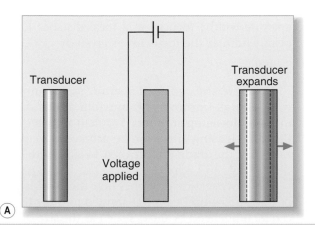

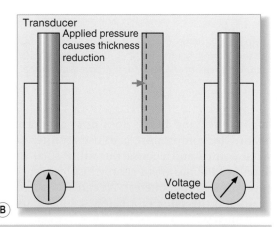

Fig 1.7 • A. Generation of ultrasound using a piezoelectric device. B. Detection of ultrasound using a piezoelectric device.

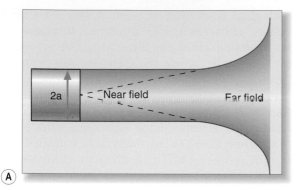

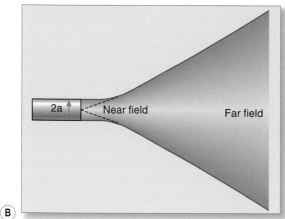

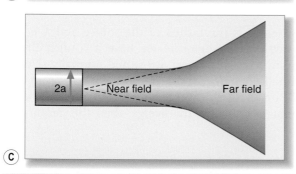

Fig 1.8 • A. Beam shape with large circular source. The radius of the source is 'a'. B. Beam shape with small source. C. Beam shape with intermediate source.

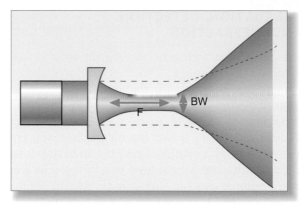

Fig 1.9 • Effect of lens focusing. The dotted line represents the beam shape with no lens present. BW, beam width and F, focal length.

used. Two basic types of focusing can be employed, lenses and mirrors. An ultrasonic lens is similar to the more familiar optical lens except that the surfaces normally curve in the opposite direction. This is because acoustic lenses are normally made of materials with a higher speed of sound than the surroundings which is not true in optics. We can see in Fig. 1.9 that the introduction of a lens has the effect of narrowing the beam at some selected depth F, although it also causes extra divergence at other depths. Thus we trade off beam width improvements at the focus for beam width degradation elsewhere. Exactly the same focusing effect can be obtained by using a curved front face on the transducer. It is just as if a curved lens was attached to its surface. If the source diameter is increased, the beam width at the focus is reduced further at the expense of still more divergence (Fig. 1.9). For a source of diameter A (sometimes known as the aperture width) focused at a focal distance F, the beam width at the focus BW is given by

$$BW = F\lambda/A$$

Therefore, the choice of aperture size is another compromise. Improved beam width at one depth means defocusing at others. We shall see later that the same lensing effect can be achieved electronically, but the trade-off between beam width and depth range still applies.

The above section describes how the dimensions of the ultrasound beam transmitted into the tissue can be influenced by factors such as the size of the source and the wavelength. However, it should be noted that the same factors also influence the

large source and hence does not create a narrow beam. The compromise is to use an intermediate-sized source and choose the value such that the length of the near field is only just long enough to cover the depth of interest. We can also see that this is aided if the value of λ is low, i.e. if we use high frequencies.

It is possible to reduce the width of the beam to a smaller dimension if focusing techniques are shape of the region from which echoes can be received. When the transducer is operating as a detector there is a zone within which any echoes generated will be detected. The shape of this zone is determined in exactly the same way. Thus focusing applies both on transmission of the beam and during detection of the echoes.

INTERACTIONS OF ULTRASOUND WITH TISSUE

As the ultrasound pulse travels through tissue, it is subject to a number of interactions. The most important of these are:

- reflection
- scatter
- absorption.

Each of these is discussed below.

Reflection in ultrasound is very similar to optical reflection. A wave encountering a large obstacle sends some of its energy back into the medium from which it has arrived. In a true reflection, the law governing the direction of the returning wave states that the angle of incidence i must equal the angle of reflection r (Fig. 1.10). The strength of the reflection from an obstacle is variable and depends upon the nature of both the obstacle and the background material. Of particular relevance is a quantity, known as the characteristic acoustic impedance and normally given the symbol Z. For our purposes we can regard Z as a quantity which is specific to the individual material and dependent upon the

density ρ (rho) and the speed of sound in the material c.

$$Z = \rho c$$

The strength of the reflection can be described in terms of a *reflection coefficient* R, which is defined as a ratio:

$$R = \left\{ \frac{\text{Energy in the reflected wave}}{\text{Energy in the incident wave}} \right\} \times 100\%$$

We can see from this that the maximum value of R is 100% and this will correspond to a perfect mirror. If we consider the interface between two materials with acoustic impedance values Z_1 and Z_2, then the reflection coefficient for the interface is given by:

$$R = \left(\frac{Z_1 - Z_2}{Z_1 + Z_2} \right)^2 \times 100\%$$

Hence the strength of the reflection depends upon the *difference* in Z values between the two materials which make up the interface. We can expand the data in Table 1.1 to include density and hence calculate the Z values for the materials as shown in Table 1.3.

It is clear that the Z values of most soft tissues are similar. Therefore we would predict that the interface between two soft tissues would result in a small reflection but with most of the energy being transmitted. This is found in practice and it is indeed fortunate because otherwise the idea of getting many echoes along each beam direction (Fig. 1.4) would not work and only the first reflector encountered would generate a detectable signal. On the other hand, it is equally clear that an interface between any soft tissue and either gas or bone involves a considerable change in acoustic impedance and will create a strong echo. It is quite probable that there would be so little energy transmitted beyond such an interface that no more echoes would be detected even if there were many targets there. This can be seen, for example, in third trimester scanning when the large calcified bones of the fetal limbs or skull can create misleading shadows behind them.

As well as this, the strong reflections caused by gas collections have other consequences. First, pockets of bowel gas can make it difficult to visualize anatomy lying posteriorly to them. In obstetric

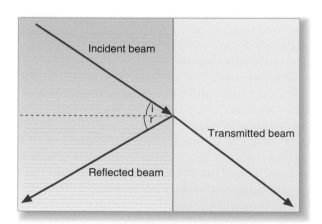

Fig 1.10 • Reflection from a large reflector. Note that the angle i equals the angle r and that some of the energy continues beyond the reflecting surface.

7

MATERIAL	SPEED OF SOUND (m s^{-1})	DENSITY (kg m^{-3}) x 10^{-3}	ACOUSTIC IMPEDANCE (kg m^{-2} s^{-1}) x 10^{-6}
Air	330	1.2	0.0004
Water	1480	1000	1.48
Steel	5000	7900	39.5
Blood	1575	1057	1.62
Fat	1459	952	1.38
Muscle	1580	1080	1.70
Cortical bone	4080	1912	7.8

Table 1.3 Speed of sound through and density and acoustic impedance values of various materials

ultrasound, for example, this can make it difficult to image certain segments of the uterus. It may be necessary either to scan through a different section, ask the woman to fill her bladder or else consider a transvaginal approach to overcome the problem. Second, it becomes important to use a coupling material between the transducer and the woman's skin. A variety of gels and oils are available for this purpose. They need an acoustic impedance value that is intermediate between that of the transducer and the skin. However, acoustically almost any material that displaces air from the transducer–skin interface would work. An important additional feature of couplants is that they act as lubricants making a smooth scanning action possible.

The reflection model above strictly applies only where the interface is large, flat and smooth on a scale comparable with the beam width. In practice, there are very few such interfaces in the body. Nevertheless the importance of acoustic impedance matching is valid and provides a useful explanation for many effects observed in routine scanning.

Scattering occurs at the opposite end of the size scale. The theories available here tend to assume that the target is not only very small (much less than a wavelength) but also not influenced by other nearby scatterers. If such a target were to exist in the body, we would expect to see a very weak interaction. In other words, most of the beam energy would pass through with no effect. The small fraction of the energy that interacted would be redistributed in almost all directions including backwards as shown in Fig. 1.11. The closest

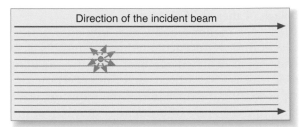

Fig 1.11 • Small scatterer (green dot) redistributing energy in all directions.

approximation to this type of scatterer in the body is the erythrocyte but even this does not really fit the model because with normal haematocrit levels, the distance to the nearest neighbour is too small to achieve independence. Multiple scattering involving many such cells is thought to occur. Nonetheless this process is critical in the generation of Doppler signals, which is discussed below.

Thus we have two models of interaction, the reflection model and the scattering model, but we are aware that neither is a good descriptor of most interactions. It is interesting to note that this is quite fortunate in one respect. If the anatomy of a particular region was similar to that of a reflector, such as in Fig. 1.10, the returning echo would miss the transducer and not be displayed. Thus no matter how strong the reflecting surface, it would not be displayed until the angle of incidence was made approximately 90°. When scanning the fetal head, for example to measure the biparietal diameter (BPD), it is often noted that structures such as

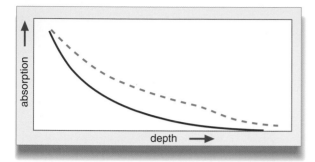

Fig 1.12 • Absorption at two frequencies. The dotted line represents a lower frequency.

the falx cerebri and cavum septum pellucidum and bodies such as the lateral ventricles are best demonstrated clearly when insonated at 90°. This should be remembered when identifying the appropriate section for measurement and/or evaluation.

In practice most interfaces are somewhat irregular, rough and curved. The interaction of the sound wave with them is complex but has elements of both of the above two descriptions. This means that it is not generally necessary to approach a structure at right angles in order to visualize it, and this happy situation makes scanning a much more practical proposition than it would otherwise be.

Absorption on the other hand has few redeeming features and is generally as undesirable as it is inevitable. It is defined as the direct conversion of the sound energy into heat and it is always present to some extent. In other words, all scanning generates some tissue heating. The extent to which this might constitute a hazard is discussed later in this chapter. At this stage we should concentrate on two other aspects of absorption. The first is that it follows an exponential law and the loss can be expressed using the same mathematics as used to describe the attenuation of x-rays in tissue. In other words, the fraction of the beam energy lost due to absorption is the same for each centimetre travelled. The second key point is that higher frequencies are absorbed at a greater rate than lower frequencies. This is illustrated in Fig. 1.12.

FRAME RATE

Users of modern ultrasound scanners stress the importance of having machines which operate in

real time. Strictly this means that any real movement in tissue must be immediately associated with a corresponding movement in the displayed image. In practice it is sufficient to satisfy two criteria:

- the image must appear to be that of a constantly moving object i.e. there must be no perceptible 'judder' such as can be seen on early cinema movies
- the object being imaged must not be able to move excessively between successive views i.e. it must not be seen to jump.

Satisfying these criteria can be achieved by maintaining a sufficiently high frame rate. This is defined in terms of the rate at which the image is updated or refreshed. In order to avoid 'judder' the human eye requires that the image be updated at a rate which is approximately 25 times a second or higher. If this is achieved, then the image is perceived to be continuously moving rather than being a series of still frames. However, if the actual object being scanned is moving slowly, or is still, then it will be sufficient to simply repeat the old frame at this rate without adding any new information. Scanners are equipped with a switch often labelled frame freeze which implements precisely this, i.e. the same image is written on to the screen about 25 times a second. In normal scanning operation, we would normally require an updated image to be displayed at this rate and this imposes some limitations on scanner operation.

If the desired frame rate is 25 frames per second, then it follows that each frame must occupy no more than 1/25 seconds i.e. 40 ms. During this 40 ms the scanner needs to build up the whole image as shown in Fig. 1.5. If the image consists of n separate ultrasound lines, then each individual line cannot take more than 40/nms. However, the time taken for each line is not within our control. If we consider that each line requires a pulse to be transmitted to the depth of interest and then for echoes generated at that depth to travel back to the receiving transducer, then it is clear that the time taken by this is determined by the distance travelled and the speed of sound in the tissue. Thus we can say that the time per line, T, is given by

$$T = (\text{Distance travelled})/\text{speed}$$
$$= (2 \times \text{depth})/\text{speed} = 2D/c$$

If there are n lines in the image, then the time taken for each frame is 2Dn/c. The corresponding frame rate F_R is 1/(time per frame) and hence

$$F_R = c/2nD$$

This has a curious consequence. If we substitute reasonable values of a speed of sound of 1540 m s^{-1} and a depth of say 15 cm, with a frame rate of 25 frames per second, we find that the maximum number of lines is 205. Limiting the number of lines on display to this kind of value would result in an image that would appear very coarse. We might think of a conventional domestic television that has 625 lines in its display and imagine how poor the image would seem if only one third of those lines were displayed. In fact the scanner manufacturers avoid this problem by introducing 'manufactured' lines which are created by assuming that the values required are intermediate between the adjacent real lines. This technique called line interpolation is widely used and results in an image that is more acceptable to the eye while not adding any real information. It does, however, illustrate the difficulties of making the scanner operate in real time. The time constraint limits other aspects of scanner performance as we shall now see.

FOCUSING

As mentioned earlier, it is common to use electronic means to narrow the width of the beam at some depth and so achieve a focusing effect which is similar to that obtained using a lens (Fig. 1.13). This improves the resolution in the plane being imaged. The reduction in beam width at the selected depth in the beam being transmitted is achieved at the expense of degradation in beam width at other depths. Similar methods can be used to achieve focusing of received echoes. The electronic lens can be set up to receive only those echoes originating from a defined region. However, there is an important distinction to be drawn. Whereas a transmitted beam consists of a single pulse travelling through the tissue, the received signal may consist of many echoes originating at a range of depths but separated in time. Thus a single transmitted pulse will normally result in the generation of many echoes. It is possible when receiving these echoes to exploit the fact that at any one

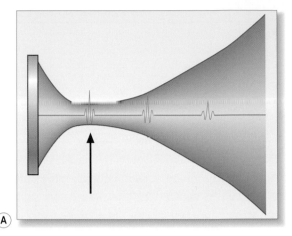

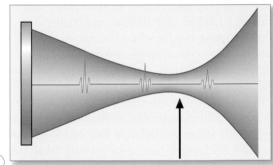

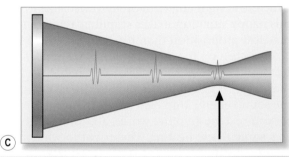

Fig 1.13 • Focusing on reception. The initial focal depth (arrow) in (A) is set up to focus echoes from superficial depths and the focal depth is swept out synchronously with the returning echoes as in (B) and then (C).

time, we know the depth from which the arriving echoes have originated. Echoes from superficial reflectors arrive early whereas those from deeper structures take longer to arrive. The focusing of these received echoes can be altered quickly so that the focal depth always corresponds to the depth of origin. We can say that the focus is swept out simultaneously with the arrival of the echoes. This technique is often called *swept* or *dynamic focusing* and adds to the quality of the image without any penalty apart from an increase in electronic complexity (Fig. 1.13).

It is also possible to consider using similar methods to improve the focusing of the transmitted beam. It was noted earlier (see Fig. 1.9) that we can reduce the beam width at the focus by using a smaller aperture. This can be done for the transmitted beam, resulting in sharper images at the selected depth. However, it is also clear that this will normally result in poorer images from other depths. One option is to begin by sending out a beam focused at, say, a superficial depth and reject echoes coming back from depths away from that focal region. This can be followed by a second pulse transmitted along the same line but this time focused more deeply. In this case early echoes would be rejected as well as very late ones. A third pulse can then be transmitted focused at greater depths and now all early echoes would be rejected and so on. In this way a composite image would be built up from the superposition of data from all the depths resulting in improved resolution throughout. However, in this case, unlike the dynamic focusing on reception, there is a penalty. Each scan line now requires three or more transmissions for its acquisition and this delays the formation of each image frame.

Thus the operator may well have to choose between high frame rates and high resolution. Many machines allow switching between different modes to allow the operator to select the optimal set up for that particular examination. Indeed there is nothing to stop the operator from swapping between a high resolution mode and a high frame rate mode during an examination.

HARMONIC IMAGING

As an ultrasound pulse travels through tissue, it changes shape. There are two main reasons for this. First, as mentioned earlier, absorption causes the wave to get smaller. In this case the overall shape is maintained but scaled down as shown in Fig. 1.4. This is why it is necessary to use the various gain controls and why there is a limit to how far the beam will penetrate. However, there is another process occurring at the same time known as *nonlinear propagation*. This is a form of distortion which alters some parts of the waveform more than others. In effect, the positive portions of the pulses travel slightly faster than the negative portions and so appear to 'catch up' with them as shown in Fig. 1.14. The extent to which this happens depends on the wave amplitude, i.e. how large a voltage is applied to the transducer. The operator can influence this by using the transmit output power control if one it is fitted.

The overall effect of this nonlinear distortion is to take some of the energy of the pulse and to convert it to new frequencies. These new frequencies are multiples of the original one. For example, if the original frequency of the pulse is 3 MHz, then the new frequencies will be 6, 9, 12 MHz and so on. These new extra frequencies are called *harmonics*.

It is possible to persuade the receiver of the scanner to 'tune in' to these higher frequencies instead of the original one. This leads to a situation in which the pulse sent out is at one frequency, say 3 MHz, while the selected received echoes are at a multiple of that frequency, say 6 MHz. This way of operating a machine is called *harmonic imaging* or *tissue harmonic imaging* (THI).

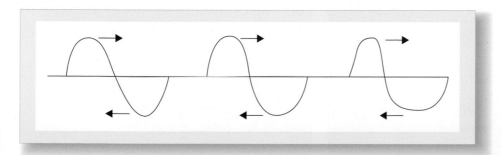

Fig 1.14 • Effect of nonlinear propagation of pulse shape. Note that the positive phases travel slightly more quickly than the negative phases and tend to 'catch up'.

The use of the higher received frequency brings with it the benefits generally expected of high frequencies, i.e. improved resolution. However, it also turns out that much of the clutter and some of the artefacts (see next section) contain less harmonic signal than the wanted echoes because they are generally smaller and are therefore selectively reduced. Overall the result is a 'cleaner', sharper image and so, in many cases, machine preset default settings have THI switched on.

ARTEFACTS

Artefact can be defined as misleading or incorrect information appearing on the display, e.g. a bright dot suggesting the presence of a structure that in fact does not exist. Ultrasound imaging is susceptible to a wide range of artefacts and it is not appropriate to discuss them all in detail in this context. However, they can be divided into the following:

- caused by the nature of the tissue
- caused by the operator
- caused by equipment malfunction.

In many cases, the problem is caused by a violation of one or more assumptions that underpin 2D scanning. These include:

- the beam being infinitely thin
- propagation being in a straight line
- the speed of sound being exactly 1540 m s^{-1}
- the brightness of the echo being directly related to the reflectivity of the target.

Two common examples of such violations are 'acoustic shadowing' and its opposite, 'flaring'. In Fig. 1.15 there appears to be a break in the outline of the posterior uterine wall where it lies posterior to the fetal head. In fact the head structures are the cause of the appearance because they reflect and absorb more of the sound energy than their surroundings. This means that any pulses which would have impacted on the uterine wall travelling through the fetal head *en route*, suffer an unexpectedly large loss and this is repeated on the return journey made by the echoes from this region. The consequence is that the signal strength reaching the receiving transducer from this part of the uterine wall is relatively weak and gives a misleading appearance. The fetal head can be correctly stated to be the cause of acoustic shadowing.

The opposite is true in Fig. 1.16 in which the posterior wall of an ovarian cyst appears to be very bright. In this case, the problem is that the path travelled by the pulse and its corresponding echoes is largely through the fluid within the cyst which absorbs very little of the beam energy. This is an example of 'flaring' or 'enhancement'. If the effect is sufficiently marked, it can result in saturation of the display at this point and hence a loss of diagnostic information.

On the other hand, these artefacts can be used to diagnostic advantage. Some solid masses are quite homogeneous and their image can be devoid of internal echoes. Such an appearance is termed

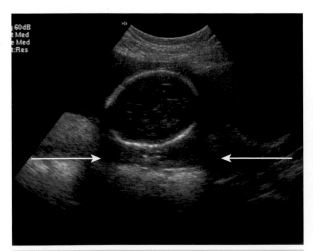

Fig 1.15 • Image showing acoustic shadowing from the fetal head (arrows).

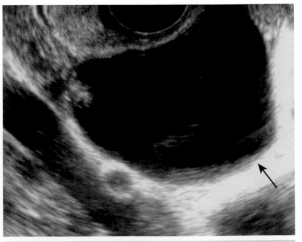

Fig 1.16 • Image showing flaring (arrow) in a benign serous cystadenoma.

hypoechoic. In this case there is potential for the solid mass to be confused with a cyst of the same dimensions which would also be expected to be hypoechoic. However, the solid mass is much more likely to be absorptive than the cyst and hence the two can normally be distinguished by the presence or absence of flaring or shadowing posteriorly.

The possibility of an operator-induced error also merits attention. The correct use of the TGC control for example is critical if the various structures are to be displayed with meaningful grey levels. Too much TGC can incorrectly create filled-in (hyperechoic) regions, whereas too little can make solid inhomogeneous regions appear clear. Similarly, the simple error of not using sufficient coupling gel can have dramatic consequences.

For further information of artefacts and their appearances the reader is referred to one of the standard ultrasound texts (Hedrick et al 1995).

3D IMAGING

The B-mode ultrasound image formation and display described so far is essentially obtained from a thin 'bacon slice' of tissue. If the transducer is held steady, then the slice is imaged many times per second producing the familiar 2D real-time moving image. If the operator wishes to image some other slice, it is necessary to manually move the transducer to the new position. Of course, operators do this many times throughout each scan without thinking too much about it. However, it is possible to arrange for the transducer to be moved automatically, thereby scanning a predetermined three-dimensional (3D) volume. Such a volume is built up of a systematic series of conventional 2D slices as shown in Fig. 1.17.

There are three advantages to this. First, the systematic nature of the scanning format ensures that no sections within the selected volume are missed. Second, having the whole examination stored in a large electronic memory allows the display of other sections which could not have otherwise been obtained. Third, it allows the use of sophisticated software techniques such as segmentation and artificial lighting to create images which seem more 'realistic,' particularly to the woman. In some cases, the 3D scanning can be carried out very quickly, allowing some movement to be seen; the term *4D* is used for this (Fig. 1.18). However, whereas the skilled operator is constantly making subtle changes to the scanning angle to highlight anatomy of interest, the angles at which the 3D slices

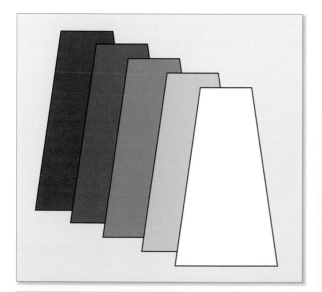

Fig 1.17 • A series of parallel two-dimensional slices are combined to form a composite three-dimensional volume.

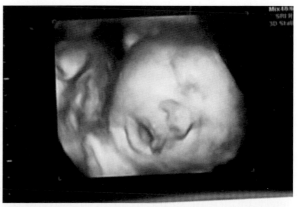

Fig 1.18 • Frozen four-dimensional image of a fetal face.

are obtained are essentially fixed. Moreover, it is important to stress that 3D delivers no new information. What is displayed is a reformatting of the various 2D slices. It is expected that any competent sonographer will develop the necessary concepts to think in 3D, even when scanning in 2D. It remains to be seen whether 3D scanning will eventually become the standard tool in obstetrics.

DOPPLER ULTRASOUND

The Doppler effect was first described by Christian Johann Doppler (1803–1853), who discussed the apparent change in the colour of the light emitted by stars caused by their motion relative to the Earth. He later investigated the closely related phenomenon that occurs with moving sources of sound and recorded a remarkable experiment in which a brass band was commissioned to play a series of notes while sitting on a moving train and observers at the track side were asked to identify the notes being played! There are many such examples in the world around us today, including the apparent change in the sound of a racing car or a train coming toward us compared with the same car or train seconds later, when it has passed us and is moving away; people on board the moving car or train do not perceive any change in the sound it makes as it passes an observer standing at the side of track. We can generalize the Doppler effect as follows. It:

- is an apparent change in the pitch or frequency of a wave due to relative movement between the source and the receiver
- can be demonstrated for any type of wave, including light, sound and ultrasound
- is direction dependent.

THE DOPPLER PRINCIPLE

The situation in which the source is stationary and the receiver is moving differs slightly from that in which the receiver is stationary and the source is moving. Let us consider the first case and assume for the moment that the receiver is moving directly towards the source (Fig. 1.19). The receiver will detect more waves per second than are actually being sent out. In other words, the receiver will detect an increase in the frequency relative to the source. If the receiver is moving in the opposite direction, then it will receive fewer waves per

second than are being generated, and hence detect a lower frequency. Note that an independent observer would conclude that it is the receiver that is 'wrong', i.e. the Doppler shift is introduced by the receiving device.

The situation is slightly different if the source is moving and the receiver is stationary. In this case, the actual wave travelling through the material is altered. If we take the case in which the source is moving towards a stationary receiver (Fig. 1.20), the physical distance between the waves is reduced by the motion. In a sense, the wave is being compressed. In other words, its wavelength is reduced. As there is a relationship between wavelength and frequency, then we would predict that this reduction in wavelength corresponds to an increase in frequency. This increase is detected by the receiver. Unlike the previous case, an independent observer would judge that the receiver is 'correct' and that it is the source that has created the change.

The importance of this is that both effects occur in medical Doppler applications. The original wave is sent out from the stationary transducer at the skin

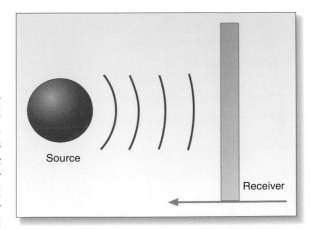

Fig 1.19 • A receiver moving towards a stationary source detects waves more rapidly than they are being generated. Hence an increased frequency is perceived.

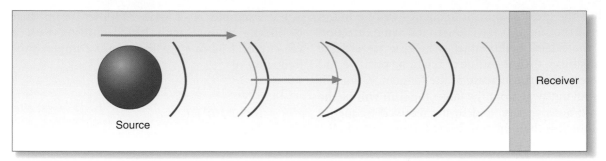

Fig 1.20 • A source moving towards a stationary receiver. The wave fronts are positioned ahead of where they would otherwise be. This is a reduced wavelength and hence an increased frequency is detected.

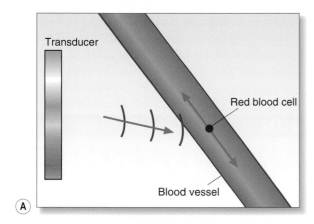

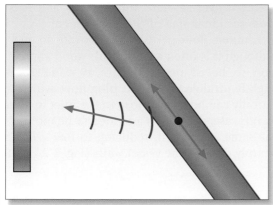

Fig 1.21 • A. A stationary source insonates a moving target. In this case, the target is a single blood cell. B. A blood cell scatters sound back towards the transducer. This is then a moving source and the transducer is a stationary receiver.

surface and arrives at some moving target or interface. The target might be an erythrocyte in a blood vessel intersected by the beam (Fig. 1.21). The fact that the target is moving means that it will experience a slightly different frequency from that which

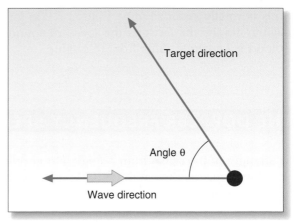

Fig 1.22 • The angle between wave and target movement.

was sent out. This target will then scatter or reflect the sound and so act as a moving source. Some of this movement will be detected at the surface by the transducer and so, on the return path, we have the moving source and the stationary receiver. Although the two Doppler shifts can be calculated and described separately, it is convenient to combine them into a single expression. In a round trip such as this, the change or Doppler shift in the frequency f_d can be shown to be given by

$$f_d = 2f_0 v \cos\theta/c$$

where f_d is the Doppler shift in the frequency; f_0 is the frequency of the emitted ultrasound; v is the velocity of the moving target; θ is the angle between the ultrasound beam and the direction of movement of the target; and c is the speed of sound in tissue (Fig. 1.22).

Note that the angle θ is important. The maximum value of $\cos\theta$ is 1, and this occurs when θ is zero.

15

Thus the greatest shift in frequency will be found when the sound is travelling in the same direction as the target. If the target is moving toward the transducer, then the value of f_d will be positive and there will be an increase in the frequency, but if it is moving away from the target the shift will be the same but negative, and so the received frequency will be less than the transmitted frequency. On the other hand, if the target is moving at right angles to the beam, θ will be 90° or 270° and $\cos\theta$ will have the value zero. We conclude that this will result in there being no Doppler shift under these circumstances. The speed of sound in this calculation is normally assumed to be 1540 m s^{-1}, as for imaging, despite the fact that the speed of sound in blood is known to differ from this value.

For example, a 4 MHz Doppler beam that is directly in line with blood moving with a velocity of 1.54 m s^{-1} will detect a Doppler shift frequency of

$$f_d = 2 \times 4 \times 10^6 \times 1.54/1540$$
$$= 8 \times 10^6/10^3 \, Hz$$
$$= 8 \, kHz$$

Doppler shifted frequencies obtained from flowing blood in the uteroplacental and fetal circulation with angles of insonation of 20–60° are typically in the audible range (up to 12 kHz). This is convenient because it means that the signals can be monitored by loudspeakers and stored on magnetic audio tape for later off-line analysis.

THE DOPPLER FREQUENCY SPECTRUM

The strength of the signal from a single blood cell is too low to be detected at the surface; its level is less than the size of the noise signal. It is thought that the signals used clinically arise from the multiple scattering from groups (or ensembles) of cells, although the erythrocytes are the major contributors. However, at any time the blood cells along a length of blood vessel (of, say, a few millimetres) will have a range of velocities. The simplest model is that of a fluid flowing in a long, straight, smooth-sided, nonbranching tube. In this case, the distribution of velocities is radially symmetrical about the centre of the tube. The velocities are greatest at the centre and tail off radially, following a parabolic law, to end with zero velocity at the tube walls. This velocity distribution is known as laminar or parabolic flow and is shown in Fig. 1.23. An important characteristic of parabolic flow is that the maximum velocity, which occurs at the centre, is twice the mean velocity. This implies that a reliable estimate of mean velocity can be obtained simply by measuring the peak velocity at the centre of the vessel and halving it. This will, of course, vary throughout the cardiac cycle, but if it is averaged over several cycles, an estimate of volume flow in the vessel can be made, assuming that the cross-sectional area of the vessel, A, is measured by ultrasound or other means

$$V = (V_{max})_{ave} A/2$$

where V is the volume flow in ml s^{-1}; $(V_{max})_{ave}$ is the maximum velocity at the vessel centre in cm s^{-1} averaged over several cardiac cycles and A is the cross-sectional area of the vessel in cm^2.

Laminar flow of this type is rare in practice, although it is often a sufficiently good approximation to be of practical clinical value. Another, slightly idealized profile is plug flow, which theoretically can be found close to the inlet to a vessel. In this case, the flow is assumed to be more or less the same at all radii, reducing to low values very sharply close to the vessel walls (Fig. 1.24). This is

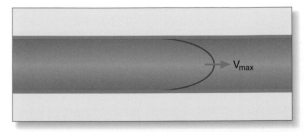

Fig 1.23 • Velocity profile associated with laminar or parabolic flow. Note that the peak velocity is at the centre, reducing parabolically to zero at the vessel walls.

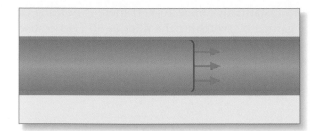

Fig 1.24 • Velocity profile for plug flow. The velocity is uniform over most of the vessel radius.

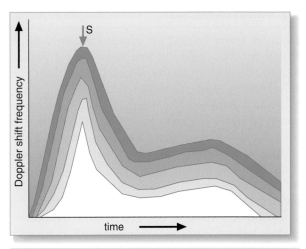

Fig 1.25 • Doppler spectrum. The horizontal axis represents time; the vertical axis is Doppler shift frequency. The shade of green is related to the strength of the signal received at that frequency. Peak systole (S) is often chosen as a reference point.

shown in Fig. 1.24. If the profile of velocities is traced along a vessel, the tendency is for it to begin as plug flow and gradually move to a more parabolic profile. The main reason for the transition is viscous drag at the interface between the vessel walls and the blood in close contact with them. In practice, the mean velocity will normally lie between the two extremes, i.e. it will be more than half of the maximum measured velocity. The pattern will be disrupted by branching, twisting and pulsatility.

In the fetal circulation, the descending aorta normally demonstrates plug flow during systolic acceleration and parabolic flow during diastole. The umbilical artery normally demonstrates parabolic flow throughout the cardiac cycle.

The consequence of the above is that any ultrasound beam irradiating a volume that includes a blood vessel will create a range of Doppler shifts in the returning echoes, as opposed to the single value of f_d that might be expected from the basic Doppler shift equation. At any point in time, this range or spread of Doppler frequencies can be described and displayed as a Doppler spectrum. The nature of the spectrum at any location will be subject to change throughout the cardiac cycle. If all of the blood cells were moving at the same speed all of the time, then the spectrum would simply consist of a single line. The factors listed above give rise to a range of Doppler frequencies that result in a band rather than a line. This is known as spectral broadening. In fact, the scanner itself, as we will see, adds further broadening to the spectrum, which is undesirable and is a misleading artefact, and this additional factor is known as intrinsic spectral broadening.

The spectrum is further complicated by the fact that the frequency shift signal at some frequencies will be stronger (i.e. have a greater amplitude) than that at others. If there is a large number of blood cells moving at one speed and a smaller number moving at another, then the strength of the Doppler signal will also be stronger at the first frequency. The spectral display therefore needs to be three-dimensional if it is to show all of the available information. It needs to show:

• time
• frequency shift
• Doppler signal strength.

This is shown diagrammatically in Fig. 1.25.

Plug flow can be recognized in the Doppler spectrum by all the frequencies being clustered close to the maximum frequency waveform, whereas parabolic flow shows frequencies evenly distributed from the level of the vessel wall filter to the maximum frequency, thus filling the waveform (Fig. 1.26).

Yet more spectral broadening originates from factors such as divergences of the ultrasound beam as it travels through different tissues or slight spectral distortion as a result of differences among the velocity directions of dispersing erythrocytes. These components of contamination, however, are minor, but the most important additional source of contamination is caused by Doppler shifts attributable to the pulsatile movements of the vessel walls.

The Vessel Wall Filter

Doppler shifts caused by vessel walls are low in frequency but high in intensity. They have an amplitude that is many times higher than the echoes from the erythrocytes because the acoustic mismatch between the vessel wall and blood is much greater than that between the red cell–plasma interface. To remove these low-frequency Doppler signals generated by the vessel walls, a high-pass filter (or wall-thump filter) can be used. Filters of 50–200 Hz are common. The most important error caused by high-pass filters is to eliminate low velocities occurring at the end of diastole. Nevertheless, manufacturers use high-pass filters for very good reasons, and whenever Doppler frequencies are substantially above 200 Hz there is nothing to be gained by switching the filter to 50 Hz because vessel motion signals might contaminate an otherwise good signal. High-pass filters should therefore be used at their highest value and only switched to 50 Hz when necessary.

DOPPLER FLOWMETERS

These are instruments for acquiring, displaying and analyzing Doppler waveforms. They can be relatively cheap stand-alone instruments or part of more sophisticated imaging systems.

The Continuous Wave Flowmeter

The simplest Doppler device is the continuous wave (CW) flowmeter, the basic elements of which are illustrated in Fig. 1.27. One important feature of this device it that it requires two transducers. However, only one is needed for imaging because once each short pulse has been generated there is no more transmission work to do and the transducer can be used as a receiver. For a CW device, the transducer must transmit all the time and hence a separate receiver is required. In fact, it is common to house both transducers in the same cover (often as concentric rings or back-to-back D shapes) and the user can be unaware that two separate transducers are involved.

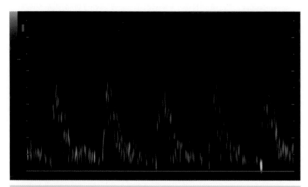

Fig 1.26 • Doppler spectral waveform from the fetal aorta. Note the change from parabolic flow within each cardiac cycle.

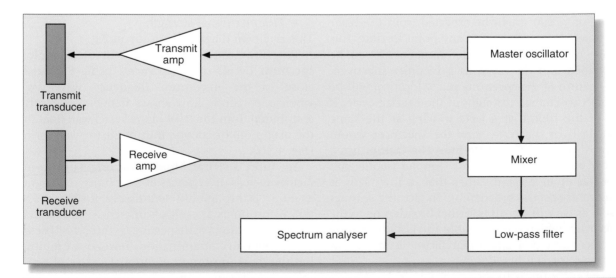

Fig 1.27 • Block diagram of a simple continuous wave flowmeter.

The master oscillator produces a steady, continuous, sinusoidal waveform that is amplified and used to drive the transmitting transducer at its resonating frequency. The consequent ultrasonic beam hits the moving targets (erythrocytes) that produce reflected and back-scattered echoes, some of which will eventually return to the receiving transducer. It also hits stationary targets, which can produce much stronger echoes, although they will not have any Doppler shift. All of these echoes are mixed together in the received signal that is amplified and presented to the Doppler demodulator. The demodulator therefore has to perform two tasks. It must identify the echoes from moving targets and reject the stationary target echoes that will be unshifted. In addition, it needs to measure the size of the Doppler shift – i.e. how large a deviation has there been from the original frequency? It does this by comparing the incoming signal with a reference signal that is in fact simply the original unshifted frequency. In one simple version the demodulator simply mixes the received signal with the reference. The outcome of this is a combination of sum and difference frequencies. At first sight this would seem to be a retrograde step because we now have an even greater variety of signals than before. However, the difference frequency will be at a much lower frequency than the rest and this is the component that is wanted. After the demodulator it can be readily identified by using a low-pass filter that will eliminate all the unwanted higher frequency signals. The signal after low-pass filtering contains only the desired Doppler shifted frequencies and can be processed and presented to the user in a variety of ways.

Display options

All of the available data can be presented to the user in the form of a spectral display. However, the clinical application might not require that level of complexity. It is possible to calculate a mean velocity as a function of time and to display this on a screen or meter. Alternatively, the maximum velocity alone can be calculated and displayed.

To give some idea of the required capabilities of Doppler flowmeters it is useful to examine the properties of the Doppler shift spectrum. Using a 5 MHz ultrasound probe to insonate the fetal aorta with an angle of about $40°$, the Doppler spectrum would be expected to extend up to a frequency of about 12 kHz, corresponding to a peak velocity of about 1.6 m s^{-1} during the maximum systolic phase. Furthermore, the blood would accelerate from almost complete rest at the end of diastole up to this peak velocity in a time interval of less than 0.1 s. The Doppler signal frequency analyzer must therefore be able to accommodate frequencies up to 12 kHz and must be capable of updating the analysis at a rate of at least 100 spectra per second. However, if lower ultrasonic frequencies are used to investigate more slowly moving venous blood, it would be better to use lower range analysis frequencies placed closer together to maintain the required frequency (and therefore velocity resolution). Thus a variable frequency analyzer is useful where multiple purpose instrumentation is needed.

Simple continuous wave flowmeters are not limited by the maximum velocity that can be measured and, as they do not usually use real-time imaging, they are relatively cheap. Their major disadvantage, however, is their inability to discriminate in range. All targets within the beam are producing echoes all the time and so the receiving transducer cannot use time to distinguish echoes from different depths as it does in imaging systems. In clinical use it is sometimes impossible to separate signals from vessels at different depths.

Pulsed Doppler Flowmeters

Pulsed Doppler combines the range discriminating capabilities of a pulsed echo system with the velocity detection properties of a Doppler system.

A block diagram of a pulsed Doppler system is shown in Fig. 1.28. The key differences between this and the CW system are that there is now a second transducer and that it uses long pulses rather than continuous waves.

The system is essentially an extended version of the CW system. There is still an oscillator, demodulator and filter. However, the pulsed Doppler system needs some form of sample and hold device. A clock is started when the initial long pulse is transmitted. The operator stops the clock at a time that is selected to be the arrival time for the echoes from the depth of interest. When this happens, an electronic 'gate' is opened; this is called the range gate. It admits echoes for a short time and then closes. It is this short burst of signal that is processed, thereby excluding echoes from all other depths. The pulsed

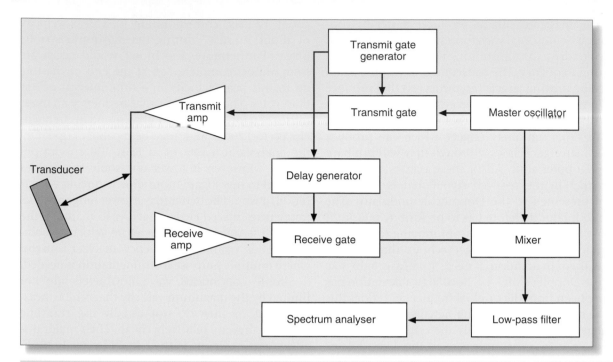

Fig 1.28 • Block diagram of a pulsed Doppler flowmeter.

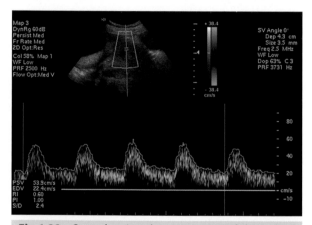

Fig 1.29 • Scan showing the range gate of the pulsed Doppler system and the spectral waveform arising from the selected depth.

Doppler arrangement can be readily combined with an imaging system. The B-scan image can then be made to show precisely where the Doppler signals are to be sampled. In this way, ambiguity arising from uncertainty in the anatomy or proximity of other vessels can be avoided. A typical pulsed Doppler display is shown in Fig. 1.29.

The sample volume

The sample volume can best be visualized as a region at some distance in front of the transducer and from which all returning echoes must have originated. The dimensions of the sample volume are defined axially by the pulse length and laterally by the beam width of the ultrasonic beam.

Limitations of pulsed Doppler

In practice, pulsed Doppler has two important limitations. The first is that there is a maximum flow velocity that it can reliably detect. The second is that because Doppler information is only collected from one sample volume, it will fail if the operator is unable to identify the correct location at which to position it.

Sampling limitations

The upper limit of frequency shift that can be detected by the pulsed Doppler flowmeter is determined by the sampling process. In pulsed Doppler mode, the sample volume is interrogated every time a pulse is sent down that specific scan line. The sampling rate can be increased by freezing the displayed image and ceasing to fire along the

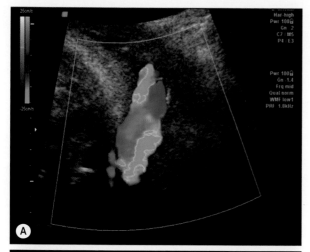

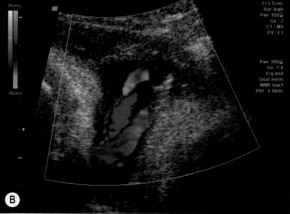

Fig 1.30 • Colour Doppler image of the umbilical cord. (A) showing aliasing in the arteries because the PRF is set too low (1.6 kHz). Increasing the PRF to 4.0 kHz as shown in (B) displays the colour in the arteries correctly, with no evidence of aliasing.

length of the array. Even then, the Doppler waveform has to be reconstructed from a series of samples taken at regular intervals and the maximum Doppler frequency that can be detected is one-half of the pulsed repetition frequency (Nyquist criterion). If higher-frequency signals are present, then the sampled waveform cannot be reconstructed correctly and a phenomenon known as aliasing occurs (Fig. 1.30). This is explained in more detail in Chapter 13.

Range–velocity limitations

Pulsed Doppler systems are subject to maximum range and maximum velocity limitations. The range restrictions occur because it is necessary to

wait for the returning echo to have been received from the most distant target before a further pulse of ultrasound is transmitted. This affects the maximum velocity because the deeper the target, the lower the pulse repetition frequency (PRF) and the lower the maximum detectable blood velocity. Major fetal vessels are generally located within 15 cm of the surface of the maternal abdomen and the peak systolic velocities recorded from the descending aorta can approach 1.5 m s^{-1}, so that with angles of insonation from 45° to 55° the optimum PRF is 5–7.5 kHz with ultrasound frequencies of 2–3 MHz. For pulse repetition frequencies of up to 2.5 kHz it is possible to interlace Doppler and real-time ultrasound such that a simultaneous real-time image can be displayed (duplex, pulsed Doppler ultrasound). To achieve higher PRF values, the real-time screen has to be frozen to record the Doppler signals. Most systems have a means of updating the real-time picture about once every second, although some modern scanners utilize ingenious techniques that allow the simultaneous presentation of real-time images and Doppler signals, albeit with a frame rate penalty. For optimum Doppler signals, however, the real-time image must always be frozen.

Real-Time Spectrum Analysis

A real-time spectrum analyzer measures the power at each frequency contained in the Doppler signal, as described above. Furthermore, it separates forward (i.e. blood flowing towards the transducer) and reverse signals. The Doppler signal is digitized and scanned rapidly (200 times per second) by a sweeping filter that measures the power of each individual frequency. The method most commonly employed is known as the Fast Fourier Transform (FFT), the details of which are beyond our scope here. The characteristics of an analyzer that are important to the user are the speed of operation and the number of separate frequencies that can be resolved. For obstetric use, a sampling time of 5 m s (200 per second) is desirable, with a frequency resolution of at least 64 frequency slots or bins per channel, although most analyzers offer at least 128 frequency bins.

Real-time spectral analysis is essential in obstetrics use because the Doppler signals are often complex and contain frequencies emanating from more than one vessel. Providing the user can see the spectrum displayed in real time, these artefacts can be detected. More importantly, as most analyzers now perform automatic calculations, the user must be able to judge whether the signal selected by the analyzer is valid or whether the reading should be discarded because of artefact.

Automatic calculations performed by the analyzer are mostly carried out on the maximum frequency outline. To recognize this, the analyzer inspects each of the frequency bins in turn and determines the highest frequency at which there is a signal. This simple approach only works on near perfect waveforms with a high signal-to-noise ratio, so in practise the analyzer's software imposes several conditions, which must be satisfied before it validates the maximum frequency. The maximum frequency is usually superimposed upon the spectral display so that the user can judge whether it is a true representation. Of course, they are still prone to error if there is too little gain to make the highest velocity components detectable, and this is an important source or error and inconsistency in obstetric Doppler measurements.

Doppler Indices

When the vascular system is subject to pulses from the heart, its behaviour is very similar to mechanical springs that are subject to a weight and some kind of damper. Everyday examples are car suspension springs and guitar strings, which perform some kind of damped oscillation in response to being disturbed. Blood velocity waveforms exhibit similar characteristics. The spring is represented in blood vessels by their compliance, and dampening by factors such as blood viscosity, vessel length and luminal diameter. Thus a typical blood velocity waveform will have a maximum at the peak of systole followed by diastolic frequencies that might, in one extreme, oscillate to the reverse flow direction before falling to zero, or in the other extreme could fall gently until the next systole. Several indices attempt to describe these variations in the waveforms and the most commonly used are illustrated in Fig. 1.31. All these indices are independent of the angle between the Doppler beam and the vessel.

The pulsatility index (PI) was originally described as the difference between the most positive (or

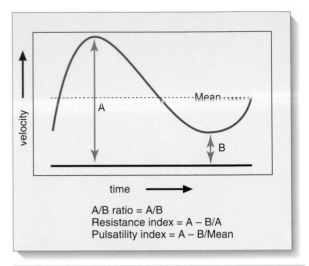

Fig 1.31 • Common indices used to describe variations in waveform.

highest) value, A or S, and the most negative (or lowest) value, B or D, over one cardiac cycle, divided by the mean value. In bidirectional waveforms the most negative value is found in the reverse channel. The mean (or time-averaged mean, TAM) is the mean frequency averaged over one cardiac cycle. The concept of this index is that the more pulsatile the waveform, the greater the difference between the positive and negative peaks and the higher the value of the PI. Flow velocity waveforms from the uteroplacental circulation are rarely (if ever) bidirectional and reverse flow in the umbilical artery occurs only when the fetus is *in extremis*, so simple indices have been more widely applied to such waveforms.

The A/B (or S/D) ratio is simple and describes the rate at which flow velocities fall away during diastole. This closely corresponds to the peripheral resistance to blood flow beyond the measurement point.

The resistance index (RI) makes use of the same two points as the A/B ratio but expresses the values in a more convenient form.

Peripheral resistance cannot be measured directly by means of Doppler waveforms but increasing peripheral resistance causes a diminution and then a loss of frequencies in end-diastole. In vessels that supply vascular beds of muscles, increasing peripheral resistance causes an increase in pulsatility and consequently a rise in the PI. In obstetric practice, reverse flow rarely occurs and, as peripheral resistance is further increased, the systolic peak decreases in amplitude, thus giving a decrease in the PI. If the values of the PI are considered in isolation, this worsening situation can result in a false sense of security. Furthermore, calculation of the PI requires a complete and accurate maximum frequency waveform to calculate the time-averaged mean frequency.

As end-diastolic frequencies disappear, point B becomes zero, so the A/B ratio becomes infinity whereas the RI becomes unity. In all situations where end-diastolic frequencies are lost it is best to describe this in words rather than using indices.

Frequency Calculations

The maximum frequency waveform is relatively simple to derive from the Doppler spectrum and describes the variation in the fastest moving red blood cells, which occupy the centre of the vessel. To calculate blood flow, an estimate of the mean of all the velocities recorded throughout the cardiac cycle is needed. This parameter is known as the intensity weighted mean frequency (IWMF). The IWMF is the sum of the product of the square of the amplitude of each frequency (a) and that frequency (f), divided by the sum of the square of the amplitudes

$$IWMF = \frac{\sum_{0}^{max} a^2 f}{\sum_{0}^{max} a^2}$$

The amplitude of the signal must be squared when making this calculation because the power or intensity of each frequency is proportional to the square of the signal amplitude or voltage. Contamination by signals from other vessels invalidates IWMF because the mean of all signals is calculated, whereas the maximum frequency waveform is much more reliable in this respect.

Velocity Calculations

If the angle between the Doppler beam and the blood vessel is known, then the frequency can be converted into actual blood velocity (see p. 16 and Chapter 13). Velocity measurements have not achieved popularity in obstetric use because of the difficulty of obtaining accurate measurements of the angle of insonation. In obstetric practice, velocity measurements are only of clinical value when obtained from the middle cerebral artery.

Volume Flow Calculations

To calculate volume flow accurately, estimation of the IWMF, the angle of insonation and the vessel diameter are required. Measuring the vessel diameter is difficult because:

- diameter measurements are usually made by means of onscreen callipers to the nearest millimetre
- the diameter has to be squared to derive the cross-sectional area of the vessel, hence any error in measurement will be squared
- the cross-section of the vessel is not necessarily round
- the cross-sectional diameter of the vessel can change between systole and diastole.

Overall, errors in the vessel diameter measurements, measurements of angle and calculation of IWMF result in errors of up to 30% in volume flow calculation in the obstetric field.

COLOUR FLOW DOPPLER ULTRASOUND

Colour flow Doppler is an attempt to overcome some of the limitations of pulsed Doppler. It was introduced in the 1980s and is now a common feature on ultrasound scanners.

The key feature is that the search for Doppler shifts is not restricted to a single volume, as in pulsed Doppler, but rather applies to a large region, possibly even the whole image. Each ultrasound line is divided into blocks (typically 50–100 blocks per line) and the echo signals returning from each block are examined for evidence of Doppler shift. If a shift is detected, then a colour (typically blue or red) is superimposed on the underlying image. However, if the Doppler signal arises from a block that is already white (because it originates from a strong reflector), then the colour signal is suppressed and the grey level is presented instead. In this way, colours are presented only in regions that would otherwise be black or quite dark. There is scope for interpretation of the rules governing this selection and this can form an operator option via a front panel control.

The task of searching such a large region for Doppler shifts in real time is demanding and requires certain compromises. To evaluate each of the blocks or sections in each line, it is necessary to send multiple pulses along each line (typically eight pulses per line). This, not surprisingly, has an effect on frame rate and hence there are further compromises for the operator to consider.

The detection of Doppler shifts is not done using Fourier spectral analysis as in pulsed Doppler. Instead, the successive pulses along each scan line are examined in pairs and evaluated for changes in phase. If we consider a single cycle of a sine wave as corresponding to a trip round a circle, then one cycle corresponds to 360°. Thus the angle of the wave can be thought of as changing from 0° to 360° during each cycle. The rate of change of phase will be greater for higher frequency waves and less for lower frequencies because the time taken for one cycle varies accordingly. Hence we can, in effect, measure frequency and frequency shifts by measuring the rate of change of phase. Of course, if many frequencies are present, then this will be more complex and the result will be some kind of mean or average shift. The calculation of the mean rate of change of phase is normally performed using a mathematical tool known as autocorrelation, although other tools have been used with some success. The outcome of each use of autocorrelation is to produce the following information for each block:

- the mean Doppler shift
- the strength of the signal
- its direction (forward or reverse)
- its variance, i.e. the amount of spread.

The size of each block is larger than the pixels used for imaging and it would be fair to say the colour Doppler has poorer spatial resolution than B-mode imaging for any selected machine.

Although the choice is arbitrary, it has become conventional to use red to designate flow towards the probe and blue for flow away from it. Typically, the shade of red or blue displayed indicates the mean velocity. Hence a deep blue often indicates low mean velocity and a very light blue high velocity. The strength of the signal can be displayed by the luminance or brightness of the colour, i.e. the shade of blue or red can remain unchanged but there can simply be more or less of it. Variance is often shown by the introduction of different

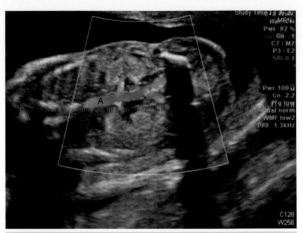

Fig 1.32 • Coronal section of the fetal abdomen using colour flow imaging to identify the fetal renal arteries (solid arrows), the aorta (A) and its bifurcation (dashed arrow). Flow within both kidneys can be seen. Note aliasing in both renal arteries.

colour, with green and yellow being common choices. The user needs to be aware that these colour options vary considerably between scanners and can normally be altered by the operator. It is a mistake to allocate quantitative meaning to the colours displayed unless the colour calibration has been conducted previously.

The great advantage of colour flow mapping is that the signal relies only upon the presence of a Doppler signal, so that small blood vessels can be visualized even though they are below the spatial resolution of the real-time image (Fig. 1.32). Errors in interpretation can occur, however, as each colour flow pixel in a single scanning line is sampled by transmitted pulses. Hence, the Nyquist theory applies and if the mean Doppler frequency is more than half the pulse repetition frequency then aliasing occurs (see p. 21 and Chapter 13). The wraparound effect leads to contamination of a red colour map in areas of very high flow towards the probe (Fig. 1.30(A)).

The disadvantages of colour flow Doppler are the absence of the spectral display that is such a valuable feature of pulsed Doppler and the absence of quantification. Despite the fact that the spectrum is absent, the limitations identified for pulsed Doppler remain. There is a similar trade-off between maximum detectable velocity, frame rate and depth of penetration. Failure to recognize this can lead to aliasing, as for pulsed Doppler. The angle dependence is the same as pulsed Doppler and hence the colours displayed are dependent on the angle of insonation. Blood moving at the same velocity can appear in different colours in differing parts of a curved vessel. Furthermore, absence of colour does not necessarily indicate absence of flow as no colour will be displayed if the beam is at right angles to the vessel.

POWER DOPPLER

A recent innovation is the introduction of power Doppler. In this mode the Doppler signal is processed differently for different reasons. You will note from the block diagrams of Fig. 1.27 and Fig. 1.28 that the signal emerging from the demodulator contains a mixture of Doppler signals from a variety of targets at each range. In the conventional colour flow system, these are then divided into separate frequency slots and displayed as a spectrum. In the case of power Doppler, no attempt is made to identify velocities. Instead, the total signal level across all frequencies at each depth is displayed. This gives a crude measure of how much energy or power there is in the local blood flow. It can be altered by changing either the local mean velocity or the total mass of moving blood in the locality. It has been described (wrongly!) as a perfusion map, although it can come close to this on occasions. A typical power Doppler image is shown in Fig. 1.33. Note that there is no longer any angle dependency because velocities are not being measured.

One advantage of power Doppler is its signal-to-noise ratio, which is normally better than that of its colour flow counterpart. At a simple level we can see why this is so. In colour Doppler, each velocity 'bin' has a signal accumulating in it that depends on the amount of energy that has been found at

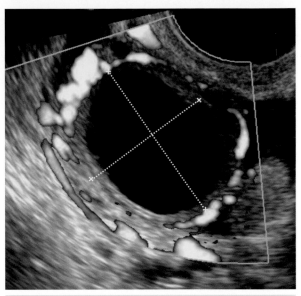

Fig 1.33 • Power Doppler image of a large hypoechoic corpus luteum demonstrating circumferential flow.

that frequency. The noise level is more or less fixed by the electronics. If all of the signals from all of the bins are put into the same bin, then the total will be many times greater and the noise level will remain the same. This improved signal-to-noise ratio will mean that small vessels can be imaged, which are otherwise invisible to ultrasound.

In general terms, the advice often given is to start a scan in B-mode and turn on the colour only when the gross anatomy has been identified. Colour used at this stage can help to separate blood vessels from other fluid collections, distinguish one vessel from another by virtue of its flow direction and find small vessels that are not seen in B-mode. Detailed hemodynamic information can then be obtained by using pulsed Doppler on selected regions.

SAFETY

The question of whether an ultrasound examination carries risks to the woman and/or operator has been the subject of considerable research for many decades and is ongoing. Readers are referred to the comprehensive review of this subject published by the British Medical Ultrasound Society (ter Haar, 2012).

It remains true that no one has ever been shown to have been damaged as a result of the physical effect of a diagnostic ultrasound examination. Of course, this is not true of the consequences of a misdiagnosis due to operator or equipment error.

It is well accepted that high levels of ultrasound are capable of producing biological damage. This includes, for example, the use of ultrasound for cell disintegration in cytology laboratories and oncological applications of ultrasound in which tumours are selectively killed.

The issue for the diagnostic user is how to operate safely while still optimizing the diagnostic potential of the tool. The modern machine provides some assistance to the operator here but the user needs to understand something of the interaction mechanisms in order to interpret the information supplied.

There are two main ways in which ultrasound can cause biological effects:

- mechanical
- thermal.

As there are still gaps in our scientific knowledge in this area, the possibility of other mechanisms also being involved cannot be excluded, but we will deal here only with the two effects stated above.

Mechanical effects occur because ultrasound consists of mechanical vibrations which are propagated through tissue. These cause stresses which create small scale movement of fluids know as microstreaming. The exact extent and significance of these is still a matter for some debate. However, the main mechanical interaction mechanism is cavitation. This is the growth, oscillation and decay of small gas bubbles under the influence of an ultrasound wave.

Small bubble nuclei are present in many tissues. When subjected to ultrasound these bubbles can be 'pumped up'. Although their detailed behaviour is complex, they often grow to some limiting size and continue to vibrate at the ultrasound frequency. Laboratory studies have shown that cells and intact tissues can be influenced by such local bubble oscillation. However, the results are difficult to predict or reproduce, and they may not necessarily be harmful. For example, under some conditions, cell growth can be enhanced. This relatively benign situation changes if the bubble oscillation becomes unstable and, under some circumstances, the bubbles can collapse. If this

occurs, there can be very high and damaging temperatures and pressures generated. It is thought that part of the reason why kidney stones can be broken by ultrasonic lithotripters is that the conditions are such as to encourage collapse cavitation. Although such dramatic events are dangerous, they are confined to a small region and will be over quickly.

Cavitation is encouraged by the following:

- low frequencies
- long pulses
- high negative pressures
- the presence of bubble nuclei.

It follows that, if we wish to minimize the risk of cavitation damage, we would select the opposite of the above conditions.

Microstreaming is enhanced in the presence of a cavitating bubble.

Thermal effects are a consequence of the absorption of the ultrasound wave by tissue. All ultrasound tissue exposures produce heating. The task is to identify where and if it is significant. Because absorption increases with increasing frequency, we would expect more heating from higher frequency probes, and generally this is true. However, the temperature rise caused by an ultrasound beam is dependent upon many factors, including:

- beam intensity and output power
- focusing/beam size
- depth
- tissue absorption coefficient
- tissue specific heat and thermal conductivity
- time
- blood supply.

There has been considerable research into the prediction of temperature increases as a result of ultrasonic exposures, and complex mathematical models have been proposed. These attempt to predict the worst case – i.e. with the specified exposure, what is the greatest temperature rise that could occur?

The guidance from the World Federation of Ultrasound in Medicine and Biology (WFUMB), (1998) is:

A diagnostic exposure that produces a maximum in situ temperature rise of no more than 1.5°C above normal physiological levels (37°C) may be used clinically without reservation on thermal grounds.

The task then is to let the operator know what temperature rise might be involved for each examination so that an informed decision can be made. The system which is now in place to facilitate this was suggested by the American Institute for Ultrasound in Medicine (AIUM) and National Equipment Manufacturers Association (NEMA) and involves on-screen labelling.

The on-screen labelling scheme, which now is effectively universal on all new machines, involves the display of two numbers on the screen in real-time. These are termed the thermal index (TI) and the mechanical index (MI).

As their names imply, the purpose of the TI is to give the operator a real-time indication of the possible thermal implications of the current examination, and similarly, the MI is designed to indicate the relative likelihood of mechanical hazard. The displayed numbers are based on real-time calculations which take into account the transducer in use, its clinical application, the mode of operation and the machine settings.

In simple terms, the TI is defined as:

$$TI = W'/W_{deg}$$

where W' is the machine's current output power and W_{deg} is the power required to increase the temperature by $1.0°C$.

Thus a TI value of 2.0 suggests that the machine temperature rise which might be induced under the current exposure conditions is $2°C$. If the TI value falls below 0.4, it need not be displayed but any scanner that is capable of producing a value in excess of 1.0 must display the TI value.

The calculation of W_{deg} is complex and depends upon the organ being scanned. This has led to the introduction of three different TI indices:

- TIS (thermal index for soft tissue)
- TIB (thermal index for bone)
- TIC (thermal index for cranial bone).

TIS is to be used for upper abdominal and other similar applications.

TIB is used when exposure to bone interfaces is likely, which is the normal expectation for obstetric and neonatal applications.

TIC is for paediatric and adult brain examinations.

The MI (mechanical index) is the counterpart for mechanical effects. These are known to be enhanced by the large negative pressure values and low frequencies and therefore it is unsurprising that the definition is:

$$MI = p_- / \sqrt{f}$$

where p_- is the maximum negative pressure in MPa (megaPascals) generated in tissue and f is the frequency in MHz.

The clinical use of MI and TI merits further discussion. It is not true that scanning under conditions that have either TI or MI in excess of 1.0 is hazardous and this is not the implication of the scheme. The purpose of the display of the index is to move the responsibility for decision-making back to the operator. If the diagnostic information obtained can be acquired using lower TI and MI values, then this is the preferred option.

Often the same image can be obtained by using better gain settings rather than increased output levels. However, if the operator concludes that the only way to reach the necessary diagnostic outcome is to use levels in excess of 1.0, then this is not contraindicated by this scheme. However, the duration of the exposure is also relevant.

The British Medical Ultrasound Society (BMUS) has released guidance suggesting time limits on ultrasound exposure for different values of MI and TI.

It should also be noted that the highest values of TI are commonly recorded when using the machine in pulsed Doppler mode. For that reason, some authors have been specifically concerned with the use of Doppler ultrasound in early pregnancy.

This subject is extensively discussed by the Safety Watchdog Committee of the European Federation of Societies for Ultrasound in Medicine and Biology (EFSUMB). Their regular updates can be found in the *European Journal of Ultrasound*.

Further reading

Barnett SB (ed) 1998 WFUMB World Federation of Ultrasound in Medicine and Biology Symposium on Safety of Ultrasound in Medicine: conclusions and recommendations on thermal and non-thermal mechanisms for biological effects of ultrasound, Ultrasound in Medicine and Biology 24 (Special Issue) S1 1–55

Deane C 2000 Doppler ultrasound: principles and practice. In: Nicolaides K H, Rizzo G, Hecher K (eds) Placental and fetal Doppler. Diploma in Fetal Medicine series. Parthenon Publishing, New York

Hoskins P, Martin K, Thrush A 2010 Diagnostic ultrasound: physics and equipment. Cambridge University Press, Cambridge, UK

Evans D H, McDicken W N, Skidmore R, Woodcock J P 1989 Doppler ultrasound: physics, instrumentation and clinical applications. Wiley, Chichester, UK

ter Haar G, ed 2012 The safe use of ultrasound in medical diagnosis, 3rd edn. British Institute of Radiology, London

Hendrick et al 1995

Guidelines for the Safe Use of Diagnostic Ultrasound Equipment (BMUS). 2009. http://www.bmus.org

Preparing to scan

This chapter addresses the issues which need to be considered before the ultrasound examination is started.

The aims of this chapter are to:

- explain the basic components of the ultrasound machine
- describe how the woman should be prepared before the scan
- describe what is required for a safe and effective environment for you as the operator.

In order to obtain maximum information from any ultrasound examination, the ultrasound equipment should be suited to the required examination and should be functioning correctly. The ultrasound technique selected should be the most appropriate for the required examination. The woman should be properly prepared and you, as the interpreter of the ultrasound information, must understand what clinical question is being asked. You must be confident that you have the technical ability and clinical knowledge to answer that question safely and correctly.

THE COMPONENTS OF THE ULTRASOUND MACHINE

The production of ultrasound images is discussed fully in Chapter 1. A brief explanation only therefore is given here.

All current equipment provides two-dimensional (2D) information and most machines now also include the additional options of three-dimensional (3D) and four-dimensional (4D) imaging, the latter being 3D imaging in real time. As almost all routine obstetric ultrasound examinations, and the vast majority of routine gynaecological ultrasound examinations, are performed using 2D imaging, this book addresses in detail the technique of 2D imaging only.

The majority of obstetric scans are performed transabdominally. However, the transvaginal ultrasound route is the preferred method of imaging pregnancies of less than 10 weeks of gestation. Furthermore there are specific clinical indications where transvaginal imaging is the preferred approach. Conversely the majority of gynaecological scans are performed transvaginally, with fewer performed transabdominally. Transabdominal scans of the nonpregnant uterus are performed either because a transvaginal scan is contraindicated or as an adjunct to the transvaginal scan. An explanation of the rationale for choosing either the transvaginal or the transabdominal approach with the respective advantages and disadvantages of both methods is discussed later in this chapter.

Real-time equipment currently available varies greatly in size, shape and complexity, but will contain five basic components:

- the probe, in which the transducer is housed
- the control panel
- the freeze control
- measuring facilities
- a means of storing images.

THE PROBE

The probe is the piece of equipment in which the transducer (or transducers) is mounted. The transducer is a piezoelectric crystal(s) which, when activated electronically, produces pulses of sound at very high frequencies – this is known as ultrasound. The crystal can also work in reverse in that it can convert the echoes returning from the body into electrical signals from which the ultrasound images are made up. In practice, however, the terms *probe* and *transducer* are used interchangeably. There are three broad types of probe: linear, sector and array. These terms refer to the way in which the crystal or crystals are arranged and manipulated to produce an image. The image field produced by the flat-faced probe is rectangular whilst that produced by the curvilinear probe is fan-shaped. The probe may be either a conventional type used externally or an intracavity type such as that used transvaginally (Fig. 2.1).

Irrespective of its type, the probe is one of the most expensive and delicate parts of the equipment. It is easily damaged if knocked or dropped and so should always be replaced in its housing when not in use. A damaged probe often causes crystal 'drop out'. This means that the signals from a small part of the probe surface are lost which in

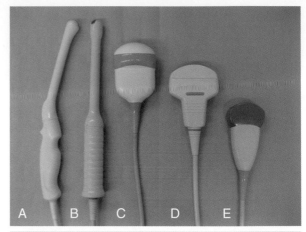

Fig. 2.1 • Ultrasound probes used for obstetric and gynaecological imaging. A, B. Transvaginal two-dimensional curvilinear. C. Transabdominal three-/four-dimensional curvilinear. D, E. Transabdominal two-dimensional curvilinear.

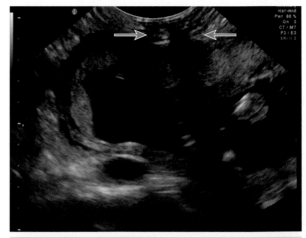

Fig 2.2 • Fan shaped image produced by a curvilinear probe. Lack of vertical information within the area of interest due to loss of contact over the umbilicus (arrows).

turn produces a vertical area within the image, which is devoid of information and therefore appears as a black vertical stripe on the ultrasound monitor. A similar appearance is produced if contact is lost between the probe surface and the maternal skin surface. This is most commonly encountered when scanning over the umbilicus or with a hirsute woman when small amounts of air become trapped in the body hair (Fig. 2.2).

Left/Right Invert Control

Which information is displayed on the left of the ultrasound monitor and which is displayed on the right is determined by a combination of the left/right invert control and the orientation of the probe.

All equipment has a left/right invert control, which, as its name suggest, reverses the left–right display on the monitor to a right–left display. All machines will display a probe orientation symbol (typically the manufacturer's logo) on the left or right side of the ultrasound monitor (Fig. 2.3). The symbol's position on the monitor is determined by whether or not the left/right invert control is activated.

Providing the invert control is not activated, one side of the probe (see point A in Fig. 2.3) always relates to one side of the ultrasound monitor. This relationship is constant however the probe is positioned. When performing longitudinal scans of the pelvis using the abdominal method, as opposed to the transvaginal method, the woman's bladder is conventionally shown on the right of the image on the ultrasound monitor (see Fig. 2.3A, left panel, and Fig. 2.3B). Holding the probe the wrong way round will alter the orientation of the image, such that the woman's bladder will be demonstrated on

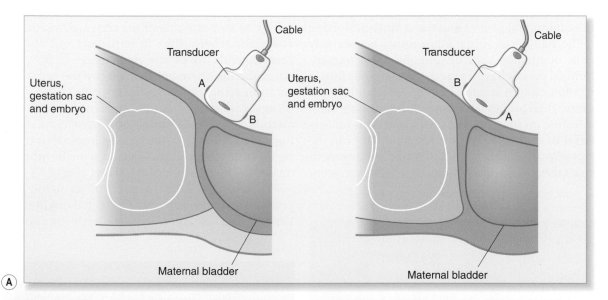
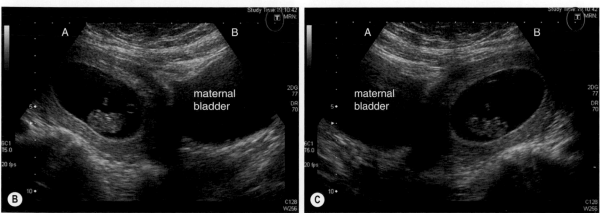

Fig 2.3 • The constant relationship between one end of the probe and one side of the screen. The end of probe 'A' relates to the left side of the screen regardless of the orientation on the maternal abdomen. The manufacturer's logo remains on the same side of the screen (red circle) indicating that the image invert control has not been activated.

31

the left side of the image (Fig. 2.3A, right panel and Fig. 2.3C). There is no convention in the United Kingdom for left/right orientation when scanning in transverse section. Many departments adopt the radiological convention, i.e. the woman's left is displayed on the right of the screen and this is the convention adopted throughout this text. Operators performing invasive techniques such as chorion villus sampling and amniocentesis have adopted the converse method and prefer to display the maternal left on the left side of the monitor. What is important for you as the operator is to maintain a consistent probe orientation in longitudinal and transverse planes, and the oblique planes in between.

The symmetrical shape and/or small size of many transabdominal probes and the symmetrical shape of the handle of some transvaginal probes may make orientation difficult initially. Most transabdominal probes have a raised mark, groove/dimple or coloured spot at one side (Fig. 2.4). Similarly all transvaginal probes have some distinguishing mark or feature on some part of the handle. This mark is useful in distinguishing the longitudinal from the transverse axis of both types of probe before experience takes over. It also provides a reference point

that you can use to ensure you always place the probe on the abdomen or into the vagina using the same orientation. Failure to understand these principles can easily lead to confusion when, for example, localizing the placenta, diagnosing fetal lie or reporting a pelvic mass. An innocuous fundal placenta may be diagnosed as placenta praevia, a cephalic presentation may be mistaken for a breech and a right-sided mass reported as left-sided if orientation of the probe is not appreciated. When performing obstetric examinations it is also important to remember that orientation of the maternal anatomy on the screen is unrelated to orientation of the fetal anatomy on the screen.

When scanning in transverse or oblique planes the relationship between one end of the transducer (point A) and one side of the screen also remains. This same relationship, in transverse and oblique planes, tends to escape the novice. It is worth remembering therefore that exactly the same orientation principle applies irrespective of the plane being scanned. A rather unscientific but easy method of confirming left and right is to run a finger over one end of the transabdominal or transvaginal transducer. The shadow seen on the monitor relates to the position of the finger (Fig. 2.5).

The left/right invert control, as its name suggests, reverses this carefully elucidated orientation. Unless you are very familiar with ultrasound

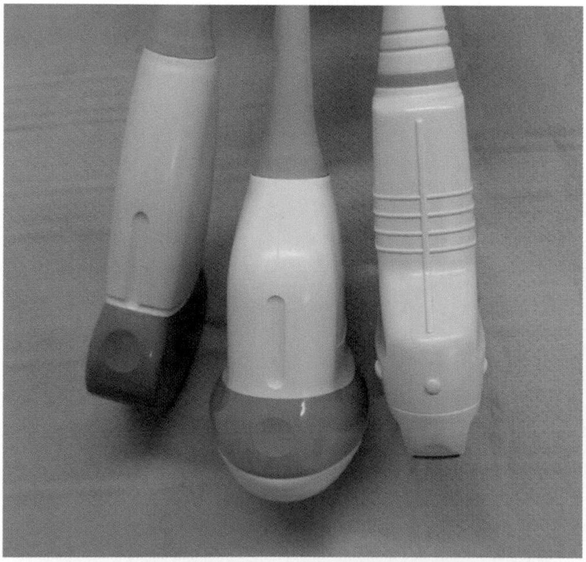

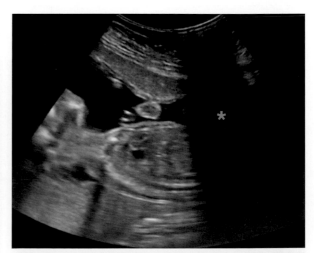

Fig 2.4 • Three types of transabdominal probes showing their identifying dimple or raised mark. This is present at one side only.

Fig 2.5 • An acoustic shadow (asterisk) produced by a finger introduced under one end of the probe can help to orientate the scan.

orientation you should always scan with this control in the same position.

The principles underpinning the orientation of the transvaginal image are the same as those that are applied when scanning transabdominally. The two techniques, however, are very different. For the novice operator it can be particularly confusing to appreciate the differences and similarities between the two methods. The orientation and acquisition of the scanning planes using the transabdominal method are explained fully in Chapter 3 and the transvaginal method in Chapter 4.

Ultrasound Frequency

Transducers transmit ultrasound over a range of frequencies but all will have a central frequency (or band of frequencies) which defines the frequency of that probe. Frequency is measured in cycles per second or hertz. Ultrasound frequencies are described in megahertz (MHz). Transabdominal probes used in obstetrics typically have central frequencies of between 3.5 MHz and 6.0 MHz, while transvaginal probes are able to utilize higher central frequencies of between 7.0 MHz and 9.0 MHz. The important principle to remember is that frequency is related to image resolution but inversely related to penetration of the sound beam into the tissue being insonated. Thus the higher the frequency of the probe, the better the resolution of the image but the shallower the depth of tissue which can be examined. Transvaginal imaging can utilize higher probe frequencies because the area of interest, e.g. the ovary, the cervical canal and the nonpregnant or the early pregnant uterus, is much closer to the transducer – and therefore the sound source – compared with the distances involved when a transabdominal probe is used.

THE CONTROL PANEL

Different manufacturers use various terms to describe what are essentially the same features on the control panel. An exhaustive description of all the knobs and buttons is not necessary. However, as the operator, you need to be aware of the most essential controls and how to manipulate them appropriately to maximize the information that can be obtained from an examination. The most important controls are power output, frequency, depth, zoom, focus, dynamic range (DR) gain and time gain compensation (TGC).

Power Output

Acoustic exposure is determined by the amount of sound transmitted into the woman and is manipulated by the power output. This should be kept as low as possible and in accordance with national and international guidelines. The information obtained from the echoes returning to, and received by, the transducer is manipulated by the gain and the time gain compensation (TGC) controls.

The power output in the manufacturer default presets is often set at 100%, i.e. maximum power output. We recommend that the power output used in any preset, including presets using colour and spectral Doppler, should be set at between 67% and 75% and not 100%. Manipulation of the gain controls should then be used to maximize the image information with an increase in the power output only applied in extreme situations.

Thermal Index and Mechanical Index

The thermal index (TI) and mechanical index (MI) provide important information, which relates to the amount of sound being transmitted into the woman when a particular combination of controls is used. Current safety guidelines recommend that the TI is kept below 0.7 and the MI is also kept below 0.7 during any obstetric ultrasound scan. The display of these two safety indices varies between manufacturers, with some always displaying both indices and others only displaying the specific index when it is above the threshold quoted in the manufacturers' regulatory guidelines of 0.4. You as the operator must be aware of where on the ultrasound monitor these indices are displayed. In addition, and, as importantly, how they change when various controls are altered, when different modalities – such as colour Doppler or spectral Doppler – are used and when specific examination presets are selected. It is your responsibility, as the user of the equipment, to perform your ultrasound examinations in accordance with national safety recommendations. The safe use of ultrasound is discussed in greater detail in Chapter 1.

Frequency

Although the probe will have a default central frequency, there is usually a control which will increase or decrease the central frequency. Decreasing the frequency is of value when more penetration is required, i.e. with a larger woman, a fibroid uterus or a posterior placenta in a late pregnancy. Conversely, increasing the frequency should be considered where the structure being examined is more superficial and greater resolution would be beneficial, i.e. scanning a second trimester pregnancy in a slim woman.

Depth and Zoom

The region of interest displayed on the monitor is manipulated by the depth and zoom controls. The depth control alters the distance from the transducer surface into the abdomen or pelvis that can be examined and is therefore also a form of image magnification. The initial survey of the pelvis or uterus requires the image depth to be set such that the full vertical extent of the structure(s) being sought can be seen (Fig. 2.6A). There is little value in scanning the uterus if its posterior wall is not included in the image – a good way of

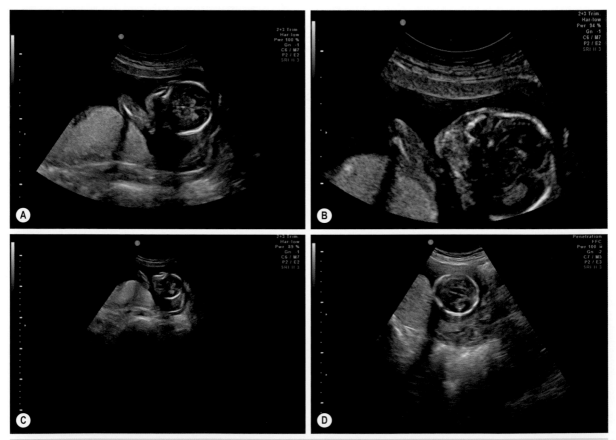

Fig 2.6 • Selecting the correct depth to perform the initial survey of the uterus. A. Correct depth control for initial uterine survey; the full depth of uterus is visible and almost fills the screen. Although the depth setting is correct, note the maximum power setting of 100% has been selected. This should be decreased to around 75% before continuing the scan. B. Depth control set too high, resulting in too little of the area of interest being imaged on the screen. Note the power setting of 94%. This should be decreased to around 75% before continuing the scan. C. Depth control set far too low, resulting in far too little of the screen displaying the area of interest. Note the power setting of 89%. This should be decreased to around 75% before continuing the scan. D. Depth control set too low. This depth setting is better than that of C but still results in too little of the screen displaying the area of interest. Note the power setting of 100%. This should be decreased to around 75% before continuing the scan.

overlooking the second twin, for example (Fig. 2.6B). Conversely, there is little value in filling the lower part of the ultrasound monitor with information produced by the woman's rectum and the scanning couch on which she is lying (Fig. 2.6C and Fig. 2.6D).

Once the initial survey of the pelvis or uterus is completed, detailed, further examination and/or measurements should be taken from images which are as large as possible. If the area of interest is close to the transducer, this can be achieved by using the depth control. If the area of interest is some distance from the probe, this can only be achieved by using the zoom control.

There are two types of zoom control, read zoom and write zoom.

Read Zoom

Read zoom is applied to a frozen image. The whole image can be magnified by the zoom control or the region of interest (ROI) box can be placed over a smaller area of the image, which requires magnification. Use the tracker ball to make sure the desired area is positioned centrally on the screen and then adjust the size of the ROI box so that only the required area will be magnified when you activate the 'select' control. When read zoom is used to magnify the image, the number of pixels from which the image is comprised remains unchanged; each pixel being simply magnified. The resultant image therefore can appear 'pixelated'.

Write Zoom

Write zoom is applied to the real-time image. The ROI box is placed over the desired area of interest and the zoom control activated. As a smaller area is selected from the original field of view, more pixels are available for the image processing. The resulting magnified area therefore has improved resolution relative to the image magnified using read zoom.

A combination of correct depth selection together with appropriate magnification of the region of interest is the preferred method of optimizing the qualitative and quantitative information within the image and reducing measurement error.

Focus

The focus control should be set at or just below the region of interest, the exact position being manufacturer-dependent. Setting the focus correctly is important as it describes the point in the image where the lateral resolution of the ultrasound beam is optimal. Focal zones can be multiple or single.

Multiple focal zones will improve resolution through the selected depth of image, at the expense of image acquisition, i.e. the frame rate. The frame rate describes the number of times the ultrasound images is refreshed per second. Multiple focal zones improve resolution as follows. When, for example, a three focal zones option is selected, the machine must transmit three separate ultrasound beams, focused at different depths, into the woman from the same point in the probe. It must then wait to receive the three sets of information before moving to the next transmission point along the probe. This takes three times as long as the single focal zone option and is therefore only an option when examining a relatively static region of interest, such as a nonpregnant pelvis. As fetal movement is a component of most obstetric ultrasound examinations, a single focal zone is usually the most practical option.

Applying too many focal zones will produce an image which does not change simultaneously with your probe movements but a fraction of time later. The resulting lag time in the image display tends to be very disconcerting and is best avoided by selecting a single focal zone.

Dynamic Range

The ultrasound image is made up of a series of dots, which range from black, through various shades of grey, to white. Dynamic range relates to the range of returning echoes that is represented by one shade of grey or, put more simply, the degree of contrast in the image (Fig. 2.7).

The dynamic range required for examinations that require a high level of contrast, i.e. those of the fetal heart (Fig. 2.7A) or nuchal translucency measurement, is lower than that required for examination of the fetal anatomy or the uterus, where more shades of grey are needed to

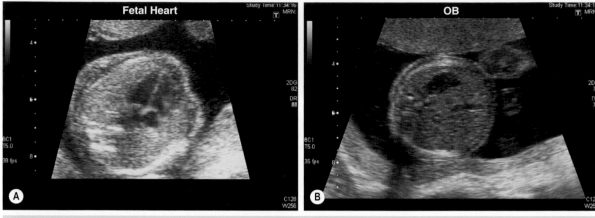

Fig 2.7 • A. A high-contrast image is desirable when examining the fetal heart. This requires a low DR setting as shown in the 'fetal heart' preset selected. B. A medium-contrast image is desirable when examining the second trimester fetal anatomy. This requires a mid DR setting as shown in the 'OB' preset selected.

appreciate the subtle differences in tissue characteristics (Fig. 2.7B).

Gain

The overall gain controls the brightness of the entire image (Fig. 2.8A–C). Too little overall gain produces a very dark image (Fig. 2.8A) whilst too much overall gain produces too bright an image (Fig. 2.8B). The overall correct gain setting is shown in Fig. 2.8C.

In addition to the overall gain control, some machines also provide the option of altering the 'near' gain and the 'far' gain independently. As their names suggest, the brightness of the upper half of the image can be altered using the near gain control, whilst the far gain control allows the lower half of the image to be altered. Gain, as used in this text, describes overall gain.

Time Gain Compensation

The brightness of horizontal slices of the image is controlled by the TGC. The TGC is manipulated by a series of sliders that relate to horizontal slices within the image field, each typically 2 cm in depth. Inappropriate setting of the TGC will produce dark (Fig. 2.9A) or light bands (Fig. 2.9B) within the image. The correct setting of the TGC tends to be manufacturer-specific, with the sliders typically raked or stacked (Fig. 2.9C).

The Resulting Image Including Presets

Manipulation of specific controls will produce an image that has, for example, more or less contrast, a higher or lower frame rate and/or high or low image persistence. Typical machine settings for a second trimester obstetric examination might include a dynamic range of 60 dB, medium persistence and a medium frame rate. Such settings produce a 'soft' image as shown in Fig. 2.7B. Examining the fetal heart is facilitated by a more contrasted image as shown in Fig. 2.7A.

The region of optimal focus can be altered to correspond to the depth of the area of maximum interest. As discussed previously, multiple focal zones improve the resolution of the image at the expense of the frame rate; thus multiple focal zones can be used during a gynaecological imaging examination as the pelvic organs will be static. These alterations can be made by the operator but most equipment has the ability to store specific combinations of machine settings provided by the manufacturer that can be recalled as preset programmes.

Presets are very useful time savers and should be explored and used fully. Remember, however, that you should also be able to adjust the controls of your machine to produce an image of the same quality as that of the preset by manipulating them yourself.

Manipulating the full range of controls, and not just the presets provided for you, is key to your

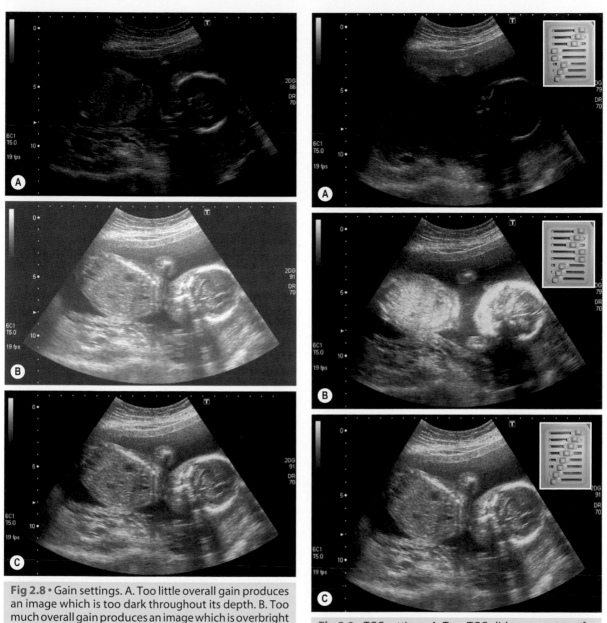

Fig 2.8 • Gain settings. A. Too little overall gain produces an image which is too dark throughout its depth. B. Too much overall gain produces an image which is overbright throughout its depth. C. The correct overall gain setting produces an image of the appropriate 'colour' throughout its depth, allowing the information it contains to be assessed properly.

Fig 2.9 • TGC settings. A. Two TGC sliders are set too far to the left resulting in a dark band in the image. This band corresponds to the depth (4 cm) controlled by this zone of the TGC. B. Two TGC sliders are set too far to the right resulting in a bright band in the image. This band corresponds to the depth (4 cm) controlled by this zone of the TGC. C. All the sliders of the TGC have been set correctly to produce an image of consistent 'brightness' throughout its depth. Note the positions of all the sliders relative to the vertical. The overall gain has also been set correctly.

ability to produce optimal images over a range of examinations irrespective of the woman's habitus.

Freeze Control

The freeze control is essential for taking measurements and for storing images. The position of the control varies; it is usually positioned on the control panel or can be provided as a foot switch.

Remember that the left hand of an experienced operator is always within instant striking distance of the control panel's freeze control.

Cine-loop

Ultrasound machines have the ability to store a specific number of frames of information, which are refreshed in real time. After the freeze control is activated, this cine-loop facility enables a portion of the examination to be 'replayed' frame by frame. This facility is invaluable for reviewing the most recent part of the examination, especially when the fetus is moving vigorously. It is also helpful for reviewing the anatomy (in both grey-scale and colour Doppler) and function (in colour Doppler) of the moving fetal heart frame by frame. It should not be used as a search facility to discover whether you have managed to image the correct section for which you were aiming. You should be able to achieve the correct section yourself, unaided by this technology.

On-Screen Measurement

All machines provide facilities for taking measurements and will typically include some or all of the following: linear, circumference, volume and area measurements.

It is a national requirement for equipment used in obstetric ultrasound examinations that linear callipers measure, and the measurement is displayed, to one decimal point of a millimetre, that is one tenth of a millimetre (0.1 mm). Circumference measurements should also provide the same facility.

The majority of calliper systems are of the rollerball type. As with all techniques, on-screen measuring requires expertise and it is therefore good practice to take several (we suggest three) measurements of any parameter to ensure accuracy.

In the obstetric setting the gestational age given will vary depending upon the equation or algorithm used for the charts programmed into the machine. We recommend that you interpret the measurements from each examination yourself rather than relying on the information produced by the machine. For example, interpreting measurements made in late pregnancy in terms of gestational age is wrong as such measurements should only be used to evaluate the pattern of fetal growth based on a previously assigned expected date of delivery.

Measurements may be displayed alone or together with an interpretation of, for example, gestational age or fetal weight when an obstetric calculation preset programme is selected.

When using spectral Doppler mode such measurements will relate to indices such as pulsatility index (PI), resistance index (RI) or peak systolic velocity (PSV). In addition to manual measurement of spectral Doppler traces automatic, continuous measurement is also available. We recommend that the automatic readout from a consistent trace is observed for several seconds to ensure that the values recorded are representative of the examination.

The Monitor

The majority of pregnant women will wish to watch their scan; therefore two monitors should be provided for all obstetric ultrasound examinations, one monitor for you the operator and a second monitor for the woman and her partner. Separate monitors allow both parties to view the examination comfortably and, more importantly, reduce considerably the risk to you of ergonomic-related repetitive strain injury (see the following discussion). Should only one monitor be available, this should be positioned directly in front of you, the operator, because you should not have to persistently rotate your neck in order to view the screen. In such a situation the monitor should only be shared with the woman once you are satisfied that you have obtained all the qualitative and quantitative information you require.

Recording Systems

Digital storage, such as picture archiving communication systems (PACS), is recommended for the permanent storage of 2D images and 3D volumes. DVD recording is the preferred method for storing 2D and 4D video clips owing to their large memory requirements. 2D images, 3D volumes and video clips can be stored on the machine's hard drive but, as the machine's capacity is limited, this does not provide a permanent archive. As with all computers, the speed of the computer is influenced by the amount of information stored. Filling the hard drive of your ultrasound machine with multiple images and clips will slow its functions down significantly and, when a certain capacity has been reached, various actions – such as the measurement functions – may not work at all.

A thermal imager is ideal for producing images for the woman as mementos from her obstetric examination. These images can also be saved on a DVD or USB which, compared with thermal images, provide a permanent rather than a time-limited record of the event. The sensitivity of thermal paper is such that small alterations of the brightness or contrast controls of either the ultrasound machine or the thermal imager will produce large differences in the quality of the thermal image. Ideally, the thermal imager controls should be set when the machine is installed. Once ideal settings have been obtained it is advisable to actively discourage over-keen colleagues from fiddling with them. Apparent deterioration in the quality of the images taken is usually due to poor gain settings, insufficient coupling gel, or dirt becoming trapped in the rollers of the thermal imaging apparatus.

Any images used for teaching purposes must be anonymized. Many ultrasound machines have the capability to store and export both anonymized individual images and complete examinations.

You should also ensure that the date and time displayed on your ultrasound machine are correct. This is particularly relevant at the start and end of British Summer Time, during leap years and when using machines which do not have an automatic date and time update feature.

THE ERGONOMICS OF SAFE SCANNING

The number of reported cases of repetitive strain injury related to ultrasound practice is increasing as the number of operators who have been scanning regularly for many years increases. It is important that the issues of operator strain, fatigue and/or injury are taken seriously both by the individual concerned and the employing department. Ideally the height of the examination couch, ultrasound machine console and any other equipment such as a computer keyboard and mouse for data entry should be adjustable. They should all be at the same height and should be placed within an arc of less than 60° from your scanning position. Such positioning together with correct height selection of your seat should enable you to access everything required during the scan without twisting, stretching or leaning. An ergonomically designed rotating chair with adjustable back support; partial, adjustable arm rests; and a foot rest should be used in preference to a stool or conventional 'office' chair. The same rules should be applied when scanning transvaginally. Most people sit to scan but your skills will be just as effective if you discover that you prefer to stand up to scan.

You should not have to persistently rotate your neck in order to view the ultrasound monitor. Thus, as stated earlier, the ergonomic needs of the operator performing the examination and those of the woman who may wish to view the examination are best served by providing two monitors, one monitor for the exclusive use of the operator and a second monitor positioned correctly for the woman's use. Should only one monitor be available, this should be positioned directly in front of you while you perform the examination and should only be shared with the woman once the clinical examination has been completed.

In many centres a room may be used for multiple types of ultrasound examinations. If you are performing both transvaginal and transabdominal examinations during a session, it is likely that you will need to change the machine's position between examinations. This should be kept to a minimum where possible, to reduce the risk, first, to you by moving bulky equipment and, second, of damage to the machine itself.

You should also make sure that you use the correct manual handling techniques when moving the ultrasound machine between its required positions to avoid damage to yourself.

The probe and electricity cables and bed controls should always be kept off the floor to minimize the risk of their damage.

The scanning room should have access to daylight and fresh air. Ideally it should be air-conditioned as the ultrasound machine produces a significant amount of heat, which, over time, is extremely debilitating for the operator, the woman and the machine's performance. If this is not possible, an electric fan and adequate ventilation are essential prerequisites.

Curtains or blinds over the windows are essential to provide dark (but not pitch black) ambient lighting levels. Scanning in either a very dark room or a room which is too light and/or with an incorrectly adjusted viewing monitor will quickly cause operator eye strain. This can be kept to a minimum by ensuring that the brightness and contrast controls of the viewing monitor are appropriate for the preferred amount of lighting. Controlled daylight, adjustable electric lighting of the room and/or the use of desk lamps, positioned to avoid reflective glare on the monitors, will ensure you the operator and the woman can see each other sufficiently well to communicate effectively during the examination.

Finally, a relaxed and informal, but informed, atmosphere will give the woman confidence not only in your scanning abilities but also to ask any questions that she may feel are important. The majority of obstetric examinations should be enjoyable, painless and reassuring to the woman. The majority of gynaecological examinations may not be enjoyable but should still be painless and reassuring when the findings are normal. The benefits of such examinations, be they medical or emotional, are directly dependent upon the quality of operator input.

PREPARING YOURSELF FOR THE SCAN

It is immaterial whether you are normally left- or right-handed as to which hand is 'better' for holding the probe. It is important that the probe is always held in the hand nearer the woman as this prevents you tying yourself in knots as you scan or, more importantly, dropping it. It is a matter of individual or departmental preference as to whether the ultrasound machine is positioned to the left or the right of the examination couch. However, the majority of manufacturers work on the right-handed scanning technique and position the probe housing and cabling accordingly.

This text assumes that you, the operator, are holding the probe in your right hand, irrespective of whether this is a transabdominal probe or a transvaginal probe, that the woman is lying to your right side and that you are facing each other.

Transvaginal scanning generally requires a slightly different arrangement of operator and machine. Ensure you are positioned in front of the perineum, holding the probe in your right hand, with the ultrasound machine close enough to operate the controls easily with your nonscanning hand. If the machine is too far away, you will jar the vagina with the probe as you stretch forward or sideways to reach the controls. Initially, many women find this method of examination embarrassing. Being able to watch the images on her dedicated monitor will often help her to relax and distract her from what you are doing.

Manual dexterity with either technique will be lacking initially, but rapidly improves with practice. Ensure that you are sitting comfortably and at the right height relative to the woman's abdomen when scanning transabdominally or to the perineum when scanning transvaginally. If your seat is too low, you will quickly develop an aching shoulder; if your seat is too high, your arm will ache from continuously stretching downwards. Try to think of the probe as an extension of your arm rather than a foreign object, and do not grip it fiercely as this will also produce a painful arm and shoulder.

The importance of the freeze control has been discussed previously. If the freeze is operated from the control panel, you should develop a technique which keeps one nonscanning finger continuously poised over the freeze button. Conversely if the freeze is operated via a foot switch, always keep your foot resting on the freeze frame foot switch so that you can instantly freeze an image if necessary. You will lose many potentially 'perfect' images if you cannot freeze the image as soon as your brain receives the message to do so.

The cine-loop is a useful tool, but you should learn to freeze optimal images rather than rely on the cine-loop because your finger or foot is too slow.

PREPARING THE WOMAN FOR THE SCAN

The clinical indication for the examination will normally determine whether the scan you are about to undertake will be performed transvaginally or transabdominally.

SELECTING THE MORE APPROPRIATE ROUTE

The majority of gynaecological ultrasound examinations should be performed using the transvaginal route with the transabdominal route being considered only when the former is inappropriate or as a complimentary technique (see the following discussion). By contrast, the majority of obstetric ultrasound examinations after 10 weeks of gestation are performed using the transabdominal approach.

We appreciate that, historically, the transabdominal approach, with a full bladder, has invariably been the first or only route used to image the nonpregnant pelvis. For those operators taught to use this method it is often initially very difficult to make the transition to scanning women who attend with empty bladders. It is worth remembering that most gynaecologists of the 'new school' have never been taught to scan using any technique other than the transvaginal route. The evidence in favour of the transvaginal route is self-explanatory when one considers the quality of the images and their clinical value compared with those obtained by the transabdominal route.

A large body of evidence now supports the fact that women find transvaginal scanning neither painful nor embarrassing. In fact, the anxiety and discomfort associated with the full bladder required for a transabdominal examination further supports the benefit of using the transvaginal route in the first instance.

In pregnancies of less than 10 weeks of gestation therefore, the transvaginal route is the preferred method of examination.

It is important to consider which of the two techniques is required on a case-by-case basis and for what reasons. Both techniques have advantages and disadvantages, the most important of which are compared in Table 2.1. The advantages and disadvantages apply primarily to gynaecological ultrasound examinations and examinations in early pregnancy. However, some are also pertinent to ultrasound examinations of later pregnancy.

As the high frequency of the transvaginal probe does not provide the penetration required to examine the uterus and fetus in its entirety in pregnancies of greater than 10 weeks of gestation, the transabdominal route is required for these examinations. However, there are also obstetric ultrasound examinations over 10 weeks of gestation where specific clinical questions are posed which also require the transvaginal route in order to maximize diagnostic accuracy and enable the clinical question to be answered. Such examinations are shown in Box 2.1.

PATIENT IDENTIFICATION

One tends to assume that the woman you are expecting to scan is the woman who enters your scanning room. Experience will show you that this is not always the case and that it is your responsibility to ensure that the identity of the woman you are about to scan correlates with the name and other details on the request form and/or case

	TRANSVAGINAL ROUTE	TRANSABDOMINAL ROUTE
Image quality in majority of gynaecological and/or early pregnancy cases	Superior	Inferior
Patient preparation	• empty bladder required • gynaecology couch with lithotomy stirrups.	• bladder sufficiently full to image uterine fundus • tilting examination couch.
Probe central frequency	7–9 MHz	3.5–6 MHz
Penetration/depth of field	• less penetration, with better resolution • the higher probe frequency reduces the depth of field that can be examined • adiposity minimal effect.	• greater penetration, with poorer resolution • the lower probe frequency allows a greater depth of field to be examined • adiposity significant effect.
Field of view	• limited by restriction of probe movements within the vagina • inability to abduct legs in the adipose or immobile woman.	• probe movements are only restricted by the symphysis pubis and the maternal ribs.
Bowel gas	Less problematic	More problematic
Pelvic masses	• adequate imaging may be compromised by probe frequency and limited field of view • need to have access to transabdominal route.	• provides an overview of the pelvis, allowing the relationship between the mass, uterus and ovaries to be determined • large masses can frequently be imaged adequately with an empty bladder.
Uterine position: • anteverted • axial • retroverted.	• imaging adequate with correct patient positioning • endometrium parallel to sound beam *so visualization compromised* • imaging adequate.	• imaging adequate with appropriate preparation • endometrium axial to sound beam (with anempty bladder) *so adequately visualised* • imaging frequently compromised, even with a full bladder.
Bleeding *per vagina*	Woman may decline (although not contra-indicated)	Woman may prefer
Chaperone required	Yes	Yes according to current guidelines
Language barrier	Contra-indicated	Only option
Paediatric patient	Contra-indicated	Only option
Virgo intacta	Contra-indicated	Only option
Mental incapacity	Contra-indicated	Only option
Woman's choice	May decline	May prefer

Table 2.1 Considerations, comparative advantages and disadvantages of imaging by the transvaginal and transabdominal routes for gynaecological and early pregnancy ultrasound scans

Clinical obstetric situations where the transvaginal route is indicated or should be considered (in italics)

Obstetric examinations where the transvaginal route is indicated:

- Early pregnancy, less than 10 weeks of gestation
- *Measurement of nuchal translucency when not possible transabdominally owing to vertical fetal position*
- *Assessment of fetal anatomy too deep in maternal pelvis to be imaged adequately using the transabdominal route*
- Cervical assessment
- Assessment of low-lying placenta in relation to the cervix
- Assessment of low-lying fibroids in relation to the cervix
- Assessment of previous caesarean section scar

notes you have in your hand. It is good practice to confirm name, date of birth and address.

Having confirmed the identity of the woman, you should enter her name and/or hospital number correctly onto the ultrasound machine. If using an electronic worklist, select the correct patient from the worklist on the ultrasound monitor and confirm that the details are correct.

Ultrasound images are as integral a part of any ultrasound examination as the written report and should, therefore, always be taken. They should also be correctly annotated where appropriate. It is vital that the patient details on the images are those of the woman being scanned and not of the previous or another patient. This mistake will be avoided if you are fastidious in the aftercare of the woman at the end of her ultrasound examination – this should include not only the cleaning of the probe, preparing the scanning couch and tidying the room, but also deleting the last ultrasound image and/or all information on the scanning monitor and computer relating to this woman before calling in the next.

PREPARING THE PROBE

Any probe should be cleaned after use and thus should be clean and ready to use at the start of the next examination. Individual soap-impregnated wipes and/or hard surface disinfectant spray are commonly employed for this purpose. It is important that advice is sought from the probe's manufacturer as some liquid preparations may adversely affect the transducer covering, making use of such products unsafe.

It is unacceptable practice to leave a gel-covered probe and/or a transvaginal probe still covered with its previous probe cover on the machine at the end of an examination. The next woman you scan should never have to watch you removing gel or, worse, a used probe cover from a previous examination from the probe with which you are about to examine her.

COUPLING MEDIUM

There are many proprietary brands of ultrasound gel or coupling medium available, the variations being in viscosity, colour and price. All fulfil the same function of providing an air-free interface between the transducer and the body to allow effective transmission (and receiving) of the ultrasound beam into the body from the probe. When using the transabdominal probe, this is achieved through direct contact, via the applied layer of ultrasound gel, between the probe surface and the woman's skin. The transvaginal route requires two layers of gel to achieve effective transmission. The first layer of gel is applied between the probe and the probe cover and the second to the outside of the probe cover, over the tip of the probe.

Ultrasound gel at room temperature feels very cold, so try to ensure the gel is warmed before starting an examination. Electric bottle warmers designed specifically for the ultrasound market are available.

PROTECTION

A successful examination requires sufficient gel to be applied such that the images obtained can be interpreted. This usually requires far less gel than the beginner feels is necessary, so apply the gel sparingly in the first instance. Too liberal an application of gel will tend to collect on the transducer cable as you move the probe over the maternal abdomen.

The examination should not result in the woman leaving your scanning room with gel-stained clothing, so you must provide protection for her clothing with, for example, disposable paper roll. One piece of roll tucked into her underwear is very unlikely to protect this from becoming soaked with gel. It will do nothing to protect her upper garments from gel, and neither will it protect your right trouser leg, dress or skirt from any excess gel collected on the transducer cable.

The Triple Sheets Technique

Adopting the triple sheets technique will provide adequate protection for both the woman's and your clothing. Take two or three sheets of paper roll, fold them double, then tuck this double-folded length into the top of the woman's underwear. Ensure that both her underwear and her skirt or trousers are protected by making sure you do not tuck the paper *between* her outer clothing and her underwear. Take another two or three sheets of paper roll, double fold it and tuck this into her upper outer clothing. Finally take a third two or three sheets, fold this and place it over your right thigh and knee. This will protect your clothing from any excess gel dripping from the cable onto your leg (Fig. 2.10).

This technique will usually provide sufficient protection for the woman's clothing. It will also allow you or her to use the lower paper pad – which is likely to be gel-dampened but should still be an intact barrier protecting her lower clothing – to remove the majority of the gel from her abdomen. The second pad – which will usually be completely gel-free and therefore dry – allows her to wipe her abdomen dry with clean paper. Meanwhile the third pad, placed over your right knee, will provide you with an instantly accessible means of wiping the probe at the end of the examination, before cleansing it with the antiseptic wipe and replacing it in its housing.

A modified process can be applied for the transvaginal examination. The woman's lower pelvis and legs will be covered by a disposable sheet during the examination but she should still be given some paper sheets to remove excess gel from her perineum once you have completed the scan. Softer tissues should also be available to her in the changing area. The paper sheets can be prepared before you start the scan, and kept within easy reach during the scan, so that they can be handed to the woman as soon as you have removed the probe from her vagina. The paper over your right knee can now be used to receive the probe cover and remove the gel from the probe, before cleaning the probe as described earlier.

PREPARING FOR A TRANSVAGINAL SCAN

You must never begin preparations for a transvaginal examination unless you are aware of the latex allergy status of the woman you are about to scan. Latex-free probe covers must be available, and if the woman is uncertain whether or not she is allergic either to latex or rubber, a latex-free probe cover must be used. Similarly, latex-free gloves must be available for you, the operator, to wear during the ultrasound examination of a woman who is allergic to latex.

Transvaginal imaging requires the woman to have a completely empty bladder as even a small amount of urine in the bladder can displace organs of interest out of the field of view. The woman should therefore be asked to empty her bladder immediately prior to her ultrasound examination.

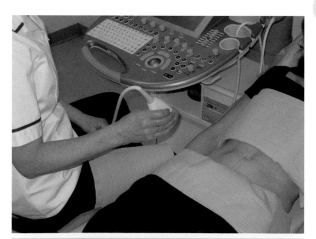

Fig 2.10 • The triple sheets technique involves one double-folded paper sheet protecting the woman's lower outer clothing, a second protecting her upper outer clothing and the third protecting the operator's right thigh.

Privacy is essential during all ultrasound examinations and is a prerequisite for all transvaginal examinations. Many women feel embarrassed and vulnerable when expected to undress in front of a stranger, be that stranger male or female. Many centres do not provide separate changing facilities so it essential that, if being asked to undress in the scanning room itself prior to her transvaginal scan, the woman is able to do so behind a curtain or screen. She must be given the courtesy of having her lower pelvis and legs covered during the examination so should be given a disposable sheet for this purpose before being asked to undress.

PREPARING FOR A TRANSABDOMINAL SCAN

Gynaecological or early ultrasound examinations should only be undertaken using the transabdominal route in cases where the transvaginal route is contraindicated or not available (see Table 2.1).

In cases where a transvaginal scan is contraindicated, the transabdominal examination will require the woman to have a full bladder. Her bladder should be full enough to allow the full length of the uterus, including the fundus, to be clearly visualized. The woman should be instructed to drink 1 litre of still water or squash 1 hour before her examination and to not empty her bladder until after the scan is completed.

She should be made to understand that 1 cup of coffee on the way to the department will not fill her bladder sufficiently and is likely to result in her having a long wait before the examination can be completed successfully. When her bladder is overfull and the woman is in obvious discomfort, partial bladder emptying is the best solution. Sufficient urine will usually be retained to make a successful examination possible. It is poor professional practice to keep a woman who has arrived correctly prepared with a full bladder for her transabdominal scan waiting past her appointment time. You should ensure therefore that you are able to keep your scanning list running to time in order that she is not kept waiting unnecessarily.

You must bear in mind that a contraindication to a transvaginal scan may not be apparent until the time of the woman's appointment. This will result in a dilemma, for which the solution is one of two options. The first option, and the option we recommend in the first instance, is to attempt a transabdominal scan as the woman may not have recently emptied her bladder. Her bladder may, therefore, be filled adequately enough for you to examine her uterus and ovaries properly. Alternatively the woman must commence drinking water or squash as soon as possible and wait for a further 30–45 minutes until her bladder is adequately filled. This is not good use of the woman's time or of your clinical time. Wherever possible therefore the requestors of such scans should be encouraged to inform you when a transvaginal scan is contraindicated and reminded why this information is important both for the woman and for the clinical department.

It is normally unnecessary for a woman attending for a scan during the late first, second or third trimesters of pregnancy to have a full bladder. Having some urine in her bladder, however, is helpful as this allows better visualization of the lower uterus and cervical canal. We recommend that such women attend with sufficient urine in their bladders to be comfortable.

Some women feel embarrassed and vulnerable when asked to reveal their abdomen to a stranger, irrespective of whether they are a male or female health professional. It is important that the woman allows you access to enough of her abdomen for the examination to be undertaken properly but equally important that you are sensitive to the discomfort she may be experiencing.

For the woman who attends for her transabdominal scan wearing a dress or skirt, a clean sheet should be provided to cover her lower pelvis and legs, in addition to the protective paper described earlier.

AFTERCARE

Incorporating the suggestions made in this chapter into your scan routine should ensure that the woman's experiences before, during and after the scan are as positive as you are able to make them. Once she is dressed again and before she leaves the scanning room, you should ensure that the woman is aware of the findings of your examination, of when and how she will receive the results or written report of the examination you have just performed and whether or not further additional examinations and/or follow-up are required.

Further reading

Dutta R, Economides D 2003 Patient acceptance of trans-vaginal ultrasound in the early pregnancy unit setting. Ultrasound Obstet Gynecol 22;503–507

NHS Fetal Anomaly Screening Programme. Available http://www.fetalanomaly.screening.nhs.uk/

Society of Radiographers 2007 Prevention of work-related musculoskeletal disorders in sonography. Available http://www.SOR.org/learning/

ter Haar G, ed 2012 The safe use of ultrasound in medical diagnosis, 3rd edn. The British Institute of Radiology, London

The Royal College of Obstetricians and Gynaecologists 1997 Intimate examinations: report of a working party. RCOG Press, London

The Royal College of Obstetricians and Gynaecologists 2002 Gynaecological examinations: guidelines for specialist practice. RCOG Press, London

United Kingdom Association of Sonographers 2008 Guidelines for professional working standards – ultrasound practice. United Kingdom Association of Sonographers

Starting to scan using the transabdominal route

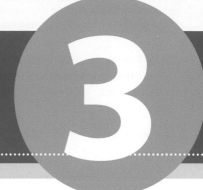

3

CONTENTS

This chapter explains the transabdominal method of imaging. As the majority of student sonographers start their training by learning to scan the second trimester fetus using the transabdominal probe, the techniques described here relate mainly to using this route to examine the second trimester fetus.

The aims of this chapter are to enable you to:

- understand the four transabdominal probe movements
- perform a survey of the uterus
- assess fetal number
- find the longitudinal axis of the fetus
- confirm the presence of heart pulsations
- identify fetal position
- obtain a midsagittal section of the fetus.
- assess situs.

Although the basic techniques of image production are the same, transabdominal and transvaginal imaging methods require the mastering of different probe movements. The transvaginal method of imaging is discussed in Chapter 4.

The first objective of the midtrimester abdominal examination is to find the fetus within the uterus. The position and movement of the fetus are unpredictable and unique to each examination, therefore you the operator must develop a methodical and systematic approach from the outset in order to provide a clinically competent examination.

PREPARING TO SCAN

Transabdominal ultrasound scans during pregnancy are an integral if not routine component of a woman's antenatal care. However, it is still important that the woman understands what her scan will entail.

The woman needs to be aware that:

- she does not need a full bladder
- she will be required to expose her abdomen sufficiently for the scan to be performed
- successful completion of the scan is dependent upon fetal position and maternal factors such as an increased body mass index (BMI), abdominal scarring and uterine fibroids

- a follow-up examination may be required if all the necessary information cannot be obtained.

THE WOMAN

The preparatory requirements that need to be considered prior to undertaking a scan have been discussed fully in Chapter 2. It is unnecessary for women to be instructed to attend for their scan appointments with a full bladder. There are methods of ensuring the lower uterus and its contents are adequately imaged which are as, if not more, effective than a full bladder, as discussed later. We recommend that the woman is instructed to arrive for her scan 'as you are' or with a bladder that is 'comfortable'. She does **not** therefore need to drink a litre of water 1 hour before her scan appointment.

The woman should lie supine with the examination couch arranged so that she lies with her head slightly raised with a pillow or head rest. Some women, especially in later pregnancy, feel dizzy in this position due to supine hypotension and it may be necessary for the woman to be tilted to one side. This is easily achieved by placing a pillow under one of her buttocks.

The woman's abdomen should be uncovered just sufficiently to allow the examination to be performed. This will always include the first few centimetres of the area covered by her pubic hair and will extend far enough upwards to allow the fundus of the uterus to be visualized.

A woman who is wearing a dress should be offered a sheet or disposable paper roll sufficient to cover her legs during the examination.

The majority of women attending for an obstetric ultrasound examination wish to see the ultrasound images on the screen. As discussed in Chapter 2, it is important to consider both the woman's wishes to 'watch her baby' and the ergonomic needs of the operator performing the examination. These needs are best served by providing two monitors, one monitor for the exclusive use of the operator and a second monitor positioned correctly for the woman's use. The woman should be positioned such that she is able to see her monitor easily, thereby removing the need for her to move frequently to see her baby better. Maternal movement is both distracting and unhelpful when trying to obtain the correct sections of the fetal target, which rarely remains still within the uterus.

Ensure that the couch, ultrasound machine, your ultrasound monitor and the scanning stool are placed in such a way so as to minimize repetitive strain injury.

Make sure also that the scanning room is stocked with gel, paper roll, thermal print paper and antiseptic wipe or spray prior to starting a scan.

PREPARING THE PROBE

The abdominal probe should have been cleaned with an appropriate antiseptic wipe or spray at the end of the preceding examination. It is also good practice to clean the probe with an antiseptic wipe at the start of your examination first, for reasons of hygiene and also to reassure the woman that she is about to be scanned with a clean probe.

PROTECTION

Ultrasound gel is usually applied to the woman's abdomen rather than to the surface of the probe as the former ensures a more even coverage across her abdomen. Apply the gel sparingly; too liberal an application of gel will tend to collect on the cable as you move the probe over the maternal abdomen. We suggest adopting the triple sheets technique previously described in Chapter 2. This is to avoid gel stains on the clothes of the woman and of you the operator.

THE SCANNING TECHNIQUE

ORIENTATION

There is no agreed convention as to whether the operator sits to the left or the right of the examination couch, whether he or she is facing the woman or looking at her feet or whether he or she holds the probe in their right or left hand.

The technique described here assumes that you, the operator, are sitting to the left of the scanning couch and are holding the probe in your right hand, that the woman is lying to your right side and that you are facing each other.

The agreed convention, when performing transabdominal longitudinal scans of the uterus, is to display the maternal bladder on the right of the image on the ultrasound monitor and the uterine fundus on the left of the image. This text adopts this principle.

There is no agreed convention as to whether the left of the woman's abdomen should be displayed on the left or on the right of the ultrasound monitor. We recommend that the radiological convention is used – that is, that the left side of the maternal abdomen is displayed on the right side of the monitor and vice versa. This text adopts this principle.

Modern probes are light and designed from the ergonomic as well as from the functional perspectives. It is important to learn quickly how to hold the probe comfortably, with a light to moderate grip and in a position which allows easy rotation of the wrist. Holding the probe incorrectly will increase the risk of your incurring a musculoskeletal injury.

As stated earlier, transabdominal longitudinal scans of the uterus conventionally display the maternal bladder on the right of the image on the ultrasound monitor and the uterine fundus on the left of the image. As discussed in Chapter 2 the transabdominal probe will have a groove or mark at one side (Fig. 2.4). This is a reference point that can be used to ensure that the correct orientation is applied to an examination. Hold the probe comfortably and place it on the maternal abdomen in the midline, immediately superior to the symphysis pubis (Fig. 3.1A). The ultrasound monitor will now display a longitudinal midsagittal section of the maternal abdomen. Note whether the probe orientation symbol is displayed to the left or to the right of the ultrasound image on the monitor. As described in Chapter 2, its position is related to whether or not the left/right invert control is activated. If you have orientated the probe correctly, the maternal bladder will be seen on the right of the monitor (Fig. 3.1B). Note whether the reference mark or groove on the probe is towards the woman's head or towards her feet when this image is displayed. If the maternal bladder is displayed to the left of the image sector, then rotating the probe through 180° will display the maternal bladder to the right on the ultrasound monitor. Note that the position of the probe orientation symbol remains unchanged. Note also how the probe cable lies relative to your scanning hand after you have reversed the position of the probe.

As most of your colleagues will use the same scanning technique, you will find that the probe

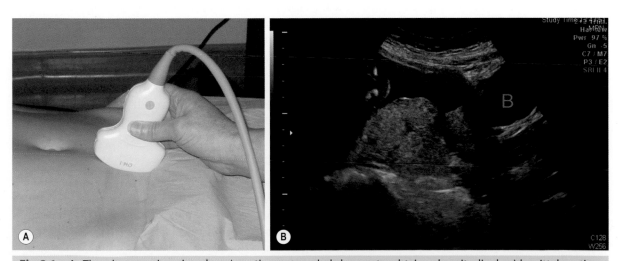

Fig 3.1 • A. The ultrasound probe placed on the maternal abdomen to obtain a longitudinal midsagittal section. B. The corresponding image obtained from the section in Fig. 3.1A. Note the maternal bladder (B) to the right of the image.

cable will tend to lie less stiffly when the probe is positioned with its reference mark either towards the woman's head or towards her feet. Hold the probe so that the cable is lying in its 'preferred' position and repeat the process described earlier to display a longitudinal midline section of the maternal abdomen. The maternal bladder should be displayed to the right of the image. If the maternal bladder is displayed to the left of the image (i.e. the orientation is incorrect), then activate the left/right invert control. The maternal bladder will then be displayed to the right of the image (i.e. the correct orientation). Note that activating the left/right invert control will change the position of the probe orientation symbol.

This method should ensure that that you are orientating the probe correctly, that the cable is not flopping over your scanning hand and that the left/right orientation control is appropriately set to produce longitudinal images in subsequent examinations which demonstrate the correct orientation, namely of the fundus on the left and the maternal bladder on the right of the image on the ultrasound monitor.

THE PROBE MOVEMENTS

There are only a limited number of ways in which a probe can be manipulated and, with the transabdominal probe, these are described by four movements. If you understand what each of these movements achieves you will quickly learn how to obtain the correct images for assessment and/or measurement. You will also understand how to move from a less than ideal section to the ideal section and when this is difficult, for example due to fetal position, you will not waste time trying to achieve the impossible.

The four possible movements of the transabdominal probe are (Fig. 3.2):

- sliding
- rotating
- angling
- dipping.

Sliding (Fig. 3.2A)

Sliding describes the movement of the probe across the maternal abdomen in a direction which is parallel to its original plane. Sliding in the sagittal plane therefore changes the position of the longitudinal sections imaged relative to the mother's midline. Sliding in the transverse plane changes the position of the cross-sections imaged, relative to the maternal symphysis pubis. As discussed below a uterine survey should be performed at the start of every scan and this is achieved using the sliding movement only.

Many beginners make the mistake of changing the angle of the probe when they think they are only sliding the probe. It is very important that you learn, as early as possible, to feel the difference between sliding, angling and a combination of the two. It is therefore helpful to look at the position of your hand before you start your sliding movement, and again once you have completed it. The angle at which you are holding the probe to the maternal abdomen should not have changed. At the start of the scan you should be holding the probe at 90° to the maternal abdomen. You should still be holding the probe at right angles to the maternal abdomen when you have finished sliding. An inability to appreciate the difference between sliding and angling causes great confusion for the novice sonographer.

Sliding is also the movement which will enable you to bring a structure which you wish to examine, but which is lying at one side of the ultrasound image, into a central position on the screen. If you are scanning in longitudinal section and the structure is seen towards the left of the screen, i.e. towards the uterine fundus, sliding your probe towards the fundus will result in your bringing the structure into the centre of the screen. If you are scanning in transverse section, and the structure is seen towards the left of the screen, i.e. towards the maternal right, sliding your probe towards the mother's right side will result in your bringing the structure into the centre of the screen.

Rotating (Fig. 3.2B)

Rotating describes rotation of the probe about a fixed point. The probe can be rotated on the maternal abdomen or by taking the probe off the skin, rotating and then replacing it onto the skin. The former movement is used when small changes in the position of the probe are required. The latter is useful when large changes, such as 90° of rotation, are required, it is the recommended method of

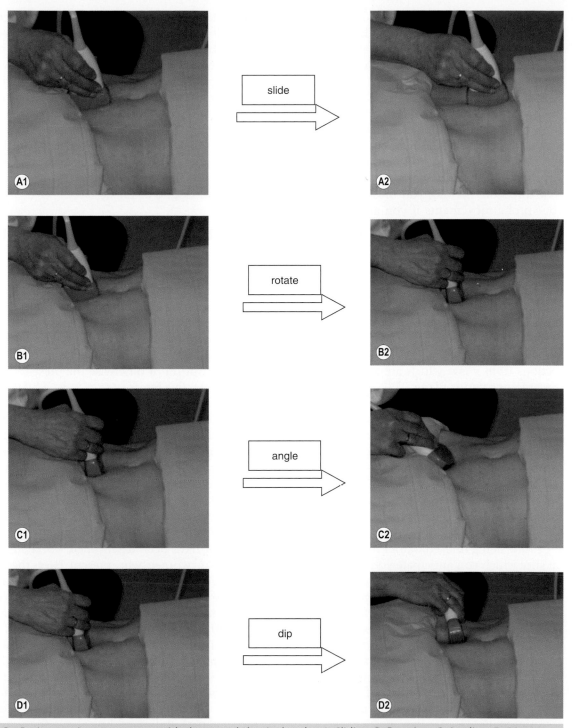

Fig 3.2 • Basic scanning movements with the transabdominal probe. A. Sliding. B. Rotating. C. Angling. D. Dipping.

rotating the probe from a longitudinal view of the fetus to a cross-sectional view. This is because it achieves the required orthogonal section more quickly and removes the temptation to stop rotating the probe before the full 90° of rotation has been reached.

Rotation of the probe to obtain a cross-section from a longitudinal section should always be performed by turning the probe in an anticlockwise direction. This is because, first, it is easier to rotate your right hand in an anticlockwise than a clockwise direction. Second, you must be consistent in your probe movements if you are to develop the innate understanding of how to move your probe to the correct section you are seeking from the incorrect section you have just obtained.

Angling (Fig. 3.2C)

Angling describes an alteration of the angle of the complete probe surface relative to the woman's skin surface. Its main use is for obtaining correct sections from views which are slightly oblique in the anteroposterior plane. This is because angling alters the angle at which a structure is 'sliced' anteroposteriorly by the ultrasound beam. Most suboptimal views of the intracranial anatomy, for example, are produced because of incorrect angling which results in a midline that is not centrally placed within the head together with discordance in the respective appearances of the anterior and posterior skull outlines. Angling while sliding results in an oblique section of the maternal abdomen under the probe being imaged, rather than the true sagittal slice which you anticipate you are producing.

As described with sliding, many beginners make the mistake of changing the angle of the probe when they are setting out to perform one of the other two probe movements. It is very important that you learn, as early as possible, to feel the difference between angling and any of the other three movements. An appreciation of what the movement feels like and the effect of angling on the image is critical if you intend to develop optimal scanning skills.

Dipping (Fig. 3.2D)

Dipping describes pressing one end of the probe into the woman's abdomen. This should not be uncomfortable and so should be done as gently as possible. The main use of dipping is to redirect the sound beam from an acute angle to the structure of interest to one of 90°. This optimizes the information produced and has the effect of moving the structure of interest so that it lies in the horizontal plane. Dipping is particularly helpful when assessing the intracranial anatomy if the midline is not lying at 90° to the ultrasound beam and when imaging the femur prior to measuring its length if, similarly, the shaft of the femur is not lying at 90° to the ultrasound beam.

THE UTERINE SURVEY AND ASSESSING FETAL NUMBER

The uterine survey should be undertaken at the start of every scan. The sliding movement is the only movement that is required to perform it.

The aims of the uterine survey are:
- to confirm or otherwise the presence of an intrauterine pregnancy
- to confirm or otherwise the presence of a single, live fetus
- to assess the longitudinal lie of the fetus
- to exclude the presence of intrauterine fibroids and ovarian pathology of significant size.

You should always be aware of the possibility that a pregnancy may be multiple rather than single. Before their second trimester scan most women will have had a dating or combined screening scan when, hopefully, the correct number of fetuses *in utero* will have been determined. For a small proportion of women who present later, the second trimester examination will be their first scan. Irrespective of whether this is or is not the woman's first scan it is good practice to begin every examination with a survey which extends from the left lateral wall of the uterus to its right lateral wall and from the symphysis pubis to the uterine fundus. Extending the survey out to the pelvic sidewalls will contribute to excluding coexisting ovarian pathology.

Start the uterine survey by placing the probe on the maternal abdomen, just above the symphysis pubis, to obtain a correctly orientated midsagittal longitudinal section as described previously. Determine whether or not this section includes the uterine fundus. If the uterus is too big to image its full length, from the internal os to the fundus, you will need to perform the uterine survey using two sets of lateral sliding sweeps rather than one. While maintaining a constant angle of the probe to the maternal abdomen, slide the probe from the midline towards the maternal left side. Keep sliding until you have imaged the left uterine wall, then slide a little further to the left to complete the survey of the left side of the maternal pelvis. Slide the probe back to the midline and then repeat this process towards the maternal right until you have imaged the right uterine wall and the right side of the maternal pelvis. Remember to keep your probe upright and its angle to the maternal skin constant.

Should you now need to perform a second set of lateral sliding sweeps, return to the midline and slide the probe towards the maternal head sufficiently that you can image the uterine fundus – this should be visible on the left of the ultrasound image. Repeat the sliding process to the woman's left side, return to the midline and repeat the sliding process to her right side to complete the uterine and pelvic survey.

During your survey of the uterus, you must note the number of fetal heads you pass, the number of fetal bodies and the presence of fetal heart pulsations within the fetal chest(s). Failing to keep your probe upright as you perform your survey, i.e. changing the angle of the probe as you slide, will frequently give you the false impression that you have seen, for example, two fetal heads and therefore that this must be a twin pregnancy. In a true twin pregnancy, you will be able to demonstrate two fetal heads in the same image. This will not be possible in a pseudo-twin pregnancy produced by incorrect manipulation of the probe.

FETAL LIE, PRESENTATION, ATTITUDE AND POSITION

IDENTIFYING THE FETAL POSITION

In the context of this text, *fetal position* describes the combination of fetal lie, presentation and attitude. Understanding the position of the fetus is an essential prerequisite for the majority of the fetal biometry and much of the anatomical assessment you need to perform. One of the skills you must achieve is the ability to manipulate your probe correctly so that you can reproduce the same section of any fetus irrespective of how it is lying within the uterus.

LIE AND PRESENTATION

The terms *lie* and *presentation* describe two different entities but are frequently used interchangeably, and therefore incorrectly, to describe the same thing.

Fetal lie describes the position of the fetus within the uterus and can be therefore be longitudinal, transverse or oblique. *Presentation* describes the part of the fetus which would be delivered first during vaginal delivery. The most common types of presentation of relevance to ultrasound examination are therefore cephalic, breech and, in later pregnancy, extended breech or flexed breech.

The lie and presentation of a fetus which is lying head down and parallel to the maternal spine are correctly described as a longitudinal lie and a cephalic presentation. The lie and presentation of a fetus which is lying head down but is not parallel to the maternal spine are correctly described as an oblique lie and a cephalic presentation. The lie and presentation of a fetus which is lying head up and parallel to the maternal spine are correctly described as a longitudinal lie and a breech presentation. A fetus which is lying across the uterus should be described simply as having a transverse lie. Describing this position in terms of presentation is incorrect for the reasons described earlier.

FINDING THE LONGITUDINAL AXIS OF THE FETUS AND CONFIRMING A LIVE FETUS

Having established the presence of a singleton live pregnancy, the next task is to establish the position of the fetus in the uterus and then to demonstrate to the woman a section of the full length of her fetus in which the heart of her fetus can be seen to be beating. Unfortunately, because the fetus can lie in any position within the uterus, a longitudinal

53

section of the uterus will not necessarily demonstrate the longitudinal axis of the fetus. If the fetus is lying transversely across the uterus, for example, a longitudinal scanning plane of the uterus will demonstrate a transverse section of the fetal head, body or trunk rather than a sagittal section. Finding the longitudinal axis of the fetus is an important precursor to performing fetal biometry accurately and assessing fetal anatomy correctly.

Finding the longitudinal axis of the fetus can be incorporated within the uterine survey but, as a beginner, it is usually less confusing to perform the survey first and then, once completed, concentrate on finding a proper longitudinal section of the fetus.

To find the longitudinal axis of the fetus, irrespective of its position within the uterus, first place the probe on the maternal abdomen to obtain a midline longitudinal section of the uterus. Slide the probe to each side of the maternal abdomen until you visualize the fetal head (Fig. 3.3A). Make sure you maintain a constant angle of the probe to the maternal abdomen as you slide. Having located the fetal head, make a mental note of the position of your right hand, which is holding the probe, on the maternal abdomen. Now slide back across the maternal abdomen, again keeping the angle of the probe constant, until you find a section of the fetal body in which heart pulsations can be seen (Fig. 3.3B). This section confirms the presence of a

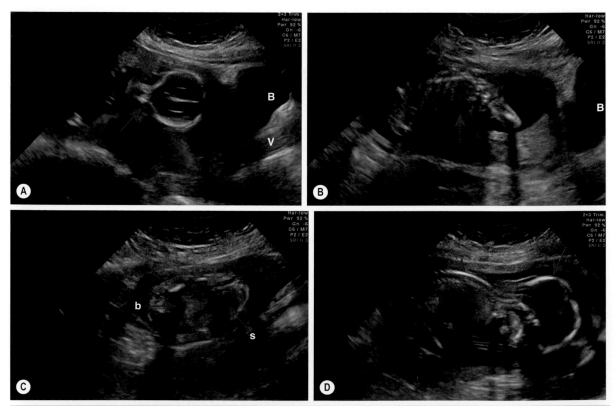

Fig 3.3 • A. Longitudinal section of the lower uterus in the midline. The maternal bladder (B) can be seen on the right, with the vagina (V) lying posterior to it. The fetal head is seen in coronal section. Both orbits (arrow) can be seen. B. Longitudinal section of the lower uterus, to the left of the midline, with the maternal bladder (B) on the right. An oblique section of the upper fetal body is obtained showing part of the heart (dashed arrow). C. Longitudinal section of the lower uterus further to the left of the midline than the section shown in Fig. 3.3B. The maternal bladder is no longer seen in this lateral section of the maternal pelvis. An oblique section of the lower fetal body is seen. Part of the stomach can be seen (s), together with the fetal bladder (b). D. The longitudinal section of the fetus is obtained by rotating the probe to link together the three sections shown in Fig. 3A, B and C. The fetus is cephalic. Note, its position has changed and it is now looking downwards with its occiput anterior (arrow). It is therefore occipito-anterior (OA) with its spine (dashed arrow) anterior.

live fetus and therefore an ongoing pregnancy. Again make a mental note of the position of your right hand, which is holding the probe, on the maternal abdomen. Keep sliding the probe across the maternal abdomen until you find the fetal bladder (Fig. 3.3C). The fetal bladder varies in size but is rarely completely empty, so provides a useful landmark for the lower end of the body. Make a third mental note of your right hand's position.

Depending on the size of the fetus you may not find all the three landmarks of the head, the heart and the fetal bladder during your survey. To find the rest of the fetus, you need to combine sliding the probe across the uterus – to the left side and to the right side – with sliding it up and down the uterus – from the symphysis pubis to the fundus.

Having remembered where your right hand was positioned when you identified each of the three fetal landmarks in the uterus, rotate the probe on the maternal abdomen until its position links the three positions of your hand described earlier in a straight line. Unless the fetal position is very curled, linking these three probe positions should produce an image of the head, the heart within the fetal chest and the fetal bladder within the fetal abdomen – namely, a longitudinal section of the fetus (Fig. 3.3D).

Once you are satisfied that the image on the ultrasound monitor demonstrates a longitudinal section of the fetus, the position of the probe and your right hand on the maternal abdomen will tell you whether the fetal lie within the uterus is longitudinal, transverse or oblique. This longitudinal section of the fetus may be sagittal, coronal or somewhere in between, depending on whether the position of the fetus is prone, supine or decubitus within the uterus.

If the fetal lie is essentially longitudinal, make sure that, when linking up the three landmarks by rotating the probe, you rotated the probe in the correct direction so that the maternal bladder remains on the right side of the screen and the fundus on the left. Similarly, if the lie is essentially transverse, make sure that you rotated the probe correctly so that the maternal left remains on the right side of the screen and her right remains on the left side of the screen.

You now need to determine whether the presentation is cephalic or breech and, if the lie is transverse, whether the fetal head is on the maternal left or on the right (Fig. 3.4).

Difficulties in Finding the Longitudinal Axis of the Fetus

Fetal position

It may be difficult to image the presenting fetal part when it lies low in the maternal pelvis. This makes it difficult to work out the accurate lie of the fetus. In such situations what is needed is to move the presenting fetal part out of the pelvis. There are various methods of encouraging the fetus to change its position. First warn the woman what you are about to do and then gently shake the maternal abdomen with the probe. If this does not produce the desired movement, ask the woman to roll right over onto her left side and then onto her right side in rapid succession. If this also fails, use the scanning couch controls to raise the foot of the scanning couch and tip the woman head down. If none of these actions is successful, the woman should be asked to go for a short walk before trying again to image the necessary sections.

Excessive fetal movement

During the course of an ultrasound scan the fetus will alternate between lying fairly still and undergoing periods of activity. It can be very frustrating to try to work out the lie of the fetus when it is being particularly active. This is because a scanning speed is required that can keep up with the fetal movements. Unfortunately, scanning effectively at speed is another skill which the novice sonographer lacks – but it will develop with practice, and patience. The best solution with a rapidly moving fetus is to defer this part of the examination for a few minutes. As an alternative, use the time to evaluate a less active component of the uterus such as the placenta, before returning to the fetus whose burst of frantic activity will usually now have slowed or ceased altogether.

DEMONSTRATING THE LIVE FETUS TO THE WOMAN

You already know that the fetus is alive because you used the position of the fetal heart within the uterus to establish the longitudinal axis of the

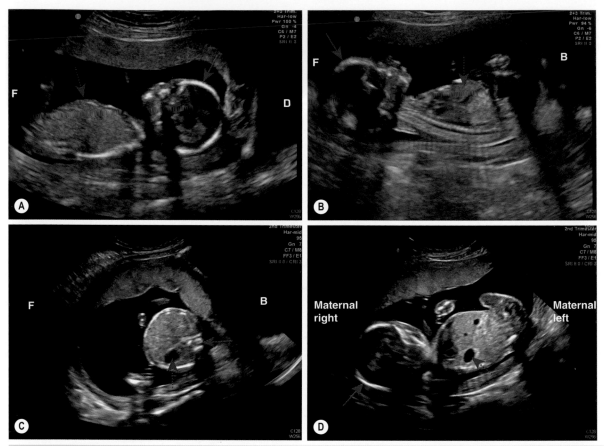

Fig 3.4 • A. Longitudinal section of the uterus in the midline showing the maternal bladder to the right (B) and the fundus (F) to the left. The fetal head (arrow) can be seen on the right of the screen and its body (dashed arrow) on the left. The fetal presentation is therefore cephalic. B. Longitudinal section of the uterus, slightly lateral to the midline, showing the maternal bladder to the right (B) and the fundus (F) to the left. The fetal head (arrow) can be seen on the left of the screen and its body (dashed arrow) on the right. The fetal presentation is therefore breech. C. Longitudinal section of the uterus, to one side of the midline, showing the maternal bladder to the right (B) and the fundus (F) to the left. A cross-section of the fetal abdomen can be seen. The fetal lie is therefore transverse. The fetal spine (arrow) is towards the maternal bladder and the fetal stomach (dashed arrow) can be seen posteriorly. The fetus is therefore lying with its spine towards the maternal bladder and, as its stomach is posterior, you would expect to find its head to the maternal right. Locating the fetal head on the maternal right will confirm normal situs. D. Rotating the probe in an anticlockwise direction from the image shown in Fig. 3.4C should produce a longitudinal section of the fetus. The mother's left side is on the right of the screen and her right side is on the left of the screen. The head (arrow) can be seen on the left of the screen, i.e., the maternal right. The fetal stomach (dashed arrow) can be seen posteriorly as expected from its position in Fig. 3.4C. The fetal spine will be imaged from this section by sliding the probe down towards the maternal bladder.

fetus. You are also aware that fetal heart pulsations will normally be obvious when the probe is aligned with the fetal chest. The next step is to demonstrate a section of the full length of her fetus to the woman in which its heart can be seen to be beating clearly. This should be done as soon as you have obtained a longitudinal section of the fetus in which the heart pulsations can be clearly seen. Do

not rush this part of the examination but take a little time to show the woman, by using the arrow cursor control, the head of her baby, its body and then its heart beating. Not only is showing the beating fetal heart to the woman extremely reassuring to her but also, by doing this early in the examination, it helps to include her in the examination from the earliest opportunity.

Cephalic or Breech Presentation

Having established that the lie is longitudinal, the presentation will therefore be either cephalic (head down) or breech (head up). Providing you have orientated your probe correctly and the maternal bladder is on the right of the screen and the uterine fundus is on the left, visualizing the fetal head on the right side of the ultrasound monitor indicates that the fetal presentation is cephalic (Fig. 3.4A). An image that demonstrates the fetal head on the left side of the ultrasound monitor indicates that the fetal presentation is breech (Fig. 3.4B).

Transverse Lie

If the longitudinal section of the uterus demonstrates a cross section of the fetus this indicates a transverse lie (Fig. 3.4C). Having established that the lie is transverse, you need to determine whether the fetus is lying with its head to the maternal left or to the maternal right. Make sure you have orientated your probe correctly and, therefore, that the maternal left is on the right side of the screen and her right is on the left side of the screen. Note the position of the fetal head on the ultrasound monitor. An image that demonstrates the fetal head on the right of the screen indicates that the fetus is lying in a transverse position with its head to the maternal left. This can be confirmed by sliding the probe towards the maternal left, as the probe moves to the maternal left more of the fetal head will appear in the image. An image that demonstrates the fetal head on the left of the screen indicates that the fetus is lying in a transverse position with its head to the maternal right (Fig. 3.4D). This can be confirmed by sliding the probe towards the maternal right, as the probe moves to the maternal right more of the fetal head will appear in the image.

Oblique Lie

If the position of the probe and your right hand on the maternal abdomen is neither longitudinal nor transverse, but somewhere between the two, then the fetal lie is oblique. You need to be able to determine whether the presentation is cephalic but the lie is not truly longitudinal, thus cephalic and oblique, or the presentation is essentially breech but the lie is not truly longitudinal, thus breech and oblique. Using the principles outlined earlier should allow you to determine whether the presentation is cephalic and oblique or breech and oblique.

FETAL ATTITUDE – PRONE, SUPINE OR DECUBITUS

You now need to determine whether the fetus is prone (looking down with spine anterior), supine (looking up with spine posterior) or decubitus (looking to the side and lying on its side) and, if decubitus, whether it is lying on its left side or its right side. This is important as understanding the fetal position is key to appreciating the success or otherwise of the anatomical assessment you are about to undertake. For example, the correct section from which to assess the fetal spine and its skin covering is from the midsagittal section of the prone fetus. Correctly applied sliding and angling of the probe will enable you to 'convert' a coronal section into a midsagittal section, but only if the fetal position is somewhere between prone and decubitus. This will not be possible if the fetal position is somewhere between supine and decubitus.

Let us start by considering the maternal abdomen and the fetal spine in terms of a clock and labelling the maternal anterior abdominal wall as 12 o'clock, the posterior uterine wall as 6 o'clock, her left side as 3 o'clock and her right side as 9 o'clock.

Let us now assume that the lie of the fetus is longitudinal and its presentation is cephalic. When the fetus is prone its spine is at 12 o'clock and when it is supine its spine is at 6 o'clock. Providing the longitudinal section you have obtained of the fetus is more or less midsagittal, this image will demonstrate the fetal spine if the fetus is either prone or supine (Fig. 3.5A and B).

If you cannot see the fetal spine in this longitudinal section, let us assume that this is because the fetus is lying on its side, in the decubitus position. Slide your probe slowly to either side of your initial longitudinal section and you should see the fetal spine in the centre of the fetal body. This section, which demonstrates the centrally positioned fetal spine, is therefore a coronal section of the fetus (Fig. 3.5C). In the decubitus position the fetal spine is at 3 o'clock when the fetus is lying on its left side and at 9 o'clock when it is lying on its right side, and imaged in cross section.

A fetal position between prone and left decubitus will result in the spine being visualized between 12 and 3 o'clock. A fetal position between prone and right decubitus will result in the fetal spine being visualized between 12 and 9 o'clock. Conversely, a fetal position between supine and left decubitus will result in the spine being visualized between 6 and 3 o'clock. A fetal position between supine and right decubitus will result in the spine being visualized between 6 and 9 o'clock.

Where the lie of the fetus is longitudinal and its presentation is breech, you will still see its spine at 12 o'clock when it is prone and at 6 o'clock when it is supine. What changes, however, is the position of its spine when it is in the decubitus position, this being the direct opposite to its position when the fetus is cephalic. In the decubitus position the fetal spine is at 9 o'clock when it is breech and lying on its left side and at 3 o'clock when it is breech and lying on its right side. Intermediate positions between prone, supine and decubitus when the presentation is breech are as follows. A fetal position between prone and left decubitus will result in the spine being visualized between 12 and 9 o'clock. A fetal position between prone and right decubitus will result in the fetal spine being visualized between 12 and 3 o'clock. Conversely, a fetal position between supine and left decubitus will result in the spine being visualized between 6 and 9 o'clock. A fetal position between supine and right decubitus will result in the spine being visualized between 6 and 3 o'clock.

When the fetal lie is transverse, the same principles can be applied but must be modified somewhat. Let us assume that the lie of the fetus is transverse with its head to the maternal left. The longitudinal axis of the fetus will therefore demonstrate the fetal head on the right of the ultrasound

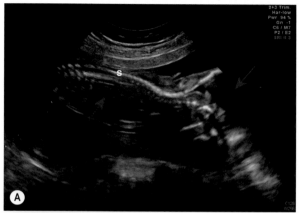

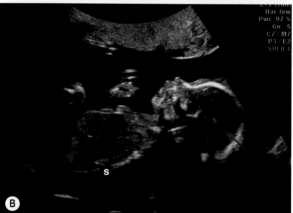

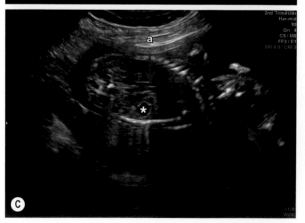

Fig 3.5 • A. A longitudinal section of the uterus slightly to one side of the midline. The fetal head (arrow) can be seen on the right of the screen, its body (dashed arrow) on the left, and its spine (s) is anterior. The fetal presentation is therefore cephalic, it is prone and OA. B. A longitudinal section of the uterus slightly to one side of the midline. The fetal head (arrow) can be seen on the right of the screen, its body (dashed arrow) on the left and its spine (s) is posterior. The fetal presentation is therefore cephalic, it is supine and OP. C. A longitudinal section of the uterus to one side of the midline. The fetal head (arrow) can be seen on the right of the screen, its body (dashed arrow) on the right. The spine is not seen in this section but the aorta (a) can be seen centrally positioned in the fetal body. The fetal presentation is therefore cephalic, it is decubitus and OT. As the stomach (*) is posterior, the fetal spine should be on the maternal left thus confirming normal situs. OA, occipito-anterior; OP, occipito-posterior; OT, occipito-transverse.

monitor, i.e. at 3 o'clock. The fetal head will be seen on the left of the ultrasound monitor, i.e. at 9 o'clock if the fetus is lying with its head to the maternal right. When the fetus is prone, the longitudinal section obtained is a sagittal section. The fetal spine will be seen at 12 o'clock. When the fetus is supine the fetal spine will be seen at 6 o'clock.

In the decubitus transverse position the longitudinal axis of the fetus is a coronal section. The fetal spine will therefore be centrally positioned in the longitudinal section obtained, irrespective of whether the fetus is lying on its left side or its right side. The fetal spine will be found by sliding from a coronal section of the fetal body towards the uterine fundus when the fetus is lying on its left side with its head to the maternal left (and therefore the fetal head will be on the right of the ultrasound monitor) or it is lying on its right side with its head to the maternal right. The spine will be found by sliding towards the symphysis pubis when the fetus is lying on its left side with its head to the maternal right (and therefore the fetal head will be on the left of the ultrasound monitor) or it is lying on its right side with its head to the maternal right.

The relationship between the position of the fetal spine and the fetal lie are summarized in Appendix 1.

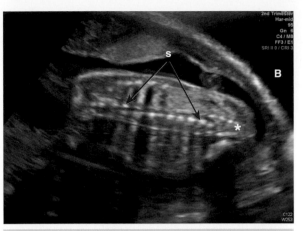

Fig 3.6 • A longitudinal section of the uterus slightly to one side of the midline, showing the maternal bladder (B) on the right of the screen. The fundus is to the left of the screen. The individual vertebrae of the fetal spine (s) can be seen centrally positioned in this section of the fetal body, which is therefore a coronal section. The fetal head (not shown) is to the left of the screen. The fetus is therefore breech and decubitus. It is also likely to be OT but this cannot be confirmed in this section. Note the tapering of the normal spine to the sacrum (*). OT, occipito-transverse.

Midsagittal and Coronal Sections

Having found the longitudinal axis of the fetus, and decided whether the fetal presentation is cephalic or breech and the lie is longitudinal, transverse or oblique (Fig. 3.6), you now also know whether its position is prone, supine or decubitus. You therefore also know whether the section you have obtained is a sagittal section or a coronal section. Understanding this is important for the following reasons. Either section is adequate as a starting point for the cross-sections you will require for the fetal biometry. The sagittal and coronal sections provide differing, but complimentary, information essential for examining the fetal anatomy. For example, a midsagittal section of the prone fetus is needed to assess the full length of the fetal spine and its skin covering, whereas a midcoronal section is more informative for the diaphragm, stomach and fetal situs. The size of the meningocele associated with an open spina bifida, for example, is best demonstrated from the midsagittal section whilst the extent of the vertebral defect itself is best demonstrated from the coronal plane.

The Midsagittal Prone Position

A midsagittal image in which the full length of the fetal spine is anterior indicates that the fetus is in the prone position (see Fig. 3.5A). Providing that the fetus does not have its head turned to one side, this midsagittal section will demonstrate the occiput of the skull anteriorly (occipitoanterior or OA) and the fetal bladder posteriorly. In this position the fetal profile will be poorly demonstrated because the fetus is looking downwards. This is because of shadowing from overlying structures together with decreasing resolution at depth. The OA position of the head is important to recognize as it effectively excludes both the taking of accurate head measurements and assessment of the intracranial anatomy at the ventricles level. This is because the landmarks used to obtain the correct section will be poorly visualized as they lie parallel to the ultrasound beam rather than at 90° to it (see Chapter 8).

The Midsagittal Supine Position

An image in which the full length of the fetal spine is posterior indicates that the fetus is in the supine position (Fig. 3.5B). Providing that the fetus does not have its head turned to one side, this midsagittal section will demonstrate the occiput of the skull posteriorly (occipitoposterior or OP) and the fetal bladder anteriorly. The profile including the forehead, nose and chin will be easily recognizable because the fetus is looking upwards. This is one of the required sections for detailed assessment of the fetal face. The OP position of the head is also important to recognize as it too effectively excludes both the taking of accurate head measurements and assessment of the intracranial anatomy at the ventricles level, in exactly the same way as the direct OA position described earlier.

In either the prone position or supine position, the midsagittal section of the fetus will demonstrate the vertebrae of the spine as two lines of parallel echoes which taper to the sacrum. These echoes originate from the ossification centre in the body or centrum of each vertebra, and from the base of one of the transverse processes, or lamina, of each vertebra. When the fetal spine is anterior, the midsagittal section will demonstrate the full length of the spine and its skin covering optimally. This is the one of the required sections for detailed assessment of the fetal spine and its skin covering. When the spine is posterior, the midsagittal section is of less value for assessing the spine and integrity of its skin covering. This is because of shadowing from overlying structures together with decreasing resolution at depth.

As the fetal bladder is centrally positioned within its pelvis, the fetal bladder will be seen in both the prone and supine midsagittal sections. As the normal fetal heart and stomach lie to the left of the midline, they will not be seen in either the prone or supine midsagittal sections. A small sliding movement of the probe towards the left side of the fetal body should demonstrate the sagittal section of the fetus in which the heart and stomach will be seen. Note that this section in which the fetal stomach and heart can be seen is not midsagittal and does not therefore demonstrate the optimal view of the spine and its skin covering.

Decubitus Position

An image in which the fetal spine is centrally positioned within the longitudinal section of the body indicates that the fetus is lying on its side, in the decubitus position (Fig. 3.6) You have therefore obtained a coronal section of the fetus. Slide the probe away from the spine and onto the fetal body to obtain a midcoronal section. Providing that the fetus does not have its head turned to one side, this midcoronal section will demonstrate a recognizably 'skull-like' image of the fetal head which includes the orbits, mandible and frontal bone. The spine is not seen in this section but the fetal ribs will be seen anterior and posterior to the fetal chest, within which the heart will be seen, slightly above or below the central axis of the chest – this being dependent on the fetal position in the uterus. The stomach should be seen on the same side of the fetal body as the heart. The fetal bladder is seen positioned centrally at the lower end of the fetal body. It is not possible to obtain the fetal profile in the decubitus position.

Coronal views of the spine can be assessed from the decubitus position with the vertebrae of the spine again appearing as lines of parallel echoes which taper to the sacrum. In this plane each vertebra is represented by three echoes rather than the two normally seen in the midsagittal view. In the coronal view the middle of these three echoes originates from the ossification centre in the body of each vertebra while the echoes on either side derive from the two laminae of each vertebra (see Chapter 10). This is one of the required sections for detailed assessment of the fetal spine and therefore the exclusion of the spinal component of an open spina bifida or in the exclusion of sacral agenesis. It is not possible to assess the skin covering of the spine in the decubitus position.

An image in which the fetal spine is neither anterior nor posterior nor centrally positioned within the longitudinal section of the body indicates that the fetus is lying in a semiprone, supine or decubitus position.

Moving from a Coronal Section to a Midsagittal Section

It will be evident from the above that both sagittal and coronal views provide important and distinct information relating to the normality of the fetal anatomy. It is therefore important that you are able to manipulate the probe to produce a prone or supine sagittal section from a coronal section and vice versa in order to obtain the differing information provided by the two scanning planes. You also need to be able to produce a sagittal or coronal section from an 'in between' section. The probe movements required are those of sliding and angling.

Let us assume that your probe is positioned in the midline of the uterus, you are holding the probe upright, at 90° to the maternal skin surface (and the scanning couch) and the longitudinal section of the prone fetus you have obtained is midsagittal. As the fetus is prone, its spine will be seen at the 12 o'clock position on the ultrasound monitor. To obtain a midcoronal section of the fetus, slide your probe out to the left, or right, side of the uterus. The distance you will need to slide the probe will depend on the size of the fetus. A midtrimester fetus is relatively small so slide only a small distance first. Do not worry if the fetus has almost disappeared from the ultrasound monitor. Now change the angle of the probe by 90°, so that it is effectively parallel to the scanning couch. The fetus should reappear on the ultrasound monitor and the longitudinal section of the fetus should now be coronal, with the spine centrally positioned within the fetal body. If your longitudinal section is coronal, then the same process of sliding then angling will produce sagittal sections of the fetus.

Following the Longitudinal Lie of the Fetus

Once you have mastered the distinct, but frequently subtle, probe movements that allow you to move between midsagittal and coronal longitudinal sections of the fetus you have one further skill to learn. Having established the fetal position within

the uterus you should be able to scan along the true length of the fetus from the top of its head to its bottom, keeping the plane in which you are imaging the fetus constant. It is a good initial aim to learn to follow the length of the spine while maintaining a proper midsagittal section of the fetal body.

If the fetal position is longitudinal, cephalic and prone, then it is a relatively straightforward procedure to place your probe above the frontal bone of the fetal skull and maintain a midsagittal image of the fetus, with the spine and its skin covering in view, simply by sliding the probe in a straight line towards the uterine fundus. This task becomes more difficult when the fetal lie is oblique and frequently much more difficult when the fetus is lying in a curled rather than a straight position. To maintain the same scanning plane in this situation requires the ability to follow the curve of the fetal spine in the horizontal plane while continuing to image longitudinal and sagittal sections of the fetus. Two probe movements are required in this instance – sliding of the probe along the length of the fetal body, combined with rotation of the probe to ensure that the sections remain longitudinal and sagittal. The degree of rotation will depend on how curled the fetus is. Too much rotation will take you from a longitudinal to a transverse or oblique section of the fetus, neither of which is what you are trying to obtain.

Following the fetal spine from top to bottom, irrespective of the position of the fetus, is a difficult manoeuvre to perform and one which is frequently overlooked in the beginner's enthusiasm to progress to 'measurements' and 'anatomy'. It is, however, worth spending time developing the skills necessary to do this properly as, once mastered, you will find that you have learnt almost all the probe driving skills you will need to find, assess and measure the fetus – irrespective of its gestational age – using the transabdominal route.

ASSESSING FETAL SITUS

Your final task is to assess fetal situs. The normal arrangement of the body organs is termed *situs solitus*. In the normal fetus, the stomach, cardiac apex and aortic arch therefore lie on the left side

of the body and the inferior vena cava lies on the right. *Situs inversus* is a mirror image of this arrangement. *Situs ambiguous* or heterotaxy is used to describe the condition where some, but not all, of the organs are incorrectly positioned. Some types of severe cardiac disease are associated with abnormal situs and identifying normal fetal situs is therefore an important precursor to excluding them. Assessing fetal situs is therefore an important final objective to the start of your examination. Confirming situs solitus is discussed in Chapter 8.

You are already aware of the importance of making sure your probe is orientated correctly and that you know which part of the woman is displayed on which side of the ultrasound monitor. It is very easy to misinterpret the arrangement of the organs and blood vessels if you are working with an incorrect orientation of the image on the ultrasound screen.

The aim of this very important exercise is to work out which side of the fetus is its left side and which is its right. This is obviously dependent on knowing accurately how the fetus is positioned within the uterus. An easy way to work out situs mentally is to place yourself in the uterus in the position occupied by the fetus. Unless you explain carefully to the woman what you are attempting to do, we recommend that you try to keep your inevitable swaying and twisting to a minimum, as the woman may find this somewhat disconcerting unless she has been forewarned.

Having established the fetal position correctly, you should now know where you expect the left side of the fetus, where its stomach and the apex of its heart should appear on the ultrasound monitor and, therefore, situs. We recommend you confirm situs from longitudinal sections first, and then confirm your conclusion from transverse sections. This is because it is easier to make sure your probe is correctly orientated from longitudinal axis views of the fetus than from cross-sectional views.

You are now ready to progress to performing fetal biometry and assessing the fetal anatomy as discussed in Chapter 8.

Starting to scan using the transvaginal route

4

CONTENTS

This chapter explains the transvaginal method of imaging.

The aims of this chapter are to enable you to:

- make the necessary preparations prior to performing a transvaginal scan
- understand the four transvaginal probe movements
- perform a survey of the pelvis
- find the uterus and ovaries.

Although the basic techniques of image production are the same, transvaginal and transabdominal imaging methods require the mastering of different probe movements. The transabdominal method of imaging is discussed in Chapter 3.

This text assumes that you, the operator, are sitting to the left of, or at the foot of, the scanning couch, holding the probe in your right hand, that the woman is lying to your right side and that you are facing each other.

The first objective of the transvaginal examination is to find the uterus and then the ovaries. Although both the uterus and the ovaries tend to be relatively immobile within the female pelvis, they do not occupy the same positions in every woman. You the operator must therefore develop a methodical and systematic approach from the outset in order to provide a clinically competent examination.

EXPLAINING THE PROCEDURE

Having made the decision that a transvaginal scan is the examination that is most likely to provide maximum information, it is important that the reasons for your decision are discussed fully with the woman in order that her 'informed' consent is given. The examination procedure obviously needs to be explained in a way in which the woman will understand, through an interpreter if necessary. Although few women will decline a transvaginal ultrasound examination if its necessity is properly explained, many find the examination and the whole procedure embarrassing, uncomfortable and potentially stressful. As a new ultrasound operator you may lack confidence in your technical abilities and may also find this type of examination challenging for a variety of reasons. You will need to be aware of all these issues when discussing the examination with the woman. Remember that the manner in which you deliver this information and in which you approach the examination is key to the woman's experience. In addition, it is paramount that you pay attention to the woman's privacy and dignity and maintain them throughout the examination.

As with any medical procedure the woman must have sufficient information about the examination she is being asked to undergo in order to give fully informed consent. How this is achieved will vary between centres; some will require written consent, whereas others will use verbal consent. It is assumed that local guidelines will be in accordance with current national recommendations and/or those from the relevant professional body or bodies.

The woman needs to be aware that:

- the examination is not contraindicated during menstruation or bleeding *per vagina*
- she will need an empty bladder
- she will be required to remove her lower outer clothes and underwear

- the examination will be carried out transvaginally
- the examination may be uncomfortable but should not be painful
- a follow-up examination may be required if all the necessary information could not be obtained.

Current guidelines recommend that every woman undergoing an intimate examination is offered a chaperone. This offer should be made irrespective of whether the examination is performed by a male or a female operator. Our recommendation therefore is that every woman undergoing transvaginal ultrasound examinations should be offered a chaperone and her decision recorded. In addition, male operators should only perform transvaginal ultrasound examinations when chaperoned, irrespective of whether the woman has accepted or declined this offer.

Ideally, there needs to be a local strategy in place to review gynaecological examination requests prior to the woman's appointment being made. A decision can then be taken as to which examination route is the more appropriate to offer. This may vary with local practice. For instance, if contraindications for a transvaginal scan are known, then a transabdominal examination, with the necessary preparatory bladder filling, can be arranged.

GETTING STARTED

GETTING INTO POSITION

It is important that you learn how to position the woman, the machine and the scanning stool correctly in order to minimize the risk to you of repetitive strain injury or work-related upper limb disorders. It is also good practice to prepare the couch and correctly position the ultrasound machine and scanning stool before you start. The ideal position for the operator is directly in front of the woman's perineum with the machine to the operator's left, appropriately positioned for manipulating the controls with the left hand, while holding the probe in the right hand. Many operators sit to the left, rather than at the end, of the scanning couch, in the position used for transabdominal examinations. When scanning transvaginally, it is easier to maintain an upright posture if you are positioned in front of the perineum. You are more likely to lean away from the recommended upright position, and also to abduct your right shoulder inappropriately, when sitting to the left of the couch. Thus, from an ergonomic perspective, sitting in front of the perineum is recommended.

PREPARING AND POSITIONING THE WOMAN

Transvaginal imaging requires the woman to have a completely empty bladder as even a small amount of urine in the bladder can displace organs of interest out of the field of view. The woman should therefore be asked to empty her bladder immediately prior to her ultrasound examination.

Privacy is of paramount importance during a transvaginal scan. As stated previously, the woman will need to remove her lower outer clothes and underwear and should be able to do this in private behind a curtain or screen. A paper or cloth sheet should be provided behind the screen for her to cover her lower body before, during and after the examination. A chair or stool should also be available for her to place her clothes on. You must also consider the aftercare of the woman once the scan has been completed. Tissues should be provided in the changing area to allow her to wipe herself after the scan. The appropriate type of refuse bin should also be provided, in accordance with local infection control guidelines, for their disposal.

One of the challenges of transvaginal imaging is positioning of the woman to obtain optimum images while ensuring her comfort during the examination. The position and orientation of the uterus and ovaries within the pelvis vary from individual to individual. The ability to acquire certain scanning planes may be compromised by patient positioning. Of particular importance is the ability to manoeuvre the probe in the anteroposterior plane so that the handle of the probe can be manipulated below the level of the woman's buttocks. This is essential when, for example, imaging an acutely anteflexed uterus.

The best imaging access is obtained by placing the woman on a gynaecological couch with her legs supported by low stirrups. Where this is not available an acceptable alternative is to use a couch in which one end can be removed or folded back through 90°. The woman should then be positioned with her bottom at the end of the couch, her feet resting on a chair placed at its end and with her heels together and her knees apart. Both these methods will allow adequate probe manoeuvrability in both lateral and anteroposterior planes. Positioning the woman's bottom on a 'wedge' or a folded pillow (with or without clenched fists under the buttocks) does *not* achieve the same access. From the woman's point of view, she may have difficulty climbing onto the wedge. She may also find it undignified and uncomfortable and the

position difficult to maintain for any length of time. Furthermore, this position will be difficult for a woman in the third trimester of pregnancy.

Having positioned the woman correctly, the sheet or paper should be placed so that her lower abdomen, pelvis and thighs remain covered throughout the examination.

PREPARING THE PROBE

No transvaginal examination should be performed without the use of a probe cover. Before preparing the probe for use, it is of critical importance to ascertain whether or not the woman has an allergy to latex. Inserting a probe covered with a probe cover into the vagina of a woman who is allergic to latex may cause her to have an anaphylactic shock, which has potentially severe consequences. Latex-free probe covers should be used for women who have a latex allergy or whose allergy status is unknown.

It is good practice to clean and prepare the probe in view of the woman as this should give her the reassurance that appropriate infection prevention is being used.

Disposable gloves should be worn throughout the procedure and we recommend that you first wash your hands, put on your gloves and then prepare the probe. The probe should first be cleaned with an appropriate antiseptic wipe or spray. The probe manufacturer's advice on the use of proprietary cleaning agents together with the advice from the local infection control team should be sought and adhered to. A small amount of either sterile jelly or ultrasound gel should be applied to the tip of the probe which is then covered with a nonspermicidal probe cover. Care should be taken to ensure that sufficient jelly or gel remains on the tip of the probe, rather than running down the shaft of the probe. This ensures that no air is trapped between the probe and the probe cover. A further application of sterile jelly onto the tip of the covered probe will facilitate easy insertion of the probe into the vagina.

Before you start scanning you will also need to prepare for the aftercare of the woman when you have finished scanning. You need to develop the technique of removing the covered probe from the vagina, offering the woman tissues with which to clean herself, removing the probe cover from the probe, wiping the probe, removing your gloves and disposing of the soiled consumables before replacing the probe in its housing on the machine and while still seated at the machine.

A modified version of the three sheets technique described in Chapter 2 works well in this situation. Place one sheet over your right leg and place a further three sheets within easy reach. Pass one sheet to the woman as you are about to remove the probe from her vagina. She can use this to wipe herself. Take the second sheet in your left hand and use it to remove the probe cover from the probe and wipe the probe while still holding the probe

under the paper or cloth sheet covering the woman's legs. Take the third sheet and use this to wrap up the soiled second sheet and probe cover. Remove this bundle and the cleaned probe from under the sheet. Place the probe back in its holder and put the bundle in the appropriate refuse bin which should be positioned within easy reach. Finally cleanse the probe with an appropriate antiseptic wipe or spray. You should then wash your hands. It is not acceptable practice to replace the probe, still covered with its used probe cover, into its housing on the machine, remove the soiled probe cover and then clean the probe.

THE SCANNING TECHNIQUE

ORIENTATION

There are various ways of displaying the transvaginal image on the ultrasound monitor. Three concepts need to be considered: First, which hand is being used to hold the probe – this text assumes that you are holding the probe and scanning with your right hand; second, the top/bottom orientation of the image on the ultrasound monitor; and third, the left/right orientation of the image on the monitor.

This text assumes that you, the operator, are sitting in front of the woman's perineum or to the left of the scanning couch, are holding the probe in your right hand, that the woman is lying to your right side and that you are facing each other.

There is no agreed convention as to whether the apex of the image should be displayed at the top of the monitor or at the bottom. Gynaecologists tend to orientate the image so that the apex of the image is at the bottom of the monitor, while ultrasound operators tend to orientate the image with its apex at the top of the monitor. The gynaecologist's orientation is more logical if the scan is being considered as an extension of the clinical examination. The rationale for the ultrasound operator's orientation comes from the familiarity with transabdominal convention, where the top of the monitor represents the anterior abdominal wall and the bottom of the monitor the scanning couch. This text uses the ultrasound operator's orientation. The techniques discussed later in this chapter all relate

therefore to the orientation of the apex of the image being displayed at the top of the ultrasound monitor.

As with transabdominal imaging, there is no agreed convention as to whether the left of the woman's pelvis should be displayed on the left or on the right of the ultrasound monitor. We recommend that the same orientation is adopted on transvaginal imaging as for transabdominal imaging. We therefore recommend that the radiological convention is used – that is, that the left side of the maternal pelvis is displayed on the right side of the monitor and vice versa. This text adopts this principle.

It must be remembered that both the top/bottom orientation and the left/right orientation of the image are influenced by two factors: how you hold the probe and whether the relevant invert buttons (left/right and top/bottom) on the machine's control panel are activated or deactivated.

The ultrasound monitor will display a logo or similar on one side of the image sector. The left/right invert control should be used to position this logo on the left of the image sector.

The majority of modern probe handles are shaped to provide a comfortable hand grip in one plane. Holding the probe in this position, with your thumb uppermost (rather than with your thumb at the side), gives you an important guide to your orientation – and one which can be 'felt' throughout the scan (Fig. 4.1). Some transvaginal probes may be symmetrically shaped. These always

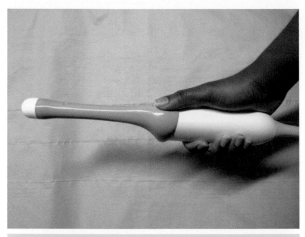

Fig 4.1 • Demonstration of how to hold the transvaginal probe. Note the thumb comfortably positioned at the uppermost aspect of the probe. Note the operator is not wearing a glove neither has a probe cover been applied.

have some means of distinguishing between one side of the handle and the other by a groove, spot or other mark. One side of the probe, be it modern or otherwise, always relates to one side of the sector displayed on the monitor. We recommend that the left side of the sector should relate to the position of your thumb or the mark on the probe. This relationship is linked to the left/right invert control.

Before starting an examination it is important to ensure that the orientation of the image sector, and of the probe, are such that the left side of the image relates to the right side of the body, as per the normal convention. It is not usually necessary to alter the invert control as the machine will normally be set up to default to the normal convention.

We recommend linking the position of the thumb of your right hand with the left-hand side of the image sector as displayed on the monitor by the following exercise:

- start with the apex of the sector at the top of the monitor. If it is not, activate the top/bottom invert button
- ensure the logo is displayed on the left side of the image sector. If it is not, activate the left/right invert button
- hold the probe comfortably and make sure your thumb is uppermost
- rub the upper edge of the probe face nearest your thumb. The resulting shadow should

be displayed on the left-hand side of the sector
- if this results in a shadow on the *right*-hand side of the image sector, rather than the left-hand side, you have two options: (a) activate the left/right invert button – this will result in left/right inversion of the image sector – or (b) rotate the probe through 180°.

The Importance of Orientation

Establishing and maintaining the relationship between your right thumb and the left-hand side of the monitor will enable you, first, to develop your spatial awareness accurately while steering the probe; second, to develop an appreciation of anatomical relationships within the pelvis; and, third, to differentiate correctly between right and left. Failing to appreciate this relationship leads to the reporting of, for example, a left-sided mass when it is right-sided, an anteverted uterus when it is retroverted and/or an anterior fibroid when it is posterior.

Putting It into Practice

Holding the probe in your right hand so that the mark and/or your thumb are uppermost (Fig. 4.1), with the apex of the image at the top of the monitor and the logo displayed on the left of the sector image will produce a sagittal image of the pelvis orientated as shown (Fig. 4.2A and B). In the sagittal plane the woman's head is at the bottom of the sector and her feet at the apex. The left side of the sector relates to her ventral surface and the right side to her dorsal surface.

The implications of correct orientation in the sagittal plane are best explained by considering the various positions of the uterus relative to the cervix. A sagittal section will display the fundus of an anteverted uterus on the left of the monitor (Fig. 4.2B) and the fundus of the retroverted uterus on the right of the monitor (Fig. 4.3).

The longitudinal and transverse scanning planes, which are perpendicular to each other, display sagittal and true transverse sections of *the pelvis*, respectively. It is possible to obtain true sagittal sections of, for example, *the uterus* by manipulation of the probe. Unfortunately the uterus and other

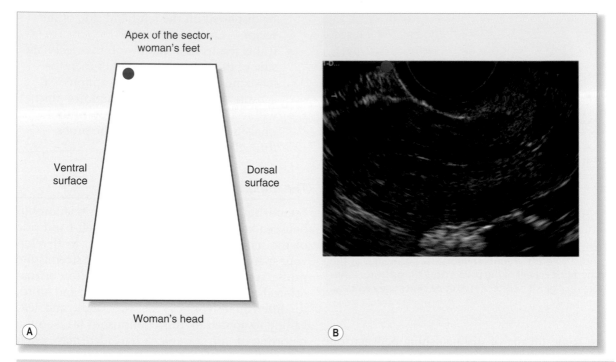

Apex of the sector, woman's feet

Ventral surface

Dorsal surface

Woman's head

(A)

(B)

Fig 4.2 • (A) is a schematic diagram of the sector; the red dot corresponds to that displayed in the real-time image of a sagittal view of the anteverted uterus shown in (B).

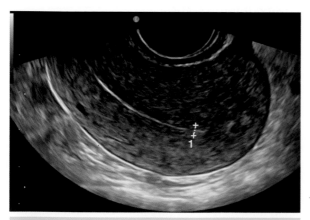

Fig 4.3 • Sagittal retroverted uterus; note that the fundus of the uterus is towards the right of the sector.

organs do not normally lie horizontally within the pelvis, but at an angle to the horizontal. Thus, true transverse planes of *the pelvis* can be obtained but, because probe movement is restricted by the confines of the vagina, true transverse planes of *the uterus* cannot be obtained, as the required probe movement is not possible.

The term 'transverse' should be considered carefully in the context of transvaginal imaging. The 'transverse section' more accurately describes a section which lies somewhere between a *true transverse* section (i.e. one that is perpendicular to the longitudinal section) and a *coronal* section. How truly transverse this section is will depend on the angle of the structure to the horizontal and the degree of probe manipulation possible. It is important that this issue is appreciated as it has implications relating to measurement accuracy. For example, the uterine endometrium or a gestation sac has a specific anteroposterior (AP) diameter. This measurement should be the same irrespective of whether it is taken from a longitudinal or a transverse ultrasound image. However, this is not the case because in practice the measurement taken from the 'transverse' plane will be oblique and not the true AP diameter. This differs from transabdominal imaging because this route allows unrestricted probe manipulation. It is therefore possible, when scanning transabdominally, to obtain transverse sections that are truly perpendicular to the longitudinal, resulting in AP measurements that

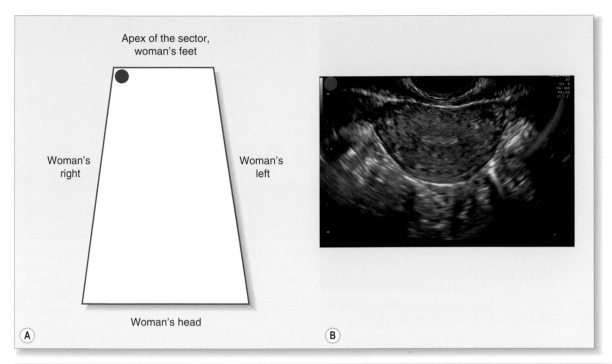

Apex of the sector,
woman's feet

Woman's
right

Woman's
left

Woman's head

(A)

(B)

Fig 4.4 • (A) is a schematic diagram of the sector corresponding to the transverse view of the uterus displayed in the image in (B).

should be the same in both longitudinal and transverse sections.

Although the term 'transverse' has been used throughout this text, it should be remembered that it describes a slightly different section depending on whether the route used is transabdominal or transvaginal.

Rotating the probe anticlockwise so that the mark and/or your thumb are now at 9 o'clock, with the apex of the image at the top of the monitor and the logo displayed to the left of the image sector will produce a transverse image of the pelvis orientated as shown (Fig. 4.4 A and B). In a transverse image, the top of the sector relates to the inferior aspect of the woman (towards her feet) and the bottom of the sector to the superior aspect of the woman (towards her head). This is a key fundamental difference between transabdominal and transvaginal imaging. In a transverse, transabdominal section, the top of the image relates to the anterior abdominal wall and the bottom of the image the posterior wall (or the couch). The left of the image, however, relates to the woman's right side

and the right of the image relates to her left side in both transabdominal and transvaginal scanning.

PROBE MOVEMENTS

There are four possible movements of the transvaginal probe:

- sliding
- panning
- angling
- rotating.

Each movement will affect the image in different ways and it is important that you appreciate what each movement does. This will enable you to use the appropriate sequence of movements to find the structure you are seeking and to obtain the optimal images of it.

Sliding

Sliding describes the forward and backward movement of the probe in the vagina (Fig. 4.5) and

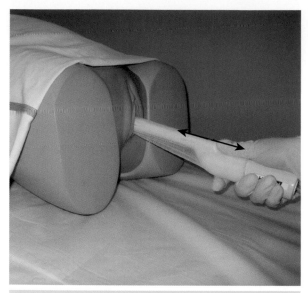

Fig 4.5 • Sliding movement of the probe. The movement is in the direction of the axis of the probe

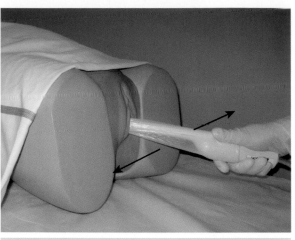

Fig 4.6 • Panning movement of the probe. The operator's hand is positioned at the woman's left thigh; therefore the tip of the probe is directed towards the woman's right. The arrow denotes the lateral arc of movement (a maximum of 130°).

is used to alter the field of view from inferior to superior. When sliding, the tip of the probe will move in the same direction as the handle of the probe.

Panning

Panning is the pivoting movement of the probe around a fixed point that enables sequential fanned slices of the pelvis to be imaged from its right side to its left side and vice versa. When panning, the tip of the probe will move in the opposite direction to the handle of the probe. The shape of the vagina restricts movement of the probe to one of panning from a pivotal point (Fig. 4.6). Panning moves the field of view through a maximum lateral arc of approximately 130°. Further movement is limited by the woman's thighs.

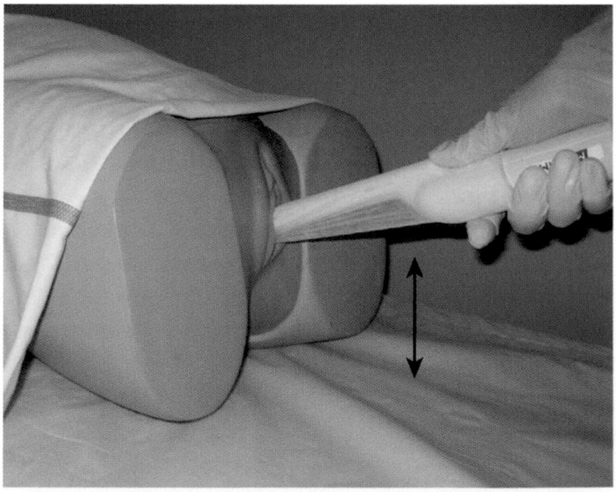

Angling

Angling (or rocking) is the same pivoting movement of the probe around a fixed point as panning, but in the orthogonal plane. Angling enables sequential fanned slices of the pelvis to be imaged in an anteroposterior plane. When angling, the tip of the probe will move in the opposite direction to

Fig 4.7 • Angling of the probe. The handle of the probe is raised; therefore the tip of the probe is directed posteriorly within the woman. The arrow denotes the direction of movement of the probe handle.

the handle of the probe. Angling moves the field of view through a maximum AP arc of 60° (Fig. 4.7). Further movement is limited by the woman's perineum posteriorly and her symphysis pubis anteriorly.

Rotating

Rotating describes the turning movement of the probe in the vagina (Fig. 4.8) and is used to alter the field of view from sagittal to transverse or oblique. The degree of rotation will normally be restricted by the amount of movement in the wrist of the operator. When rotating, the tip of the probe will move in the same direction as the handle of the probe.

Sliding, panning and angling can all be undertaken in both sagittal and transverse planes.

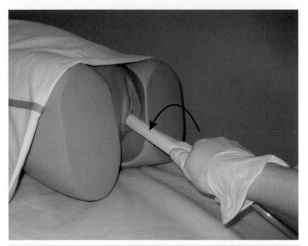

Fig 4.8 • Rotation of the probe is manoeuvred by a rotating action of the operator's wrist. The arrow denotes the rotation usually through a maximum of 90°.

FINDING THE UTERUS

The first image you should aim to obtain is that of the uterus in sagittal section. Confirm the identity of the woman, ensure that the controls of the machine are set up appropriately and hold the prepared probe correctly, with your thumb at 12 o'clock. To provide an image of the appropriate orientation, insert the prepared probe gently into the vagina with a sliding movement. It is likely that you will slide the probe too far into the vagina to image the cervix and the first structure you will see will be part of the uterus. Pan the probe slowly to the right or left to obtain a view of the uterus in sagittal section (Fig. 4.2B). As the uterus is typically dextrarotated, panning to the woman's right side is usually more successful. You must retain your sliding position while optimizing your panning position. You now need to obtain an image that combines the maximum length of the uterus with that of the cervix – this usually requires angling anteriorly or posteriorly. If the uterus is anteverted, you will need to angle gently anteriorly (handle down, probe tip up). If the uterus is retroverted, you will need to do the reverse – that is, angle posteriorly (handle up, probe tip down) as in Fig. 4.7. You must retain your sliding and panning positions while optimizing your probe angle. Finally you should rotate your probe slightly in either direction to obtain the optimal view of the endometrium and to compensate for the lateral tilt that the uterus adopts in the pelvis. This more often than not requires a slight rotational movement in an anti-clockwise direction bringing your thumb to the 11 o'clock position.

Having achieved the optimal image of the cervix, uterus and endometrium in sagittal section, you should then survey the uterus by panning slowly out to either side while maintaining the slide, angle and rotation positions of the probe. If the uterus is acutely ante- or retroflexed, it may not be possible to image its entire length in one sagittal section. A similar problem may be encountered if the uterus is enlarged. In such situations you will need to examine the uterus by obtaining two or more sagittal sections by sliding and/or panning from one to the next.

Rotating the probe through 90° while maintaining your slide, pan and angle positions, will produce a transverse section of the uterus and endometrium. Your thumb is now likely to be at 8 o'clock. Surveying the uterus in the transverse plane is achieved by gently angling the probe from anterior to posterior. If the uterus is anteverted, you

71

will need to angle gently anteriorly (handle down, probe tip up) to image the fundus and posteriorly to image the cervix. If the uterus is retroverted, you will need to do the reverse, that is angle posteriorly (handle up, probe tip down) to image the fundus and anteriorly to image the cervix.

The following text describes in detail how to acquire the basic planes when examining the nonpregnant pelvis – namely, those of the uterus and ovaries. Explanation of how to examine the uterus and ovaries in early pregnancy is given in Chapter 5. Similarly, transvaginal examination of the low-lying placenta and cervix is given in Chapter 14. The fundamental principles are the same with regard to orientation and probe movements.

FINDING THE OVARIES

The ovaries can be sought either by panning in a sagittal or in a transverse plane. Both are equally acceptable as a complete examination requires imaging in both planes. The novice may find it easier to adopt the sagittal, or iliac vessels, technique.

THE ILIAC VESSELS TECHNIQUE

The ovaries usually lie medial and anterior to their respective internal iliac artery (superior) and vein (inferior). Using the iliac vessels as a landmark will focus your search of the pelvis. As the vessels run in a roughly superior/inferior plane through the pelvis they will appear as tubular structures in sagittal sections of the pelvis and round structures in transverse sections of the pelvis (Fig. 4.9). The ovaries will be easier to locate by panning out to the pelvic sidewall in the sagittal plane rather than the transverse plane. First, obtain a sagittal view of the uterus, then pan out to either left or right to image the iliac vessels which lie at the outer limit of the panning arc (Fig. 4.6). The woman's contralateral thigh may obstruct the handle of the probe, hindering your ability to pan the probe sufficiently laterally to visualize the vessels. This tends to be more problematic when the woman is positioned on a pad and far easier when the recommended positioning is adopted. Once you have found the iliac vessels, panning in a medial direction should reveal the ovary in an approximately parasagittal section. It is unlikely that this first image will demonstrate the optimal sagittal section of the ovary. You will thus need first to appreciate this fact and then apply the correct sequence and degree of probe movements. In addition to the subtle changes in panning and angling, you may find that a degree of rotation is helpful. Once a sagittal section of the ovary is obtained, the ovary should be assessed completely by panning parasagittally from one side through to the other.

Having assessed the ovary in sagittal plane, rotate the probe 90° anticlockwise to visualize it in transverse section (Fig. 4.9). Angling slowly from anterior to posterior will allow you to interrogate the ovary in its transverse plane and to complete a thorough examination. As previously, do not lose the correct slide, pan and rotational movements of the probe while angling.

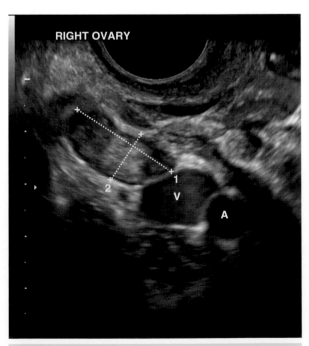

Fig 4.9 • Transverse view of a postmenopausal, right ovary. Note the round shapes of the internal iliac vein (V) and artery (A).

A common error is to 'lose' the ovary whilst moving the probe from a sagittal to a transverse plane or vice versa.

Strategies which might help include:

- moving the probe very slowly whilst performing this manoeuvre – until you gain in confidence. As the normal ovary is the size of a walnut, it is very easy to move the probe off the ovary so that it is no longer visualized and your scanning hand becomes disorientated
- keeping the area of interest, i.e. the ovary, in the centre of the screen. The rotational movement of the probe is, in effect, pivoting on the region of interest, i.e. the ovary, so it is logical that it is placed in the centre of the screen
- ensuring that the depth of the field is increased sufficiently so that the ovary is not too small. Conversely, a zoomed image of the ovary may be too large in size, making the rotational manoeuvre difficult.

Return to the sagittal section of the uterus and repeat the process to examine the contralateral ovary.

Theory has a habit of failing to work consistently in practice. The success of the previously described method is dependent on the position of the ovaries being adjacent to the iliac vessels. The position of the ovaries can be very variable and when one or both lie in a more superior and/or anterior position than normal in the pelvis the slide and pan technique described later is likely to be more successful.

SLIDE AND PAN TECHNIQUE

This technique is useful to locate the ovary which is more superior and/or anterior than normal, is in close proximity to the uterus or lies in the pouch of Douglas. To access a superiorly located ovary requires positioning the probe in the ipsilateral fornix. The novice may be reluctant to slide the probe into the vagina sufficiently to reach this position. However, a gentle sliding movement into the lateral fornix is usually well tolerated by the woman. Once positioned in the fornix, further panning movement of the probe may be necessary to locate the ovary and image it optimally. To access an anterior ovary requires a more acute anterior angling of the probe than normal. An anteriorly positioned ovary that is also superior in the pelvis requires a combination of both probe movements. An ovary that lies superior and/or anterior to the uterine fundus is unlikely to be adequately imaged by the transvaginal route because it frequently lies beyond the field of view of the high-frequency transvaginal probe. However, an ovary in either of these positions can often be imaged perfectly adequately using the transabdominal route (with an empty bladder).

The ovary that lies in close proximity to the lateral wall of the uterus may be overlooked as your initial search will tend to be concentrated in the adnexae. An ovary in this position is best sought as follows. Obtain a transverse view of the uterus and pan towards its lateral margin on the relevant side. Keeping the edge of the uterus in view, slowly angle in an AP direction. The ovary will appear as a rounded mass, adjacent to the uterus. It should demonstrate a positive 'sliding sign', i.e. it should move independently to the uterus when gentle pressure is applied to it with the tip of the probe. This is helpful in distinguishing an ovary adjacent to the uterus from a serosal fibroid arising from the uterine wall. This will demonstrate a negative sliding sign. Rotating the probe clockwise should enable a sagittal view of the ovary to be obtained. In practice, however, this is often problematic because of the difficulty in defining, and distinguishing between, the boundaries of the uterus and of the ovary.

An ovary can also lie in the pouch of Douglas. Imaging this area requires partial withdrawal of the probe by sliding it backward towards the introitus. This will enable the cervix and lower uterine body to act as reference points for location of an ovary in this position. With experience, an ovary lying in the Pouch of Douglas will be recognized from the initial images of the uterus in sagittal section.

PROBLEMS IN IMAGING THE UTERUS AND OVARIES

ADIPOSITY

Adiposity is traditionally considered only to be a problem with transabdominal imaging. However, it can also hinder visualization when scanning transvaginally because the panning arc of the probe is reduced by the size of the woman's thighs. Reduced mobility may also be an issue in the obese woman. This may result in the woman's inability to abduct her thighs sufficiently to enable the required lateral probe movement to take place. Positioning an obese woman on a pad, rather than in the recommended position, compounds this panning problem.

BOWEL GAS

Although bowel gas is known to be a problem with transabdominal imaging, it can also affect visualization, particularly of the ovaries, when scanning transvaginally. Bowel gas has the same appearance when imaged transvaginally or transabdominally, namely high-level echoes with acoustic shadowing behind. The net effect is the inability to visualize the structures lying posterior to the air-filled bowel. It tends to be more problematic on the left side of the pelvis than the right due to the position of the sigmoid colon. Applying gentle but firm pressure with your nonscanning hand to the woman's anterior abdominal wall may cause displacement of the bowel, enabling improved visualization of the structures previously obscured.

FIBROIDS

Fibroids are the most common pathological condition in women of reproductive age that will be seen on ultrasound. The effect that one or more uterine fibroids may have on the quality of the examination will depend on their size, position and consistency.

Where fibroids enlarge the size of the uterus it may be difficult to complete the interrogation of the uterus because the uterine size may be such that it extends outside the field of view. Similarly, it may be difficult to interrogate or even identify large fibroids themselves as they may lie partially or completely outside the field of view.

The ultrasound appearance of a fibroid is typically that of a circular, well-circumscribed mass with a homogeneous echo pattern. As fibroids are more dense than surrounding tissue, there is reduced transmission of sound through them. This adversely affects the diagnostic quality of the examination posterior to the fibroid.

The presence of subserosal fibroids within the uterus may mimic ovarian tissue. This tends to be more problematic in suboptimal examinations of the pelvis which are compromised by bowel gas and/or adiposity resulting in suboptimal images of the pelvis. Fibroids typically are circular, well-circumscribed structures with a homogeneous echo pattern, whereas the ovary is oval with a heterogeneous echo pattern due to the presence of follicles.

BOWEL LOOPS

It is always important to interrogate a structure in multiple planes as it will have differing characteristic features in the various planes. Fluid-filled bowel imaged in cross-section may be mistaken for ovary, but rotating the probe through 90° will reveal the typical tubular appearance of bowel in longitudinal section. Peristalsis will usually be seen if it is observed for a few seconds, confirming the presence of bowel rather than ovary.

Non-fluid-filled loops of bowel in cross-section can also be mistaken for ovarian tissue. This is most likely to occur when trying to locate a small and atretic postmenopausal ovary rather than the larger and active ovary of the reproductive woman.

BLOOD VESSELS

In a similar fashion to bowel loops, a blood vessel imaged in transverse plane may have the appearance of a cyst or follicle within ovarian tissue. Rotating the probe through 90° will reveal the typical tubular appearance of the blood vessel in longitudinal section. Applying colour flow will help to confirm that this structure is a blood vessel. Pulsations will be observed if the vessel is arterial.

CLINICAL INFORMATION

Knowledge of the menstrual status of the woman, the menstrual phase in the premenopausal woman, the contraceptive used and the hormone replacement therapy status will help you anticipate the appearances that you are most likely to be seeking. The postmenopausal ovary may be more difficult to locate and visualize than the functioning ovary because it will generally be atretic, i.e. smaller than the premenopausal ovary.

It is also useful to be aware of any previous gynaecological surgery, especially if hysterectomy and/or oophorectomy have taken place.

The information given here should provide you with the technical ability to address the clinical question being asked. Practice will give you the confidence to answer that question safely and correctly.

Further reading

Royal College of Obstetricians & Gynaecologists 2002 Gynaecological Examinations: Guidelines for Specialist Practice. RCOG Press; London

Assessing the early intrauterine pregnancy

5

This chapter explains the technique for examining intrauterine pregnancies of between 4 and 10 weeks of gestation.

The aims of this chapter are to enable you to:

• examine an early intrauterine pregnancy using the transvaginal and transabdominal approaches

• describe the normal findings of early pregnancy

• report the findings of the early pregnancy scan.

ASSESSING THE LENGTH OF THE PREGNANCY

The gestational age describes the length of pregnancy and was, historically, always calculated from the first day of the last menstrual period (LMP). For reasons that will become clear, it is now accepted that a more accurate method is to calculate gestational age from ultrasound measurements. The gestational age, and therefore the expected date of delivery (EDD) or full term, of a pregnancy should only be calculated once. This is because changing the date of delivery, either by recalculating the date using the same method or by using more than one method which each produce different dates, is clinically unhelpful and confusing for the woman.

It would seem reasonable to assume that the most accurate way to calculate the length of pregnancy is from the date of conception. Full-term delivery would then be expected to occur 266 days or 38 weeks later. It would therefore also be reasonable to assume that the dating of a pregnancy which results from assisted conception would give the most accurate EDD, compared with that from a spontaneously conceived pregnancy. The literature indicates that ovulation takes place between 10 and 22 days after the last menstrual period in women with regular cycles, and between 7 and 60 days in women with irregular cycles. The length of time between ovulation and implantation also varies, with a time difference of between 6 and 12 days in spontaneous conceptions. In addition, there is debate as to whether it is correct to assume that the length of pregnancy should be 266 days in all cases. These issues then raise the questions of whether the length of the pregnancy should be calculated from the date of ovulation, conception or implantation, and how many days should be added to this date to calculate the EDD.

Until such time as these challenges of very early pregnancy and length of gestation have been resolved, we recommend using the following traditional assumptions:

- that the date of ovulation also describes the date of conception
- that full term is 38 weeks or 266 days after the date of conception.

EARLY EMBRYOLOGICAL DEVELOPMENT AND TERMINOLOGY

At ovulation the oocyte, or egg, is released from the ovary and swept into the Fallopian tube by the fimbriae surrounding the end, or infundibulum, of the tube. The oocyte continues to move down the Fallopian tube and is normally fertilized in the ampulla, which is the longest and widest part of the tube. Fertilization describes the fusion of a sperm and an oocyte and takes approximately 24 hours. The resulting cell is called a zygote and is the beginning of the human being. The zygote divides and, by day 3, has formed a solid ball of 12–16 cells which is called the morula. The morula continues to travel down the Fallopian tube into the uterine cavity where fluid passes into its centre, thus forming a hollow ball of cells called the blastocyst. The blastocyst is composed of three parts:

- the inner cell mass, from which the embryo will develop
- the cavity called the blastocyst cavity

- an outer layer of cells called the trophoblast, from which the placenta will develop.

The blastocyst lies free in the secretions of the uterine cavity for about 2 days. Between 5 and 6 days after fertilization the blastocyst starts to attach itself to the endometrium of the uterus, initiating the invasion of the endometrium by the cells of the trophoblast. By day 7, or 1 week after fertilization, the blastocyst is superficially implanted into the endometrium and is fully covered by endometrium by day 12 or day 13 after fertilization. All of this therefore has taken place 1 or 2 days before the first period has been missed.

As the blastocyst is implanting, the inner cell mass begins to differentiate and produces a layer of cells, called the embryonic endoderm. A second layer of cells, called epiblast (the future ectoderm and endoderm of the three-layered, or trilaminar, embryo), also differentiates. This results, by about day 8 after fertilization, in a two-layered, or bilaminar, embryonic disc.

The correct use of the term *embryo* should be to describe the bilaminar embryonic disc and therefore should not be used until the beginning of the 2nd week, or day 8 after fertilization. It is acknowledged that this term is frequently used incorrectly in the clinical setting of assisted conception. For this reason embryo is used in this text, incorrectly at times but in keeping with clinical practice.

The embryonic period extends until the end of the 7th week following fertilization, by which time all the major structures required for functional life have started to form.

The fetal period extends from the beginning of the 8th week following fertilization to birth.

USING EMBRYOLOGICAL AGE

As discussed earlier, embryonic life starts at fertilization or conception and 'embryological age' describes the number of days or weeks which have followed this event. Embryological age is equivalent to postconception age. They are both calculated from the date of fertilization or conception. A pregnancy based on conceptual age is 38 weeks, or 266 days, in length and reflects the true length of pregnancy, namely from conception to delivery.

It is correct, but confusing, therefore that embryological age and postconception age are numerically 14 days or 2 weeks *less* than the gestational age. This is because embryological age and post-conception age are based on the date of conception whilst the gestational age is historically based on the LMP. The EDD as calculated from both methods will be the same.

In this text all reference made to 'weeks of gestation' is based on gestational age and not conceptual or embryological age unless otherwise stated.

USING THE LMP

As most women who conceive spontaneously are unaware of their date of conception, the first day of their LMP has traditionally been used to calculate their EDD. This method assumes that ovulation takes place 14 days after the first day of the last menstrual period and that the first day of the next menstrual period would take place 14 days after ovulation if conception had not occurred. It therefore assumes that the menstrual cycle is always 28 days in length. The method also assumes that ovulation and conception occur on the same day. Using this method, the EDD can be calculated by applying a derivation of Naegele's formula to the LMP as follows:

- add 7 to the days
- add 9 to the months
- add 1 to the years.

For example, if the LMP is 01.04.2016, then the EDD is $(01 + 7 = 8) : (04 + 9 = 13$ [i.e. January]) : $(16 + 01 = 17)$, that is 08.01.2017. This means that pregnancy is 40 weeks (280 days) long and assumes that conception occurs 2 weeks after the LMP.

As stated previously, there are many reasons why using Naegele's formula to calculate the EDD is unreliable. These include situations where:

- the date of the LMP is not accurately known
- the menstrual cycle is regular but is not 28 days long
- the menstrual cycle is irregular
- the woman has stopped taking the combined oral contraceptive pill ('the pill') within the last 3 months
- the woman has had vaginal bleeding in early pregnancy
- the woman is breastfeeding or has been pregnant in the preceding 3–6 months.

USING A GESTATION CALCULATOR WHEEL

You will be pleased to learn that there are quicker methods at your disposal to calculate the EDD rather than using Naegele's formula. One method is to use a gestation calculator wheel. This is a pocket-sized wheel with the calendar dates displayed around the circumference. The inner wheel is marked out in week intervals, normally from 0 to 43. The inner wheel is rotated so that various landmarks during the pregnancy can be aligned to a calendar date. For example, if the LMP is 01.04.2016, the inner wheel is rotated so that the point marked LMP (week zero) is aligned to the respective calendar date – in this case, 1st April. Level with the 40th week is the point marked EDD. In this example case the EDD point on the inner wheel will now be aligned to the calendar date 8th January. You will note that gestation calculator wheels are not year specific.

USING THE COMPUTER DATABASE

Another method for calculating the EDD is via the computer database used to produce the ultrasound report. Depending on the package, the software may enable calculation of the EDD. For an individual patient record there is often a field titled LMP, which requires the relevant calendar date to be entered. The software will then apply Naegele's formula, i.e. add 280 days to the LMP date to calculate the EDD.

As mentioned earlier in this chapter, the gestational age and EDD is best made from the ultrasound measurements. Operators need to be aware that an EDD calculated from the LMP either using the gestation calculator wheel or using the computer database may change once dated from ultrasound measurements.

USING ASSISTED CONCEPTION DATES

Where the pregnancy is a result of an assisted conception the gestational age can easily be calculated, as the date of ovulation /conception is certain.

Where in vitro fertilization (IVF) has taken place, the day of egg collection is taken as the day of ovulation. As this is the day when the oocytes were inseminated with sperm, it is also taken as the day of conception. The fertilized egg(s) or embryo(s) will be transferred back into the uterus between 2 and 5 days after egg collection. Any remaining embryos may be frozen. Currently, the most common time for embryo transfer to take place is 5 days after the egg collection, at the blastocyst stage. In the past, IVF units transferred embryos, which were 2 or 3 days old, but latterly have achieved higher pregnancy success rates transferring blastocysts, which are 5 days old.

When calculating the gestational age of an assisted conception pregnancy it is important to know both the date of egg collection and the date of embryo transfer if the pregnancy results from a fresh cycle. The age of the embryo(s) at transfer will provide a check that the two dates provided correspond appropriately. Where the pregnancy has resulted from the use of one or more frozen embryos, then the date of transfer and the age of the embryo(s) when frozen is the information that is required.

USING THE DATE OF EGG COLLECTION

Let us assume that the date of egg collection was 15.04.2016 and that this was a 'fresh' cycle. The EDD can be calculated as follows:

The date of ovulation/conception is taken as the date of egg collection, namely 15.04.2016.

Method 1

Using the gestation calculator wheel, find the point on the inner wheel, which is marked date of ovulation/conception. If it is not labelled as such, it corresponds to week 2 or day 14. Align the point marked date of ovulation/conception (or week 2) to the calendar date 15th April. In this example case the EDD point on the inner wheel will now be aligned to the calendar date 8th January.

Method 2

Using the computer database, enter 15.04.2016 into the field titled date of conception. The software will add 266 days to the conception date to calculate an EDD of 08.01.17. If there is no option to date of conception, the LMP field will need to be entered. The LMP is 'artificially' created as

having occurred 14 days before the date of egg collection, namely 01.04.2016. The software will add 280 days to the conception date to calculate an EDD of 08.01.17. It is likely that the woman's true LMP was in fact more than 14 days earlier as stimulation of the ovaries to produce multiple follicles during IVF may be prolonged.

USING THE DATE OF EMBRYO TRANSFER

Let us assume that this was a 'fresh' cycle and that a day 5 blastocyst was transferred on 15.04.2016. The EDD can be calculated as follows:

As a day 5 blastocyst was transferred, the date of egg collection was 5 days before the date of embryo transfer. As the blastocyst was transferred on 15.04.2016, the date of egg collection was 10.04.2016. The date of ovulation/conception is taken as the date of egg collection, namely 10.04.2016. Therefore the EDD can be calculated, as previously, using 10.04.2016 as the date of ovulation/conception.

These calculations apply irrespective of whether the egg was collected from the woman herself or was a donor egg.

USING THE DATE OF EMBRYO TRANSFER IN A FROZEN CYCLE

Let us now assume that this was a 'frozen' cycle and that a day 5 blastocyst was transferred on 15.04.2016. The calculations are essentially the same as for a fresh cycle. The EDD can be calculated as follows:

As a day 5 blastocyst was transferred, the date of egg collection would have taken place 5 days earlier, had this been a fresh cycle. As the blastocyst was transferred on 15.04.2016, the 'date of egg collection' is assigned as 10.04.2016. The date of ovulation/conception is taken as the assigned date of egg collection, namely 10.04.2016.

These calculations apply irrespective of whether the egg was collected from the woman herself or was a donor egg.

AGE OF THE WOMAN OR DONOR AT THE TIME OF EGG COLLECTION

The age of the woman at the time of her egg collection is of no importance when calculating gestational age but is extremely important when calculating the risk of maternal age-related chromosomal abnormalities such as Down's syndrome. This applies whether the egg was collected from the woman herself or from a donor. It is the age of the provider of the egg which is important when calculating these risks, and not the age of the woman into whom the fertilized egg has been transferred. This is described in greater detail in Chapter 7.

ASSIGNING THE EDD

It is clear therefore that using the LMP to assess the length of pregnancy will be inaccurate in a high proportion of cases. It is also accepted that accurate measurement of the embryo/fetus between 7 and 12 weeks of gestation is the best method of assessing gestational age using ultrasound. It is further accepted that the agreed EDD should be that calculated from an ultrasound examination in which the appropriate measurement(s) are correctly taken.

Although it can be argued that the optimal time to measure the length of the conceptus is before 12 weeks, the need for optimal accuracy of the EDD needs to be considered in the context of the clinical management of potentially many thousands of pregnancies within a routine obstetric service. Current recommended practice is to date the pregnancy and assign the EDD at the routine 'dating' or the 'combined screening' scans, which are normally offered to all women at around 12 weeks of pregnancy. As all women participating in a screening programme should be placed on the same pathway of care, and as not all women will be scanned in early pregnancy, ultrasound examination in early pregnancy should be used to assess the length of pregnancy but not to formally date the pregnancy or assign the EDD. Correct measurement of CRL and pregnancy dating are discussed in Chapter 7.

ESTIMATING THE LENGTH OF PREGNANCY

Although the pregnancy should normally not be formally dated before the 12-week scan, it is helpful to have some estimation of the expected length of pregnancy prior to starting your scan. Normally the only relevant information available to you will be the LMP and this should therefore be used as a guide, remembering that it can be unreliable for the reasons outlined previously. The LMP will help you to decide in the first instance whether the transvaginal or the transabdominal approach is more appropriate for the scan you are about to perform. It will also help you in advising the woman on the ultrasound appearances you are anticipating – for example, equivocal findings due to the very early gestation, the small 'empty' gestation sac of a very early pregnancy or the live embryo in the gestation sac of the early pregnancy. Where no LMP data are available, the woman may recall the date of her first positive pregnancy test. As a positive pregnancy test cannot occur any earlier than 4 weeks of gestation, this can be used as a rough estimate of gestational age, in lieu of the LMP.

THE POSITIVE PREGNANCY TEST

A pregnancy test detects a specific pregnancy hormone, human chorionic gonadotropin (hCG), in either blood or urine.

Following the start of implantation at around day 7 (range 6–12 days), the trophoblast begins producing intact β hCG, which then enters the maternal bloodstream. It is first detectable with current assays in maternal serum about 2 days later – that is, around day 9. The hCG in the maternal blood is filtered through the woman's kidneys and subsequently will first be detectable with current assays in her urine 2–3 days later, approximately on day 11–12.

As detection of hCG in the maternal serum or urine depends on the timing of implantation, hCG can normally be detected in the maternal serum

81

8–14 days postconception and in the maternal urine, and therefore in a urinary pregnancy test, 10–17 days postconception. Home pregnancy urine tests will give a 'positive' result at a level of hCG of 25 IU/L. This level usually coincides with that in the maternal urine at the time of the first missed period, i.e. around 14 days postconception.

Much is made of the behaviour of maternal serum hCG assays in early pregnancy, with many centres using a level between 1000 IU/L and 2000 IU/L to describe 'the discriminatory zone'. This level is cited in many publications as describing the threshold above which a pregnancy would be expected to be visualized within the uterus by transvaginal ultrasound. Clinically, therefore, hCG assays are used as a guide in the requesting of ultrasound investigations, in the expectant management of ectopic pregnancies and in the subsequent management of women with a positive pregnancy test but where a gestation sac cannot be identified on ultrasound. These pregnancies are described as pregnancies of unknown location (PUL) and are an important component in the management of possible ectopic pregnancy (see Chapter 6).

ULTRASOUND PARAMETERS

In early pregnancy the ultrasound parameters most commonly used to estimate the length of pregnancy are:
- mean sac diameter (MSD)
- crown rump length (CRL).

ASSESSMENT OF EARLY PREGNANCY

There are no clinical reasons why the ultrasound examination of the early pregnant uterus should not be performed transvaginally.

The transvaginal approach is normally the preferred method of imaging the early pregnant uterus because of its superior image quality compared with the transabdominal route. The higher frequencies of 7–9 MHz used in transvaginal imaging have a greater ability to resolve very small structures, such as the 2–5 mm diameter gestation sac typical of the 4^+–5 week pregnancy, and to image larger structures with better resolution than the lower frequencies of 3.5–6 MHz used in transabdominal imaging.

The only clinical situation where the transabdominal approach is likely to provide superior imaging of the pregnant pelvis prior to 10 weeks of gestation is in the presence of one or more fibroids that lie between the probe and the gestation sac, thus increasing the distance between the transducer face and the pregnancy. In such situations the lack of penetration associated with imaging at higher frequencies affects the normally superior resolution of the transvaginal approach. The transabdominal approach may be preferable where the uterus is axial, and therefore very difficult to insonate effectively with the transvaginal probe. In cases where there are large ovarian cysts these may displace the pregnant uterus so that it is beyond the field of view of the transvaginal probe.

Some women may be concerned that the placing of the probe into the vagina may be dangerous and/or cause harm to their pregnancy. It is important therefore that you are able to reassure the woman that a transvaginal ultrasound examination is a safe procedure both for her and her baby. Furthermore, you should be able to explain that the transvaginal approach is more likely to give a more accurate assessment of her pregnancy because of its superior image quality than the transabdominal approach. Should the woman decline to consent to a transvaginal scan following this discussion, a transabdominal examination should be performed. It is important you record clearly in your report that the woman declined a transvaginal scan and the reason(s) for her decision.

Ultrasound practitioners tend to hold very specific, but not necessarily evidence-based, views regarding the gestational age above which the transabdominal approach should be used. We suggest that before 10 weeks of gestation the transvaginal approach should be the default method. Transabdominal scanning can be then used as an adjunct if clinically indicated. In follow-up early-pregnancy scans performed at gestations between 8 and 10 weeks, a transabdominal scan will normally suffice – although this will be dependent upon the clinical indication.

For the reasons discussed earlier, this chapter concentrates primarily on the transvaginal method of assessing early pregnancy, with the transabdominal approach being included for completeness.

The criteria and algorithms for diagnosis and management of early pregnancy problems have been formulated using the transvaginal and not the transabdominal approach. This should be borne in mind if you are performing an early pregnancy examination using the transabdominal approach.

THE TRANSVAGINAL METHOD

This text assumes that you, the operator, are sitting to the left of, or at the foot of, the scanning couch, holding the probe in your right hand, that the woman is lying to your right side or directly in front of you, and that you are facing each other. The image is orientated so that the apex of the image is displayed at the top of the ultrasound monitor, that the left side of the maternal pelvis is displayed on the right side of the ultrasound monitor and the right side of the maternal pelvis is displayed on the left side of the ultrasound monitor when imaged in transverse section.

EXAMINING THE UTERUS

The preparation and technique required for a transvaginal examination have been described in detail in Chapter 4. As a small amount of urine in the bladder can displace the organs of interest out of the field of view, it is important to confirm with the woman before starting the scan that her bladder is empty. The clinical value of scanning an asymptomatic woman with a negative pregnancy test in order to search for ultrasound features of an early pregnancy is highly debatable. Asking the woman to empty her bladder prior to her ultrasound examination therefore provides your clinical colleagues with the opportunity to confirm that the pregnancy test is positive before confirming that an ultrasound examination is clinically indicated.

Establish whether the uterus is anteverted, axial or retroverted in orientation. Examine the uterus and cervix in sagittal, parasagittal and transverse planes. It is important that a complete survey of the uterus and its endometrium is carried out. This is because the earliest evidence of a normal intrauterine pregnancy, namely a gestation sac of 2–3 mm in diameter, can easily be missed. It is also important to confirm that there are no uterine anomalies

such as a bicornuate or septate uterus, and also that a pregnancy is not interstitial or cornual in location.

If no obvious gestation sac is apparent, the endometrium should be assessed and measured (see Chapter 16). This is because thickened endometrium is more likely to be associated with an early pregnancy than thin endometrium. There is no agreed 'normal range' for endometrial thickness associated with early pregnancy; we suggest that 5.0 mm would not normally be considered to be 'thick' but 15.0 mm would. Visualization of the endometrium can be improved by ensuring the sound beam is orthogonal to the axis of the endometrium, zooming up or magnifying the image, using multiple focal zones, increasing the frequency and/or narrowing the sector width.

Thickened Endometrium

Thickening of the endometrium is a normal precursor to visualization of the gestation sac. It cannot be taken as diagnostic of pregnancy as the differential diagnosis for thickened endometrium includes:

- the late secretory phase of the menstrual cycle
- a very early intrauterine pregnancy, i.e. before the gestation sac can be resolved
- a decidual reaction in association with ectopic pregnancy
- retained products of conception within the uterine cavity.

The Intrauterine Gestation Sac

The early gestation sac can be seen within the uterus from approximately 4^{+4} weeks of gestation. It appears as a circular, hypoechoic or black area surrounded by a thick, hyperechoic or white ring and measures 2–3 mm in diameter. The position of the gestation sac reflects the implantation site of the blastocyst within the endometrium. As the blastocyst moves from the cavity of the uterus into, most frequently, either the anterior or posterior endometrium, the gestation sac is seen in an eccentric position within the endometrium, respectively above or below the 'cavity line'. The cavity line is the thin, regular, hyperechoic line produced by the apposition of the anterior and posterior endometrial layers. The hyperechoic, thick ring and the eccentric position of the gestation sac are important features in distinguishing between an intrauterine pregnancy (Fig. 5.1) and the so-called pseudosac (see below).

The hyperechoic, thick ring of the early gestation sac corresponds to a rim of invading chorionic villi from the trophoblast together with the underlying decidual reaction of the uterine endometrium. The decidual reaction describes the enlargement of the endometrial stromal cells around the conceptus and their accumulation of glycogen and lipid together with additional vascular and glandular changes within the endometrium. These changes occur locally, around the implantation site initially, but soon spread throughout the endometrium.

The circular hypoechoic area of the gestation sac corresponds to two separate fluid-filled compartments, namely the inner amniotic cavity surrounded by the amniotic membrane and the outer chorionic (or exocoelomic) cavity surrounded by the chorionic membrane.

In very early pregnancy the chorionic cavity predominates and the resolution of the equipment is not sufficient to identify the amniotic cavity developing within it. By about 8 weeks of gestation the amniotic membrane, which defines the border of the rapidly expanding amniotic cavity, can be identified within the gestation sac (Fig. 5.2). Because the amniotic cavity grows more rapidly than the chorionic cavity, the two cavities reach equivalent size by the end of the first trimester or early in the second trimester. This leads to the fusing of the amniotic and chorionic membranes and the complete obliteration of the chorionic cavity. This is normally completed by 14–16 weeks of gestation.

Some authors place importance on the relative sizes of the gestation sac, or chorionic cavity, and the amniotic sac or cavity within it. Reference ranges for both mean gestation sac diameter and mean amniotic sac diameter are available. Only mean gestation sac diameter is included in this text, as measurement of mean amniotic sac diameter normally is not used in routine practice.

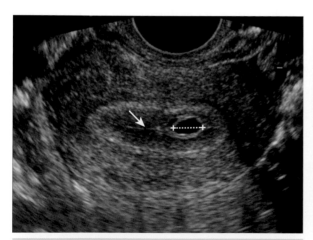

Fig 5.1 • A transverse section of the uterus demonstrating an intrauterine gestation sac at 5 weeks of gestation. The gestation sac is eccentrically located within the anterior endometrium. Note the hyperechoic rim of the gestation sac. The cavity line is denoted by the arrow.

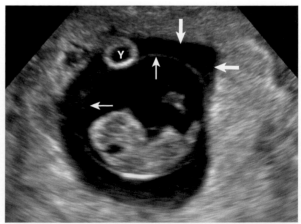

Fig 5.2 • Intrauterine gestation sac demonstrating the inner amniotic cavity (thin arrows) and outer chorionic cavity (thick arrows) at 8⁺ weeks. The amnion completely surrounds the embryo. The yolk sac (Y) lies outside the amniotic cavity.

The Very Early Gestation Sac (4–5 Weeks)

As described earlier, the typical appearance of the early gestation sac after 5 weeks of gestation is distinctive and specific. The characteristic hyperechoic and thick ring surrounding the early gestation sac is produced from the trophoblast and local decidual reaction. As the thick, bright ring takes some days to develop, the white rim of the gestation sac of less than 5 weeks of gestation is frequently not thick and bright but thin and bright. The ultrasound appearance of the very early gestation sac therefore has the same ultrasound attributes as other simple cystic structures.

Small cystic areas can sometimes be seen within the pregnant or nonpregnant endometrium and are thought to be due to glandular activity within the tissue. Their appearance is indistinguishable from that of the very early gestation sac. Although the appearances are the same, if this cystic area is a gestation sac, only one such area will normally be present within the endometrium. By contrast, multiple cystic areas will be present if the appearance is due to glandular activity

Extreme caution should be applied in the interpretation of a single thin, rimmed cystic area within the endometrium as confirmation of an intrauterine pregnancy. The experience of the operator and the resolution of the ultrasound machine both affect the ability to correctly identify true early intrauterine gestation sacs. A repeat examination performed in no less than 10 days may demonstrate features of an early pregnancy at the subsequent scan, i.e. a yolk sac with or without an embryo if it is an ongoing pregnancy. However, early pregnancy units may choose to adapt a policy of describing these findings as a pregnancy of unknown location (PUL) and managing these women using the PUL pathway (see Chapter 6).

The Pseudosac (Fluid Within the Cavity)

Pseudosac is a historic term, which, as its name suggests, was – and continues to be – used to describe fluid that has collected within the uterine cavity. As it is fluid, the area appears black or hypoechoic. As the fluid collection lies within the uterine cavity, it is centrally placed within the uterus and is circumscribed not by the thick hyperechoic ring seen in the gestation sac but by a thin white line. This thin

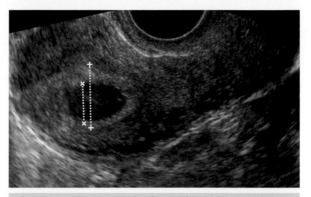

Fig 5.3 • Fluid centrally located within the uterine cavity. There was a left tubal ectopic gestation. The depth of fluid has been measured, excluding both layers of the endometrium (x) and including both layers of endometrium (+).

white line represents the separation of the 'cavity line' generated by the opposing borders of the anterior and posterior endometrium into their component parts, namely the medial borders of the anterior and posterior endometrium, respectively. The shape of the fluid collection reflects that of the uterine cavity and therefore will not be circular (Fig. 5.3). In an attempt to discourage the continuing use of a clinically unhelpful and incorrect term we recommend that fluid within the uterine cavity is reported as *fluid within the uterine cavity* and not as a *pseudosac*.

Fluid can collect within the uterine cavity for a number of reasons including missed miscarriage and ectopic gestation. It is therefore important to be able to distinguish between the typical appearance and features of fluid within the uterine cavity and those of the early intrauterine gestation sac. This topic is discussed further in Chapter 6.

Implantation Bleed

A frequently triangularly shaped, echo-poor area may be visualized adjacent to, and often inferior to, the gestation sac is described as an *implantation bleed* (Fig. 5.4) and is typically seen between usually 5 and 8 weeks of gestation. It is good practice to measure the area of bleed in three planes to provide a baseline for comparison of size if required later in pregnancy.

The clinical significance of an implantation bleed is debatable as the association between the presence and extent of an implantation bleed and

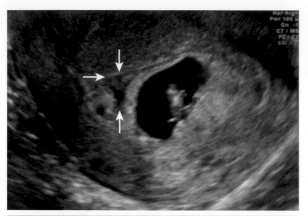

Fig 5.4 • Sagittal view of a retroverted uterus with an intrauterine gestation sac containing a live embryo (8 weeks of gestation). There is an implantation bleed located at the inferior aspect of the gestation sac (arrowed). Note the triangular shape, which is typical of an implantation bleed.

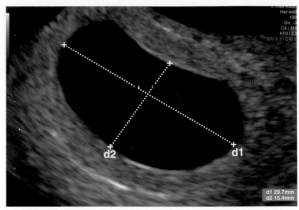

Fig 5.5 • Sagittal section of the uterus demonstrating the longitudinal and anteroposterior diameters of the gestation sac (29.7 × 15.4 mm)

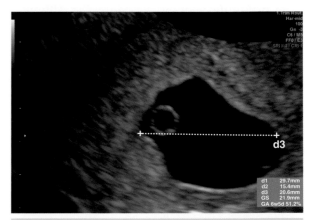

Fig 5.6 • Transverse section of the uterus demonstrating the transverse diameter of the gestation sac (20.6 mm). A yolk sac is present.

vaginal bleeding appears weak. For example, an implantation bleed can be visualized, and can be extensive in size, in a woman who has had no vaginal bleeding, whereas, by contrast, there can be no evidence of an implantation bleed in a woman who reports vaginal bleeding.

FINDING AND MEASURING THE GESTATION SAC

First you must obtain a true sagittal section of the uterus. If the gestation sac is not immediately visible, pan the probe gently from side to side until the whole of the endometrium has been examined. Now return to the section which displays the maximum length of the gestation sac. Additional very small rotational and/or angling movements of the probe will allow you to determine whether altering the plane of the image slightly produces a longer length of the sac. Freeze the image and measure the maximum longitudinal diameter (L), in millimetres, together with the maximum anteroposterior diameter (AP), in millimetres, of the gestation sac (Fig. 5.5). The longitudinal and AP diameters should be at 90° to each other and the intersection of the cross of the linear callipers should be placed on the inner borders of the sac, thus producing an 'inner to inner' measurement in each case.

Rotate the probe through 90° in order to obtain a transverse section of the gestation sac. This is most easily obtained by keeping the gestation sac in view as you rotate the probe. Make sure you have rotated the probe through the full 90°. If the gestation sac disappears from view as you rotate, pan the probe across the width of the uterus until it reappears. Angle the handle of the probe until the maximum diameter of the sac is obtained in this plane. Freeze the image and measure the maximum transverse diameter (T), in millimetres (Fig. 5.6), by placing the intersection of the cross of the linear callipers on the inner borders of the sac to obtain an 'inner to inner' measurement. Calculating the mean gestation sac diameter is discussed in the next section.

When the uterus is very anteflexed or retroverted, it may not be possible to angle the probe sufficiently to obtain a true transverse section of the gestation sac. As discussed in Chapter 4, an AP diameter measured from a transverse section is not accurate. We therefore recommend that the AP diameter is measured from the sagittal section.

Every effort should be made to optimize the image of the intrauterine gestation sac employing the same methods as described previously for the endometrium. The size of the gestation sac and what can be seen inside it are key factors in the differentiation between an ongoing and a failing or failed pregnancy.

Finally note whether the inner contour of the gestation sac is regular or irregular. The contour of a healthy gestation sac in an ongoing pregnancy is typically regular and smooth, whereas an irregular contour is more frequently associated with a poor outcome.

The normal gestation sac grows by approximately 1.0 mm in mean diameter per day. The early gestation sac is essentially spherical and therefore circular in both sagittal and transverse planes. The sac becomes more elliptical as it grows and this contributes to the increasing inaccuracy of the mean sac diameter as a method of assessing the length of pregnancy. This will also affect the accuracy, and therefore the reliability, of serial measurements of the mean gestation sac diameter undertaken to determine whether or not a pregnancy is ongoing.

Calculation of Mean Gestation Sac Diameter

The calculation of the mean gestation sac diameter is useful to assess the length of pregnancy before the embryo can be visualized. Once the embryo can be seen and measured, the mean gestation sac diameter is of limited value.

The mean gestation sac diameter is calculated using the following formula:

Mean sac diameter (mm)

$= [L (mm) + AP (mm) + T (mm)]/3$

The diameters are measured using the 'inner to inner' method of caliper placement.

The literature contains a number of data sets linking mean gestation sac diameter and gestational age. They vary in their methodologies and in the relationship between the two parameters. For example, the method used to calculate gestational age includes the LMP in women with regular menstrual cycles, dating from IVF and retrospective dating from the CRL at 11–13 weeks. In addition, there are few data relating length of pregnancy and mean gestation sac diameter below 5^{+0} weeks and/ or 4.0 mm mean gestation sac diameter. Table 5.1 shows the length of pregnancy estimated from the mean gestation sac diameter, together with crown rump length measurement. The data shown in Table 5.1 are derived from data sets from different sources, all of which are based on certain menstrual dates and resulted in the delivery of a normal singleton infant at term.

Threshold Values for Mean Gestation Sac Diameter

In normal pregnancy the gestation sac must reach a certain size before the yolk sac and then the embryo will be visualized within it. There is therefore a threshold mean gestation sac diameter below which the normal finding is of an 'empty' sac and above which the normal finding is of a gestation sac within which the yolk sac is seen. This value varies between authors, but we recommend that a yolk sac should always be seen in a gestation sac of mean diameter of 10.0 mm and above.

Current guidelines indicate that the yolk sac and a live embryo should always be seen in a gestation sac of mean diameter of 25.0 mm or greater. The value of 25.0 mm is therefore the recommended threshold of the (empty) mean gestation sac diameter above which the diagnosis of delayed miscarriage can be made (see Chapter 6).

The Yolk Sac

The yolk sac is the first structure that can be identified within the gestation sac and can be seen from about 37 days of gestation. It appears as a circular, hypoechoic mass with a thin, hyperechoic rim and, depending on the technique used, measures 3–4 mm in diameter (Fig. 5.6). At this stage the yolk sac is significantly larger than the embryo,

MEAN GESTATION SAC DIAMETER (mm)	GESTATIONAL AGE (weeks + days)	RANGE (weeks + days) 5th and 95th centiles	CROWN RUMP LENGTH (mm)	FETAL HEART RATE (beats/min)
2.0–4.0	4^{+4} to 4^{+6}	Not provided	**Not visible**	
4.0	5^{+0}	Not provided	**Not visible**	
5.0	5^{+1}	Not provided	**Not visible**	
6.0	$5^{+2\dagger}$	3^{+6}, 6^{+6}	2.0	100
7.0	5^{+3}	4^{+0}, 7^{+0}	2.0	
8.0	5^{+4}	4^{+1}, 7^{+1}	3.0	105
9.0	5^{+5}	4^{+2}, 7^{+2}	3.0	
10.0	5^{+6}	4^{+3}, 7^{+3}	4.0	110
11.0	6^{+0}	4^{+3}, 7^{+3}	4.0	
12.0	6^{+1}	4^{+4}, 7^{+4}	5.0	120
13.0	6^{+2}	4^{+5}, 7^{+5}	5.0	
14.0	6^{+3}	4^{+6}, 7^{+6}	6.0	130
15.0	6^{+4}	5^{+0}, 8^{+0}	6.0	
16.0	6^{+5}	5^{+1}, 8^{+1}	$7.0^{\ddagger}$	130
17.0	6^{+5}	5^{+2}, 8^{+2}	8.0	135
18.0	6^{+6}	5^{+3}, 8^{+3}	9.0	145
19.0	7^{+0}	5^{+4}, 8^{+4}	9.0	
20.0	7^{+1}	5^{+5}, 8^{+5}	10.0	150
21.0	7^{+2}	5^{+5}, 8^{+5}	11.0	
22.0	7^{+3}	5^{+6}, 8^{+6}	12.0	
23.0	7^{+4}	6^{+0}, 9^{+0}	13.0	
24.0	7^{+5}	6^{+1}, 9^{+1}	14.0	
25.0*	7^{+6}	6^{+3}, 9^{+3}	15.0	
26.0	8^{+0}	6^{+4}, 9^{+3}	16.0	
27.0	8^{+1}	6^{+5}, 9^{+4}	17.0	
28.0	8^{+2}	6^{+5}, 9^{+5}	18.0	
29.0	8^{+3}	6^{+6}, 9^{+6}	19.0	
30.0	8^{+4}	7^{+0}, 10^{+0}	20.0	

Table 5.1 Association between length of pregnancy (weeks + days), MSD and CRL using data combined from several authors

Data from Coulam (FHR), Grisolia (GSD and age, GSD and CRL) and Papaioannou (yolk sac).

*Threshold mean gestation sac diameter at and above which the diagnosis of delayed miscarriage can be made when no yolk sac or embryo can be identified within the sac.

†Threshold gestational age above which the yolk sac is normally seen within the gestation sac.

‡Threshold CRL above which the diagnosis of delayed miscarriage can be made when no heart pulsations are seen.

CRL, crown rump length; FHR, fetal heart rate; GSD, gestation sac diameter; MSD, mean sac diameter.

which explains why it is seen within the gestation sac some days before the embryo can be clearly identified.

The yolk sac is derived from the inner cell mass of the conceptus. Its identification is confirmatory evidence of the presence of an intrauterine pregnancy. This can be compared to fluid within the uterine cavity, a pseudosac indicating a possible ectopic pregnancy, or glandular activity within part of the nonpregnant endometrium. We recommend that the presence of the yolk sac should be used in the confirmation of the early intrauterine pregnancy before the embryo can be identified. Once the embryo is visualized, assessment of the pregnancy should be based primarily on the appearance and size of the embryo rather than any other features of the gestation sac.

In the early stages of development, the yolk sac and the embryo lie very close to each other within the gestation sac. Identifying the yolk sac therefore should lead to the embryo, which at this stage will measure approximately 2 mm in length. As the vitelline duct, which connects the yolk sac to the gut of the embryo, grows, the close association between them is rapidly lost. In addition, the embryo develops within the amniotic sac, whereas the yolk sac lies outside the amniotic sac, within the chorionic sac. The amniotic membrane therefore can be seen lying between the embryo and the yolk sac. The increasing size of the amniotic sac compresses the yolk sac against the wall of the chorionic cavity, making identification of the yolk sac difficult after 12–13 weeks.

Correlation between yolk sac morphology and the outcome of pregnancy is not clear. Some authors report an association between a yolk sac, which is 'absent' (or not visualized on ultrasound), before 8 weeks and abnormal pregnancy, even when the embryo is alive. Miscarriage is commonly reported in this situation. Furthermore, in cases of delayed miscarriage with a visible embryo, the yolk sac tends to be larger and its wall thinner than in normal pregnancies. Other authors are unable to demonstrate any significant correlation between size and shape of the yolk sac and pregnancy outcome.

The yolk sac increases only minimally during the first trimester, from a mean diameter of 3.0 mm at approximately 5 weeks to a maximum mean diameter of 5.0–6.0 mm at 10 weeks of gestation.

As with mean gestation sac diameter, different authors report differing values for yolk sac size and also report using different methods of calliper placement in its measurement. Measuring the yolk sac diameter is of limited clinical value, we therefore recommend that its presence should be noted and reported when performing an early pregnancy examination but that it is not necessary to measure or report its mean diameter.

Should you wish to calculate the mean yolk sac diameter, we recommend using calliper placement as described for the gestation sac diameter, namely taking 'inner to inner' measurements. The yolk sac is essentially circular and therefore the mean of two diameters is sufficient to calculate the mean yolk sac diameter rather than three.

The mean yolk sac diameter is calculated using the following formula:

$$\text{Mean yolk sac diameter (mm)} = L\,(mm) + AP\,(mm)/2$$

The Embryo

The embryo can be identified within the gestation sac from about 37 days or 5^{+2} weeks of gestational age. It is first seen as a hyperechoic linear echo, adjacent to the yolk sac, and measures around 2 mm in length. This measurement is described as crown rump length (CRL), although reference to an embryological text will indicate that implying the embryo has either a crown or a rump at this stage of its development is somewhat optimistic. The measurement of the length of the embryo before 7 weeks of gestation, more correctly, describes the neck-to-rump length. The resolution of the equipment is such that it can often be difficult to identify such a small structure and it is visualization of heart pulsations which leads to confirmation of an ongoing pregnancy.

CRL Definition

The CRL is defined as the sagittal section of the whole embryo or fetus, in a neutral position and with the end points of the crown, or neck in the very early embryo, and rump clearly visible. The embryo should be imaged in a plane that is horizontal to the ultrasound beam and should be measured using linear callipers.

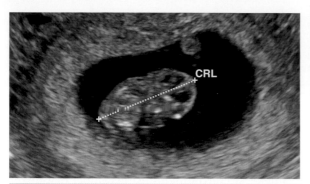

Fig 5.7 • Embryo with CRL measurement of 22.8 mm, equivalent to 8^{+6} weeks

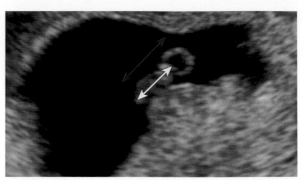

Fig 5.8 • The embryo lies close to the yolk sac. Failure to identify the yolk sac separately may result in an overestimation of the CRL measurement (denoted by the red arrow). This can be compared to the correct CRL measurement denoted by the yellow arrow.

CRL Measurement

Once the embryo can be seen within the gestation sac, the length of pregnancy should be assessed from measurement of the CRL and not from calculation of the mean gestation sac diameter. It should be remembered that the gestational age and therefore the EDD for the pregnancy should only be calculated once and, where combined screening for Down's, Edwards' and Patau's syndromes is offered, this should be done at the time of screening, namely at around 12 weeks of gestation.

Owing to movement of the embryo or fetus there can be no standardized technique for obtaining a CRL. First, obtain a longitudinal section of the uterus and gestation sac. Pan the probe slowly to each side of the sac until heart pulsations from the embryo can be seen. Slowly rotate the probe, keeping these pulsations in view, until the long axis of the embryo is obtained. Freeze this image. The maximum length of the embryonic pole is measured using the on-screen callipers (Fig. 5.7).

It is important to ensure that you are imaging the longest length of the embryo before taking your measurements. To confirm this, continue to pan, angle or rotate the probe past your intended optimal section. If the selected section is optimal, then the subsequent CRLs should reduce in size. Return to the original section, freeze the image and measure the optimal CRL.

The CRL should be measured from three different images. There are no national recommendations defining an 'acceptable' range of error for comparative CRL measurements. We recommend

that the difference between the measurements should be no greater than 5% of the mean between the three. This will equate to approximately 0.5 mm in the embryo, or approximately 1 day of gestation before 10 weeks of gestation. We also recommend that the measurement from the image which displays the best section and which has also been measured correctly is selected for the reported CRL. On no account should the three measurements be averaged to produce the CRL.

CRL measurements may be inaccurate before 10 weeks of gestation, and thus estimation of the length of pregnancy inaccurate, for the following reasons:

- the full length of the embryo has not been obtained – this will produce an underestimated CRL
- the end points of the embryo have not been clearly identified as separate from the closely adjacent yolk sac or the wall of the gestation sac and one or both have been included in the measurement – this will produce an overestimated CRL (Fig. 5.8).

Once the fetal spine can be easily identified, i.e. from about 9 weeks of gestation, this should be used as a guide in assessing the true length of the embryo. The aim is to examine the embryo with the full length of its spine positioned directly anteriorly or posteriorly, thereby enabling you to assess any degree of flexion. As the early embryo has no flexion, this only becomes problematic in the fetus after 10 weeks of gestation. Dating the pregnancy by accurate measurement of the CRL is discussed in more detail in Chapter 7.

Ongoing Pregnancy, Heart Pulsations, CRL Threshold, Miscarriage Risk

The pregnancy can only be said to be ongoing when cardiac pulsations from the embryo can be demonstrated within the gestation sac. The embryonic heart begins to 'beat' by 22 days after conception – that is, 5^{+1} weeks of gestational age. Initially an ebb and flow circulation is established, progressing to a unidirectional circulation by the end of the 6th week of gestation. The embryo can be first visualized with ultrasound at approximately the same time as the heart starts to beat. This has clinical significance as it provides a potential threshold above which the diagnosis of embryonic death, and therefore a failed pregnancy, can be made. Conversely, the same threshold determines the CRL below which this diagnosis should not be made.

As it is good clinical practice to err on the side of caution, current guidelines indicate that heart pulsations should always be visible in an embryo with a CRL of 7.0 mm or greater. The value of 7.0 mm is therefore the recommended threshold for CRL used in the diagnosis of delayed miscarriage (see Chapter 6).

As shown in Table 5.1, normal ranges for fetal heart rate in pregnancy have been described. It has been shown that a late onset of cardiac activity and a decreased heart rate in the first trimester are associated with a higher rate of spontaneous miscarriage.

Pulsed Doppler ultrasound – that is, spectral Doppler, power Doppler and colour flow imaging – should not be used in the routine assessment of heart activity in the early pregnancy. This is due to the risk of biological damage from the heating effect of pulsed Doppler on the developing embryo. Heart activity is best assessed by direct visualization using the grey-scale image only. Alternatively, M mode can demonstrate the movement of the embryonic heart in a wavelike display across time. The display can be stored electronically or as a hard copy image. Furthermore, if the heart rate needs to be calculated, this can be done from the M mode display.

Care should be taken when confirming cardiac activity in the very early stages of pregnancy as movement caused by the maternal pulse can be falsely identified as pulsations from the embryo's heart.

Once an embryo with normal cardiac activity is seen, the chance of the pregnancy ending in miscarriage decreases from 12% to 1%, as shown in Table 5.2.

Physiological Herniation of the Gut at 8–10 Weeks

Rapid changes can be observed in the appearance of the embryo after 7 weeks of gestation. One of the most significant changes which you must be aware of is the physiological herniation of the gut into the base of the umbilical cord, which takes place between 8 and 10 weeks of gestation. The bowel starts to elongate within the abdominal cavity but, because there is insufficient room within the abdomen for the rapidly growing midgut, it projects into the base of the umbilical cord (Fig. 5.9). The

ULTRASOUND APPEARANCE	GESTATIONAL AGE	% MISCARRIAGE RISK
Early gestation sac	4^{+3}–6^{+0} weeks	12%
Live embryo < 5.0 mm	6^{+0}–7^{+0} weeks	7%
Live embryo > 10.0 mm	>7^{+0} weeks	1%

Table 5.2 Percentage chance of miscarriage associated with ultrasound appearances in early pregnancy
<, less than; >, more than.

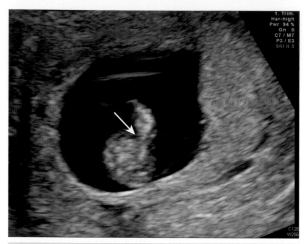

Fig 5.9 • Normal physiological herniation of the fetal gut.

shortage of space is due primarily to the relatively massive liver and kidneys. Between 8 and 10 weeks of gestation therefore the bowel develops both within the abdominal cavity and within the base of the umbilical cord. The latter is termed the *physiological herniation of the gut* and is a normal finding in all embryos at this gestation. The herniation appears as a hyperechoic mass in the base of the umbilical cord. The bowel should always have returned completely into the abdominal cavity by the end of the 11th week of gestation. Failure of the bowel to return to the abdominal cavity results in the abnormality of omphalocele or exomphalos (see Fig. 7.12). Detection or exclusion of abdominal wall defects should therefore not be attempted until after 12 weeks of gestation (see Chapter 7).

Twin Pregnancies

Multiple gestation sacs can be identified as early as singleton sacs, i.e. from 4^{+4} weeks of gestation. The presence of two separate gestation sacs before 6 weeks is compatible with the diagnosis of a dichorionic pregnancy. This may be either dizygotic or monozygotic. As both sacs may contain more than one embryo, the number of sacs should not be used as a conclusive indication of either the number of future embryos at this early gestation or of the chorionicity of the twin pregnancy.

You must remember that the presence of a gestation sac does not indicate an ongoing pregnancy, but merely confirms an intrauterine pregnancy. An apparently empty sac(s) in a multiple pregnancy may regress spontaneously before the embryo can be identified within it. This 'vanishing twin' phenomenon has been reported to affect up to 20% of multiple pregnancies. These phenomena further support delaying the diagnosis of a definitive multiple pregnancy until multiple live embryos have been identified.

Finally, not all live twin pregnancies confirmed in early pregnancy will go on to deliver twin infants. The conception rate of a twin pregnancy is approximately double that of the twin delivery rate and the overall loss rate of one embryo or fetus in the first trimester is approximately 30%.

These points are important to remember when discussing early ultrasound findings with the parents.

Zygosity, chorionicity and amnionicity, together with the ultrasound appearances and management of monochorionic and dichorionic twin pregnancies in the first trimester, are discussed in Chapter 15.

OVARIES AND ADNEXAE

An early pregnancy scan is not complete without assessment of the ovaries and adnexae. The transvaginal technique for examination of the ovaries is described in Chapter 4. You need to be aware that ovarian pathology may be encountered. This may be an incidental finding or may include findings that are relevant and pertinent to the clinical presentation of the woman at the time of your examination.

A normal physiological finding of the ovary in pregnancy is the presence of a corpus luteum. Identification of the corpus luteum and recognition of the different appearances of corpora lutea are useful for three reasons:

- to differentiate confidently the corpus luteum from ovarian pathology
- ectopic gestations are most likely to occur on the same side of the pelvis as the corpus luteum (approximately 75% of cases)
- to improve your confidence in differentiating the corpus luteum from an ectopic gestation.

The primary function of the corpus luteum is to secrete progesterone and oestrogen during the early stages of pregnancy. These hormones are essential for the maintenance of the pregnancy before the placenta is sufficiently developed to provide this role – that is, from approximately 12 weeks.

The corpus luteum lies within the ovary and is surrounded by a rim of ovarian parenchyma. It is essentially a unilocular functional cyst of variable ultrasound appearances which can be broadly divided into three groups:

- anechoic
- haemorrhagic
- collapsed.

The corpus luteum is surrounded by a peripheral vascular network which produces the so-called 'ring of fire' when interrogated with colour or power Doppler. This provides very useful confirmation of the presence of a corpus luteum and helps identify its position within the remaining ovarian tissue.

Anechoic Corpus Luteum

The hypoechoic corpus luteum appears as a dark, rounded mass and contains no internal echoes (see Fig. 1.33). It is typically thick-walled with a mean diameter of less than 3.0 cm and with a range of 2.0–8.0 cm.

Haemorrhagic Corpus Luteum

A haemorrhagic corpus luteum arises when fragile vessels within the wall of the newly vascularized corpus luteum rupture and bleed into the luteal fluid (Fig. 5.10A). This is a common appearance of the corpus luteum. The appearances of haemorrhage vary depending on the extent of the bleed and, because the appearance of blood changes over time, the length of time which has elapsed since the bleed occurred. Haemorrhage can produce a complex mass of mixed echo pattern, with focal areas of brighter echoes due to blood clot or clot retraction and lower-level echoes due to debris within the hypoechoic serum. In these instances, without the help of colour or power Doppler, it can be difficult to distinguish the corpus luteum from the surrounding ovarian tissue and therefore it can easily be overlooked.

Collapsed Corpus Luteum

A collapsed corpus luteum loses its rounded shape, this frequently being replaced by a less well-delineated mass with a hypoechoic centre. The wall of the corpus luteum also loses its relatively smooth inner surface and becomes crenulated (Fig. 5.10B).

The collapsed corpus luteum can be mistaken for an ectopic gestation because the adnexal ring

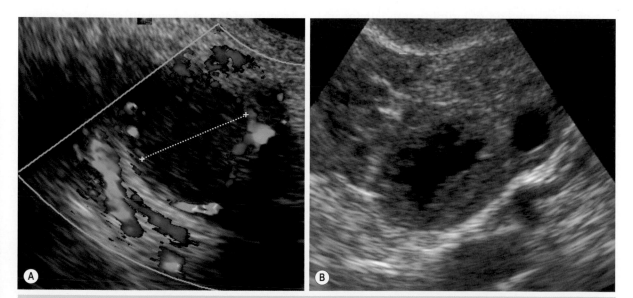

Fig 5.10 • A. Right ovary. Haemorrhagic corpus luteum (circumferential ring of flow demonstrated with colour Doppler). Note that the corpus luteum is isoechoic compared with the surrounding ovarian cortex. B. Left ovary. There is a small collapsed anechoic corpus luteum. Note the crenulated wall compared to the smooth wall shown in A.

of an ectopic gestation can be similar in appearance to that of a collapsed corpus luteum. Both may also demonstrate circumferential blood flow when interrogated with colour Doppler. As most ectopic pregnancies are extraovarian in location, identification of ovarian tissue surrounding the collapsed corpus luteum should exclude an ectopic gestation.

The Ovaries Following In Vitro Fertilization

The formation of normal corpora lutea may be impaired by the medication required in the first key stage of IVF treatment, namely the down-regulation process, and also by the oocyte collection procedure. The second key stage in the standard IVF cycle is to induce ovarian super-ovulation. This is achieved by hyperstimulating the ovaries with gonadotropin injections of either pure follicle stimulating hormone (FSH) or a mixture of FSH and luteinizing hormone (LH). The aim is to stimulate multiple follicular development of, on average, 10 or more follicles in each ovary. When the mean diameter of the largest follicles is at least 18 mm, maturation of the oocytes is induced, with an injection of hCG, prior to their collection. At oocyte collection each follicle is punctured and aspirated, with the resulting formation of multiple corpora lutea.

This drug regimen produces a distinctive 'IVF' appearance of the ovaries, which will be recognized in subsequent scans in early pregnancy, even though egg collection occurred several weeks earlier. The ovaries are enlarged and contain the multiple corpora lutea. The corpora lutea show the same range of (three) appearances as described earlier. The ovaries will return to normal size and appearance over time but, even at the 12-week dating scan, may frequently exhibit the typical features of stimulated IVF ovaries.

The ovaries will not appear hyperstimulated if an assisted conception is as a result of a donor egg or of the woman's own frozen embryo.

THE TRANSABDOMINAL METHOD

The preferred method of examining the uterus in early pregnancy should always be via the transvaginal approach. We describe the transabdominal method to enable an appropriate examination to be carried out in the woman who is adamant in her refusal to consent to a transvaginal ultrasound examination.

It is important to remember that the ability to visualize structures using the transabdominal approach is delayed by approximately 1 week when compared with the transvaginal approach. The earliest that a gestation sac would therefore normally be seen using the transabdominal approach is 5^{+3} weeks and the embryo at 6^{+3} weeks. This can be compared with 4^{+4} weeks for the gestation sac and 5^{+2} weeks for the embryo using the transvaginal approach. The lower frequency of the transabdominal probe, which results in inferior resolution of the structures visualized, also means that the quality of the information obtained is often poorer than from the transvaginal approach.

Examining the nonpregnant or early pregnant uterus using the transabdominal approach usually requires the woman to fill her bladder. This is because her bladder ideally must be full enough to allow the full length of the uterus, including the fundus, to be clearly visualized. Depending on departmental protocol, the woman's decision to decline a transvaginal scan may only be made on the day of her attendance at the early pregnancy unit or ultrasound department. Therefore the woman will have to fill her bladder. She should be asked to drink one litre of still water or squash and not empty her bladder until after the scan is completed.

This text assumes that you, the operator, are sitting to the left of the scanning couch, holding the probe in your right hand, that the woman is lying to your right side and that you are facing each other. The image is orientated so that the apex of the image is displayed at the top of the ultrasound monitor, the left side of the maternal pelvis is displayed on the right side of the ultrasound monitor and the right side of the maternal pelvis is displayed on the left side of the ultrasound monitor.

EXAMINING THE UTERUS

Place the transabdominal probe on the maternal abdomen in the midline, superior to the symphysis pubis to obtain a longitudinal section of the pelvis. The maternal bladder will be seen to the right of the screen. The vagina is usually visualized as three bright parallel lines posterior to the bladder. If only the lower part of the uterus is seen, rotate the probe slightly towards the right side of the woman, to compensate for the dextrorotation of the uterus. The section should clearly demonstrate the uterine fundus.

The cervical canal may be difficult to define because of the angle at which the cervical canal lies relative to the sound beam. This is a problem irrespective of whether the uterus is anteverted or retroverted. The position of the internal os can be gauged as it lies directly beneath the point at which the posterior wall of the bladder appears to change direction. This change in direction occurs because the lower part of the bladder (the trigone) is fixed to the cervix and cannot change position as the bladder fills. The external os is not seen transabdominally.

Subtle sliding, rotational and angling movements are required to gain the optimum longitudinal view of the uterus. Ideally the vagina, cervical canal, endometrium and the uterine fundus should all be visualized in this plane (Fig. 5.11).

Examination of the uterus longitudinally in a parasagittal fashion is accomplished by sliding the probe to the woman's right and left in turn to visualize the right and left lateral margins of the uterus, respectively. The sliding movement of the probe should be made without alteration of the degree of rotation, angulation and dipping of the probe.

Returning to the midline longitudinal section of the uterus, cross-sectional views of the uterus are obtained by rotating the probe through 90° in an anti-clockwise direction whilst keeping the cavity line in view. Sliding the probe up and down the abdomen will produce transverse sections of the uterus (Fig. 5.12) from fundus to cervix. Oblique sections of the uterus, rather than transverse

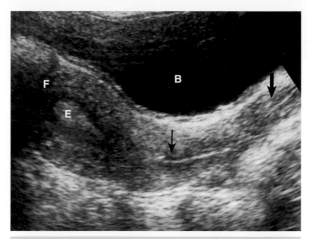

Fig 5.11 • Transabdominal scan. Sagittal section of a nonpregnant uterus demonstrating the fundus (F), endometrium (E), cervical canal (thin arrow) and vagina (thick arrow). Note that the maternal bladder (B) extends above the uterine fundus.

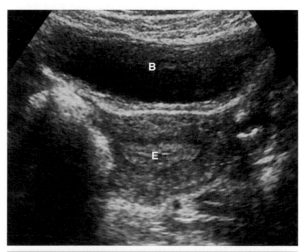

Fig 5.12 • Transabdominal scan. Transverse section of a nonpregnant uterus demonstrating the endometrium (E). The maternal bladder (B) is anterior to the uterus.

sections, will be obtained if the angle of the probe on the woman's abdomen is not at 90° to the longitudinal axis of the uterus or is altered during the examination.

PROBLEMS

The fundus of the uterus will not be visualized unless the bladder is filled sufficiently to cover it.

A retroverted uterus occurs in about a third of women and is more common after pregnancy. The uterine fundus and the upper part of the uterine body may not be visualized in this situation because it is impossible to direct the ultrasound beam at right angles to them. Further filling of the bladder is of little help except to displace the bowel that lies between the bladder and the uterus. If transvaginal scanning is not an option, then little can be done in this situation except to review the findings at a later date. In such situations clinical management must be decided without the benefit of an ultrasound examination.

Finding the Gestation Sac

Locate the longitudinal axis of the uterus as described previously. The gestation sac should be visualized towards the uterine fundus. By sliding the probe and/or rotating slightly to either side, the maximum longitudinal axis (L) of the sac will be obtained. Rotate the transducer through 90°. If the sac has now disappeared, slide the probe either up or down the abdomen until you find it again. Obtain the section demonstrating the maximum transverse diameter (T) of the sac. Remember to maintain the correct angle of the probe to the maternal abdomen. Freeze the image and measure the maximum transverse diameter (T) of the sac. The maximum anteroposterior diameter (AP) can be measured from either the longitudinal or transverse section, as it is common to both views. The mean gestation sac diameter can be calculated as described previously (p. 87).

The ultrasound appearances of the yolk sac and early embryo are essentially similar whether imaged using the transabdominal or the transvaginal approach, although more detail will usually be obtained by the latter.

If there is no evidence of an intrauterine gestation sac, measure the endometrium and assess the cavity. You should explain to the woman that a transabdominal scan on this occasion is not able to provide clinically useful information regarding her pregnancy.

OVARIES AND ADNEXAE

Assessment of the ovaries and adnexae should be included in the transabdominal scan just as in the transvaginal examination. It may not be possible to visualize both ovaries in every examination as overlying bowel gas is more problematic using this approach.

As with the transvaginal approach, a systematic approach to examination of the pelvis is required to locate the ovaries transabdominally. The ovaries may lie in the pouch of Douglas, superior to the uterine fundus or very close to the uterine lateral margins. They will always lie medial and anterior to their respective internal iliac artery and vein so the iliac vessels provide a useful landmark to assist you in locating the majority of them.

Place the probe in a transverse position so that a midline transverse section of the uterus is obtained. Maintain this transverse plane and slide the probe down to the level of the cervix. Now slide the probe in a caudal to cranial direction from the cervix to the level of the fundus. This sweep will allow you to interrogate the locations where the ovaries are most likely to be found, namely lateral to the uterus and medial and anterior to the iliac artery and vein. The iliac vessels will be visualized as two hypoechoic, rounded structures in this transverse plane; the artery will be seen to pulsate, anterior to the vein. Rotating the probe through approximately 90° clockwise should produce two longitudinal structures, confirming that these are the iliac vessels. Focusing the search for the ovaries anterior and medial to the iliac vessels should ensure success in locating the majority of them.

When the ovaries are located in a relatively anterior position, they are usually easy to locate and image. Where the ovaries are located in a more posterior and lateral position, you will need to use the urine filled bladder as an acoustic window. If we consider examination of the right ovary, for example, slide the probe towards the left iliac crest whilst maintaining the same degree of angulation and rotation. The right lateral aspect of the probe face is gently dipped into the woman's abdomen. The ultrasound beam is in effect directed across the full bladder and towards the right adnexa (Fig. 5.13).

Once the ovary is located in transverse plane a caudal-cranial sliding movement of the probe is needed to visualize the ovary in transverse section through its length. As the ovaries tend to lie in an oblique plane to transverse plane of the pelvis, once you have located one ovary you may need to

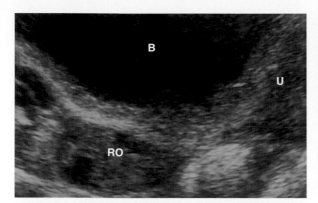

Fig 5.13 • Transabdominal scan. Transverse section of the right ovary (RO), the probe has been dipped towards the right adnexa in order to use the bladder (B) as an acoustic window. The uterus (U) is visualized on the right of the image.

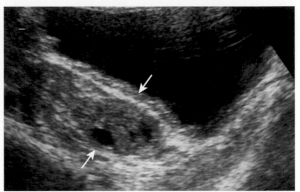

Fig 5.14 • Transabdominal scan. Sagittal section of the right ovary (arrowed).

rotate the probe slightly to obtain a true transverse section of it (Fig. 5.13) rather than the oblique transverse section you obtained initially. To view the ovary in longitudinal section, rotate the probe in a clockwise manner through 90°. Again, as the ovaries tend to lie in an oblique plane to the sagittal plane of the pelvis, you may need to change the angle of the probe to obtain a true sagittal section of the ovary (Fig. 5.14) rather than the oblique longitudinal section you obtained initially. Once the ovary is visualized in the sagittal plane, make small sliding the probe to visualize the ovary in sagittal section through its width. Again it is important to maintain the same degree of dip and angulation applied to the probe.

It is often possible to identify the corpus luteum, which will demonstrate the same features as described with the transvaginal approach, namely hypoechoic, collapsed or haemorrhagic.

WRITING THE REPORT

Many ultrasound departments use a computer database, which allows the ultrasound report to be recorded and archived. Many software packages have templates for obstetric reporting including early pregnancy. The template facilitates a consistent and structured approach to the report so that all relevant features and measurements are included and then summarized in a conclusion. If a template is not available, it is important to be aware of what the clinician requires in a report.

Writing of the report for commonly encountered early pregnancy problems is discussed in Chapter 6.

We suggest the following template of information that should be included for an early pregnancy scan report:

- the reason for the examination
- the approach used, whether transvaginal, transabdominal or both
- verbal consent for a transvaginal scan obtained from the woman
- reason(s) for only performing a transabdominal scan
- recording of a latex allergy and documentation of appropriate management
- confirmation of the presence of an intrauterine gestation sac or multiple sacs
- measurement of the mean gestation sac diameter (mm)
- interpretation of the size of the gestation sac relative to whether or not, in a normally developing pregnancy, a yolk sac and/or embryo should be visible within it
- presence or absence of the yolk sac
- presence or absence of an embryo
- measurement of the CRL
- confirmation of the presence or absence of heart pulsations

- interpretation of whether or not, in a normally developing pregnancy, heart pulsations should be visible in an embryo of the reported CRL
- presence and site of the corpus luteum, with measurement of the mean diameter (mm)
- documentation that the ovaries are of normal appearances as this may prove useful later in the pregnancy
- a conclusion of the scan findings
- documentation of any other relevant management following the scan
- recommendations for the purpose and timing of a further scan
- the name and professional role of the operator/supervisor
- the name and status of a trainee if performing any aspect of the examination
- the name and status of the chaperone.

Further reading

Bourne T, Condous G S, eds 2006 Handbook of early pregnancy care. Informa UK Ltd

Coulam C B et al 1996 Early (34–56 days from the last menstrual period) ultrasonographic measurements in normal pregnancies. Human Reprod 11:1771–1774

Goldstein S et al 1994 Endovaginal ultrasound measurement of early embryonic size as a means of assessing gestational age. JUM 13:27–31

Grisolia C et al 1993 Biometry of early pregnancy with transvaginal sonography. Ultrasound Obstet Gynecol 3:403–411

International Society of Ultrasound in Obstetrics and Gynecology 2013 ISUOG practice guidelines: performance of first trimester fetal ultrasound scan. Ultrasound Obstet Gynecol 41:102–113

National Institute for Health & Clinical Excellence 2012 Ectopic pregnancy and miscarriage. Diagnosis and initial management in early pregnancy of ectopic pregnancy and miscarriage. NICE Clinical Guideline 154, www://guidance.nice.org.uk/cg154 2012

Papaioannou et al 2010 Normal ranges of embryonic length, embryonic heart rate, gestational sac diameter and yolk sac diameter at 6–10 weeks. Fetal Diagn Ther 28:207–219

Rossavik et al 1988 Conceptual age and ultrasound measurements of gestational sac and crown rump length in in vitro fertilization pregnancies. Fertil Steril 49:1012–1027

Royal College of Obstetricians and Gynaecologists 2006 RCOG green top guidelines: the management of early pregnancy. RCOG Press, London

Problems of early pregnancy

6

CONTENTS

This chapter addresses the technique for examination of commonly encountered problems in early pregnancies of between 4 and 10 weeks of gestation.

The aims of this chapter are to enable you to

- describe the ultrasound findings of the more commonly seen problems of early pregnancy:
  - subchorionic haematoma
  - pregnancy of unknown viability
  - miscarriage
  - pregnancy of unknown location
  - ectopic pregnancy
  - trophoblastic disease
  - pregnancy with an intrauterine contraceptive device
  - uterine fibroids and ovarian cysts
- report the findings of the scan
- consider how to communicate sensitively with a woman in the early pregnancy setting.

Early pregnancy disorders are one of the most common indications for referral to hospital emergency services and they account for approximately three quarters of acute gynaecological admissions. The most common reasons for referral are vaginal bleeding, abdominal pain or both. The primary role of the ultrasound examination in the management of these pregnancies is to distinguish between an ongoing, intrauterine pregnancy, miscarriage and an ectopic pregnancy. The ability to do this will depend on the gestational age of the pregnancy and the rigour with which you are able to examine the pelvis.

Miscarriage is the most common complication of pregnancy, with 20% of pregnancies resulting in miscarriage. Clinical symptoms of miscarriage are often dramatic and include pelvic pain and bleeding. This, compounded by a woman's fear of losing her pregnancy, contributes to her readiness of accessing the nearest Accident and Emergency department or Early Pregnancy Unit. During your ultrasound examination you should attempt to establish the cause of the woman's pain or bleeding, although the reasons for this are not often evident from the scan findings. The opportunity to observe the examination on the ultrasound screen is welcomed by most women, thus ideally two monitors should be provided, as discussed in Chapter 2.

As discussed in Chapter 5, the ultrasound appearances of the normal early intrauterine pregnancy are sequential, change rapidly and are dependent on gestational age. Before starting the scan, therefore, it is important that the woman is aware that the aim of the examination is, first, to confirm the presence of an intrauterine pregnancy and, second, to confirm that the pregnancy is ongoing. Your ability to do this will depend primarily on the anticipated gestational age of the pregnancy. The woman must understand that you may not be able to give her this reassurance if the gestational age of her pregnancy is below the threshold for cardiac activity in the embryo.

TERMINOLOGY

HISTORICAL TERMINOLOGY

The following terms were used in the past to classify various types of miscarriage and to describe ultrasound appearances:

- *missed miscarriage:* pregnancy which had failed but in which there had been no vaginal bleeding
- *inevitable miscarriage:* pregnancy associated with vaginal bleeding and in which the external os was open
- *blighted ovum:* gestation sac in which no yolk sac or embryo could be identified
- *anembryonic pregnancy:* more recent description of blighted ovum.

CURRENT TERMINOLOGY

These historical terms have now been replaced by the following:

- *miscarriage*
  - early embryonic demise
  - early fetal demise
  - delayed miscarriage
  - incomplete miscarriage
- *empty sac*
- *threatened miscarriage.*

Threatened miscarriage refers to a pregnancy associated with vaginal bleeding in which the external os is closed. In practice the term is often used to refer to a pregnancy associated with vaginal bleeding in which it is not known whether the os is open or closed. Assessment of the cervix would need to be done visually via a speculum examination.

It is widely accepted that the term *abortion* should never be used.

SELECTION OF WOMEN FOR SCANNING IN EARLY PREGNANCY

Opinion is divided as to what basis should be used for deciding when a transvaginal scan should be offered to symptomatic and asymptomatic women in early pregnancy.

LENGTH OF PREGNANCY

Some departments may not scan women whose pregnancies are anticipated to be less than 6 weeks of gestation. This is because of the differential diagnosis of uterine findings in pregnancies of less than 6 weeks. These women need to be monitored with serum biochemistry and rescanned at timings according to the trend and levels of those results before a definite diagnosis can be made. However, women with ectopic pregnancies often present with symptoms of pain and bleeding at less than 6 weeks of gestation.

This method of triage therefore may result in the diagnosis of a potentially dangerous ectopic pregnancy being delayed unnecessarily. One could also argue that if ectopic pregnancies are detected earlier they will be smaller and potentially more safely managed.

SERUM hCG

Other units may only scan women with a serum human chorionic gonadotropin (hCG) level greater than 1000 IU/L. Many authors report this level as corresponding to the discriminatory, or cut-off, level above which an intrauterine gestation sac should be seen with transvaginal ultrasound imaging. However, ectopic gestations can be visualized in women in whom the serum hCG level is less than 1000 IU/L.

This method of triage therefore may also result in the diagnosis of a potentially dangerous ectopic pregnancy being delayed unnecessarily.

PREGNANCY TEST

Other units may offer a scan to any symptomatic woman with a positive pregnancy test, irrespective of gestational age. This is beneficial to the significant group (15–45%) of women who may not recall their last menstrual period or have conceived whilst taking a nonbleed form of contraception. Therefore many units scan symptomatic women with a positive urinary pregnancy test, which corresponds to an hCG level of 25 IU/L. Adopting such a policy is likely to yield a larger number of inconclusive scans. It does, however, provide an opportunity for the earlier identification of women with ectopic pregnancies and those who require closer monitoring if resources allow.

CLINICAL QUESTION

Other units may triage their scanning policy based on the woman's clinical symptoms and therefore the clinical question being asked. Thus where the clinical suspicion is of an ectopic pregnancy, the clinical question posed is whether a gestation sac can be seen within the uterus. By contrast, where the clinical suspicion is of a miscarriage, the clinical question posed is whether a live embryo can be seen within the gestation sac.

A gestation sac can normally be seen within the uterus from 5^{+3} weeks or often earlier, and a live embryo from 6^{+3} weeks. A possible way of allocating often limited resources may be to manage the scanning of symptomatic early pregnancies on the basis of the anticipated findings – that is, to defer ultrasound until 6^+ weeks if a miscarriage is suspected and scan earlier, at 5^+ weeks, if an ectopic gestation is suspected. However, clinical symptoms can vary and be nonspecific. An ultrasound scan that is timed on the basis of expected dates can be of a significantly earlier or later gestation than anticipated. Once again this method of triage therefore may also result in the diagnosis of a potentially dangerous ectopic pregnancy being delayed unnecessarily.

It should be remembered that it is the appearance of the thick trophoblastic ring surrounding the eccentrically placed gestation sac which confirms an early intrauterine pregnancy. Visualizing the yolk sac provides further reassurance that the structure seen is the gestation sac, rather than confirming that it is an ongoing pregnancy.

ASYMPTOMATIC WOMEN

Although the majority of women attending for assessment of early pregnancy will be symptomatic, a proportion of asymptomatic women may be referred for reassurance that they have an ongoing, intrauterine pregnancy because of their previous history. Such women normally fall into three groups, namely those who have had one of the following:

- a previous ectopic pregnancy
- a previous molar pregnancy
- three or more previous miscarriages.

The clinical question being posed for asymptomatic women is whether or not a live embryo can be seen within the intrauterine gestation sac. Ultrasound scans of asymptomatic women with a previous early pregnancy problem are best timed at later than 6^{+3} weeks in order to increase the likelihood of visualizing a live embryo provided that the subsequent pregnancy is developing normally.

SCANNING THE SYMPTOMATIC EARLY PREGNANCY

There are no clinical reasons why the ultrasound examination of a pregnant woman presenting with vaginal bleeding, abdominal pain or both should not be performed transvaginally.

This text assumes that you, the operator, are sitting to the left of, or at the foot of, the scanning couch, holding the probe in your right hand, that the woman is lying to your right side and that you are facing each other. The image is orientated so that the apex of the image is displayed at the top of the ultrasound monitor, the left side of the maternal pelvis is displayed on the right side of the ultrasound monitor and the right side of the maternal pelvis is displayed on the left side of the ultrasound monitor.

The recommended method of finding and measuring the intrauterine gestation sac is described in Chapter 5.

SUBCHORIONIC HAEMATOMA

Subchorionic haematoma (SCH) describes a bleed that lies between the chorionic membrane and the inner wall of the uterus (Fig. 6.1). Usually the woman will have experienced vaginal bleeding. The SCH often adopts a crescent-like shape. The ultrasound appearances of the SCH can vary from hypoechoic to hyperechoic dependent upon the time that has elapsed from the initial bleed. The SCH should be measured in three planes orthogonal to each other. This can be difficult as the SCH often extends around the sac so that the haemorrhagic area is not easily defined in three dimensions. The location of the SCH relative to the intrauterine gestation sac should be described – for example, whether it lies below, level (to the right or left) or above the gestation sac. An SCH which is less than 20% of the size of the sac is considered small, whereas an SCH which is greater than 50% of the size of the sac is considered large.

An SCH can be present with live intrauterine pregnancies, pregnancies of unknown viability and miscarriage. The presence of an SCH increases the background risk of miscarriage. The majority of SCH will resolve. Larger SCH are often monitored at a repeat scan, particularly if there is a history of previous miscarriage.

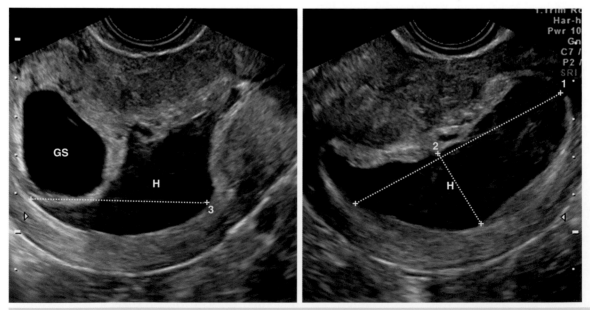

Fig 6.1 • A large subchorionic haematoma (H) located below the gestation sac (GS) measured in three planes orthogonal to each other.

There are five principle differential diagnoses which you will need to consider when performing an early pregnancy scan. These are the following:

- pregnancy of unknown viability
- miscarriage
- pregnancy of unknown location
- ectopic pregnancy
- trophoblastic disease.

Each of these has characteristic ultrasound appearances but, as with many ultrasound appearances, they may be associated with more than one diagnosis. It should therefore be remembered that in some situations it may not be possible to reach a definitive conclusion from the ultrasound findings and that a follow-up scan may be required in order that a clinical diagnosis can be made.

PREGNANCY OF UNKNOWN VIABILITY

Pregnancy of unknown viability (PUV) describes two distinct ultrasound appearances of the intrauterine gestation sac. Namely:

- a gestation sac the size of which is below the threshold for imaging the yolk sac and embryo
- a gestation sac containing an embryo, the length of which is below the threshold for identifying cardiac activity.

A pregnancy cannot be confirmed as 'ongoing' until a live embryo can be visualized within the intrauterine gestation sac. The yolk sac is not normally visible in a gestation sac of less than 10.0 mm mean diameter. Cardiac pulsations and the embryo itself are not normally visible in a gestation sac of less than 18.0 mm mean diameter. Therefore a normal very early pregnancy scan will not infrequently demonstrate an intrauterine gestation sac in which neither a yolk sac nor live embryo can be seen.

Current guidelines indicate that a yolk sac and embryo should always be seen in a gestation sac of 25.0 mm mean diameter or greater. Pregnancies in which an empty sac of diameter less than 25.0 mm is present should be reported as a PUV.

Cardiac pulsations will often, but not always, be seen in an embryo as soon as the embryo itself can be visualized, namely from 2–3 mm in length. Current guidelines indicate that heart pulsations should always be seen where the crown rump length (CRL) is 7.0 mm or greater, whereas a pregnancy in which a CRL less than 7.0 mm is present but heart pulsations cannot be identified should be reported as a PUV.

Irrespective of the clinical indications for the scan, and the anticipated gestational age, of the pregnancy, it is important that you apply the same systematic approach to the scan, consider the current local and nationally recommended guidelines and include all the relevant information in your ultrasound report.

Identifying a PUV

First, ensure that the typical appearances of the intrauterine gestation sac are present, namely the bright trophoblastic ring and the eccentric location of the sac within the endometrium.

Second, it is necessary to apply the necessary diagnostic criteria to distinguish between a PUV and miscarriage.

As described earlier, the ultrasound appearances of a PUV are typical of pregnancies of between 5 and 6 weeks of gestation when it is too early to visualize the embryonic landmarks necessary for confirmation of a live intrauterine gestation. These appearances can also be seen in intrauterine gestations which are failing, or have failed, and will subsequently miscarry. The differential diagnosis for these similar ultrasound appearances will result in very dissimilar outcomes.

Every effort should be made to ensure that the mean gestation sac diameter is measured correctly and accurately in order to reduce the intra- and interobserver error. You must remember that the last menstrual period can be unreliable, and bleeding in early pregnancy does not always herald an adverse finding.

You must not assume that a woman who is experiencing vaginal bleeding, is certain that she is, for example, 8 weeks pregnant and in whom the ultrasound findings are of an empty intrauterine gestation with a mean gestation sac diameter of 12.0 mm has had a miscarriage. In such a situation it should be explained to the woman that the scan has not demonstrated a live embryo of a size consistent with her anticipated 8 weeks of gestation. However, her scan has demonstrated an empty intrauterine gestation of a size more consistent with a 6 weeks of gestation and that she therefore has a pregnancy of unknown viability or PUV. A follow-up scan will be required to determine whether or not this is an ongoing pregnancy of an earlier than anticipated gestational age or whether it is a failing pregnancy.

Various ultrasound features or symptoms have been reported to be associated with an increased risk of miscarriage. Such features include the absence of a yolk sac, a yolk sac diameter greater than 5.0 mm, heavy vaginal bleeding and increased maternal age. Clinicians may use these features to raise their index of suspicion of a miscarriage. You should not use these findings to influence your interpretation of the likely outcome of your scan findings when your findings are consistent with a PUV.

A proportion of women will experience a significant worsening of their symptoms before their scheduled rescan appointment. Women should be warned that this may occur and in this event they are advised to attend an Accident and Emergency department or the Early Pregnancy Unit. In these situations, if clinically indicated, an ultrasound scan can confirm whether a miscarriage has occurred.

Follow-up Scan and Diagnosis

In order to establish whether the PUV is ongoing or has failed, a further transvaginal scan is required with a minimum interscan interval of 7 days. The follow-up scan requires the following:

- assessment of the growth of the gestation sac
- visualization or not of the yolk sac and/or embryo
- growth of the embryo if present initially
- confirmation or otherwise of heart pulsations in the embryo.

It is sensible to delay arranging the follow-up scan until the empty gestation sac, which you have just visualized and measured correctly and which normally grows at 1.0 mm in diameter per day, would be expected to reach a mean diameter of at least 25.0 mm.

Where an embryo smaller than 7.0 mm is present but heart pulsations cannot be identified, the follow-up scan should be arranged for 7 days' time.

The diagnosis of an ongoing pregnancy can obviously be made at the follow-up scan if a live embryo is present.

Where the follow-up scan has been arranged with too short an interscan interval and the gestation sac has grown as expected (~1.0 mm/day) but is still less than 25.0 mm in mean diameter, or an embryo is now present but is less than 7.0 mm in length and heart pulsations cannot be seen, the scan findings are suggestive of an ongoing pregnancy but they must be reported as a PUV.

Writing the Initial Report for PUV

In addition to the information included in the report template (see Chapter 5), we suggest the following additional information should be included in the initial reporting of a PUV:

- explanation that an empty gestation sac may be a normal finding where mean sac diameter is less than 25.0 mm
- reporting of the absence of heart pulsations and explanation that this may be a normal finding where the CRL is less than 7.0 mm
- conclusion of the scan findings and a recommendation for a follow-up scan, timed for between 7 and 14 days, depending on time interval required to make diagnosis, to include the following statement: *'The findings are consistent with a pregnancy of uncertain viability (PUV). A follow-up scan has been made in ___ days to review today's findings'.*

The diagnosis of a failed pregnancy or miscarriage can be made at the follow-up scan if the following occur:

- the mean diameter of the gestation sac is equal to or greater than 25.0 mm and no yolk sac or embryo is present
- the CRL is 7.0 mm or greater and no heart pulsations are seen
- the mean diameter of the gestation sac has increased, but negligibly, and remains less than 25.0 mm
- the CRL has increased, but negligibly, and remains less than 7.0 mm, and no heart pulsations are seen.

There is lack of clarity as to management of pregnancies in which there is growth in the gestation sac but the mean sac diameter is less than 25.0 mm at the repeat scan and no embryo can be identified within it, or there is an increase in the CRL but it measures less than 7.0 mm and no heart pulsations are present. Some units will arrange a third scan before making a diagnosis of a delayed miscarriage, whereas others will base their clinical decision on the comparative findings of the first two scans. Women often find it difficult to understand that the diagnosis of a delayed miscarriage can be made based on the insufficient growth rate of the sac, although the sac has increased in size.

Most women struggle to remember the information given to them at the time of their scan. All units should provide a patient information leaflet for each specific early pregnancy problem with an explanation of their scan findings, details of what happens next, contact details and, importantly, what to do if they experience worsening of their symptoms.

Writing the Follow-up Report for PUV

In addition to the information included in the report template (see Chapter 5), we suggest that the following additional information should be included in the reporting of the follow-up scan for PUV where the diagnosis is of a failed pregnancy:

- measurement of the mean gestation sac diameter (mm), reporting of suboptimal growth based on expected growth of approximately 1.0 mm per day (assuming that no yolk sac or embryo are present in the sac) and an explanation that this is indicative of a failed pregnancy
- presence or absence of a yolk sac and embryo
- measurement of the CRL and reporting of suboptimal growth if embryo was visualized at first scan
- reporting of the absence of heart pulsations and explanation that this is indicative of a failed pregnancy where CRL is 7.0 mm or greater
- explanation that an empty gestation sac 25.0 mm or larger is indicative of a failed pregnancy
- conclusion of the scan findings, to include the following statement: 'The findings are consistent with a failed pregnancy'.

MISCARRIAGE

Threatened miscarriage occurs in approximately one third of pregnancies. The definition of threatened miscarriage is of vaginal bleeding with or without abdominal pain before 24 weeks of pregnancy. Clinical assessment alone is rarely sufficient to establish a correct diagnosis in women with a threatened miscarriage. Ultrasound examination is routinely used in these cases. It is important to remember that miscarriages can occur in asymptomatic women. A proportion of early scans performed for indications such as a history of recurrent miscarriages, assisted conception or an underlying medical condition such as diabetes may demonstrate a miscarriage.

Some women may reach 12 weeks of gestation with no indication that their pregnancy is not progressing normally. It may be only at the time of their dating scan that they learn that their pregnancy has resulted in miscarriage. It is particularly difficult to convey adverse findings when they are not suspected and they are a shock to both the woman and the operator performing the scan.

The main role of the ultrasound examination is to make the definitive diagnosis of miscarriage and to provide the information which can assist in the selection between conservative and surgical management options.

Ultrasound Diagnosis of Miscarriage

The classification of miscarriage is based on the ultrasound findings and includes the following:

- early embryonic demise
- early fetal demise
- delayed miscarriage
- incomplete miscarriage
- complete miscarriage.

What You Should Look for, Measure and Include in Your Report for Miscarriage

The reader of your report needs to be confident that your diagnosis of miscarriage has been made correctly. Therefore it is important that reference is made in the report to the ultrasound parameters measured and the criteria applied to reach the diagnosis. If the gestation sac is irregular in shape, for example, or there is any evidence of haematoma, these findings should be documented in the report. Any coincidental findings, such as one or more fibroids or an ovarian cyst, should be described, measured and documented in the report.

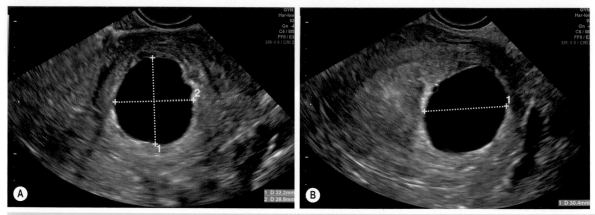

Fig 6.2 • A and B. Sagittal and transverse sections of the uterus demonstrating an empty gestation sac. The mean sac diameter was 30.4 mm. The woman was 12^{+5} weeks by her menstrual dates and had attended the Early Pregnancy Unit with pain and bleeding. The ultrasound appearances are consistent with a miscarriage, early embryonic demise.

The type of miscarriage should be deducible from your description of your findings. However, a conclusion should always be made to the effect that the ultrasound findings are consistent with a miscarriage and the classification stated.

If a woman opts for conservative management of her miscarriage, all relevant information needs to be included in the report so that comparison can be made with any subsequent scans.

Miscarriage, Early Embryonic Demise

The transvaginal ultrasound findings of early embryonic demise include an intrauterine gestation sac of mean diameter equal to or greater than 25.0 mm and in which there is no evidence of a yolk sac or embryo (Fig. 6.2). The empty gestation sac may appear collapsed and elongated. It may also lie more towards the body of the uterus than towards the fundus.

Although it may not be possible to identify a yolk sac or an embryo within the sac, the amniotic membrane, surrounding the amniotic cavity, may be seen within the gestation sac. The membrane may have contracted within the gestation sac and it is easy to mistake this for a large yolk sac. Remember that the yolk sac lies outside the amniotic cavity, in the chorionic cavity (Fig. 6.3). If only one sac like structure is seen, it is much more likely, from an embryological developmental viewpoint, to be the amniotic membrane rather than a yolk

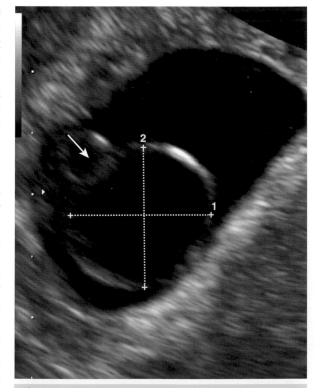

Fig 6.3 • Intrauterine gestation sac containing an amniotic sac (with callipers) and yolk sac (arrowed). Note that the yolk sac lies outside the amniotic cavity. There is no evidence of an embryo – this is a PUV. A rescan was arranged and a miscarriage was diagnosed at the second scan.

sac lying in what you are therefore presumably assuming must be the chorionic cavity. The presence of a yolk sac also means this should not be reported as a miscarriage, early embryonic demise.

The transvaginal ultrasound criteria of a miscarriage, early embryonic demise, are as follows:

- mean gestation sac diameter equal to or greater than 25.0 mm
- no yolk sac or embryo visible within the sac.

Although no evidence of the embryo can be seen with ultrasound in a miscarriage, early embryonic demise, there is often histological or biochemical evidence of early embryonic death. Some units refer to this type of miscarriage as a delayed miscarriage as they choose not to classify the miscarriage on the basis of the ultrasound criteria.

Early embryonic demise was previously referred to as a blighted ovum or an anembryonic pregnancy.

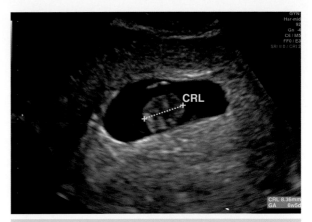

Fig 6.4 • Intrauterine gestation sac containing an embryo with no evidence of cardiac activity. The crown rump length (CRL) measured 8.4 mm, equivalent to a gestation of 6^{+5} weeks. Appearances consistent with a miscarriage, early fetal demise. Note the amorphous appearance of the embryo.

Writing the Report for Miscarriage, Early Embryonic Demise

In addition to the information included in the report template (see Chapter 5), we suggest the following additional information should be included in the reporting of a miscarriage, early embryonic demise:

- explanation that an empty gestation sac 25.0 mm or greater is indicative of a failed pregnancy
- conclusion of the scan findings, to include the following phrase: *'The findings are consistent with a miscarriage, early embryonic demise'.*

Miscarriage, Early Fetal Demise

Because the term *fetus* correctly refers to a conceptus of 10 weeks or greater gestational age, using the term of *early fetal demise* to describe a failed pregnancy of less than 10 weeks' of gestational age and in which a dead conceptus is present is incorrect. However, because this is the phrase that is commonly used to describe this type of miscarriage, we have used it in this text to avoid confusion.

The transvaginal ultrasound findings of early fetal demise are of an embryo or fetus of 7.0 mm or greater in length and in which no cardiac activity

is present (Fig. 6.4). It is also important to calculate and report the mean gestation sac diameter. Units will use threshold levels of CRL and mean sac diameter to determine which management options they offer to their women.

Depending on the length of time which has elapsed between death and the scan, the embryo may appear amorphous and ill-defined. There is also often a disparity between the size of the gestation sac and the dead embryo, with the size of the gestation sac being disproportionately large compared with the length of the embryo.

Where a definitive diagnosis is not possible because of poor image quality for whatever reason, a repeat scan should be arranged.

The transvaginal ultrasound criteria of a miscarriage, early fetal demise, are as follows:

- embryo with a CRL 7.0 mm or greater
- no cardiac activity present.

Some units choose to refer to this type of miscarriage also as a delayed miscarriage. Early fetal demise was previously referred to as a missed miscarriage.

Writing the report for Miscarriage, Early Fetal Demise

In addition to the information included in the report template (see Chapter 5), we suggest the following additional information should be included in the reporting of a miscarriage, early fetal demise:

- reporting of the absence of heart pulsations and explanation that this is indicative of a failed pregnancy when CRL is 7.0 mm or greater
- conclusion of the scan findings, to include the following phrase: *'The findings are consistent with a miscarriage, early fetal demise'.*

Many units stipulate and current guidelines recommend that a second operator should always confirm a diagnosis of miscarriage, either early embryonic or early fetal demise. Unfortunately, resources often do not allow the close and immediate availability of a second experienced operator, making obtaining a second experienced opinion impractical within a busy clinical service where the relevant staff may be in geographically separate and distant locations.

If there is no second operator available, units need to take a local decision on how they undertake miscarriage diagnoses. An option would be to arrange a rescan for women so that a second operator performs the scan. If resources do not allow this, it is imperative that a less experienced operator who has any uncertainty regarding the absence or presence of cardiac activity always ask a more experienced colleague to provide a second opinion.

Incomplete Miscarriage

Incomplete miscarriage describes the ultrasound findings of products of conception within the uterine cavity and/or retained products of conception within the uterine cavity. The term incomplete miscarriage is commonly used as an umbrella term to cover the range of findings. However, their ultrasound appearances are on the whole different and are therefore described separately.

Products of conception

As *products of conception* within the uterine cavity may include placental tissue, a collapsed gestation sac (Fig. 6.5), embryonic or fetal tissue, clotted blood and unclotted blood, the ultrasound appearances are varied. With the exception of unclotted blood, the typical appearance, however, is of a

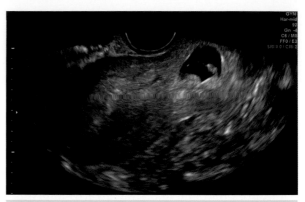

Fig 6.5 • Sagittal section of the uterus. The gestation sac is collapsed, irregular and lies close to the cervix. Within the gestation sac the amnion is collapsed and there is an embryo with no cardiac activity. A scan 2 weeks previously had demonstrated a live intrauterine gestation. The appearances are therefore of an incomplete miscarriage.

well-defined area of mixed or heterogeneous echoes within the distended uterine cavity. Unclotted blood is homogeneous in echopattern and therefore essentially black in colour. This appearance can also be seen with an ectopic pregnancy, where it is commonly described as a 'pseudosac'.

You will note that products of conception within the cavity tend to slide up and down inside the cavity, particularly if gentle pressure is applied with the transvaginal probe. Gentle pressure applied to unclotted blood in the uterine cavity, however, does not have this effect. As the products in the uterine cavity no longer have an endometrial blood supply, you will see no evidence of blood flow in the products if you apply colour Doppler to them.

To measure the products, first obtain a sagittal section of the uterus and distended uterine cavity. Ensure you have obtained the maximum length of the products with small rotational and panning movements of the probe. Measure their maximum longitudinal diameter together with their maximum anteroposterior diameter of the products. Rotate the transducer through 90°, repeat the small rotational and panning movements in order to obtain the maximum cross-section of the products and measure their transverse diameter. *All measurements should be 'inner to inner' and recorded in millimetres.*

Writing the report for products of conception

In addition to the information included in the report template (see Chapter 5), we suggest the following additional information should be included in the reporting of products of conception within the distended uterine cavity:

- description of the uterine cavity distended with the measured area of clot/tissue/blood (L × T × AP mm)
- the conclusion of the scan findings, to include the following phrase: *'The findings are consistent with an incomplete miscarriage with products of conception present within the uterine cavity'.*

Retained products of conception

Retained products of conception are, as their name suggests, the trophoblast or placental remnants of a failed pregnancy, which remain within the uterine cavity. A surgical procedure to remove a previously diagnosed delayed miscarriage may not successfully remove all tissue. In these cases the pregnancy test will remain positive and an ultrasound scan may be indicated, if bleeding continues for more than a week after the procedure, to exclude retained products of conception. The typical ultrasound appearance of retained products is one of a discrete area of echoes which are brighter than the surrounding endometrium. The application of colour Doppler will often demonstrate flow within and to this area, confirming that some endometrial blood supply to the retained tissue remains. The three maximum diameters (L, AP and T [mm]) should be measured, using the 'outer to outer' calliper placement, and reported as described earlier (Fig. 6.6). Ultrasound examinations to exclude retained products of conception are also performed after delivery if it is suspected that not all of the placental tissue has been delivered. As vaginal bleeding within the first week after delivery is a normal finding, scanning for retained products is likely to be of little clinical value in this period and is better performed at least 7 days after delivery.

Writing the report for retained products of conception

In addition to the information included in the report template (see Chapter 5), we suggest the

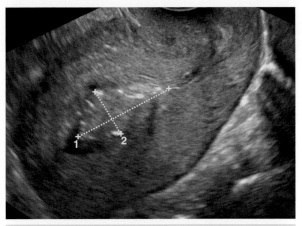

Fig 6.6 • Sagittal section of the uterus with the maximum longitudinal and anteroposterior diameters of the retained products of conception measured.

following additional information should be included in the reporting of retained products of conception within the endometrium:

- confirmation of the absence of an intrauterine gestation sac and/or live embryo
- description of the area within the uterine cavity with measurements
- recording of the presence or absence of blood flow with colour Doppler within and to the area
- the conclusion of the scan findings, to include the following phrase: *'The findings are consistent with an incomplete miscarriage with retained products of conception'.*

It is important that you also consider the possibility of a molar or partial pregnancy – that is, trophoblastic disease – in your differential diagnosis of incomplete miscarriage. Trophoblastic disease is discussed later in this chapter. Although the classic signs of a molar pregnancy and partial molar pregnancy are distinct from the typical appearances of incomplete miscarriage, they can also present with very similar appearances. It is not unusual for a partial mole to be incorrectly diagnosed as an incomplete miscarriage and vice versa.

Complete Miscarriage

The findings of an empty uterus with a thin endometrium in women who have experienced

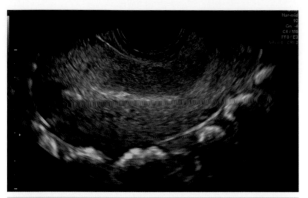

Fig 6.7 • The findings of an empty uterus with thin endometrium in a woman who has experienced heavy vaginal bleeding with clots is consistent with a complete miscarriage. This ultrasound diagnosis can be made as a previous scan demonstrated a failed intrauterine gestation.

heavy vaginal bleeding with clots is consistent with a complete miscarriage (Fig. 6.7). A subjective assessment of the uterine cavity should always be undertaken to ensure that there are no retained products of conception. However, this ultrasound diagnosis should *only* be made if a previous scan demonstrated either a live or failed intrauterine gestation. Women who have not had their pregnancy confirmed at a previous scan should be treated as having a pregnancy of unknown location (see following section). They should be followed up with serial hCG measurements to establish the outcome of their pregnancy.

Management of miscarriage

A failed pregnancy can be clinically managed in one of three ways, namely the following:

- surgical management
- medical management
- expectant management.

Surgical management

Over the last 50 years, surgical evacuation of retained products has become universally accepted as the method of choice for the management of miscarriage. The initial rationale for the use of curettage was a perceived risk of sepsis and haemorrhage associated with spontaneous miscarriage. It is likely that a number of complicated miscarriages at that time represented retained products after illegal terminations, which contributed to the severity of clinical presentation. The improvement of women's general health and the legalization of termination in many developed countries now result in most infections being effectively treated using antibiotics.

Surgical management can be performed by manual vacuum aspiration in the outpatient setting under local anaesthetic or by surgical removal in theatre under general anaesthetic.

Medical management

Medical management of miscarriage involves vaginal or oral medication to initiate a miscarriage. Vaginal bleeding, followed by miscarriage, will normally start within 24 hours of the required drug being administered. In cases of early fetal demise medical management may not prove effective and surgical management may be required.

Expectant management

In recent years there has been a growing concern about the unconditional and nonselective use of surgery for the treatment of miscarriage. There is also concern about morbidity caused by surgical and anaesthetic complications. *Expectant management* of incomplete miscarriage is an attractive option in this context. It follows the natural history of the disease, uses no treatment and therefore avoids iatrogenic problems associated with both medical and surgical treatment and as such is likely to be cost-effective. The expectation is that the miscarriage will normally be completed within 7–14 days after the ultrasound diagnosis of the pregnancy failing, during which time the bleeding and pain associated with the miscarriage will have resolved.

The pathway may include transvaginal scans at two-weekly intervals to assess changes in the ultrasound appearances of the uterus, the findings being used to determine whether or not the expectant management pathway is still clinically safe.

As discussed above in cases of early fetal demise expectant management may similarly prove ineffective. It may be suitable only for highly motivated women or those who have difficulty in accepting the diagnosis of a failed pregnancy and feel unable to make a rapid decision about surgical treatment. In cases of early fetal demise, both medical and expectant management are relatively ineffective and may be suitable only for individual, highly motivated women or those who have difficulty in accepting the diagnosis of a failed pregnancy and feel unable to make a rapid decision about surgical treatment.

PREGNANCIES OF UNKNOWN LOCATION

A *pregnancy of unknown location (PUL)* describes the situation in which there are no transvaginal ultrasound signs of either an intra- or an extrauterine pregnancy or retained products of conception in a woman with a positive pregnancy test. It should be remembered that all women with a PUL could have an ectopic pregnancy until the location of the pregnancy is determined.

The transvaginal ultrasound appearances of a PUL (Fig. 6.8) include the following:

- a uterus in which no gestation sac can be seen. The endometrium can vary in thickness from very thin (~3.0 mm) to very thick (>15.0 mm)
- normal appearance of both ovaries. The presence of a corpus luteum should be carefully sought
- no adnexal mass on either side
- no free fluid in the pelvis.

As has been discussed previously, the ability to identify a pregnancy with ultrasound is critically dependent on the gestational age of the pregnancy and also on its location. The expertise of the opera-

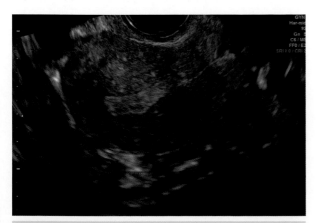

Fig 6.8 • Sagittal section of the uterus. The pregnancy test was positive and there was no evidence of an intrauterine gestation sac. There were no adnexal masses. The endometrium measures 6.4 mm. Appearances are of a pregnancy of unknown location. A repeat scan 1 week later demonstrated an early intrauterine gestation sac.

tor influences the detection rate of early intrauterine and ectopic gestations. This is supported by the reporting by various authors that the ultrasound diagnosis of a suspected abnormal early pregnancy cannot be made at the initial visit in up to 30% of cases.

There are four main explanations for a PUL:

- a very early, failing intrauterine or ectopic pregnancy. This will resolve spontaneously
- a very early pregnancy which cannot yet be visualized on ultrasound. Women requesting reassurance of their pregnancy as early as possible, women with uncertain dates and a unit's policy of scanning very early in pregnancy contribute to the likelihood of performing scans at a gestation before which any ultrasound evidence of an intrauterine pregnancy can be expected
- an ectopic pregnancy. In addition to being gestational age dependent, it is also operator dependent as an experienced operator will be able to detect and identify the appearances seen in an ectopic pregnancy more often than a less experienced operator
- a persisting PUL. A very small percentage of women will have a persisting PUL on repeat ultrasound examination. Biochemically these pregnancies behave as ectopic pregnancies and most likely represent early, asymptomatic ectopic pregnancies that are not visualized with ultrasound.

Management of PUL

Early Pregnancy Units should have specific guidelines to manage women with PULs using measurement of serum hCG or progesterone levels. Serum hCG levels reflect proliferation of the trophoblast, whereas progesterone levels reflect whether support of placental development is adequate.

In normal early pregnancy current guidance suggests that the increase in the serum hCG level should be greater than 63% after 48 hours and that a decrease of more than 50% after 48 hours indicates that the PUL is most likely to be failing. In the presence of a PUL a serum progesterone level of less than 20 µmol/L is predictive of a spontaneous pregnancy resolution.

A suboptimal rise, or plateauing, of the serum hCG levels can be indicative of an ectopic pregnancy.

Monitoring of women should be stratified on an individual case basis. Expectant management will be appropriate for the majority of women, including those with failing PULs and those with an early intrauterine pregnancy. Closer monitoring can be reserved for those women whose serum hCG levels indicate a higher index of suspicion of an ectopic pregnancy. However, caution needs to be applied to interpretation of serum biochemistry as there are always exceptions to the rule. Furthermore it should be remembered that twin and heterotopic pregnancies will behave differently to singleton pregnancies.

Writing the Report for a PUL

In addition to the information included in the report template (see Chapter 5), we suggest the following additional information should be included in the reporting of a PUL:

- confirmation of the absence of an intrauterine gestation sac and/or live embryo
- measurement of the endometrial thickness
- document the presence or absence of free fluid in the pelvis
- the conclusion of the scan findings, to include, for example, the following phrase: *'There is no evidence of an intrauterine or extrauterine gestation. No free fluid present. The findings are therefore consistent with a PUL'*
- documentation of any other relevant management following the scan, such as *'serum hCG levels required and review by early pregnancy unit'.*

ECTOPIC PREGNANCY

Ectopic pregnancy is defined as the implantation of the fertilized ovum outside the uterine cavity. The site of approximately 93% of ectopic pregnancies is within the Fallopian tube, with 70% of all ectopic pregnancies implanting in the ampullary region of the tube. Isthmic and fimbrial ectopic pregnancies account for a further 12% and 11%, respectively. The remaining sites are rare and include interstitial, ovarian, abdominal, cervical and a previous Caesarean scar.

Ectopic pregnancies classically present with abdominal pain, with or without vaginal bleeding. In the last few decades a dramatic rise in the incidence of ectopic pregnancy has been reported worldwide, although the incidence in the United Kingdom has remained essentially unchanged with an incidence of 11.3/1000 pregnancies reported in 2006–2008, compared with an incidence of 11.1/1000 pregnancies reported in 2003–2005. Although the incidence of ectopic pregnancy in the United Kingdom has remained stable over the last triennium, the maternal mortality rate has almost halved from an estimated 31.2/100 000 estimated ectopic pregnancies during 2003–2005 to 16.9/100 000 during 2006–2008.

The clinical signs and symptoms of ectopic pregnancy are very similar to miscarriage and women are often urgently referred to hospital in order to establish a correct diagnosis. In addition, ectopic pregnancy is often portrayed as a life-threatening condition unless diagnosis is made early, before serious complications occur.

Women with previous tubal pathological conditions or surgery and those with an intrauterine contraceptive device in situ have an increased risk of ectopic pregnancy. The possibility of an ectopic pregnancy should always be considered in such women with a high risk of ectopic pregnancy and who present a positive pregnancy, even in the absence of symptoms.

As discussed previously, some ectopic pregnancies will resolve spontaneously and it is now well recognized that not all ectopic pregnancies require surgical intervention. It is also apparent that many ectopic pregnancies are being detected at a much earlier stage than, for example, a decade ago. A proportion of these would have spontaneously miscarried without the woman or her clinician ever being aware that this had occurred.

Ultrasound Findings of Ectopic Pregnancy (Tubal)

Traditionally, the findings of a positive pregnancy test and a uterus in which no gestation sac can be seen at the time of ultrasound scan have been synonymous with the presence of an ectopic pregnancy. Many women would be referred for laparoscopy on the basis of these findings. It is no longer acceptable to suggest that 'an ectopic pregnancy cannot be excluded' on a report. If there is no evidence of an intrauterine or extrauterine pregnancy, the pregnancy should be reported and managed as a PUL. The advent of high-resolution, transvaginal ultrasound has resulted in an increase in the proportion of ectopic pregnancies, currently approximately 85% of cases, that can be directly visualized at the initial ultrasound scan.

Assessing the endometrium and uterine cavity

The first step in establishing the location of a pregnancy is assessment of the uterus for evidence of an intrauterine gestation sac within the endometrium.

If there is no evidence of an intrauterine gestation sac, examine the uterine cavity carefully to determine whether there is any evidence of fluid, blood or other products within the cavity. Fluid or blood within the uterine cavity is commonly reported as a 'pseudosac'. As discussed in Chapter 5, in an attempt to discourage the continuing use of a clinically unhelpful and incorrect term, we recommend that fluid within the uterine cavity is reported as 'fluid within the uterine cavity' and not as a 'pseudosac'.

Fluid within the uterine cavity is visible within the uterus in up to 30% of ectopic pregnancies and represents the accumulation of nonclotted blood within the uterine cavity. As discussed previously in Chapter 5, this finding should not be mistaken for an early gestation sac. Because the fluid lies within the uterine cavity, it is surrounded by the endometrium, which appears as a thin, bright edge surrounding the centrally positioned fluid. The shape of the fluid collection reflects the shape of the uterine cavity and therefore, in longitudinal section, often resembles a teardrop in shape. Alternatively the cavity may be distended with blood, which is clotted and therefore appears hyperechoic (Fig. 6.9).

On colour Doppler examination, the fluid collection/pseudosac will typically appear avascular. This can be contrasted with the early gestation sac, which is eccentrically placed within the endometrium and is surrounded by a thick, bright rim of trophoblast, which would demonstrate high-velocity flow if interrogated with colour Doppler.

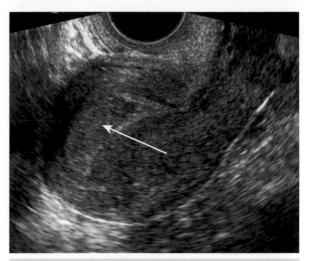

Fig 6.9 • Sagittal section of the uterus of a woman with a tubal ectopic pregnancy. The thin, bright edge of the endometrium surrounds the centrally positioned blood (arrow).

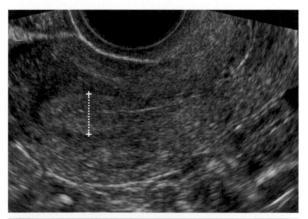

Fig 6.10 • Sagittal section of the uterus. The anterior and posterior layers of the endometrium are in apposition. The thin central line represents the cavity line. The callipers are placed to measure the endometrium (6.8 mm).

If the uterine cavity is empty, the endometrium should be measured as described in Chapter 16. The endometrium is composed of the anterior layer and the posterior layer, which are in apposition. The interface between the opposing layers – and which therefore represents the empty uterine cavity – can be seen as a fine, bright line. This is referred to as the cavity line (Fig. 6.10).

If you are unable to visualize an intrauterine gestation sac and the uterine cavity is empty, you must now make a very careful assessment of the ovary and adnexal region on both sides and the Pouch of Douglas in order to diagnose or exclude an ectopic pregnancy.

Assessing the ovaries

Identification of the corpus luteum can aid detection of an ectopic pregnancy because around 75% of ectopic pregnancies will be ipsilateral to the corpus luteum. Once you have identified the corpus luteum, it may therefore be prudent to focus your search for an ectopic pregnancy on the side of the corpus luteum initially, as statistically that is more likely to be the side on which an ectopic pregnancy (if present) will be demonstrated.

Assessing the adnexae

Although an ectopic pregnancy will very rarely implant in the ovary, it can sometimes be difficult to differentiate between a corpus luteum in the ovary and a suspected ectopic pregnancy, which is more likely to be fimbrial or tubal in origin but is lying directly adjacent to the ovary. The 'sliding organs sign' is helpful in this situation to distinguish between a bulging corpus luteum and an extraovarian ectopic pregnancy.

Apply gentle pressure to the mass with the tip of the probe. A positive sliding sign describes movement of the mass that is separate from any movement of the ovary. A negative sliding sign is the converse, where there is no movement of either the mass or the ovary or, if movement is seen, both the mass and the ovary move together. Your report should include reference to either a positive or negative sliding sign.

Care must be taken not to confuse a static loop of bowel, hydrosalpinx, adhesions or an endometrioma with an ectopic pregnancy. These appearances are described in Chapter 18.

Occasionally it may be difficult to image and assess one or both adnexae because of the presence of large fibroids. In such cases, if you can find no evidence of ectopic pregnancy using the transvaginal route, you should consider using the transabdominal route. A transabdominal scan may enable demonstration of an ectopic pregnancy, which is positioned beyond the focal zone of the transvaginal probe.

Adequate visualization can also be compromised by the technical difficulties associated with the transvaginal imaging of the pelvis in a woman with a high body mass index. In this situation, it is unlikely that a transabdominal scan will provide images of the pelvis that are better than those already obtained transvaginally.

Assessing the ectopic pregnancy

Having identified a mass in the adnexa and decided that the chances of it being an ectopic pregnancy are high, the diagnosis is likely to be of a tubal ectopic pregnancy if the mass is described by one of the following appearances:

A *complex mass*, which is most commonly round in shape. This is the most common appearance of an ectopic pregnancy and is the most difficult to identify. The mass may be hyperechoic or bright and homogeneous in appearance or of a mixed echo pattern. The mass represents the miscarried or ruptured ectopic pregnancy together with the associated haematosalpinx. The mass should be measured in three orthogonal planes ('outer to outer'), in millimetres, and its dimensions included in your report. This is important because the size of the adnexal mass is a consideration in the management options of ectopic pregnancy. Peripheral blood flow may be present, although this is not a constant finding. It should be remembered that this 'ring of fire' is also seen in association with a corpus luteum or a normal maturing follicle.

A *tubal ring*, which is the second most common appearance of an ectopic pregnancy and is reported in 40–68% of cases. Its typical ultrasound appearance is of a hyperechoic, bright ring surrounding a hypoechoic centre. The ring is derived from the trophoblast of the pregnancy and the wall of the tube. The dark centre represents the chorionic cavity of the gestation sac (Fig. 6.11). Some authors describe this appearance as a 'bagel sign'.

A *gestation sac* in which a yolk sac and/or an embryo can be seen. This is the least common appearance of an ectopic pregnancy, being reported in around 15%

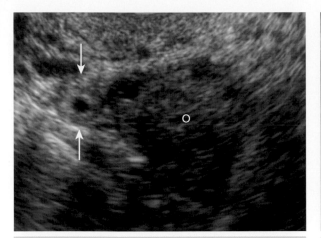

Fig 6.11 • Transverse section of the left ovary. Left tubal pregnancy (arrowed) visualized medial to the ovary (O). The hyperechoic ring represents the trophoblast surrounding the hypoechoic chorionic cavity (bagel sign). A positive sliding sign confirmed movement of the mass separate to movement of the ovary.

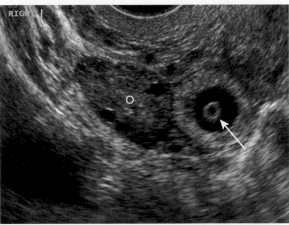

Fig 6.12 • Right tubal pregnancy. A yolk sac is clearly identified within a gestation sac (arrow). The ectopic pregnancy is separate to the ovary. (O) A positive sliding sign confirmed movement of the mass separate to movement of the ovary. A corpus luteum was identified in the contralateral ovary.

of cases, but the easiest to visualize. Heart activity may be seen within the embryo – this confirms the diagnosis of a live ectopic. In the absence of heart activity within the embryo, the diagnosis is of a nonviable ectopic pregnancy (Fig. 6.12).

Where no adnexal mass is identified you must remember that there is still a risk (approximately 5%) of an unruptured ectopic pregnancy being present. This occurs in 15–35% of women with ectopic pregnancies. The incidence is related to the gestational age at the time of the scan and operator expertise.

Assessing the Pouch of Douglas

Clear free fluid in the Pouch of Douglas is not uncommonly seen in normal on-going pregnancies. The presence of blood or clot is suggestive of leakage of blood from the fimbrial end of the Fallopian tube or of a ruptured ectopic. Blood appears as low level, homogenous echoes whereas the appearance of clot tends to be more heterogenous and will vary depending on the age of the clot. Blood in the Pouch of Douglas may also be seen in a woman with a ruptured corpus luteum cyst.

The amount of free fluid in the pelvis is difficult to quantify. We recommend that the following terms are used to describe the amount of fluid visualized in the Pouch of Douglas posterior to the uterus in a sagittal section of the pelvis:

minimal: a vertical depth of 5.0 mm or less and confined to the Pouch of Douglas

noticeable: a vertical depth greater than 5.0 mm but confined to the Pouch of Douglas

significant: free fluid extending from the Pouch of Douglas to around the uterine fundus. The maximum vertical depth, and its location in the pelvis should be included in the report (Fig. 6.13)

extensive: free fluid extending from the Pouch of Douglas into Morrison's pouch when the abdomen is examined using a transabdominal probe. The maximum vertical depth, and its location, should be included in the report.

Management of ectopic pregnancy

As with miscarriage of an intrauterine pregnancy, there are three options for management of an ectopic pregnancy, namely surgical, medical and expectant. There are several factors which affect the choice of management pathway. These include the morphology of the ectopic pregnancy, whether the woman is haemodynamically stable, the severity of her symptoms, sequential hCG levels and the woman's future fertility wishes.

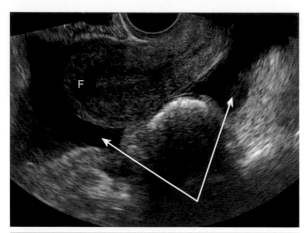

Fig 6.13 • Sagittal section of the pelvis. There is significant free fluid (arrows) which extends from the Pouch of Douglas around the uterine fundus (F).

What should be included in the report for ectopic pregnancy

The morphology of the ectopic pregnancy as described by ultrasound needs to be considered when deciding upon the best management option for a woman. It is therefore important to include the following points in your report:

- describe the morphology (i.e. whether a complex mass, a tubal ring or a gestation sac is present)
- provide the size of the ectopic pregnancy. Measurement of the ectopic mass in three planes orthogonal to one another, using the 'outer to outer' measurement technique, should be included
- when a gestation sac is present, include the presence or absence of the yolk sac and embryo
- when an embryo is present, measure the CRL and state whether heart activity is present
- document the presence or absence of free fluid present
- where free fluid is present, describe its appearance and document whether the appearance therefore is consistent with fluid/unclotted blood or clotted blood
- measure the free fluid and qualify as minimal, noticeable, significant or extensive

- comment on whether the woman experiences pain during the ultrasound examination.

Management of Ectopic Pregnancy

Expectant management

Expectant management is becoming increasingly important as the ability to detect small ectopic pregnancies and tubal miscarriage increases. Exclusion criteria include the presence of haemoperitoneum, a live ectopic pregnancy and an ectopic mass larger than 3.0 cm. These would be considered unsuitable for all but surgical management. Women on expectant management are managed on an outpatient basis and attend for serial hCG levels and monitoring of the ectopic pregnancy with ultrasound.

At the follow-up ultrasound examination, the ectopic mass should be measured as described previously, and any evidence of an associated haematosalpinx or haematoperitoneum should be documented.

Expectant management is not always successful because women need to be compliant with their management and/or many women may need additional treatment with methotrexate or surgery.

Medical management

Medical management is the treatment of ectopic pregnancy with methotrexate. Methotrexate is a folic acid antagonist, which leads to interference with DNA synthesis and cell multiplication in the conceptus. Methotrexate may be given either intramuscularly or by direct injection into the ectopic pregnancy under laparoscopic/ultrasound guidance.

The use of methotrexate is contraindicated when the diameter of the ectopic mass is 35.0 mm or greater, a live embryo is present, the hCG level is 5000 IU/L or greater or the woman is experiencing significant pelvic pain.

The success rate for treatment of ectopic pregnancy with methotrexate varies between 74% and 94%. Fertility rates after methotrexate therapy are compatible with surgical treatment. Women are monitored on an outpatient basis and may require a rescan if clinically indicated – for example, if tubal rupture is suspected.

Surgical management

Surgical management is used in women in whom a live ectopic has been identified. Surgery is the management option of choice for those women who are haemodynamically unstable or experiencing severe symptoms (i.e. there is evidence of, or they are clinically suspected of having, a ruptured ectopic pregnancy).

Surgical options include salpingectomy or salpingostomy, performed either as an open procedure or laparoscopically. Laparoscopy has been found to be superior to laparotomy in haemodynamically stable patients. In the laparoscopic approach there is less blood loss, less analgesic requirement and shorter hospital stays. However, persisting trophoblast is a complication and this occurs more often after laparoscopic surgery.

Postoperative follow-up with monitoring of weekly serum hCG levels is necessary in all women after salpingotomy and tubal conservation.

In the absence of an obvious tubal ectopic pregnancy, extratubal locations should be considered. Although rare, it is important that you are aware of their ultrasound appearances in order that you can exclude them in your differential diagnosis.

Interstitial Ectopic

Interstitial pregnancy describes the implantation of the pregnancy in the interstitial portion of the Fallopian tube (Fig. 6.14). Interstitial pregnancy occurs in 2–6% of all ectopic pregnancies. Implantation of the fertilized ovum is more likely to occur in the interstitial part of the Fallopian tube after IVF and previous salpingectomy.

You should consider this diagnosis if there is no gestation sac in the normal position within the endometrium but you identify a gestation sac towards the uterine fundus, in an abnormal lateral location and surrounded by only a very thin layer of uterine tissue, which, in this condition, is myometrium.

Traditionally, interstitial pregnancies were treated surgically by laparotomy, as diagnosis was usually not made until after rupture. Earlier diagnosis has allowed more conservative management to be used. Methotrexate is effective for the treatment of early interstitial pregnancies. Surgery is reserved for those cases complicated by rupture.

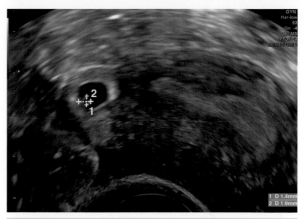

Fig 6.14 • Transverse section of the uterus. An interstitial pregnancy is located in the right interstitial portion of the Fallopian tube. The gestation sac contains a yolk sac. It is in an abnormal lateral location and is surrounded by a thin layer of myometrium and is separate to the uterine cavity. This scan has been performed with the apex of the image at the bottom of the screen.

Cervical Pregnancy

Cervical pregnancy describes the implantation of the pregnancy below the level of the internal os. The incidence is quoted as less than 1% of all ectopic pregnancies.

You should consider the diagnosis of cervical pregnancy if there is no evidence of a gestation sac within the endometrium but you can identify ballooning of the cervical canal. Examine the cervical canal carefully for the presence of a gestation sac or placental tissue. Peripheral blood flow is likely to be present around the gestation sac when interrogated with colour Doppler. The internal os should be closed. The diagnosis of a cervical pregnancy may only be made easily if a live embryo is present within the gestation sac when heart activity will be seen.

The difficulty is in distinguishing a cervical pregnancy from an inevitable miscarriage. An inevitable miscarriage will demonstrate an intrauterine gestation sac that has detached from the endometrium into the uterine cavity and has then been retained within the cervical canal before being expelled. Gentle pressure with the probe will demonstrate sliding between the gestation sac and cervical canal. This sign is absent in true cervical pregnancies.

Management options for cervical pregnancy may include surgery with dilation and curettage, but this carries the risk of uncontrollable haemorrhage and a high rate of hysterectomy. Alternatively, local injections of methotrexate or potassium chloride under ultrasound control can be used. Systemic therapy with methotrexate is also effective.

Caesarean Scar Pregnancy

Caesarean scar pregnancy describes the implantation of the pregnancy into the myometrium of a dehiscent scar secondary to a previous Caesarean section. The incidence is quoted as in the region of 1 in 2000 of all pregnancies and is increasing. This increase is attributed to the rising Caesarean section rate and the more frequent use of high-resolution transvaginal ultrasound.

You should consider the diagnosis of a Caesarean scar pregnancy if there is no evidence of a gestation sac within the endometrium but you can identify a gestation sac at the level of the internal os or at the site of the previous lower segment Caesarean section scar (Fig. 6.15). Peripheral blood flow is likely to be present around the gestation sac when interrogated with colour Doppler. The gestation sac should demonstrate a negative sliding sign – that is, you are unable to displace the gestation sac from its position at the level of the internal os when you apply gentle pressure with the transvaginal probe.

Treatment options include medical, surgical or expectant management. Medical treatment includes methotrexate administered systemically and/or locally. Surgical options include laparotomy and excision of the gestational mass, suction curettage or laparoscopy.

Ovarian Pregnancy

The incidence of ovarian pregnancy is between 0.5% and 6% of all ectopic pregnancies and relies on the presence of a gestation sac or gestation sac like mass – that is, a cyst with an unusually bright and thickened border within the ovarian tissue (Fig. 6.16). It is important to identify the corpus luteum separately from a suspected ovarian ectopic pregnancy to avoid misinterpreting the corpus luteum as an ovarian pregnancy. Because the differential diagnosis therefore includes a corpus luteum and other ovarian pathological conditions, the specific diagnosis of ovarian pregnancy is very difficult. The sliding sign in an ovarian pregnancy, relative to the ovary, will be negative – as indeed will the sliding sign with a corpus luteum.

Ovarian ectopic pregnancies are usually treated by local excision.

Abdominal Pregnancy

Abdominal pregnancy is a rare form of ectopic pregnancy which occurs in about 1% of all ectopic pregnancies. Abdominal pregnancy describes an intraperitoneal implantation of the pregnancy within the peritoneal cavity excluding the uterus,

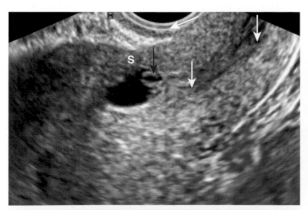

Fig 6.15 • Caesarean scar pregnancy. Sagittal section of the uterus. The gestation sac contains a yolk sac (red arrow) and embryo located within the scar (S). The cervix is arrowed. The empty endometrium lies to the left of the image and therefore is not visible.

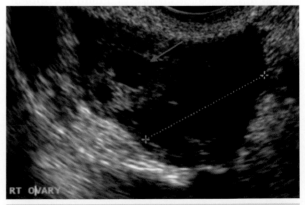

Fig 6.16 • Right ovarian ectopic pregnancy. A yolk sac (arrow) is identified within the gestation sac. A negative sliding sign was demonstrated as the ectopic mass is contained within the ovarian capsule. The dotted line demonstrates normal ovarian tissue.

ovaries or the Fallopian tubes. To make a first trimester diagnosis, a gestation sac or fetal parts are usually seen behind the uterus in the Pouch of Douglas or laterally within the broad ligament.

Heterotopic Pregnancy

Heterotopic pregnancy is the combination of an intrauterine and an ectopic pregnancy. The incidence of heterotopic pregnancy in the general population is around 1 in 6000 and is particularly high, on the order of 1–3%, in women who undergo some form of assisted conception. The diagnosis of a normal intrauterine pregnancy thus cannot rule out a concomitant ectopic pregnancy, and every effort should be made to exclude this in a symptomatic patient.

TROPHOBLASTIC DISEASE

Trophoblastic disease covers the spectrum from benign hydatidiform molar pregnancy to malignant choriocarcinoma. Molar pregnancy is commonly referred to as a mole and can be 'complete' or 'partial'. Early diagnosis enables appropriate management and counselling to be planned. However, diagnosis in the first trimester is difficult as the clinical presentation, sonographic findings and pathologies are variable.

Complete Hydatidiform Mole

Complete hydatidiform mole describes the generalized swelling of the villous tissue of the placenta and diffuse trophoblastic hyperplasia in the absence of any embryonic or fetal tissue.

A complete mole arises in one of two ways. More commonly an 'empty' ovum devoid of DNA is fertilised by one sperm which has duplicated and therefore has a 46XX diploid chromosome complement. Less commonly the 'empty' ovum is fertilised by two sperm each of which has a haploid chromosome complement of either 23X or 23Y. The resulting diploid chromosome complement is therefore either 46XX or 46XY.

The ultrasound appearances of a complete mole are of a uterus which is enlarged for gestational age and within which are multiple small, round, dark, hypoechoic areas measuring 2–10 mm in diameter. These cystic areas represent vesicles,

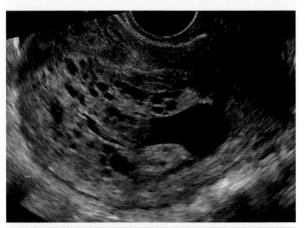

Fig 6.17 • Complete molar pregnancy. There are multiple hypoechoic cysts occupying the endometrium.

which result from the abnormal proliferation of the trophoblast (Fig. 6.17). The molar tissue fills the endometrial cavity but does not invade the myometrium. These ultrasound appearances are most readily identified between 9 and 12 weeks of gestation. The villous hydatidiform changes are less apparent in earlier pregnancy, making the diagnosis earlier in gestation more difficult. The presenting complaint is normally vaginal bleeding.

Serum hCG levels will be high in these women, usually more than 2.5 multiples of the median, and will continue to increase as the pregnancy advances. Theca-lutein cysts are usually found in association with high levels of circulating hCG and therefore may be present with a molar pregnancy. Theca-lutein cysts are usually bilateral, multiple, multilocular and may be large.

Management of complete hydatidiform mole is by surgical evacuation of the pregnancy with follow-up serial measurements of hCG levels.

Partial Hydatidiform Mole

Partial mole describes the focal swelling of villous tissue and focal trophoblastic hyperplasia of the placenta in the presence of embryonic or fetal tissue.

Partial hydatidiform moles have three sets of chromosomes and therefore have a triploid karyotype which is either 69XXX, 69XXY or 69XYY. The partial mole results from fertilisation of a normal ovum by either two sperm, each with a normal haploid complement of 23 chromosomes (23X or 23Y) or one sperm in which the haploid complement of 23 chromosomes has duplicated producing a diploid complement of 46 chromosomes (46XX or 46YY) in a manner similar to that of a complete mole.

The ultrasound features of a partial mole include both abnormal placental and fetal appearances. The placental appearances are similar to those of a complete mole as described earlier. Major structural abnormalities and/or severe intrauterine growth restriction are almost always present in the fetus of a partial mole. As with a complete mole, the placental changes are less obvious in early gestations before 12 weeks as a partial mole may not demonstrate any obvious macroscopic vesicular changes, although the placenta may be moderately enlarged. The fetal appearances suggesting the diagnosis of a partial mole are unlikely to be detectable in the first trimester of pregnancy. Thus the ultrasound diagnosis of a partial mole is difficult, with a detection rate of only approximately 30%.

When molar changes are identified within the placenta, the differential diagnosis is of a partial mole or a twin pregnancy where one conceptus is normal and the other a complete mole. In the case of a partial mole, the molar changes within the placenta are dispersed throughout the placental mass. By contrast, in a complete mole coexisting with a fetus, one placenta is molar and the other is normal. Thus the ultrasound appearances will be of an abnormal placental mass adjacent to but distinct from the normal placenta of the coexisting fetus.

Invasive Mole

A small percentage of complete and partial hydatidiform moles will become invasive. In this condition the trophoblastic tissue penetrates and invades the myometrium with metastatic spread to other organs. It is important therefore that you evaluate carefully the junction between the molar tissue and the myometrium to ensure that the interface is smooth and regular. Any areas of irregularity at the interface should be treated with suspicion and a more experienced opinion sought.

As discussed earlier, it is important you remember that molar pregnancy, and particularly partial molar pregnancy, and incomplete miscarriage can present with very similar ultrasound appearances. It is not unusual for an incomplete miscarriage to be incorrectly diagnosed as a partial mole and vice versa.

PREGNANCY AND AN INTRAUTERINE CONTRACEPTIVE DEVICE

Where an intrauterine pregnancy occurs with an intrauterine contraceptive device (IUCD) in situ, removal of the IUCD is the preferred option. Leaving the device in situ is associated with a high rate of miscarriage and an increased risk of haemorrhage, sepsis, preterm delivery and stillbirth.

A transvaginal ultrasound examination should be performed as early as possible in order to determine whether the device is still within the uterus. Where this is the case, the most common position for the IUCD is directly below the gestation sac, as IUCD malposition is the most common cause of its failure.

If the threads are visible and the IUCD can be seen to be separate from the gestation sac, then the IUCD should be removed. If the threads are lost or the IUCD appears embedded in the gestation sac, removal should not be attempted because of the risk of causing a miscarriage.

Whilst ectopic pregnancies are more commonly seen when an IUCD is present, IUCDs do not increase the overall risk of an ectopic pregnancy when compared to controls, namely women not using any contraception. However, an early ultrasound is warranted in every woman who conceives with an IUCD in situ to confirm the presence of an intrauterine pregnancy and, by assumption, to exclude an ectopic pregnancy.

UTERINE FIBROIDS

Fibroids, or leiomyomata, are benign tumours of the smooth muscle of the uterus. They are composed mainly of smooth muscle which is arranged in concentric rings, and it is this dense arrangement of the muscle fibres which produces the characteristic ultrasound appearance of a fibroid. The ultrasound appearance of a fibroid is of a rounded, homogeneous mass of echoes, which are typically slightly brighter than the surrounding myometrium.

Up to 4% of pregnancies are associated with fibroids, and fibroids are reported in up to 40% of women older than 40 years of age.

Fibroids should be described in terms of their size and their site, which defines their type. There are four possible types of fibroid:

- submucosal
- subserosal
- intramural
- pedunculated.

The most common type of fibroid is intramural. The fibroids need to be further identified by their location; for example, an intramural fibroid can be located within the anterior or posterior uterine wall or at the fundus or low towards the cervix. Assessment of fibroids is discussed in more detail in Chapter 18. The maximum diameter of the fibroid should be measured in three planes orthogonal to each other.

The presence of fibroids may lead to difficulties in visualizing, and therefore obtaining accurate measurements of, the gestation sac or embryo. They may also compromise the ability to image and assess the ovaries and adnexae to such an extent that the transabdominal route may be required as an adjunct to the transvaginal examination when exclusion of ovarian and/or adnexal pathological conditions is clinically indicated.

Fibroids may increase in size during pregnancy because of the high levels of circulating oestrogen. Their measurement therefore allows comparison to be made at subsequent scans in order to assess whether they are increasing significantly in size. Their position is important, as a fundal fibroid is unlikely to affect labour and delivery irrespective of its size, whereas a much smaller cervical fibroid may.

OVARIAN PROBLEMS IN EARLY PREGNANCY

The more liberal use of transvaginal ultrasound in early pregnancy has increased the number of incidental findings of adnexal masses. The majority of these masses are normal physiological ovarian findings or incidental findings of ovarian pathological conditions which are not contributing to the woman's symptoms. However, careful assessment should be made of all adnexal masses.

Ovarian Cysts in Pregnancy

The ovarian mass that is most commonly seen in pregnancy is the corpus luteum. The majority of corpora lutea resolve spontaneously by the end of the first trimester. As discussed in the previous chapter, corpora lutea can exhibit a spectrum of appearances, which can be readily identified.

Common ovarian pathological conditions encountered in early pregnancy include dermoid cysts, benign cystadenomas and endometriomas. These various cysts may give rise to symptoms of pain in a pregnant woman but are more commonly identified as a coincidental finding in the asymptomatic pregnant woman. The typical ultrasound appearances of these pathological conditions are generally distinct from each other and therefore easily recognized. They are discussed in more detail in Chapter 18.

Theca-lutein cysts are usually found in association with high levels of circulating hCG. Thus they may be present with molar pregnancy or ovarian hyperstimulation syndrome or can be seen with normal intrauterine pregnancies. These cysts are usually bilateral, multiple and multilocular. As with other functional cysts, they will usually resolve spontaneously by 16 weeks of gestation, although this is dependent on their origin, and the mean time for resolution is 8 weeks.

Expectant management is the option of choice for benign pathological conditions in the pregnant woman, with ultrasound monitoring being often performed towards the end of pregnancy in order to plan the best method of delivery. The risk of ovarian malignancy in women of reproductive age is low. As an ultrasound examination in experienced hands is often able to differentiate accurately between benign and malignant cysts, surgical removal via laparotomy is less often performed in asymptomatic women during pregnancy.

Difficult-to-Assess Ovarian Cysts

Assessment of complicated ovarian cysts in pregnancy should be undertaken systematically by an experienced operator and a scoring system applied to assess whether there is any evidence of malignancy or borderline changes. In case of any doubt a sonographer or clinician with a specialist expertise in gynaecological ultrasound should repeat the ultrasound to assess the ovarian mass. Suspected cases of ovarian malignancy should always be discussed at a multidisciplinary team meeting in order to best plan management. The same systematic scoring system and methodology is applied to these cysts irrespective of whether they are identified in the pregnant or nonpregnant woman and are discussed in Chapter 19.

Further reading

Bolaji I, Singh M, Goddard R 2012 Sonographic signs in ectopic pregnancy; update. Ultrasound 20:192–210

Bourne T, Condous G S (eds) 2006 Handbook of early pregnancy care. Informa UK, London

Condous G, Okaro E, Bourne T 2003 The conservative management of early pregnancy complications: a review of the literature. Ultrasound Obstet Gynecol 22:420–430

National Institute for Health & Clinical Excellence 2012 Ectopic pregnancy and miscarriage. Diagnosis and initial management in early pregnancy of ectopic pregnancy and miscarriage. NICE Clinical Guideline 154, www://guidance.nice.org.uk/cg154

Grudzinskas J G, O'Brien P M S (eds) 1997 Problems in early pregnancy: Advances in diagnosis and management. RCOG Press, London, p 160–173

Royal College of Obstetricians and Gynaecologists 2004/2010 RCOG green top guideline number 21. In: The management of tubal pregnancy. RCOG, London

CONTENTS

This chapter explains the techniques for dating the pregnancy using the transabdominal approach and how to screen the pregnancy for Down's syndrome, Edwards' and Patau's syndromes and structural abnormalities between 10 and 14 weeks of gestation.

The aims of this chapter are to enable you to do the following:

- measure the crown rump length, head circumference and biparietal diameter
- date the pregnancy and assign the expected date of delivery (EDD)
- measure the nuchal translucency
- understand the elements of screening for Down's syndrome and Edwards' and Patau's syndromes
- examine the fetus for structural abnormalities
- report the findings of the dating scan and of the combined screening scan.

Examinations undertaken between 10 and 14 weeks of gestation will normally be performed using the transabdominal approach, with the transvaginal route only being required in addition in a very small number of cases. This chapter therefore addresses the transabdominal route only.

This text assumes that you, the operator, are sitting to the left of the scanning couch, holding the transabdominal probe in your right hand, that the woman is lying to your right side and that you are facing each other.

The first objective of the examination is to find the fetus within the uterus. As the position and movement of the first trimester fetus is unpredictable and unique to each examination, you must be aware of the need to develop a methodical and systematic approach to measuring the crown rump length (CRL), measuring the nuchal translucency (NT) and examining the fetus from the outset.

This chapter assumes that you are already able to locate the longitudinal axis of the first trimester fetus and assess its attitude and are able to manipulate the transabdominal probe to obtain a sagittal section of the fetus as described in Chapter 3. It also assumes, as described in Chapter 3, that you have performed, or will perform before the end of your examination, longitudinal and transverse sweeps of the uterus and pelvis to exclude the presence of uterine fibroids and/or significant ovarian pathological conditions.

As of the relatively small size of the first trimester fetus and the speed of its movements, applying these skills often requires a quicker assessment of the fetal section obtained and a faster scanning speed to produce the correct section for measurement than those required with the larger and usually less agile second trimester fetus.

THE VALUE OF AN ACCURATE EDD

One of the most important contributions that routine ultrasound screening has made to obstetric care since the 1980s has been the ability to date the pregnancy, and therefore assign the EDD, accurately. Knowledge of the gestational age is important for the woman herself, for ensuring tests are arranged at the optimal time and for assessing the clinical progress of the pregnancy. In addition, because the EDD is known, appropriate management decisions when clinically indicated can be made around preterm, term and post-term delivery.

Historically, the first trimester has been the optimal time within which to take measurements to date the pregnancy and assign the EDD. The British Medical Ultrasound Society (BMUS) currently recommends that measurement of the CRL should be used to date a pregnancy from 6 weeks + 0 days to 13 weeks + 0 days, with the head circumference (HC) or femur length (FL) being used to date the pregnancy from 13 weeks + 1 day to 25 weeks + 6 days.

However, the need for optimal accuracy of the EDD must be considered in the context of a modern routine obstetric screening service that incorporates both assessing the gestational age and, often, screening for Down's syndrome. The current national recommendation is to offer all pregnant women an ultrasound scan between 10 and 14 weeks of gestation in order to determine gestational age and assign the EDD. All spontaneously conceived pregnancies therefore are now dated using ultrasound criteria rather than the woman's last menstrual period (LMP). The dating of pregnancies resulting from assisted conception is discussed later in this chapter.

In addition, it is routine practice to offer all women a screening test for Down's syndrome or trisomy 21. In England, women are also offered screening for Edwards' syndrome, or trisomy 18, and Patau's syndrome, or trisomy 13. Edwards' and Patau's syndromes conditions are screened for together rather than separately, with a single risk being reported for the two conditions. The recommended screening test for the three aneuploidies is the combined screening test. This is best carried out at around 12 weeks of gestation. In practice, therefore, most pregnancies are dated, and the EDD assigned, towards the end of the first trimester by measurement of the CRL or, where accurate measurement of the CRL is not possible, by measurement of the HC. As the biparietal diameter (BPD) rather than the HC is used in some departments and laboratories to date the pregnancy, we also include discussion of this measurement for completeness.

ULTRASOUND PARAMETERS

Between 10 and 14 weeks, the ultrasound parameters which should be used to date the pregnancy and assign the EDD are the following:
- crown rump length
- head circumference

and, for the reasons stated earlier,
- biparietal diameter.

CROWN RUMP LENGTH

A correctly performed measurement of CRL is the most accurate means of estimating the gestational age, and it is preferable to the parameters of HC or FL used to date a pregnancy which is scanned for the first time in the second trimester.

THE CORRECT SECTION

The CRL is defined as the sagittal section of the whole fetus, in a neutral position and with the end points of the crown and rump clearly visible (Fig. 7.1A).

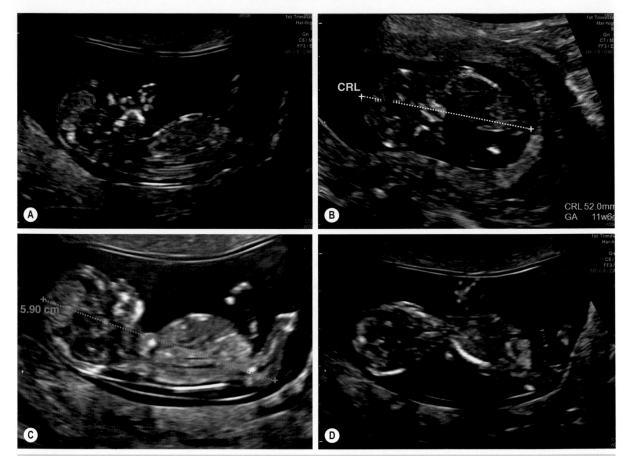

Fig 7.1 • A. CRL measurement (56.6 mm). Midsagittal section of the whole fetus, in a neutral position and with the end points of the crown and rump clearly visible. Neutral position – neither hyperextended nor flexed. A useful way of assessing one component of the neutral position is to compare the pocket of amniotic fluid between the fetal chin and chest to the width of the bright 'cheekbone' or palate seen in the same section. CRL is horizontal to the ultrasound beam and should be measured by placing the linear callipers correctly on these defined endpoints. B. Fetus is too flexed. If the fetus is not in a neutral position and the chin is on its chest, no pocket of fluid will be visible and the fetus will be too flexed to measure accurately. Failing to appreciate that the position of the fetus is not neutral and, therefore, that a degree of flexion is present is one of the main reasons for inaccuracy of CRL measurements between 10 and 14 weeks of gestation. We recommend that a fetus which has its sacrum above the level of its chin, when imaged in the horizontal plane, is too flexed to measure as this will produce an underestimate of the CRL. C. Fetus is too extended. Conversely, if the fetal head is extended there will be a large difference in the size of the pocket of fluid and the width of the cheek bone. In this position the fetus will be too extended to measure accurately. The fetal spine is straight, with no curvature. D. Fetus is extended with lateral rotation of the head to one side. CRL, crown rump length.

The fetus should lie, or the image be manipulated, such that the fetal length is as close as possible to the horizontal. Thus the angle of insonation by the ultrasound beam to the CRL is 90°. Measurement between the two end points of the crown and rump should be taken using linear callipers (see Fig. 7.1A).

NEUTRAL POSITION

The neutral position is one in which the fetus is neither hyperextended nor flexed. Defining neutral position is difficult to do in any other than qualitative terms and is therefore open to personal and/or departmental definition. Fetal extension and flexion increase with increasing gestation, compounding the difficulty of obtaining a sagittal section of the whole fetus, in a neutral position.

A useful way of assessing one component of the neutral position is to compare the pocket of amniotic fluid between the fetal chin and chest to the width of the bright 'cheekbone' or palate seen in the same section (see Fig. 7.1A). If the fetus has its chin on its chest, no pocket of fluid will be visible and the fetus will be too flexed to measure accurately (Fig. 7.1B). Conversely if the fetal head is extended there will be a large difference in the size of the pocket of fluid and the width of the cheekbone. In this position the fetus will be too extended to measure accurately (Fig. 7.1C).

If the fetus is not in a neutral position, you should wait until it moves into the required position before attempting to take a measurement of the CRL. Failing to appreciate that the position of the fetus is not neutral and, therefore, that a degree of flexion or extension is present is one of the main reasons for inaccuracy of CRL measurements between 10 and 14 weeks of gestation (Fig. 7.1B, C and D).

DEGREE OF CURVATURE OF THE LOWER SPINE

There is much debate as to what defines an acceptable degree of curvature of the lower spine in the neutral position and, to date, this remains unquantifiable. It is accepted that it is incorrect to measure the CRL if the fetal spine is straight, with no curvature (Fig. 7.1C), as this will produce an overestimate of the CRL. It is more difficult to be precise in describing the range of positions that demonstrate the 'correct' degree of curvature.

We recommend that a fetus which has its sacrum above the level of its chin, when imaged in the horizontal plane, is too flexed to measure as this will produce an underestimate of the CRL (Fig. 7.1B).

IDENTIFYING THE END POINTS

It is important that you can clearly identify the end points of the crown and the rump if you are to place your callipers accurately. Ideally, a pocket of fluid should be visible between the end point(s) of the fetus and the wall of the gestational sac or the edge of a lateral placenta (Fig. 7.1A).

When the fetus is lying directly adjacent to the wall of the gestational sac or a lateral placenta, using the dipping movement of the probe to change the angle at which you are insonating the fetus may improve your ability to visualize the outer limit of the crown and/or rump. Alternatively, ask the woman's permission first and then encourage the fetus to move by gently shaking the probe on the maternal abdomen. You must then be ready to use the freeze control quickly if you are to capture the required image.

FINDING THE MAXIMUM LENGTH

Having established that the fetus is in a neutral position, it is important to ensure that you are imaging the maximum length of the fetus before taking your measurement. To confirm you have obtained what will be the longest CRL, continue to slide or rotate the probe past your intended optimal section. If the selected section demonstrates the maximum length, then the subsequent CRLs should reduce in size. Return to the original section, freeze the image and measure the CRL.

MEASURING THE CRL

Having obtained the correct section for measurement, select the linear callipers, making sure they display either a '+' or an 'x' at each end. The intersection of the cross of the linear callipers should be placed on the outer border of the crown and of the rump to provide the CRL (Fig. 7.1A).

The CRL should be measured from three different images. There are no national recommendations defining an 'acceptable' range of error for comparative CRL measurements. We recommend that the difference between the measurements should be no greater than 5% of the mean between the three. This will equate to approximately 1 mm in the fetus, or approximately half a day of gestation after 10 weeks of gestation.

We also recommend that the measurement from the image which displays the best section and which has also been measured correctly is selected for the reported CRL.

On no account should the three measurements be averaged to produce the CRL.

REPORTING THE CRL MEASUREMENT TO ONE DECIMAL PLACE

The CRL should be reported in millimetres, corrected to one decimal place. Thus calliper readings of, for example, 65.50 mm, 65.51 mm, 65.52 mm, 65.53 mm and 65.54 mm give a CRL measurement of 65.5 mm, whereas calliper readings of 65.55 mm, 65.56 mm, 65.57 mm, 65.58 mm and 65.59 mm give a CRL measurement of 65.6 mm. This method of correcting to one decimal place should be used for all ultrasound measurements where calliper measurements are given to two decimal places.

PROBLEMS

CRL measurements may be inaccurate for the following reasons:
- the full length of the fetus has not been obtained; this will produce an underestimated CRL
- the full length of the fetus has been obtained, but its attitude is flexed, with lateral rotation of the head to one side (Fig. 7.1B); this will produce an underestimated CRL
- the full length of the fetus has been obtained but its attitude is extended, with lateral rotation of the head to one side; this will produce an overestimated CRL (Fig. 7.1D)
- one or both end points of the fetus have not been clearly identified as separate from the walls of the gestation sac or the placental edge; this may produce either an under- or overestimated CRL (Fig. 7.2)
- the fetal lie is decubitus and therefore the spine is lateral and the degree of flexion is estimated incorrectly; this will produce an underestimated CRL (Fig. 7.3).

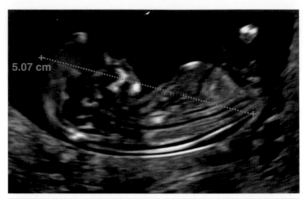

Fig 7.2 • The fetal rump is not clearly identified as it is close to the uterine wall. This will result in an underestimation of the crown rump length.

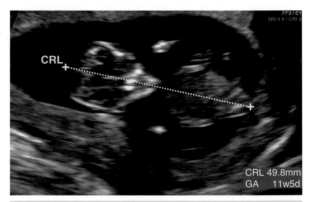

Fig 7.3 • The fetal lie is decubitus; therefore the spine is lateral and the degree of flexion is estimated incorrectly. This will produce an underestimated crown rump length (CRL).

When the fetus remains obstinately in the wrong position to measure an accurate CRL, you have a number of choices, of which four are reasonable to consider:
1. encourage the fetus to move or wait until it does, then measure the correct CRL section accurately using linear callipers
2. measure the flexed length using on-screen nonlinear measuring facilities. This is likely to produce an overestimated CRL measurement (Fig. 7.4)
3. use two sets of linear callipers to measure the parts of the fetal length that are in straight sections, and then add them together. The accuracy of this method will depend on the degree of flexion (Fig. 7.4)

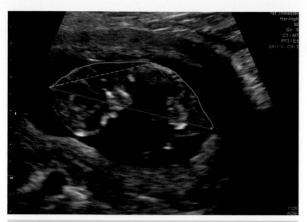

Fig 7.4 • Three methods of measuring a flexed CRL, hand tracing the flexed length using the nonlinear measuring facility (blue solid line, 74.5 mm), applying two sets of linear calipers (green dashed lines, 38.4 mm + 31.7 mm = 70.1 mm) and using one set of linear calipers to measure the flexed length (red solid line, 60.2 mm). CRL, crown rump length.

5 use one set of linear calipers to measure the flexed length of the CRL (see Fig. 7.4). *This method is not recommended under any circumstances but is included to illustrate the reason why the CRL will be significantly underestimated if applied.*

Obviously method 1 is the preferred choice but, in the reality of a busy, often time-limited screening service, this is not always the feasible option.

The accuracy of methods 2 and 3 will depend on your perception of the degree of flexion of the fetus. In theory, method 2 should be the more accurate of the two methods. However, the calliper system is often very sensitive or obstinate (or both) and you will tend to overestimate the true measurement because of the difficulty in keeping the calliper line on the curve of the fetus while tracing its length.

Method 3 horrifies all purists (usually quite rightly) but is actually often a better, although less scientific, option than method 2. The alternative is to date the pregnancy using the HC or, if still the preferred measurement, the BPD.

Under no circumstances should you use method 5 because the underestimate of the CRL will underestimate the gestational age. Where Down's syndrome and/or Edwards' and Patau's screening has been requested, the underestimated CRL and the underestimated gestational age will both contribute to reducing the sensitivity of *all* the components of the combined screening or of the quadruple test screening for the three aneuploidies.

4 date the pregnancy by measuring the HC, or the BPD if this remains your department's standard practice. You will need to be aware of the implications of dating the pregnancy by either the HC or BPD if screening for Down's syndrome is also requested, as discussed later

HEAD CIRCUMFERENCE AND BIPARIETAL DIAMETER

The techniques for obtaining the correct section of the fetal head and measurement of the HC and BPD are described in detail in Chapter 8.

Owing to the developmental time line of the intracranial anatomy, the structures that can be identified within the HC section at 12–14 weeks are more limited than at 18–22 weeks. In the normal fetus, the cavum septum pellucidum and cerebellum, for example, should always be seen at 18–22 weeks. One or both may be seen in the normal fetus at 12–14 weeks but cannot always be clearly identified. It should also be remembered that the normal skull shape at 12–14 weeks will often appear more angular or 'lemon-shaped' than the normal skull shape at 18–22 weeks.

THE CORRECT SECTION AT 12–14 WEEKS

The image selected to date the pregnancy using the HC should include the following features:
- a rugby football-shaped skull, rounded at the back (occiput) and more pointed at the front (synciput)
- a continuous skull outline

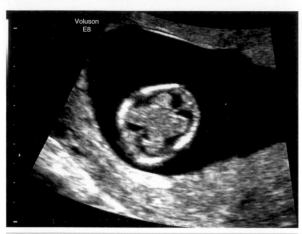

Fig 7.5 • Transverse section of the head demonstrating the complete cranium at 12 weeks. Note the small spaces between the bones of the skull, which represent the sutures.

- a midline echo, equidistant from the proximal and distal skull echoes
- where the cavum septum pellucidum is visible, interruption of the midline one third of the distance from the synciput to the occiput
- the butterfly-shaped choroid plexus (Fig. 7.5).

MEASURING THE HC

As described in Chapter 8, the HC can be calculated using three basic methods. We recommend the ellipse method.

MEASURING THE BPD

As described in Chapter 8, the BPD can be calculated using two methods of calliper placement. We recommend the 'outer to inner' technique.

PROBLEMS WITH HC AND BPD MEASUREMENTS

HC and BPD measurements at 12–14 weeks may be inaccurate for the following reasons:
- *incorrect angle*

    If the angle of the probe on the maternal abdomen is incorrect, the midline echo does not lie centrally within the fetal skull. Similarly the echoes from the choroid plexus will not be visualized symmetrically about the midline. The angle of the probe to the maternal abdomen should be altered, without sliding or rotating the probe

- *incorrect rotation*

    This is readily recognized because the shape of the fetal skull is not that of a rugby football and/or the correct landmark features are not seen.

    Visualizing the orbits together with only the posterior portion of the choroid plexus seen – producing an incomplete 'butterfly' – indicates that your selected level at the front of the head is too low. Alternatively, visualizing only the anterior portion of the choroid plexus (together with the cerebellum in the same section, if visible) indicates that your selected level at the back of the head is too low.

    Rotating the probe – in the correct direction – should produce the correct information both anteriorly and posteriorly within the skull, together with the correct shape of the skull. You must be careful to maintain the correct angle of the probe while rotating it

- *incorrect level*

    Sliding movements of the probe will alter the level of section. The inability to demonstrate the normal butterfly shape of the choroid plexus together with a continuous midline indicates that your selected level is too high. A section demonstrating the orbits and the cerebellum (if visible) or no, or minimal, choroid plexus posteriorly indicates that your selected level is too low. Be careful not to rotate or change the angle of the probe as you slide it

- *midline not horizontal*

    Measurement of the HC and BPD ideally should only be taken when the fetal head is in the occipitotransverse (OT) position – that is, when the midline echo is at 90° or orthogonal to the ultrasound beam. At 12–14 weeks, the landmarks you are seeking relate to the head shape, the midline and the symmetrical butterfly shape produced by the choroid plexus. Dipping one end of the probe gently into the maternal abdomen should bring the head into a more OT position. If this is unsuccessful, ask the woman's permission first and then encourage the fetus to move by gently shaking the probe on the maternal abdomen.

Should both these, and any other methods, be unsuccessful in producing the required movement, we consider it acceptable at this gestation to measure the HC and BPD when the head is not in an OT position, providing all the required features are satisfactorily demonstrated (see Fig. 7.5).

SIZE CHARTS AND DATING CHARTS

Having obtained the correct section and correctly measured the CRL, HC or BPD you must now use the correct chart, graph or look-up table to interpret the biometric information correctly.

Each published chart, graph or look-up table should be described by its own equation. This equation has been derived from a data set that, hopefully, was collected correctly and analyzed appropriately by the correct statistical tests. There are two types of data sets that can be used in interpreting CRL, HC, BPD and FL measurements, namely size charts and dating charts.

A size chart compares the ultrasound parameter measured or calculated to its normal range at a specific gestational age. Size charts are commonly, and incorrectly, also called growth charts. This term is incorrect because a proper growth chart describes an increase in size over time, rather than the size itself, which is the parameter described by a size chart. Proper growth charts are not used in routine clinical practice.

Dating charts, unsurprisingly, use the ultrasound parameter measured to predict gestational age.

All data are plotted on graphs in the following way. The known variable is plotted on the horizontal or *x*-axis. The unknown variable is plotted on the vertical or *y*-axis.

SIZE CHARTS

You will be familiar with size charts as these are the 'charts' used to plot fetal growth or, more correctly as these are size charts, an increase in size with gestation. They are used throughout pregnancy, once the pregnancy has been dated and the gestational age established.

Size charts plot the known variable of gestational age on the horizontal or *x*-axis and the

unknown variable of the size of, for example, the HC on the vertical or *y*-axis.

DATING CHARTS AND LOOK-UP TABLES

A dating chart uses the known variable of the ultrasound measurement to estimate the unknown variable of gestational age. Dating charts therefore plot the CRL, HC or BPD on the horizontal or *x*-axis and the unknown variable of gestational age on the vertical or *y*-axis. The plotting of measurements on a dating chart is not only confusing but clinically unhelpful. Should you try to attempt this you will discover that the measurement plot 'goes the wrong way'.

As a measurement to date the pregnancy is acquired only once, we recommend that look-up tables are used for dating purposes in preference to dating charts or dating graphs.

Using the Correct Data Set Correctly

In order to date the pregnancy from the CRL, HC or BPD and assign the EDD, you must use a dating chart or table.

You must be aware that, first, different authors have used the same measurement to produce different equations to assess gestational age and, second, different sections and/or techniques may be used to describe the same measurement. Thus you must know which data set you are using and must use the methodology described by the author for that data set. Finally, you should also be aware that different parameters measured during the same examination (e.g. the CRL and the HC) will not always give the same estimation of gestational age. This can be problematic from a philosophical point of view and also, more importantly, in your discussions with the woman.

131

THE IMPACT OF DIFFERING EQUATIONS FOR PREGNANCY DATING

CROWN RUMP LENGTH

The original equation for the estimation of gestational age from the CRL was published by Robinson in 1975. A modification of this equation was published by BMUS in 2009. The implication of this modification was to change the gestational age calculated from the same CRL by between 1 and 2 days.

An example of this difference can be seen when considering the gestational age equivalents for the CRL range of 45.0–84.0 mm. As will be seen later, this CRL range defines the limits for the assessment of the Down's screening risk using NT. The original 'Robinson' equation used in the estimation of gestational age from CRL calculated a gestational age of 11^{+0} weeks from a CRL of 45.0 mm and of 13^{+6} weeks from a CRL of 84.0 mm. The modified 'BMUS' equation as currently recommended by the national guidelines for England and Wales, calculates a gestational age of 11^{+2} weeks from a CRL of 45.0 mm and of 14^{+1} weeks from a CRL of 84.0 mm. Although these differences may seem small, they affect the accuracy and sensitivity of any test or combination of tests that rely on gestational age.

The publication date of the literature and the country of origin of its authors will normally indicate which gestational age range the CRL range refers to. It is important that you remember this when consulting the literature.

The modified equation, together with the look-up table for estimating gestational age from the CRL as recommended by current national guidelines are provided in Appendix 2.

The electronic package into which you input your ultrasound measurements and from which you produce your reports will have within it a programme for the estimation of gestational age from the CRL. If you are participating in the national United Kingdom screening programme, it is important that you use the nationally recommended equation for pregnancy dating when assigning the gestational age in your report. Your electronic reporting package therefore must also use the recommended equation.

A calculation of the gestational age, based on, for example the CRL, is shown on the ultrasound monitor of the machine when the CRL programme is selected from the machine's calculations package. You should be aware of whether or not your ultrasound machines use the nationally recommended equation. If they do not, it is likely that the gestational age estimates that they display will differ from that produced using the current national guideline. This can cause confusion to the woman when the gestational age she has seen on the ultrasound monitor differs from that assigned from the CRL measurement in her ultrasound report.

HEAD CIRCUMFERENCE

As with the equation used to date the pregnancy from the CRL discussed earlier, it is important that the correct equation is used to date the pregnancy from the HC. The equation that should be used to calculate the gestational age from the HC is given in Appendix 3 together with the nationally recommended HC dating table.

It will be noted that the authors of the dating table only provide a calculation of gestational age from an HC of 80.0 mm or greater. This HC is equivalent to a gestational age of 12 weeks and 4 days and therefore a CRL of 61.0 mm.

BIPARIETAL DIAMETER

Historically gestational age was calculated from the BPD rather than the HC. This method has now been superseded, and dating by HC is recommended because of its superior accuracy irrespective of fetal position. We include the Chitty data set for the calculation of gestational age from the BPD, using the 'outer to inner' method, in Appendix 4 for completeness.

DEALING WITH THE DIFFERENCES IN GESTATIONAL AGE EQUIVALENTS

When examining the post 12 week fetus, we recommend, as discussed later, that not only are the appearances of the fetal skull and intracranial anatomy assessed but the HC is also measured. You will discover when measuring the CRL and HC that the same gestational age equivalents from the two measurements will not always equate precisely. If the gestational age equivalents differ between the CRL and HC by more than a few days, you should review your HC and CRL sections and measurements to ensure that both are correct and both have been correctly measured. Do not be tempted to use a technically poor CRL image to date the pregnancy.

Where you are satisfied that the section taken and measurements of your CRL and HC are acceptable but they are producing differing gestational ages, then it is most likely that the differences in gestational age equivalents between the measurements being compared are due to the variations between the charts or tables used. You should also consider whether the differences could be due to an underlying clinical problem.

ESTIMATION OF GESTATIONAL AGE IN A SPONTANEOUSLY CONCEIVED TWIN PREGNANCY

The same criteria for measurement of the CRL, HC and BPD apply irrespective of whether the gestation is single or multiple.

In a spontaneously conceived twin pregnancy the pregnancy should be dated and the EDD should be calculated using the ultrasound measurements as with a singleton pregnancy. The CRL of both fetuses should be measured. The larger CRL should be used for assigning the gestational age in the same way as described for the singleton pregnancy.

A difference in the CRL measurement of 25% or greater between the fetuses should be noted and monitored with further ultrasound scans. Although the discrepancy is often due to constitutional differences, early-onset intrauterine growth restriction (IUGR), early twin to twin transfusion in monochorionic twin pregnancies and structural and/or karyotypic abnormalities need to be excluded.

The same criteria apply if the HC or BPD is used to date the pregnancy. The management of twin pregnancy is discussed in Chapter 15.

ESTIMATION OF GESTATIONAL AGE IN AN ASSISTED CONCEPTION PREGNANCY

As also described in Chapter 5, it is customary to date the pregnancy and assign the EDD in an assisted conception pregnancy using the date of egg collection and/or embryo transfer.

Most women can provide accurate information relating to the day of egg collection, the day of embryo transfer and the age of the embryo(s) – or more correctly the blastocyst(s) – at transfer. Blastocysts are commonly transferred at 5 days of age, although transfer at 2 or 3 days of age may also take place.

The date of egg collection is taken as equivalent to the date of conception.

Providing the age of the embryos at transfer is known, the date of conception can also be calculated by subtracting the age in days of the embryos at transfer from the date of the transfer. The resulting date of conception should be the same as the reported date of egg collection.

In cases of assisted conception, therefore, the ultrasound measurements are used first to confirm normal growth of the fetus or fetuses rather than assign the gestational age. Second, the measurements are used to confirm the EDD as calculated from the date of egg collection/date of conception rather than to assign the EDD.

Additional calculations must be made if the pregnancy resulted from a frozen embryo or embryos.

SCREENING FOR DOWN'S SYNDROME AND EDWARDS' AND PATAU'S SYNDROMES IN THE FIRST TRIMESTER

As stated earlier, the current national recommendation in England is to offer all pregnant women a screening test for Down's syndrome and a screening test for Edwards' and Patau's syndromes together, in addition to an ultrasound examination to date their pregnancy. Some women may wish to have screening for all three conditions, some for Down' syndrome only, some only for Edwards' and Patau's syndromes together; some may decline screening for all three conditions.

DOWN'S SYNDROME

Down's syndrome, or trisomy 21, occurs when three rather than two copies of chromosome 21, or of a segment of the long arm of chromosome 21, are present in a cell. This occurs because of one of three different mechanisms, namely nondisjunction, translocation or mosaicism. Most – approximately 95% – cases of trisomy 21 are caused by *nondisjunction*. This is the failure of separation of the chromosome pair during the third phase (anaphase) of the first meiotic division in the ovum. Thus 95% of cases are maternal in origin.

The remaining cases are due to translocation or mosaicism. *Translocation* describes the transfer of genetic material from one chromosome, such as chromosome 21, to another, such as chromosome 15. A reciprocal translocation occurs when a break occurs in each of two chromosomes and the broken segments are exchanged between the two chromosomes to form two new chromosomes. The total amount of genetic material is the same between the two new chromosomes as before the breaks, but it is now arranged differently between the two chromosomes.

Robertsonian translocation is a particular type of translocation where the breakpoints occur very close to, or at, the constriction point or centromere of the chromosome. Robertsonian translocations occur in chromosomes 13, 14, 15, 21 and 22 and, in cases involving chromosome 21, result in approximately 3% of cases of Down's syndrome.

Mosaicism describes the presence of two or more cell lines which differ genetically from each other but are derived from the same fertilized egg. Mosaicism is normally the result of nondisjunction during a mitotic division in the very early embryo and accounts for 2–3% of clinically recognized cases of trisomy 21.

Approximately 30% of cases of trisomy 21 will be lost spontaneously between 12 and 40 weeks of gestation.

EDWARDS' SYNDROME

Edwards' syndrome, or trisomy 18, occurs when three rather than two copies of chromosome 18 are present in a cell. The great majority – in the order of 85–90% – of cases of trisomy 18 are caused by maternal meiotic nondisjunction during, uniquely, the second meiotic division in the ovum. Mosaicism accounts for approximately 5% of cases of trisomy 18.

The condition is associated with a range of structural and often multiple abnormalities. Approximately 80% of cases will be lost spontaneously between 12 and 40 weeks of gestation. The life expectancy is short, with approximately 45% of live-born infants dying within the first week of life and only 5% surviving to 1 year of age.

PATAU'S SYNDROME

Patau's syndrome, or trisomy 13, occurs when three rather than two copies of chromosome 13 are present in a cell. Approximately 90% of cases of trisomy 13 are caused by maternal nondisjunction during the first meiotic division in the ovum. Translocation, usually of the unbalanced Robertsonian type between chromosomes 13 and 14, accounts for 5–10% of cases of trisomy 13, with mosaicism accounting for a smaller proportion of cases.

The condition is associated with a range of structural, typically midline, abnormalities. Approximately 80% of cases will be lost spontaneously between 12 and 40 weeks of gestation. The median survival of affected infants has been reported as 7–10 days, with only 5–10% surviving to 1 year of age.

COMBINED SCREENING

The recommended screening test for Down's syndrome is the combined screening test, so named because it combines the risk for Down's syndrome generated by the measurement of the NT with that generated from measuring the levels in the maternal serum of pregnancy-associated plasma protein (PAPP-A) and the free beta subunit of human chorionic gonodatropin (βhCG).

Similarly, the risk for Edwards' syndrome and Patau's syndrome together can be calculated using the same combination of NT, PAPP-A and free βhCG. The risk for each of these two conditions can be calculated separately, but it is common practice in most laboratories, and national policy, to report a single risk for both conditions.

Using the measurement of NT as a screening tool for Down's syndrome arose from the observation that fetuses with chromosomal abnormalities, and in particular trisomy 21, demonstrated an increased collection of subcutaneous fluid, or nuchal translucency, behind the neck. This was most marked between 11 and 14 weeks of gestation. In addition to its association with chromosomal abnormalities, increased NT has also been described in association with a range of structural abnormalities, and in particular cardiac abnormalities, and a range of genetic conditions.

Screening programmes that include NT may focus primarily on Down's syndrome or, as now in England, also include screening for Edwards' and Patau's syndromes. It is important that the association between NT, the serum analytes and a range of problems including these and other abnormal karyotypes, structural abnormalities and poor outcome is appreciated by both the providers and the users of such screening programmes.

In order to standardize interpretation of maternal serum analytes, the quantity of an analyte measured in the maternal blood is compared with the laboratory's own reference range and reported as a multiple of the median (MoM) relative to that reference range. The reference MoM value for both PAPP-A and free βhCG in a normal pregnancy is 1.0 MoM (Table 7.1). Because MoMs can be used with the reference range of any measurement, they can also be applied to NT as can be seen in the combined screening reports issued by laboratories.

In a twin pregnancy the level of both serum analytes will be higher in the maternal blood compared with the levels in a singleton pregnancy. In a dichorionic twin pregnancy, a Down's syndrome risk is calculated for both fetuses separately. In a monochorionic twin pregnancy a Down's syndrome risk is calculated for the pregnancy (see Chapter 15).

In a pregnancy affected with Down's syndrome the median level of PAPP-A is reduced and the median level of free βhCG is increased compared with the karyotypically normal pregnancy. In the same way, NT is used with a different combination

CONDITION	KARYOTYPE	PAPP-A MoM	FREE βhCG MoM
Normal male or female	46XY or 46XX	1.0	1.0
Down's syndrome	Trisomy 21	0.5	2.19
Edwards' syndrome	Trisomy 18	0.19	0.21
Patau's syndrome	Trisomy 13	0.25	0.51
Diandric triploidy	69XXY or 69XXX	0.16	8.74
Digynic triploidy	69XXY or 69XXX	0.06	0.74

Table 7.1 Association between median MoM values for PAPP-A and free βhCG measured at 12 weeks of gestation, and abnormal karyotype

From Spencer K 2005. First trimester maternal serum screening for Down's syndrome: an evaluation of the DPC Immulite 2000 free beta-hCG and pregnancy-associated plasma protein-A assays. Ann Clin Biochem 42:pt 1. 30–40.
Data from SURRUSS 2003, Kagan 2008, and Goodburn 2009.
βhCG, free beta human chorionic gonodotropin; MoM, multiple of the median; PAPP-A, pregnancy-associated plasma protein A.

of PAPP-A and free βhCG levels to calculate the risk for Edwards' syndrome (trisomy 18) and Patau's syndrome (trisomy 13) together. An increased NT and further combinations of abnormal serum analytes are associated with triploidy.

TRIPLOIDY

Triploidy is the condition in which three copies of each chromosome are present rather than two copies. Thus 69 chromosomes are present rather than the normal number of 46. There are two types of triploidy, namely diandric and digynic.

Diandric or paternal triploidy occurs when the double contribution of 46 chromosomes is from the father, usually because two sperm fertilize a single egg. Digynic or maternal triploidy occurs when the double contribution is from the mother, usually because of nondisjunction in the egg. Both diandric and digynic types of triploidy give rise to both male and female conceptuses as the fertilizing sperm contributes either an X or a Y chromosome to the X of XX arising from the ovum. Approximately 60% of triploid pregnancies have a 69XXY karyotype, with around 40% demonstrating a 69XXX karyotype. The 69XYY karyotype is rarely seen.

The typical combinations of PAPP-A and free βhCG seen at 12 weeks in the karyotypically abnormal pregnancies described earlier are shown in Table 7.1.

AGE-RELATED, BACKGROUND AND ADJUSTED RISKS

Because advancing maternal age predisposes to nondisjunction, a woman's risk of her pregnancy being associated with one of the three trisomies, namely Down's, Edwards' and Patau's syndromes, increases with her age at conception.

For ease of reading, the following text refers to Down's syndrome only. The same principles apply to Edwards' syndrome and Patau's syndrome.

Although the risk of the three trisomies originates at conception, it is the risk calculation based on the woman's age at term (i.e. 38 weeks after conception) which is used. This risk is termed the 'age-related risk' (see Appendix 5).

Where the pregnancy was conceived using the woman's own frozen egg, then it is the age of the woman when her egg was collected which provides the age-related risk of Down's syndrome for the pregnancy.

Where the pregnancy was conceived using a donor egg, it is the age of the donor when her egg was collected which provides the age-related risk of Down's syndrome for the pregnancy.

The mother's risk of her pregnancy being affected by Down's syndrome is described as the 'background', 'prior' or *a priori* risk. Because most women have not had a previous pregnancy associated with trisomy 21, the mother's background risk is normally the same as her age-related risk.

A woman who has had a previous pregnancy affected with Down's syndrome has an increased risk of having another pregnancy affected with trisomy 21. This woman's background risk will therefore differ from her age-related risk. The background risk of this woman is calculated by using her age-related risk at term together with the previous Down's syndrome risk. With nondisjunction trisomy 21, the recurrence risk, over and above the maternal age-related risk, is on the order of 0.5% to 1.0%, with 0.75% specifically being quoted by various authors.

The background risk associated with a donor egg should be equivalent to the age-related risk of the donor because eggs from a woman who had had a previous karyotypically abnormal pregnancy would not be used for donation.

The adjusted risk is the risk produced by multiplying the background risk by factors derived separately from each of the NT, PAPP-A and free βhCG.

THRESHOLD RISK AND TERMINOLOGY

The threshold between what is considered to be a screen positive and a screen negative result has altered since screening for Down's syndrome was introduced. The original threshold risk that was used was a risk of 1 in 250, with a high-risk result being a risk of 1 in 250 or higher – for example, 1 in 200 or 1 in 50. A low-risk result was therefore a risk of 1 in 251 or lower – for example, 1 in 300 or 1 in 1000.

The current threshold risk uses a risk of 1 in 150. The recommended terminology varies, with some providers using *higher* and *lower* and others using *high* and *low*. These terms are preferable to *screen positive* and *screen negative*. A higher- or high-risk result is a risk of 1 in 150 or higher – for example,

1 in 100 or 1 in 50. A lower or a low-risk result is a risk of 1 in 151 or lower – for example, 1 in 200 or 1 in 1000.

The screen positive rate, the screen negative rate and the detection rate for a test will vary depending on where the threshold risk is set. Thus the sensitivity of tests which used the threshold of 1 in 250 differed from those which use the current threshold of 1 in 150.

- *the screen positive rate* is the proportion of women having the test who have an adjusted risk of 1 in 150 or higher
- *the true positive rate* is the proportion of women who have an adjusted risk of 1 in 150 or higher and who have an affected pregnancy
- *the false positive rate* is the proportion of women who have an adjusted risk of 1 in 150 or higher but who do not have an affected pregnancy
- *the screen negative rate* is the proportion of women having the test who have an adjusted risk of 1 in 151 or lower
- *the true negative rate* is the proportion of women who have an adjusted risk of 1 in

151 or lower and who have an unaffected pregnancy
- *the false negative rate* is the proportion of women who have an adjusted risk of 1 in 151 or lower but who have an affected pregnancy
- *the detection rate* or *'sensitivity'* is the proportion of women who have an affected pregnancy and who have an adjusted risk of 1 in 150 or higher
- *the positive predictive value* (PPV) is the number of women who have an affected pregnancy with an adjusted risk of 1 in 150 or higher divided by the total number of women with an adjusted risk of 1 in 150 or higher
- the odds of having a pregnancy affected with Down's syndrome given a positive result, or *OAPR*, is equivalent to the PPV. It is the ratio of affected pregnancies to unaffected pregnancies within the group of pregnancies with an adjusted risk of 1 in 150 or higher.

SCREENING FOR DOWN'S SYNDROME USING NT

Measuring NT allows a more sensitive estimation of the risk of trisomy 21 to be made than that derived from the maternal age alone.

The NT risk can be evaluated using a simple numerical threshold or cut-off such as 3.0 mm, a simple numerical cut-off related to the CRL such as 2.5 mm at 45.0 mm and 2.8 mm at 65.0 mm or a calculation based on the combination of the maternal age-related risk, CRL and NT.

The calculation of risk from NT is only possible within the CRL range of 45.0 to 84.0 mm, because accurate data have not been collected outside these limits. Using the nationally recommended dating equation from the CRL, this CRL range is equivalent to a gestational age range of 11^{+2}–14^{+1} weeks. Note that the risk conferred from the NT is based on the CRL and not the gestational age.

A more sensitive estimation of the risk of trisomy 21, with a lower false positive rate, can be made by

calculating an adjusted risk based on the combination of the age-related risk, CRL, NT, PAPP-A and free βhCG. This describes the combined test, and its risk calculation requires a computer program.

GETTING THE CORRECT SECTION FOR MEASURING THE NT

Obtain a sagittal section of the fetus demonstrating the profile anteriorly and the spine posteriorly. Ensure that the lie of the fetus is as horizontal as possible on the screen. Dipping the probe therefore may be necessary. Although the NT can be measured from a fetus in the prone position, we do not recommend you attempt this until you are confident in obtaining the required landmarks from the supine fetus.

A true sagittal section should demonstrate the bright, hyperechoic tip of the nose, the bright,

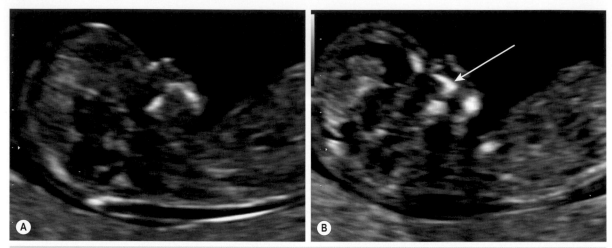

Fig 7.6 • A. A sagittal section of the fetus showing the profile anteriorly and spine posteriorly. A true sagittal section should demonstrate the bright, hyperechoic tip of the nose; the bright, hyperechoic rectangular block of the palate; the dark, hypoechoic diencephalon of the forebrain; and the nuchal membrane. B. Not a true sagittal section as the nasal tip is not clearly defined and the orthogonal osseous extension at the front end of the maxilla is visible (arrow).

hyperechoic rectangular block of the palate, the dark, hypoechoic diencephalon of the forebrain and the nuchal membrane (Fig. 7.6A). If you cannot see the tip of the nose, and/or can see the orthogonal osseous extension at the front end of the maxilla (Fig. 7.6B), you have not achieved a true sagittal section and will usually need to decrease the angle of the probe to the maternal skin.

Alternatively, you may have the correct angle but the section is not quite sagittal – that is, it is parasagittal. If this is the case, a minimal sliding movement of the probe towards the middle of the fetus should produce the correct section. As with the correct section for the CRL described earlier, the fetal neck should be neither flexed nor extended.

The strong linear echo produced by the nuchal membrane is very similar in appearance to that produced by the amnion. Because your aim is to measure the nuchal translucency and not the distance between the fetal neck and the edge of the amniotic cavity, you must make sure that you can distinguish between the two. This can be problematic if the fetus is lying directly adjacent to the amniotic membrane. If it is not possible to distinguish one from the other, you must wait until the fetus moves away from the amnion to allow you to be certain of the depth of the nuchal translucency before attempting its measurement.

The image you have obtained should demonstrate the nuchal membrane in continuity with the skin of the skull and extending, as an unbroken line, through the neck region and into the upper thorax. The depth of the translucency should be roughly the same through its length and the translucency itself should be homogeneously hypoechoic (or black) throughout. If the nuchal membrane in your image appears broken or interrupted and/or the depth of the translucency is very variable through its length, it is likely that the fetus is lying with its head turned slightly to one side. This makes trying to obtain a sagittal section of both the head and the upper thorax very difficult because of your probe's inability to image more than two structures that are not in a straight line. Very small rotational movements of the probe may enable you to obtain a better section, but this will depend on how rotated the head is away from the body.

The image selected for measurement should include only the fetal head and upper thorax. It is easier to search for the true sagittal section using an image size in which the whole fetus can be seen, only increasing the magnification of the image to include just the head and upper thorax once you have achieved the correct section for measurement.

GETTING THE CORRECT SECTION IN PRACTICE

We recommend the following.

If your machine has a preprogrammed NT setting or, failing this, a first trimester setting, select this before going any further. Because the area of interest when measuring the NT is essentially made up of strong white echoes and black echoes, with very few shades of grey in between, a low dynamic range should be selected.

There is ongoing debate as to whether or not harmonic imaging should be used when measuring the NT as the original data set was produced before this imaging process was a standard option. It is questionable whether it is preferable to work with a possibly suboptimal image produced using the fundamental frequency only or with a clearer image produced using some level of harmonic imaging. Our view is that a better image is more likely to produce a more accurate NT measurement, and so we recommend using harmonic imaging if this provides the better image.

Make sure the read zoom control is set to zero. Adjust the depth control so that the uterus fills the screen (Fig. 7.1A). Having surveyed the uterus and identified the fetal pole, apply the write zoom box over the fetal pole such that the length of the box is slightly longer than the length of the fetus and the height of the box is approximately three times the anteroposterior depth of the fetus.

Activate the write zoom box and, using this image magnification, obtain an approximate sagittal section of the fetus. Now, using the read zoom control, magnify the image so that only the fetal head and upper thorax occupy the screen (Fig. 7.6A).

As the thickness of the nuchal membrane is affected by the gain settings, reduce the gain setting as much as is possible while still maintaining your ability to see the required landmarks. Providing the fetus remains quiescent, you can now make your small probe movements to achieve the perfect sagittal section.

If the fetus moves, your carefully sought section is likely to have disappeared off screen and, unfortunately, you will have to start the process again. As such fetal movements tend to be both rapid and short-lived, employing the cine-loop facility will make recapturing the optimal section much easier.

WHEN OBTAINING A CORRECT SECTION IS NOT POSSIBLE

When the correct section from which to measure an accurate NT cannot be obtained within a timely fashion, the following options are available:

- option 1: Attempt to alter the position of the fetus by (a) asking the woman to change her position (rolling onto her left side and then onto her right side several times) on the couch; (b) lifting the foot of the scanning couch to tilt the woman head down; and/or (c) asking her to get off the couch and move around briefly in the scanning room
- option 2: Rescan the woman after an interval of time, within the same scanning session
- option 3: Give the woman a second appointment within the required CRL/ gestational age window for combined screening
- option 4: Advise the woman that combined screening will not be possible and that her Down's screening risk should be calculated from a quadruple test at around 16 weeks (see Chapter 8).

The option which you choose will depend on the availability of resources. Rescanning the woman within the same scanning session will affect not only your scanning session but also, potentially, those of your colleagues. Many departments do not have sufficient resources to offer a second appointment for NT measurement and therefore the quadruple test will be the only option available to a proportion of women.

It is important that women understand the limitations associated with the ultrasound component of combined screening if an accurate and high-quality screening service is to be provided.

WHEN OBTAINING A CORRECT SECTION IS NOT POSSIBLE IN THE LARGER WOMAN

As discussed in Chapter 1, it is an unfortunate but unavoidable fact of ultrasound imaging that there is a steady decline in amplitude of the incident sound wave with increasing depth. You will therefore know that this occurs for two reasons. First, each reflection at successive tissue interfaces removes some energy from the pulse leaving less for the generation of later echoes further into the tissue. Second, tissue absorbs ultrasound strongly and so there is a steady loss of energy simply because the ultrasound pulse is travelling through tissue. Thus the greater the tissue mass lying between the probe and the fetus, the greater will be the attenuation of the sound wave on its inward path from the probe and on its outward path from the section of the fetus you are trying to image.

The assumption therefore is that image quality from a pregnant woman of a lower body mass index (BMI) is likely to be superior to that from a woman with a higher BMI. This is generally true although it is incorrect to assume that the image quality from overweight or obese women will automatically be poor, just as it is incorrect to assume that the images from a woman with a low BMI will automatically be wonderful.

The difficulties often encountered of trying to obtain diagnostic images in the large, overweight or obese woman are compounded when trying to measure an accurate NT.

This is due to the combination of the following factors:

- the acute positioning of the wrist often required to obtain the correct section
- the additional downward pressure of the scanning hand and arm required to reduce the large distance between the probe face and the fetus
- the lateral pressure on the scanning hand and arm required to find, and maintain, an acoustic window on the maternal abdomen inferior to the fold, or folds, of her fat.

As a sonographer performing similar physical tasks repeatedly you are at risk of developing or acquiring a repetitive strain injury and it is important that you learn to minimize this risk from the start of your ultrasound career. It is not sensible to perform, or continue to perform, an examination which causes you pain in your hand, wrist, arm, shoulder or neck. Should this happen, you should complete the examination as soon as reasonably possible, giving due consideration to both the needs of the woman and to you.

In situations where the image quality is compromised by maternal size, it is sensible to measure the CRL first, before attempting to measure the NT. Thus if the examination has to be curtailed before a satisfactory NT can be obtained and measured, quadruple testing at the appropriate time can be offered because, as you have already measured the CRL, the gestational age can be calculated.

Where maternal size is affecting image quality such that the correct section for NT cannot be obtained, offering the woman a further appointment is of limited value and is arguably a poor use of limited resources. This is because the image quality is unlikely to improve simply because the fetus is a few days larger. We suggest that quadruple testing at the appropriate time should be the preferred option in this situation.

It is sensible to make sure that every woman you are about to scan is aware of the limitations of the test before you start her examination, including the fact that image quality is often affected by size of the mother, with poorer images being obtained from larger mothers. If you explain these issues to every woman, you will become confident in dealing with the range of reactions you will receive. This in turn will give you confidence when discussing these issues with overweight or obese women for whom this understanding is particularly relevant.

The sensitivities surrounding maternal size are well-recognized, and it is unfortunate that many larger women come for their first scan with very little understanding of the association between ultrasound image quality and maternal size or the impact that maternal size can have on the health of the sonographer.

CALLIPER PLACEMENT

The required calliper placement for measuring the NT differs from that used in all other fetal biometry employed routinely.

Measurements described elsewhere in this text require the centre of the intersection of the cross, either the 'x' type or the '+' type, of the measuring system to be placed on the border of the structure being measured. This is because the measurement displayed by the machine is calculated from the distance between the central points of the intersection of the crosses of the two callipers. The required placement of the intersection of the cross should normally be on the inner or the outer border of the relevant structure. As discussed previously, the mean gestational sac diameter measurement, for example, is obtained from three *inner-to-inner* measurements; the HC is measured by placing the ellipse around the outer skull border, whereas the BPD can be obtained from either an *outer-to-inner* calliper placement or from an *outer-to-outer* calliper placement.

By contrast the correct measurement of the NT requires what is called the *on-to-on* placement of the callipers (Fig. 7.7). Assuming the fetus is lying supine, this technique describes the placement of the leading edge of the horizontal bar of the '+' type calliper over the outer edge of the echo from the fetal neck anteriorly and over the inner edge of the nuchal membrane posteriorly. This means that the centre of the intersection of the callipers does not lie at the anterior and posterior borders of the NT, respectively, but the width of half the thickness of the horizontal bar of each calliper into the echo from the fetal neck anteriorly and the nuchal membrane posteriorly. Thus the measurement of the NT displayed is the depth of the

translucency plus half the thickness of each calliper bar, i.e. the depth of the translucency plus the thickness of one calliper bar. This is of no significance to risk associated with the NT measurement because the calculation is based on the calliper placement as described by the originating authors. It is only raised here for completeness and to provide an answer to the enquiring mind of the ultrasound student.

MEASURING THE NT

The NT should be across the widest part of the translucency, using the on-to-on technique described earlier. As a novice, it is good practice to measure the NT, delete the callipers and repeat the process twice more from the same image as this will increase your awareness of your own intraoperator variability. As with measurement of the CRL, we recommend that you take and measure three separate images of the NT. The measurements should all agree to ±0.1 mm. The largest measurement of a correctly measured sagittal image should be recorded and used for risk assessment.

The effects of correctly selecting the widest part of the NT to measure but then placing one or both callipers across the NT incorrectly are shown in Fig. 7.8.

The effect of placing the callipers correctly but selecting the incorrect part of the NT to measure is shown in Fig. 7.8.

The Impact of NT on Risk

As the Down's risk conferred by the NT is determined by the CRL, a certain combination of NT and CRL measurements will affect a woman's background risk to the same extent irrespective of her age.

Let us consider a pregnancy of 12 weeks' gestation, dated from a CRL of 56.0 mm. The NT is 1.5 mm, which lies on the 50th centile for the CRL.

As the NT-related risk is based on the CRL, an approximately fivefold reduction in the background risk is conferred on the pregnancy by a 50th centile NT, irrespective of maternal age. As can be seen from Table 7.2, the change in risk is the same irrespective of whether the mother is 20, 30, 40 or 44 years of age at term.

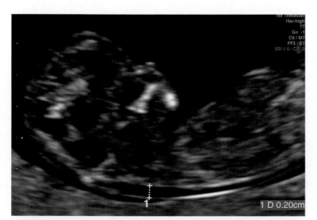

Fig 7.7 • The correct measurement of the nuchal translucency requires what is called the 'on-to-on' placement of the callipers. Assuming the fetus is lying supine, this technique describes the placement of the leading edge of the horizontal bar of the + type calliper over the outer edge of the echo from the fetal neck anteriorly and over the inner edge of the nuchal membrane posteriorly as demonstrated here.

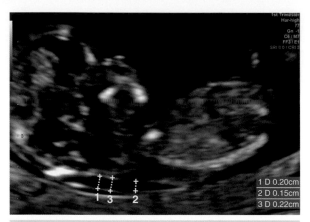

Fig 7.8 • The effects of correctly selecting the widest part of the NT to measure but then placing one or both callipers across the NT incorrectly are shown. Measurement 1 demonstrates the correct placement of the callipers with an on-to-on measurement. Measurement 2 demonstrates an inner to inner measurement and is also not measuring the widest part of the NT. Measurement 3 demonstrates an outer to outer measurement. This results in an overestimation of the NT by 0.2 mm. NT, nuchal translucency.

The relationship remains across the NT range. Thus an NT of 2.3 mm, at the upper end of the normal range for the same CRL of 56.0 mm, confers an approximate doubling of risk irrespective of maternal age, as can be seen from Table 7.3.

The impact of very small increases in NT is large towards, and above, the upper end of the normal range. As can be seen from Table 7.4, an NT of 2.2 mm, which lies just below the 95th centile for the CRL of 56.0 mm is risk-neutral – that is, it confers a risk which is approximately the same as the background risk.

By contrast, and as we have seen previously, an NT that is only 0.1 mm larger, and on the 95th centile, will double the background risk. Adding a further 0.2 mm to give an NT of 2.5 mm brings the NT outside the normal range, with the resulting approximately fourfold increase in risk (Table 7.4).

This underlines the impact that your intraoperator variability will have on the sensitivity of the

MATERNAL AGE (YEARS)	AGE-RELATED RISK AT TERM	ADJUSTED RISK AT TERM NT 1.5 mm	CHANGE IN RISK
20	1:1528	1:7877	5.15 × decrease
30	1:906	1:4667	5.15 × decrease
40	1:112	1:571	5.10 × decrease
44	1:37	1:188	5.10 × decrease

Table 7.2 Maternal age and the age-related risk, the risk at term adjusted from an NT measurement of 1.5 mm and a CRL of 56.0 mm, and the resultant change. The NT lies on the 50th centile for the CRL
CRL, crown rump length; *NT*, nuchal translucency.

MATERNAL AGE (YEARS)	AGE-RELATED RISK AT TERM	ADJUSTED RISK AT TERM NT 2.3 mm	CHANGE IN RISK
20	1:1528	1:764	2.00 × increase
30	1:906	1:454	1.99 × increase
40	1:112	1:56	2.00 × increase
44	1:37	1:19	1.95 × increase

Table 7.3 Maternal age and the age-related risk, the risk at term adjusted from an NT measurement of 2.3 mm and a CRL of 56.0 mm, and the resultant change. The NT is at the upper end of the normal range for the CRL
CRL, crown rump length; *NT*, nuchal translucency.

MATERNAL AGE (YEARS)	AGE-RELATED RISK AT TERM	ADJUSTED RISK AT TERM			
		NT 1.5 mm	NT 2.2 mm	NT 2.3 mm	NT 2.5 mm
20	1:1528	1:7877	1:1378	1:764	1:363
30	1:906	1:4667	1:817	1:454	1:216
40	1:112	1:571	1:101	1:56	1:27
44	1:37	1:188	1:34	1:19	1:10

Table 7.4 Maternal age and the age-related risk, the risk at term adjusted from NT measurements on the 50th centile, just below, at and above the 95th centile for a CRL of 56.0 mm

CRL, crown rump length; NT, nuchal translucency.

NT MEASUREMENT (mm)	ADJUSTED RISK AT TERM
1.4	1:1641
1.5	1:1569
1.6	1:1384
2.1	1:469
2.2	1:275
2.3	1:153

Table 7.5 The effect of an intraoperator variability of 0.1 mm on the risk at term from NT measurements on the 50th centile and just below the 95th centile for a CRL of 56.0 mm in a 36 year old woman with an age-related risk at term of 1:305

CRL, crown rump length; NT, nuchal translucency.

screening test risk assessment. We have recommended that your aim should be for a personal intraoperator variability of ±0.1 mm when taking NT measurements.

Consider, therefore, what this means to the risk your NT measurements of 1.5 mm and 2.2 mm are actually conferring to a woman of 36 years of age with a fetus of CRL 56.0 mm. The woman's age-related risk at term is 1:305. As can be seen from Table 7.5, the 50th centile NT measurement of 1.5 mm in theory produces, as expected, an approximate fivefold reduction of risk, to 1:1569. In reality, your NT measurement of 1.5 mm combined with your intraoperator variability of 0.1 mm means that the measurement lies between 1.4 mm and 1.6 mm. The adjusted risk therefore lies somewhere between 1:1641 and 1:1384. As these risks are all very low, your variability around 1.5 mm will have little clinical consequence.

It does, however, have a much more marked effect towards and above the 95th centile, as can be seen by considering your NT measurement of 2.2 mm. The adjusted risk here produces an increase in risk from the age-related risk of 1:305 to the adjusted risk of 1:275. Although increased, this risk remains well below the risk threshold of 1:150. In reality, however, your NT measurement of 2.2 mm combined with your intraoperator variability of 0.1 mm means that the measurement lies between 2.1 mm and 2.3 mm. The adjusted risk therefore lies somewhere between 1:469 and 1:153, one an encouraging reduction in the age-related risk and the other coming very close to the threshold risk of 1:150, although still just remaining a lower risk result.

These examples again emphasize why measuring the NT properly is so important when assessing the risk of Down's syndrome with combined screening.

THE IMPLICATIONS OF NT ABOVE THE 95TH CENTILE

By definition the NT measurement obtained from 5% of chromosomally normal fetuses will lie above the normal range – that is, above the 95th centile. We have established that the risk of Down's syndrome increases with increasing NT, as do the risks of other chromosomal abnormalities. In addition to the increasing risk of abnormal karyotypes,

143

NT	ABNORMAL KARYOTYPE	FETAL DEATH	MAJOR FETAL ABNORMALITY EXCLUDING CARDIAC	CARDIAC ABNORMALITY
<95th centile	0.2%	1.2%	1.4%	0.2%
95th–99th centile	3.7%	1.3%	1.5%	1.0%
3.5–4.4 mm	21.1%	2.7%	7.0%	3.0%
>6.5 mm	64.5%	19.0%	16.2%	30.0%

Table 7.6 Percentage association among NT and abnormal karyotype and major fetal and cardiac abnormalities
NT, nuchal translucency; <, less than; >, more than.

the risks of poor outcomes, including fetal death and structural abnormalities, also increase with increasing NT, as shown in Table 7.6.

Historically there has been much debate as to what size of NT should be used to provide a risk threshold above which further follow-up should be offered, over and above that which would be provided because of the resulting high Down's risk. Many experts consider a 3% risk to be one which warrants further investigation. As can be seen from Table 7.6, an NT of 3.5–4.4 mm is associated with a 10% risk of major structural abnormalities, of which 3% are cardiac, together with a 2.7% risk of fetal death. These data underpin the current national recommendation to use 3.5 mm to define the 'abnormal' NT, at and above which referral for further investigations should be offered. This cut-off applies irrespective of whether or not combined screening for Down's syndrome constitutes part of the examination.

You should therefore manage the finding of any NT of 3.5 mm in a similar way as the finding of, for example, anencephaly or fetal demise, namely refer to a fetal medicine specialist for the appropriate further management.

It should be remembered, however, that once chromosomal abnormalities have been excluded, about 90% of pregnancies in which an increased NT of less than 4.5 mm is present will result in a healthy live birth. The corresponding figures for 4.5–6.4mm and 6.5 mm and above are 80% and 45%, respectively.

Due to the association between structural cardiac abnormalities and NT of 3.5 mm or greater, women with pregnancies in which an NT of this size is detected should be offered referral for detailed fetal cardiac screening, over and above that which is normally offered at the routine anomaly scan. Detailed cardiac screening is typically offered between 16 and 18 weeks, with a follow-up examination at around 22 weeks. The expectation of the earlier scan is the detection of those major cardiac abnormalities which would initiate discussion around surgery/intervention in the first year of life or, alternatively, termination of pregnancy. We recommend that the first scan is performed nearer to 18 weeks than 16 weeks. This is because the 16 week fetus is more frequently in a vertical position and/or lies with its chin on its chest than the 18 week fetus. Thus obtaining the correct sections of the heart in a small fetus in this position is therefore correspondingly more challenging, even for the most experienced of operators. The expectations of the later scan are to confirm the normal findings of the first scan, possibly to identify features of a progressive abnormality or to identify minor abnormalities, such as a small ventricular septal defect (VSD), which would be unlikely to result in any significant morbidity after delivery.

Finding an NT of 3.5 mm or greater is therefore a reason for tertiary referral for detailed cardiac screening irrespective of its impact on the Down's risk for the pregnancy and irrespective of whether or not the woman requests or declines Down's screening, as discussed on page 154.

THE IMPACT OF THE CRL MEASUREMENT ON COMBINED SCREENING RISK ASSESSMENT

Accurate assessment of the Down's risk is dependent on accurate measurement of the CRL for the following reasons.

First, the gestational age is calculated from the CRL. Second, the age of the mother at conception, and therefore her Down's risk at term, is calculated from the gestational age of her pregnancy. Third, the serum analyte MoMs are calculated from the gestational age. Finally, the risk conferred from the NT is based on the CRL rather than the gestational age.

Thus if the CRL is measured incorrectly and is underestimated, the true gestational age of the pregnancy will be underestimated (Fig. 7.1B). The mother will therefore be thought, incorrectly, to be older at the time of conception than she actually in fact was. As the risk of Down's syndrome increases with increasing maternal age, the mother's age-related risk of Down's syndrome will therefore be increased, resulting in an increase in the false-positive rate of the test.

The level of PAPP-A increases and the level of free βhCG decreases with gestational age. As the risk calculated from each is based on gestational age, underestimating the gestational age by underestimating the CRL will affect their MoMs.

As can be seen from Table 7.7, underestimating the CRL by 5.0 mm, for example, will increase the PAPP-A MoM from 1.0 MoM to 1.17 MoM and decrease the free βhCG MoM from 1.0 MoM to 0.93 MoM. The change in both MoMs away from the Down's pattern will therefore decrease the detection rate for Down's syndrome but also decrease the false-positive rate of the test.

Conversely, overestimating the CRL by 5.0 mm will decrease the PAPP-A MoM from 1.0 MoM to 0.87 MoM and increase the free βhCG MoM from 1.0 MoM to 1.07 MoM. The change in both MoMs towards the Down's pattern will therefore increase the detection rate for Down's syndrome but also increase the false-positive rate, as can be seen in Table 7.7.

CLINICAL MANAGEMENT OF THE SCREEN POSITIVE RESULT

The threshold risk is used to provide a cut-off above which the implications of a screen positive result should be discussed with the woman. Such a discussion currently will normally revolve around whether or not the woman wishes to proceed with a diagnostic test, which may be either a chorionic villous sampling (CVS) test or an amniocentesis test. As both involve putting a needle into the uterus, to remove placental tissue in the case of a CVS or the fetal cells contained within the amniotic fluid in the case of amniocentesis, both tests carry a miscarriage risk. This procedure-related risk is normally quoted as 1%. This 1% risk is in addition to the background miscarriage risk at the time that either test is performed.

CRL ERROR (mm)	MEDIAN MoM		DETECTION RATE	FALSE-POSITIVE RATE
	PAPP-A	FREE βhCG		
0	1.00	1.00	85%	2.7%
−5	1.17	0.93	80%	1.4%
−3	1.10	0.96	82%	1.9%
+5	0.87	1.07	89%	5.5%
+3	0.92	1.04	87%	4.1%

Table 7.7 Effects of under- and overmeasuring the CRL on MoM values for PAPP-A, free βhCG, the detection rate for Down's syndrome and the false-positive rate for the combined screening test

βhCG, beta human chorionic gonodotropin; CRL, crown rump length; MoM, multiple of the median; PAPP-A, pregnancy-associated plasma protein A.

The data set used in this example has a detection rate for the condition of 85% for a false-positive rate of 2.7% and a cut-off between high and low risk of 1 in 250.

The CVS test can be performed at any time after 11 weeks of pregnancy and amniocentesis after 15 weeks of pregnancy. Although the background miscarriage risk is higher in the first trimester than the second trimester, it is important that the woman is aware that CVS does not put her pregnancy at any greater risk of miscarriage than amniocentesis. This is because the procedure-related risk of 1% is the same for both tests.

The first method of fetal karyotyping required culturing of the fetal cells contained within the amniotic fluid sample. This process took 2–3 weeks and provided analysis of the full chromosomal complement of the cells examined, using visual examination of the stained individual chromosomes under a microscope. This process is still carried out for conditions that cannot be detected using the more modern technique of quantitative fluorescence polymerase chain reaction (QF-PCR).

After removal of either the placental or amniotic fluid sample, QF-PCR is used to assess a specified subset of chromosomes, most commonly the three common trisomies, namely 21, 18, 13, although testing of the sex chromosomes, primarily for 45XO, can also be carried out. This test provides what is termed rapid diagnosis, as the results are normally available within 48 hours of the sample being taken.

With the increasing sophistication of DNA analysis techniques, the landscape of prenatal diagnostic testing is changing rapidly, with microarray analysis of specific genes or gene groups within individual chromosomes becoming more readily available.

A noninvasive alternative to CVS and amniocentesis has recently become available, namely noninvasive prenatal testing (NIPT). This test determines the chromosomal status of the fetus from various types of fetal material within the maternal serum, the specific type of NIPT applied being determined by the type of material being tested. The test is currently used primarily to assess the probability of the fetus being affected with trisomy 21. The results are typically reported in the following way: 'the detection rate for Tri 21 being greater than 99% for a false-positive rate of less than 0.1%'.

The risks for trisomies 18 and 13 can also be calculated. The sensitivity of the test for trisomy 18 is slightly lower than for trisomy 21, at 98%; for trisomy 13 it is around 80%. The quoted false-positive rate of <0.1% is the same as for trisomy 21.

Until NIPT has been validated by screening-based studies, its provision as a routine alternative to invasive diagnostic testing remains outside the remit of hospital-based care in this country.

As discussed earlier, where the NT is 3.5 mm or greater, a further discussion regarding detailed cardiac screening should take place. For a woman who has decided to have a diagnostic test, it may be preferable to delay making the arrangements for cardiac screening until the karyotypic status of her pregnancy is known.

Some departments may offer women with a screen positive result for Down's syndrome, and who decline diagnostic testing, an early anomaly scan at 16–18 weeks. The purpose of this examination is to look for appearances in the fetus which are associated with Down's syndrome, such as a cardiac abnormality, increased nuchal fold, echogenic bowel and/or short femur lengths. When identified, these appearances may alter the woman's initial decision regarding diagnostic testing.

The same principle may apply for women with a screen positive result for Edwards' and Patau's syndromes. The characteristic appearances associated with Edwards' syndrome are flexion deformities of the hands, overlapping fingers, omphalocele, cardiac abnormalities and rocker bottom feet. The characteristic appearances associated with Patau's syndrome are holoprosencephaly and other midline facial abnormalities (see Appendix 11).

It should be remembered that, although normal appearances of the fetus are reassuring, only approximately 50% of fetuses with Down's syndrome will have features that can be detected on ultrasound in the second trimester. This is not because these features are overlooked in 50% of Down's fetuses due to poor technique, but rather that these features are not present in this proportion of Down's fetuses.

The current national recommendation is that only one screening test should be offered for a specific condition. It is perhaps interesting to consider the rationale behind offering an anomaly scan with a detection rate of around 50% for Down's syndrome rather than a quadruple screening blood test, with a detection rate of around 75% for Down's syndrome, as a second screening test, following 1st trimester combined screening.

The percentage of fetuses with Edwards' or Patau's syndromes that have features that can be detected on ultrasound in the second trimester is reported as around 80%. For this reason, the second trimester screening test of choice for trisomies 18 and 13 is the routine anomaly scan rather than the quadruple test.

It should also be remembered that excluding abnormalities in a 16 week fetus may not be as effective as in a larger fetus. This is due first to size – the 16 week fetus and its corresponding anatomical parts being noticeably smaller than its older comparators. Second, and often more significant, is fetal position. The longitudinal axis of the younger fetus is much more likely to be vertical within the uterus, rather than the more horizontal plane adopted by the older fetus. It is extremely difficult, if not impossible, to obtain the required transverse sections of the vertical fetus because this requires being able to position the probe effectively parallel to the scanning couch. Of the three possible scanning planes, this is usually only possible in the third trimester fetus when the dome of the larger uterus provides the necessary access.

INFORMATION REQUIRED FOR ACCURATE RISK ASSESSMENT FROM COMBINED SCREENING

In pregnancies affected with Down's syndrome, PAPP-A levels are about 50% lower than those seen in unaffected pregnancies and free βhCG is a little more than twice as high as levels seen in unaffected pregnancies. By contrast, both markers are about 80% lower in pregnancies affected with Edwards' syndrome. In Patau's syndrome, PAPP-A levels are about 75% lower and free βhCG about 50% lower than those seen in unaffected pregnancies. The mean MoM values for PAPP-A and free βhCG for trisomies 21, 18 and 13 are given in Table 7.1.

The need for accurate measurements of the CRL and NT and an accurate knowledge of the age of the biological mother at ovulation has already been discussed. Knowledge of whether the pregnancy is singleton or multiple is obviously necessary. Trisomy screening in multiple pregnancy is discussed in Chapter 15.

In addition, the pregnant woman's weight, ethnicity and smoking status since conception/embryo transfer should be known in order that the most accurate assessment of risks can be calculated from the combined screening test. This information is required for the following reasons.

Maternal Weight

There is an inverse relationship between maternal weight and first trimester biochemical marker levels. This means that in heavier women biochemical marker levels will tend to be lower because of the dilution effect of their larger blood volume and, conversely, marker levels will tend to be more concentrated in lighter women because of their smaller blood volume.

Failure to correct maternal weight will result in inaccurate assessments of risk for all three trisomies, as shown in Table 7.8.

Ethnicity

PAPP-A levels are approximately 60% higher and free βhCG approximately 20% higher in Afro-Caribbean women compared with Caucasian women. In South Asian women, PAPP-A and free βhCG are lower at 2% and 8%, respectively. Without appropriate correction for ethnicity there would be a decrease in detection rate for all three trisomies in Afro-Caribbean women and an increase in false-positive rate for South Asian women.

Smoking

Both PAPP-A and free βhCG levels are lower in smokers compared with nonsmokers. Failing to correct for smoking will result in an increase in false-positive rate for all trisomies.

Other factors

Other factors taken into account when calculating the risk of aneuploidy are insulin-dependent diabetes, in vitro fertilization treatment, and multiple pregnancies.

AFTERCARE

Having successfully measured the CRL and the NT and recorded the information required by the laboratory for the accurate measurement of the

	HEAVIER WOMEN		LIGHTER WOMEN	
	LEVEL OF ANALYTE	SCREENING EFFECT	LEVEL OF ANALYTE	SCREENING EFFECT
DOWN'S SYNDROME				
PAPP-A	Lower	Increase FPR	Higher	Decrease DTR
Free βhCG	Lower	Decrease DTR	Higher	Increase FPR
EDWARDS' AND PATAU'S SYNDROMES				
PAPP-A	Lower	Increase FPR	Higher	Decrease DTR
Free βhCG	Lower	Increase FPR	Higher	Decrease DTR

Table 7.8 The effect of maternal weight on PAPP-A and free βhCG in the detection rate and false-positive rate of Down's, Edwards' and Patau's syndromes

βhCG, beta human chorionic gonadotropin; *DTR*, detection rate; *FPR*, false-positive rate; *PAPP-A*, pregnancy-associated plasma protein A.

maternal serum analytes, you must make sure the woman is aware that she should have her blood taken immediately after the scan. The woman's blood should therefore be taken before she leaves the hospital or, if phlebotomy services are not available in the same location as the ultrasound department, as soon as possible and ideally within the next 24 hours.

You should also inform the woman of the length of time that will elapse before she receives her combined screening result, whether this differs depending on whether her risk is a lower risk result or a higher risk result, how she will receive her result and that she should keep the result in her personal maternity record if the result is sent to her in paper format.

A delay in having her blood taken may decrease the accuracy of the woman's overall screening test. It may also mean that the gestational age of the pregnancy falls outside the gestational window for combined screening.

WHEN MEASURING AN ACCURATE CRL IS NOT POSSIBLE

The ability to date a pregnancy accurately requires accurate measurement of the CRL or, if this is not possible, of the HC. The ability to calculate a combined screening risk for Down's syndrome requires accurate measurement of the CRL. It therefore

stands to reason that combined screening will not be an option for the woman in whom an accurate CRL cannot be measured, even if an accurate NT measurement can be obtained. Such women should have their EDD assigned from the HC measurement and should be offered quadruple test screening for Down's syndrome. Quadruple test screening is discussed in Chapter 8.

It can be seen from Appendix 3 that an HC of 80.0 mm and greater can be used to date the pregnancy and that the gestational age equivalent of this measurement is 12 weeks and 4 days. It can also be seen from Appendix 3 that the gestational age equivalent of 101.0 mm is 14 weeks and 1 day, which is the also the gestational age equivalent of a CRL of 84.0 mm.

There will be a small number of women in whom you are unable to measure an accurate CRL but in whom the HC measurement gives a gestational age of less than 14 weeks and 1 day. It is important that these women understand that they cannot be offered combined screening because the CRL is greater than 84.0 mm. They are therefore being offered quadruple screening even though the gestational age of their pregnancy is still within the window for combined screening.

Table 7.9 summarizes our practical recommendations for dating pregnancies with and without screening for Down's, Edwards' and Patau's syndromes.

PARAMETER (mm)	DOWN'S SYNDROME SCREENING	MEASURE NT	SCREENING METHOD	PARAMETER FOR DATING & EDD
CRL 45.0–84.0	Requested	Yes	Combined	CRL
CRL 45.0–84.0	Declined	n/a	n/a	CRL
CRL > 84.0	Requested	No	Quadruple	HC (do not use or report CRL)
CRL > 84.0	Declined	n/a	n/a	HC (do not use or report CRL)
HC < 101.0 and CRL > 84.0	Requested	No	Quadruple test (ideally at 16 weeks)	HC
HC < 101.0 and CRL > 84.0	Declined	n/a	n/a	HC
HC 101.0–172.0 and CRL > 84.0	Requested	No	Quadruple	HC
HC 101.0–172.0 and CRL > 84.0	Declined	n/a	n/a	HC

Table 7.9 Range of CRL and HC measurements that should be used to date pregnancies and recommended screening method for Down's syndrome when requested

From Chudleigh T, Loughna P, Evans T 2011 A practical solution to combining dating and screening for Down's syndrome. Ultrasound 19:154–1570.

CRL, crown rump length; *EDD,* expected date of delivery; *HC,* head circumference; *n/a,* not applicable; *NT,* nuchal translucency. <, less than; >, more than.

EXAMINING THE FETUS FOR STRUCTURAL ABNORMALITIES

The primary purpose of the 10–14-week scan is to date the pregnancy. The secondary purpose is to measure the NT in those pregnancies for which Down's, and/or Edwards' and Patau's syndromes screening is requested.

Thus your primary objective is to produce, assess and/or measure the appropriate sections that will enable you to assign the gestational age and, as an additional examination to which consent has been given, measure the NT.

The woman whom you are scanning must be aware that you may identify additional findings, including fetal abnormalities, during her scan that she is neither anticipating nor has necessarily consented to. It is hoped that the health professionals with whom the woman has already interacted will have informed her of these facts. It is your responsibility to ensure she understands that you have a professional duty to inform her of the relevant findings of the scan you are about to undertake.

At the current time there is debate as to the extent of the anatomical survey of the fetus that it is reasonable to include within the routine 10–14 week examination, irrespective of whether this examination is to date the pregnancy only or also to measure the NT. The woman should appreciate that a small number of fetal abnormalities can be identified within this gestational age range.

Some abnormalities, such as acrania (Fig. 7.9), may be apparent during the measuring of the CRL from a true sagittal section of the fetus. Others, such as alobar holoprosencephaly, may be apparent if the HC is measured (Fig. 7.10). Others, such as omphalocele (Fig. 7.11) or limb abnormalities, may be apparent if a more extended anatomical survey of the fetus is performed. The woman must

149

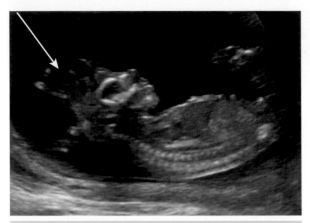

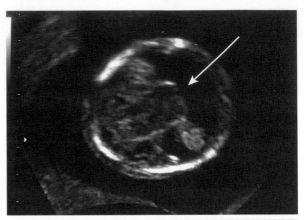

Fig 7.9 • Sagittal section of a 13 week fetus taken to measure the CRL. The cranial bones are absent and the remaining abnormal brain tissue (arrow) can be seen above the fetal orbits, exposed to the amniotic fluid. This fetus therefore has acrania. Compare these appearances to those of the normal fetuses of similar gestations shown in Fig. 7.1 and throughout this chapter.

Fig 7.10 • A cross section of the head of a 13+ week fetus with alobar holoprosencephaly. An abnormal cystic structure occupies the front portion of the skull (arrow). This is the sickle shaped single ventricle which is a classic feature of this condition.

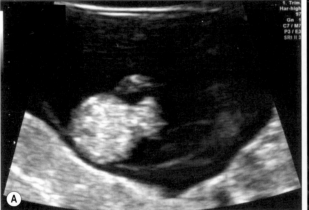

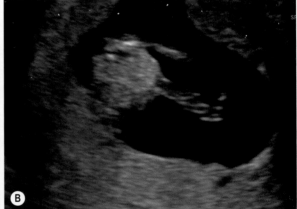

Fig 7.11 • Cross sections of the abdomen, at the level of the cord insertion, of two fetuses both between 12 and 13 weeks of gestation. There should be no abdominal contents still present in the base of the cord at this gestation. A. The appearance is strongly suggestive of an omphalocele as bowel can still be seen in the base of the cord. Compare with the normal appearance of the cord insertion shown in Fig. 7.11B.

understand that is your professional duty to tell her of these findings if present.

The abnormalities that can be detected within a routine ultrasound service carried out between 10 and 14 weeks, with transabdominal imaging, are discussed in the following section. These, therefore, are the abnormalities that you should be able to identify or exclude during the scans you perform between 10 and 14 weeks.

ACRANIA/EXENCEPHALY/ANENCEPHALY

The correct term to describe absence of the cranial bones or the vault is *acrania*. In acrania the fetal brain is present and may be normal in appearance or may demonstrate varying degrees of distortion and therefore be abnormal in appearance.

Acrania is the first stage of a progression through exencephaly to anencephaly.

Exencephaly describes the condition in which the absent cranial vault is accompanied by the progressive degeneration and disruption of the brain tissue because of its continuing exposure to the amniotic fluid. This is the most commonly seen appearance between 10 and 14 weeks of gestation.

Anencephaly is the final stage of the process in which the cerebral hemispheres have been eroded away, producing what is commonly described as the 'frog's eyes' appearance of true anencephaly. Progression to anencephaly does not normally occur until the second or third trimester.

Anencephaly is commonly used, incorrectly, to describe any one of these three conditions. We recommend that the term *acrania/exencephaly* be used to describe the typical first trimester appearances of an absent cranial vault in the presence of abnormal brain tissue.

The ultrasound detection of acrania is dependent on the ossification of the bones that comprise the vault.

Ossification of the skull begins at 10 weeks of gestation, and by 11 weeks it is normally possible to differentiate the hyperechoic bones of the vault from the brain tissue they surround (Fig. 7.5). By 12 weeks of gestation, the ossification of the fetal skull is normally complete and therefore sufficient to provide a continuous bright border around the fetal brain. This means that acrania can be excluded after 12 weeks of gestation and therefore should not be overlooked after this gestation. It also means that screening for acrania can be undertaken after 12 weeks. For this reason we recommend that the integrity of the fetal skull should always be assessed during measurement of the CRL after 12 weeks of gestation.

Ossification of the skull bones can and should be observed from the sagittal section used for the CRL. However, this is not the best section to confirm the normal appearances of the frontal, parietal and occipital bones of the vault. We consider it good clinical practice therefore also to obtain, assess and record a cross-section of the head at the level of the lateral ventricles, irrespective of whether an HC measurement is recorded. The integrity of the skull can be assessed properly from this section and acrania/exencephaly excluded (Fig. 7.9). Alobar holoprosencephaly and cystic hygroma can also be excluded from this section, as described later.

ALOBAR HOLOPROSENCEPHALY

Holoprosencephaly describes a spectrum of abnormalities associated with incomplete cleavage of the forebrain. The most severe type, alobar holoprosencephaly, is characterized by a single ventricular cavity and fusion of the two lobes of the thalamus. The normal butterfly shape of the two choroid plexuses is absent and is replaced by a sickle-shaped, single ventricular cavity in the anterior half of the skull (Fig. 7.10). Identifying the single ventricle may be difficult at 10–14 weeks, but failure to identify the normal 'butterfly' appearance should prompt suspicion and referral for more experienced review, as this appearance has a strong association with trisomy 13.

CYSTIC HYGROMA

Cystic hygroma (plural *hygromata*) is a large fluid-filled swelling that occurs in the posterolateral aspect of the fetal neck due to a failure in the connection between the lymphatic and venous systems. It is characterized by a sagittal septum extending across the depth of the hygroma from the cervical spine to the skin. Other septa, radiating out from the spine rather like the spokes of a wheel, may also be present. The skull is intact (Fig. 7.12).

These features distinguish cystic hygroma from nuchal translucency, which is not septated, and from an occipital encephalocele in which a defect in the skull is present.

Cystic hygroma is often associated with generalized hydrops – that is, skin oedema and ascites. It has a strong association with Turner's syndrome or 45XO. It has a weaker, but still significant, association with trisomy 21 and trisomy 18.

OMPHALOCELE

As discussed in Chapter 5, the physiological herniation of the bowel into the base of the umbilical cord takes place between 8 and 10 weeks of gestation (Fig. 7.13). The growth of the abdominal cavity is such that the bowel starts to return into the abdomen of the embryo at around 10 weeks of gestation. This process is normally completed approximately 1 week later.

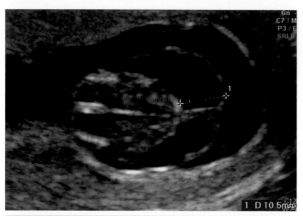

Fig 7.12 • A cystic hygroma can be identified from the head circumference section. It is characterized by a sagittal septum extending across the depth of the hygroma from the cervical spine to the skin. Other septa, radiating out from the spine rather like the spokes of a wheel, may also be present. The depth of fluid within the hygroma has been measured as 10.5 mm. The skull is intact.

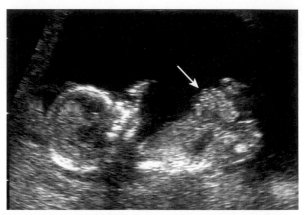

Fig 7.14 • Sagittal section of a 13 week fetus in which the frond-like appearance of the bowel, free floating in the amniotic fluid (arrow), can be seen. This is the typical appearance of the small bowel herniation in a case of gastroschisis.

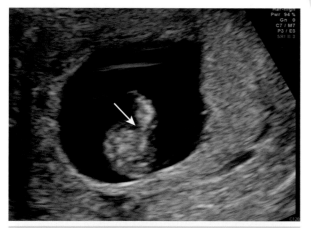

Fig 7.13 • A cross section of the abdomen of a 10 week fetus showing the normal physiological herniation of the gut into the base of the umbilical cord (arrow).

GASTROSCHISIS

The second abdominal wall defect amenable to diagnosis during this gestational age window is gastroschisis. As discussed in Chapter 11, this abnormality describes the herniation of usually small bowel only through a defect below, and to the right of, the cord insertion. Its origins therefore differ from those of an omphalocele, as does its typical appearance (Fig. 7.14).

As with omphalocele, we recommend that the diagnosis of gastroschisis is not made until 12 weeks of gestation, although its exclusion can be made from 10 weeks providing the cord insertion and abdominal wall are normal in appearance.

MEGACYSTIS

The fetal bladder can be identified from 10 weeks of gestation and is seen in approximately 95% of fetuses from 13 weeks of gestation. Confirmation of its presence will obviously depend on its fullness at the time of examination (Fig. 7.15).

The upper limit of the longitudinal diameter of the bladder between 10 and 14 weeks of gestation is 6.9 mm. Megacystis is defined as a longitudinal diameter of the bladder within this gestational age range of 7.0 mm and above (Fig. 7.16).

Omphalocele can therefore be excluded if a normal appearance of the cord insertion is obtained after 10 weeks. However, we recommend that the diagnosis of omphalocele should not be made until after 11 weeks of gestation at the earliest. We also recommend incorporating a safety margin of 1 week and for this reason suggest using 12 weeks as a cut-off (Fig. 7.11).

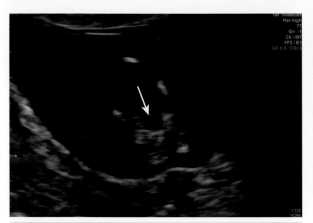

Fig 7.15 • Cross section of a 12 week fetus demonstrating the appearance of a normally full bladder (arrow).

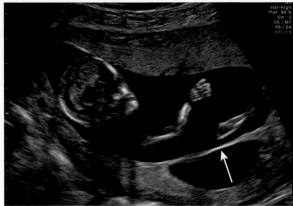

Fig 7.17 • Longitudinal section of the arm and hand of a 13 week fetus. Part of the humerus and one bone, the radius, of the lower arm together with the bones of the hand and the four extended fingers can be seen. This is a dichorionic twin pregnancy. Part of the dividing membrane can be seen (arrow).

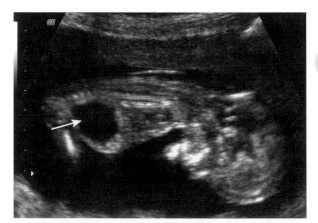

Fig 7.16 • Sagittal section of a prone, 13+ week fetus demonstrating an abnormally large bladder (arrow), the maximum longitudinal diameter of which was 9.8 mm.

ABSENT LIMB(S)

The incidence of severe skeletal dysplasias is extremely low. Thus the chance of appearances between 10 and 14 weeks of gestation raising the suspicion of one of this group of conditions is very small.

Detecting the absence of a whole limb or the distal portion of a limb is, however, within the capabilities of an examination at this gestation. Identifying the characteristic appearances of the limbs caused by the drug thalidomide, for example, would have been a realistic possibility had ultrasound screening been routinely available at the time of its use to treat morning sickness during the 1960s.

Although the hands and feet of the 10–14-week fetus are very small, detecting the absence of a whole hand or foot is, again, within the capabilities of the careful sonographer.

As the fetus tends to keep its hands open with its fingers extended at this gestation (Fig. 7.17), examination of the fingers to exclude gross abnormalities of the digits such as absent or fused whole digits, polydactyly and severe overlapping fingers is a possibility. However, we do not consider that exclusion of digital abnormalities should be an expectation of the routine service. As the toes are shorter, less splayed and therefore more difficult to examine, we do not consider their assessment for

Although the majority of cases of megacystis of 7–12 mm will resolve, megacystis can also be associated with chromosomal abnormalities and/or bladder outlet obstruction. Cases of megacystis should therefore always be referred to a fetal medicine specialist for discussion of their further management.

It is important to remember that, in contrast to the second and third trimester pregnancy, the amount of amniotic fluid present in the first trimester gestational sac cannot be used as an indicator of the normality or otherwise of the fetal urinary tract.

any of these conditions at this gestation to be a realistic expectation.

We also recommend that you evaluate the stomach and heart during your examination, as described in the following section.

STOMACH

The stomach can be identified in the majority of fetuses at 12 weeks of gestation. It appears as a circular, black or hypoechoic structure on the left side of the abdomen (Fig. 7.18). You should ensure that the stomach is positioned on the same side of the fetus as the heart and that this is the left side. Anatomically the stomach lies below the diaphragm and the heart above. The diaphragm may be difficult to visualize at this gestation, but you should attempt to confirm that the position of the stomach is below that of the heart.

HEART

Although it is optimistic to undertake a detailed examination of the heart at this gestation, you should be able to confirm the correct position of

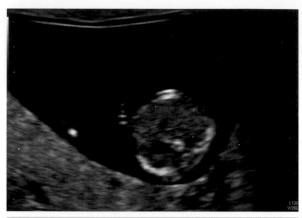

Fig 7.18 • Cross section of a 12 week fetus in which the stomach can be clearly identified within the abdomen; however, confirmation of its presence will obviously depend on its fullness at the time of the examination.

the heart, in the left side of the chest. We also recommend that you attempt to obtain a four-chamber view of the heart. You will discover that in many fetuses this is not an impossible task and that, in fact, you are often also able to image the outflow tracts.

SCAN MENUS

A woman should have decided whether she wishes to have a dating scan or combined screening for Down's, Edwards' and Patau's syndromes before she reaches your scanning room. The extent of the anatomical survey which you will attempt to include in either her dating scan or her scan for combined screening will depend on the guidelines agreed and recorded within your department for each of the three respective examinations.

The woman must understand that each type of scan includes a set menu of images that you will seek and assess. Let us consider each menu in turn.

THE 'DATING MENU'

During a 10–14-week dating scan there are a number of questions that will automatically be answered when examining the fetus before measuring the CRL.

These include the following:
- is an intrauterine pregnancy present?
- is the pregnancy a singleton or twin (or higher order of multiple) pregnancy?
- is the fetus alive?
- what is the gestational age based on the CRL?

The abnormalities that you may detect, and are wishing to exclude, during measurement of the CRL only are acrania/exencephaly, enlarged nuchal translucency, cystic hygroma and megacystis.

MANAGING THE WOMAN WHO DECLINES SCREENING FOR DOWN'S, EDWARDS' AND PATAU'S SYNDROMES

It is particularly important that a woman who does not wish to have screening for Down's, Edwards' and Patau's syndromes is aware of what is included in the 'dating menu'. She must understand that, irrespective of the fact that you will not be taking formal measurements of the NT, there may be abnormal appearances present that are associated with a number of conditions, and these include the three trisomies.

The association between an NT of ≥3.5 mm and structural cardiac abnormalities has been discussed previously. The woman who declines trisomy screening needs to be aware that, unless you are superhuman and able to distinguish between an NT of, for example, 3.2 mm and 3.6 mm by eye only, there may be the need to take measurements of the NT to decide whether or not the NT is ≥3.5 mm and therefore whether referral for detailed cardiac screening is necessary.

Some women find it difficult to understand that taking a measurement of the NT does not equate to trisomy screening so need to be reassured on this point. They also need to understand that Down's, Edwards' and Patau's syndromes are all conditions associated with a large NT so, although they do not want trisomy screening, it is correct that these associations should be discussed with them after referral to a fetal medicine specialist.

You should have this discussion with the woman before you start your examination. If the woman does not wish to accept all of what is included in the 'dating menu', then she must understand that you will be unable to offer her a scan.

THE 'COMBINED SCREENING MENU'

In addition to the questions posed during measurement of the CRL to date the pregnancy, the following question will automatically be answered when taking measurements of the NT.

- is the NT below or above 3.5 mm?
- is referral for detailed cardiac screening indicated?

AN 'ANATOMICAL SURVEY MENU'

The anatomical survey menu is an additional survey of the fetus that can be added to the dating menu or the combined screening menu.

We recommend that an anatomical survey scan includes the following:

- measurement of the HC
- assessment of the fetal anatomy in transverse section from the top of the fetal skull to the fetal rump, paying particular attention to the following:
  - the integrity of the skull
  - the normal appearance of the intracranial anatomy
  - the position of the heart in the left side of the chest, above the diaphragm if visible
  - the normal four-chamber view of the heart
  - the position of the stomach in the left abdomen, below the diaphragm if visible
  - the integrity of the abdominal wall
  - the normal appearance of the cord insertion
  - the presence and size of the fetal bladder
  - the presence and normal appearance of the four limbs
  - the presence and normal appearance of both hands including the fingers if possible
  - the presence and normal appearance of both feet.

The abnormalities that you may detect, and are wishing to exclude, during an anatomical survey are acrania/exencephaly, alobar holoprosencephaly, enlarged nuchal translucency, cystic hygroma, omphalocele, gastroschisis, megacystis, absence of a whole or part of a limb, absence of one or both hands and absence of one or both feet.

AMNIOTIC FLUID AND THE PLACENTA

The main purposes of this scan are to measure and assess the embryo or fetus, date the pregnancy, measure the nuchal translucency if requested, and exclude a range of structural abnormalities. The amniotic fluid and the placenta are also important features of the pregnant uterus, although their significance is of less relevance at this gestation than later in pregnancy.

AMNIOTIC FLUID VOLUME

Assessing amniotic fluid volume is of importance in the second and/or third trimester pregnancy because of its association with specific fetal structural abnormalities, growth problems and premature rupture of membranes. These relationships do not exist in the first trimester pregnancy. Furthermore, amniotic fluid volume at specific gestational ages in the first trimester shows minimal variation.

We suggest, therefore, that commenting on amniotic fluid volume in the first trimester pregnancy is of limited relevance.

PLACENTAL SITE

Identifying the position of the placenta within the uterus is of importance for diagnostic testing with CVS in the first trimester pregnancy. The position of the leading edge of the placenta relative to the internal os is of clinical significance in determining whether or not the pregnancy is at risk of placenta praevia. The relative positions of the cervix and uterus do not necessarily remain constant between the 10–14 week scan and the 18–22 week anomaly scan and this can affect the apparent placental site between the time frames. For this reason we do not recommend reporting the placental site at the routine 10–14 week scan.

REPORTING THE FINDINGS OF THE DATING SCAN AND OF THE COMBINED SCREENING SCAN

Having successfully completed your scan, you must now record your findings in the report. The woman should have a copy of this to place in her own handheld record and a further copy should be filed in the hospital medical record. The latter may be either a paper or an electronic copy.

We suggest the following template of information that should be included for a dating scan report:

- the date of the examination
- the reason for the examination
- the approach used, whether transabdominally, transvaginally or both
- recording of latex allergy and documentation of appropriate management if the transvaginal probe was used
- the number of fetuses present (for twin pregnancy, see Chapter 15)
- confirmation that the fetus was alive
- measurement of either the CRL, HC or both as appropriate

- gestational age as calculated from either the CRL or HC
- the EDD
- confirmation of the normal appearance, for the gestational age, of the fetal skull and brain as assessed during measurement of the CRL or as assessed during measurement of the HC
- confirmation of the normal appearance of the fetal bladder if visible
- documentation that the ovaries are of normal appearance (see Chapter 5) as this may prove useful later in the pregnancy
- a conclusion of the scan findings
- documentation of relevant management after the scan, such as referral if indicated and arrangements for the routine 18–22 week anomaly scan
- the name and professional role of the operator/supervisor

- the name and status of the trainee if performing any aspect of the examination.

In addition to these, we suggest the following template of information should be included for a combined screening scan report:

- measurement of NT
- arrangements for further management if NT ≥3.5 mm
- arrangements for taking of maternal blood for the completion of the combined screen.

Where an anatomical survey is also performed, we suggest the following template should be included in addition to the dating report or combined screening report template:

- confirmation of the normal appearances, for the gestational age, of the fetal stomach, abdominal wall, each of the four limbs, both hands and both feet.

Further reading

Altman D G, Chitty L S 1997 New charts for ultrasound dating of pregnancy. Ultrasound Obstet Gynecol 10:174–191

Loughna P, Chitty L, Evans T, Chudleigh T 2009 Fetal size and dating: charts recommended for clinical obstetric practice. Ultrasound 17:161–167

NHS Screening Programmes 2012 Measuring the NT and CRL as part of combined screening for trisomy 21 in England. In Manual for Ultrasound Practitioners. NHS Screening Programmes Fetal Anomaly. Version 2.

Robinson H P, Fleming J E E 1975 A critical evaluation of sonar crown rump length measurements. Ultrasound Obstet Gynecol 82:702–710

Salomon L J, Alfirevic Z, Timor-Tritsch I, et al 2013 ISUOG practice guidelines; performance of first-trimester fetal ultrasound scan. Ultrasound Obstet Gynecol 41:102–113

Souka A P, et al 1998 Defects and syndromes in chromosomally normal fetuses with increased nuchal translucency thickness at 10–14 weeks of gestation. Ultrasound Obstet Gynecol 11:391–400

CONTENTS

This chapter explains the techniques for taking measurements to date or assess growth in the second trimester and how to approach screening the pregnancy for structural abnormalities.

The aims of this chapter are to enable you to do the following:

- develop a checklist that addresses the measurements and sections of the fetus required to perform a routine second trimester scan
- measure the head circumference (HC), biparietal diameter (BPD), posterior horn of the lateral ventricle (PH), transcerebellar diameter (TCD), abdominal circumference (AC) and femur length (FL)
- assess fetal growth velocity or date the pregnancy and assign the expected date of delivery
- understand the elements of the routine second trimester anatomy scan
- assess the amniotic fluid volume

- localize the site of the placenta relative to the internal os
- understand the elements of quadruple test screening for Down's and other karyotypic abnormalities
- report the findings of the scan.

Examinations undertaken in the second trimester of pregnancy will normally be performed using the transabdominal approach, with the transvaginal route only being required in addition in a small number of cases. This chapter therefore addresses the transabdominal route only.

This text assumes that you, the operator, are sitting to the left of the scanning couch, holding the transabdominal probe in your right hand, that the woman is lying to your right side and that you are facing each other.

This chapter assumes that you are already able to locate the longitudinal axis of the second trimester fetus, to confirm it is alive and to determine its lie, presentation, and attitude as described in Chapter 3.

APPROACHING THE SECOND TRIMESTER SCAN

You will already be aware of the importance of the methodical approach to ultrasound examinations.

All ultrasound examinations should be associated with a 'tick list' which encompasses all the sections of the fetus that need to be obtained, all the measurements that need to be taken and all the parts of the anatomy that should be assessed. The purpose of this chapter is to help you develop your own second trimester tick list. It assumes that the scan you will be performing will be a routine second trimester anomaly scan.

You will obviously need a different tick list for a woman who is having her routine anomaly scan which succeeds an earlier dating or combined screening scan compared with the tick list for a first scan of the pregnancy. This is primarily because in the former situation you will be using the fetal measurements to assess the growth velocity of the fetus, whereas in the latter situation you will be using the fetal measurements obtained to date the pregnancy.

You will need a further tick list which can be used for the woman who has declined screening

for Down's and/or Edwards' and Patau's syndromes, as the interpretation of some findings will differ depending on whether the pregnancy has a low, a high or an unknown risk for one or more of these conditions.

We do not address the tick list required to perform a second trimester anomaly scan in a woman with an increased risk of Down's, Edwards' or Patau's syndrome, as a scan of this type is beyond the aims of this book.

The second trimester fetus provides you with an ideal opportunity to develop your methodical approach because, although the fetus is unlikely to remain completely still throughout the entire scan, it is usually sufficiently quiescent for you to open your mental checklist and work through it in a logical and efficient manner.

The main purpose of the majority of second trimester scans is to examine, and measure where appropriate, the fetal anatomy and to determine whether the appearances you have obtained are within the range of normal appearances expected for the gestational age, are clearly abnormal or – as often is the case – are equivocal. Equivocal findings may arise because the appearances you have identified are described in both normal pregnancies and potentially abnormal pregnancies. One such example is echogenic bowel.

By contrast, it may be that one or more measurements you have taken are outside the normal range – for example, a femur length below the third centile or a posterior horn of the lateral ventricle measurement greater than 10.0 mm. A short femur could be a normal finding as 3% of the normal population will, by definition, have an FL measurement below the third centile. However, a short femur is also associated with some skeletal dysplasias and Down's syndrome. A posterior horn measurement of, for example, 10.2 mm could also be a normal finding as this measurement is considered to be just above the normal range. Alternatively, it could represent the early stages of progressive ventriculomegaly.

You will also experience situations where you are unable to obtain the sections required to assess the anatomy properly, caused either by a persistently unhelpful fetal position or your inexperience. In such situations you must obviously seek help. It is your responsibility to decide whether the findings are normal, and should therefore be reported as such, or whether the woman needs to be referred for more detailed examination by a more experienced colleague or referred to a fetal medicine specialist. When you have obtained what are acceptable sections but you are not sure whether the appearances are normal or not, you must always seek advice.

Knowing how to make these decisions appropriately requires not only expertise and experience in the scanning technique itself but also a depth and breadth of appropriate ultrasound-related clinical knowledge. In addition, you need to gain experience and confidence in being able to communicate your findings verbally to the woman, irrespective of whether they are normal, abnormal, equivocal or uncertain, and in being able to prepare a written report for the referring health professional and others as appropriate.

Developing the depth and breadth of knowledge needed to provide an effective, informed and empathetic service to the women you scan takes time. As you are discovering, ultrasound scanning looks far easier than it is in practice, so do not become too disheartened as practice should eventually make perfect.

SCREENING STANDARDS

The first standards for routine second trimester anomaly screening were introduced into the English health care system in 2010. The standards recommend that all women should be offered a fetal anomaly scan between 18^{+0} and 20^{+6} weeks of gestation. More specifically, these standards recommend that the routine anomaly scan should include a prescribed set of measurements together with a standardized examination of the fetal anatomy. This combination of fetal biometry and anatomical assessment constitutes the components of the 'minimum standard' routine anatomy examination that every woman in this county can now expect.

One of the objectives of the national programme is to identify serious fetal abnormalities that are either incompatible with life or associated with long-term postnatal morbidity or would benefit from immediate postnatal intervention. It should be remembered that screening for trisomy 21, trisomy 18 and trisomy 13 has already been performed through the screening programme for Down's, Edwards' and Patau's syndromes offered to all women before the anomaly scan. The conditions screened for, and their current expected detection rates within the national screening programme, are detailed in Appendix 5.

In order to screen for an abnormality, it must be possible to image consistently the normal appearance of the relevant structure. It is important that you understand that being able to identify an abnormal appearance of a structure requires the ability to image consistently the appearance of the structure in all normal cases, in addition to being able to identify the abnormal appearances of that structure.

Thus, it is possible to screen for cleft lip because the normal upper lip can be routinely imaged in

161

the second trimester. Conversely, although a cleft palate can certainly be diagnosed in the second trimester, the difficulties in consistently imaging the normal palate mean that its assessment should not be a component of a screening programme. Thus it is not possible to screen for abnormalities of the palate, namely cleft palate.

On a more philosophical level, it is not possible to 'make sure everything is normal' during your routine anomaly scan because most cases of, for example, postnatal deafness, blindness and brain damage do not have physical sequelae that can be suspected or identified prenatally. Such conditions are therefore neither amenable to antenatal screening nor, in the majority of situations, to antenatal diagnosis.

We suggest that you take some time to consider these issues and think through, and around, the implications of the possibly misinformed expectations of many women attending for their routine anomaly scan. You will need to develop the challenging skills of placing the woman's expectations, which may be unrealistic but are nonetheless very real to her, within the actuality of the diagnostic capabilities of the screening examination you are performing.

Although the 18^{+0} to 20^{+6} week routine anomaly screening programme applies only to England, most countries across the world which offer obstetric ultrasound screening programmes will provide a second trimester examination that combines fetal biometry and anatomical assessment. Such examinations are normally performed between 18 and 22 weeks of gestation. These programmes may differ in some of the measurements taken and in some of the specifics of their individual tick lists. They are, however, broadly similar in the range of abnormalities screened for and the options available when abnormal findings are suspected or diagnosed.

The second trimester anomaly scan described in this text relates to the gestational age range of 18–22 weeks, unless otherwise specified.

ROUTINE ANOMALY SCREENING

This text assumes that the majority of women whom you are about to scan in the second trimester will already have had screening for Down's, Edwards' and Patau's syndromes earlier in their pregnancy and, as they are attending for a routine second trimester scan, also assumes that the Down's risk and Edwards'/Patau's risk after their screening test were both low. The text therefore also assumes that the pregnancy was dated at the time of the combined screening. A proportion of women, however, will attend for their first ultrasound scan in the second trimester. Management of these women is addressed later in this chapter.

Here we provide a scanning sequence which we recommend that the experienced sonographer adopts. Our aim is to ensure that you are able to provide as extensive an examination as is possible at this gestation, in a logical and efficient manner, irrespective of current national guidance. We therefore make no apology for recommending the following 24 point scanning sequence:

1 Determine the number of fetuses.
2 Determine the longitudinal axis of the fetus and more specifically its lie, presentation and attitude.
3 Confirm that the fetus is alive.
4 Show the woman a longitudinal section of her baby, in which its heart can be seen clearly beating, on the screen.
5 Confirm situs solitus.
6 Measure the HC, BPD and PH from the lateral ventricles plane. Measure the TCD from the suboccipito-bregmatic plane. Evaluate the intracranial anatomy, skull integrity and nuchal area from the two sections obtained.
7 Return to a longitudinal section, which demonstrates the fetal spine positioned anteriorly. Evaluate the full length of the spine including the sacrum and its skin covering in sagittal section. Slide and angle the probe to evaluate the fetal spine

in coronal view. Note the position of the fetal stomach below the diaphragm in both views.

8 Rotate the probe through 90° to obtain a transverse section of the fetal chest. Evaluate the 4 chamber view, the left and right outflow tracts, the 3 vessel view (3VV) and the 3 vessel and trachea view (3VT).

9 Slide the probe down the fetus in transverse section. Confirm a single stomach 'bubble'. Measure the AC.

10 Continue sliding the probe down the fetus in transverse section examining the spine down to the sacrum. Evaluate the normal appearances of the cord insertion and abdominal wall, both kidneys including both renal pelves, the bladder and a 3 vessel cord.

11 Find the femur and measure the FL.

12 Confirm the presence of three long bones in each limb.

13 Confirm the presence of two feet and that the carrying angle of each is normal. Obtain a plantar view of each foot to assess the toes.

14 Confirm the presence of two hands and obtain a view of the fingers, preferably outstretched, of each hand.

15 Evaluate the fetal profile in sagittal section of the fetal skull, the lips in coronal section of the fetal face and the alveolar ridge in transverse section of the fetal skull.

16 Observe the fetus for body and limb movements.

17 Evaluate amniotic fluid volume.

18 Localize the position of the placenta relative to the internal cervical os.

19 Assess the uterus for evidence of fibroids and the pelvis for any evidence of ovarian pathological conditions. See Chapter 6.

20 Confirm normal growth velocity, or assign gestational age and the estimated date of delivery (EDD) if this is the first scan after 10 weeks of pregnancy.

21 Decide whether any further follow-up is necessary.

22 Discuss the findings with the woman.

23 Issue a written report accompanied by graphical representation of the biometric data.

24 Arrange further follow-up as appropriate.

We recommend that, as a beginner, you start with learning how to measure the HC, BPD, PH, TCD, AC and FL and how to assess the relevant sections properly. This chapter addresses these tasks. Once you have acquired all these skills we then suggest you progress to assessing the rest of the fetal anatomy. How to acquire these skills is addressed in Chapters 9, 10, 11 and 12.

We therefore recommend that the novice sonographer begins with the following 16 point scanning sequence:

1 Determine the number of fetuses.

2 Determine the longitudinal axis of the fetus and, more specifically, its lie, presentation and attitude.

3 Confirm that the fetus is alive.

4 Show the woman a longitudinal section of her baby, in which its heart can be seen clearly beating, on the screen.

5 Confirm situs solitus.

6 Measure the HC, BPD and PH from the lateral ventricles plane. Measure the TCD from the suboccipito-bregmatic plane. Evaluate the intracranial anatomy, skull integrity and nuchal area from the two sections obtained.

7 Return to a longitudinal section which demonstrates the full length of the fetal spine. Note the position of the fetal stomach below the diaphragm.

8 Rotate the probe through 90° to obtain a transverse section of the fetal chest. Slide the probe down the fetus in transverse section. Confirm a single stomach 'bubble'. Measure the AC.

9 Continue sliding the probe down the fetus in transverse section to the sacrum. Find the femur and measure the FL.

10 Observe the fetus for body and limb movements.

11 Evaluate amniotic fluid volume.

12 Localize the position of the placenta relative to the internal cervical os.

13 Assess the uterus for evidence of fibroids and the pelvis for any evidence of ovarian pathological conditions.

14 Confirm normal growth velocity, or assign gestational age and the EDD if this is the first scan after 10 weeks of pregnancy.

15 Ask your mentor to confirm that the images you have taken are correct and that you have taken the measurements correctly.

16 Your mentor may wish to repeat your measurements to confirm they are correct. He or she will also wish to complete the examination by assessing the fetal anatomy, discussing the findings with the woman and issuing the signed report of the examination.

It is good practice to include both your and your mentor's names in the report. From a medicolegal perspective, whoever signs the report is responsible for its contents. It is therefore not appropriate for you, as a trainee, to issue a report which is not countersigned by a qualified ultrasound practitioner.

As discussed in Chapter 3, your first actions must be to determine the number of fetuses. Assuming only one is present you should then find the longitudinal axis of the fetus and confirm it is alive. Having obtained this section of the fetus it is important to show the woman her baby, with its heart clearly beating, on the screen.

CONFIRMING SITUS SOLITUS

The basic requirements for assessing situs are discussed in Chapter 3. You should then confirm

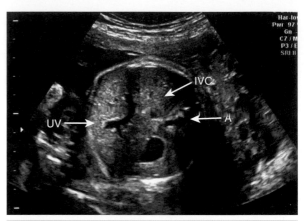

Fig 8.1 • The abdominal circumference section of a cephalic fetus confirming *situs solitus*. The descending aorta lies slightly to the left of the spine and the IVC lies slightly to the right of the spine. The aorta is more posterior than the IVC. Note the UV curving away from the stomach, to the right side. A, aorta; IVC, inferior vena cava; UV, umbilical vein.

normal fetal situs as described here before proceeding to perform the fetal biometry:

- the fetal stomach is positioned on the left side of the fetal abdomen, below the diaphragm
- the intrahepatic portion of the umbilical vein curves towards the right side of the fetus. This is best assessed in transverse section
- the descending aorta lies slightly to the left of the spine and the inferior vena cava (IVC) lies to the right of the spine. The aorta is more posterior than the IVC. These relationships are best assessed in transverse section (Fig. 8.1).

MEASURING THE HC AND BPD

Historically the BPD has been the most widely used ultrasound parameter in the estimation of gestational age. The current national recommendation is that dating a pregnancy in the second trimester should be performed by using the HC rather than the BPD. The HC is also of more clinical value in assessing fetal growth than the BPD. However, we consider measuring both the HC and the BPD to be good clinical practice and therefore both measurements are discussed here.

The section that should be selected for measurement and assessment should be that described by the authors of the data set or 'chart' which you are using. The reference plane for HC and BPD recommended by the national programme is the lateral ventricles section and is commonly known as the Chitty section, after one of the two authors of the 1997 publication. This is the same plane as that first described by Campbell and Thoms in 1977. A second plane, favoured by our transatlantic and European colleagues, is the thalami section, also known as the Hadlock section, after the author of the 1981 publication. Although the HC and BPD measurements derived from the Chitty and Hadlock sections are very similar, the anatomy displayed in the two sections differs considerably.

The section that your department uses for measurement must reflect the charts that you use. If you are participating in the national screening programme in England, you should be using Chitty reference charts for HC and BPD. You should therefore be using the lateral ventricles section and not the thalami section. The thalami/Hadlock section is included for completeness.

Lateral Ventricles/Chitty Section for HC and BPD

The correct section is demonstrated in Fig. 8.2 and should include the following features:
- a rugby football-shaped skull, rounded at the back (occiput) and more pointed at the front (synciput)

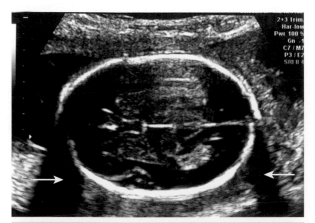

Fig 8.2 • Lateral ventricles section of the fetal brain (Chitty section) for measurement of the head circumference and biparietal diameter. Note the acoustic shadowing (arrows) arising from the normal ossification of the skull. Also note the loss of information in the upper hemisphere due to reverberation artefacts as discussed in chapter 1, see Fig. 1.15.

- a continuous midline echo equidistant from the proximal and distal skull echoes and positioned horizontally on the monitor
- the cavum septum pellucidum (CSP) interrupting the midline one third of the distance from the synciput to the occiput
- the linear echo of the lateral aspect of each of the two anterior horns of the lateral ventricles, symmetrically placed about the midline
- all or part of the posterior horn of the more posterior lateral ventricle.

In earlier gestations (15–20 weeks) the optimal view of the posterior horn is usually obtained in the lateral ventricles section (see later). At later gestations (20–24 weeks) the optimal section for visualizing and measuring the posterior horn may be slightly lower than the HC/BPD section.

Finding the Correct Section for HC and BPD

Obtain a longitudinal section of the fetus. As the section you are seeking should demonstrate the midline in a horizontal position on the monitor, you require the fetus to be in an occipitotransverse (OT), rather than an occipitoanterior (OA) or occipitoposterior (OP), position (see Problems in Obtaining the Correct Sections for HC and BPD later). Providing the lie is more or less OT, a longitudinal section of the fetal head which demonstrates a strong midline echo will be obtained if small sliding movements of the transducer to each side of the fetal spine are performed.

By rotating the transducer through 90°, a transverse section of the fetal head is obtained. If the midline is not exactly equidistant between the anterior and posterior parietal bones of the section, alter the angle of the probe slightly on the maternal abdomen. This corrects for the angle of asynclitism. Once the midline is centrally placed relative to the parietal bones, do not alter the angle of the probe relative to the maternal abdomen.

Now assess the shape of the fetal skull. The required shape is that of a rugby football with the more pointed end at the synciput. As the CSP lies one third of the distance from the synciput to the occiput, identifying the CSP will allow you to determine which is the front and which is the back of the head. If the section is not the required ovoid shape, make minor rotational adjustments.

If the landmark features listed here are not evident when the midline and shape are correctly imaged, then the level of the section is wrong and should be corrected by small sliding movements of the probe up or down the fetal head. A continuous midline which is not broken by the CSP indicates that the section you have obtained is too high in the fetal head. Slide the probe down towards the fetal body (inferiorly) to reach the correct level. A section in which both the orbits and the cerebellum can be seen is too low. Slide the probe up towards the top of the fetal head (superiorly) to reach the correct level.

As structures are best visualized when they lie at 90°, or orthogonal, to the sound beam the midline, the anterior and posterior walls of the CSP and the medial walls of the lateral ventricles will be optimally identified when they are in the horizontal plane. If the midline is not orthogonal to the incident sound beam, dip one end of the probe gently into the maternal abdomen. This action should bring the head into a more OT position and therefore the midline, CSP and lateral ventricles into the required horizontal position. This is discussed further in Problems in Obtaining the Correct Sections for HC and BPD.

Once you have obtained the correct section (Fig. 8.2), freeze the image.

Measuring the HC

Measurement of the HC should be taken from an image with the midline echo lying as close as possible to the horizontal plane, such that its angle of insonation by the ultrasound beam is 90°. The HC can be calculated using three basic methods:

- the *ellipse method*

    This is the most commonly used method and the method we recommend. The 'outer-to-outer' technique is used.

    The intersection of the cross of the first ellipse calliper is placed on the outer table of the skull at the occiput. The intersection of the second ellipse calliper is then placed on the outer table of the skull at the synciput. Using the appropriate control, a preformed ellipse of dots or crosses is moved out from between the two cursors until it matches the outline of the fetal skull (Fig. 8.3A). Adjustment of the position of both ellipse callipers can be made after the ellipse is formed to achieve a more exact match

- the *two-diameter method*

    The mathematical formula for calculating the circumference of a circle is $2\pi r$ or 'πd' where r is the radius of the

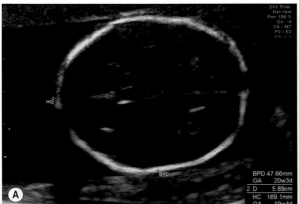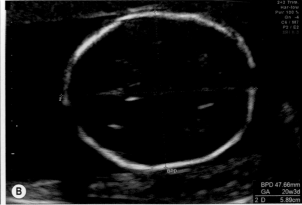

Fig 8.3 • A. Lateral ventricles section of the brain demonstrating the ellipse method of measurement of the HC with the ellipse tracing the outer border of the skull, and giving an HC measurement of 169.1 mm. B. The two diameter method of measurement for the HC using the 'outer-to-outer' calliper placement for the BPD (47.7 mm) and the OFD (58.9 mm) giving an HC of 167.4 mm. BPD, biparietal diameter; HC, head circumference; OFD, occipito-frontal diameter.

circle, d is the diameter of the circle and $\pi = 3.14$. The ultrasound machine's software calculates the HC using two diameters of the fetal skull which are orthogonal to each other, namely the BPD and the occipitofrontal diameter (OFD) using the expression

$$HC = \pi(BPD + OFD)/2 \text{ or } 3.14(BPD + OFD)/2$$

Both diameters are measured using the 'outer-to-outer' technique.

The OFD is always measured using the 'outer-to-outer' calliper placement. As is discussed later, the BPD can be measured in two ways, using either the 'outer-to-outer' calliper placement or the 'outer-to-inner' calliper placement. When using the BPD to calculate the HC, the 'outer-to-outer' calliper placement must be used (Fig. 8.3B)

- the *plot method*

The intersection of the cross of the first calliper mark is placed, where it can be easily visualized, on the outer table of the skull. The correct position is then recorded in the machine's software by pressing the calliper 'enter' control. Sequential marks are plotted and recorded around the whole circumference. In some equipment a continuous trace is produced rather than a series of dots or crosses. On many machines adjustment of the last positions of the cursor can be made in case of error.

Growth of the HC is illustrated in Appendix 6.

Measuring the BPD

The BPD describes the maximum diameter of a transverse section of the fetal skull at the level of the parietal eminences. The BPD can be measured by using either the 'outer-to-inner' calliper placement or the 'outer-to-outer' calliper placement. Both methods require placement of the intersection of the cross of the linear callipers on the outer border of the proximal parietal bone. The difference between the two methods lies in whether or not the width of the distal parietal bone is included in the measurement. The two techniques will produce

BPD measurements that differ typically by 2–3 mm in the second trimester, approximately equivalent to 1 week of gestation in midpregnancy.

There is no international consensus regarding which technique is more acceptable, although the 'outer-to-inner' method finds greater favour with physicists. This is because the anterior or 'leading' edge of the parietal echo is less influenced by the equipment's controls than the posterior or 'trailing' edge. The 'outer-to-inner' placement is thus a more accurate representation of the true distance selected for measurement than the 'outer-to-outer' placement. What is critically important is that the technique used (including the section selected for measurement) corresponds to that employed by the authors of the reference data being used.

The national recommendation is that the 'outer-to-inner' method, as described by Chitty, should be used.

'Outer-to-inner' measurement

On the frozen image, place the intersection of the cross of the first linear calliper on the outer aspect of the proximal skull surface. Place the intersection of the cross of the second linear calliper on the inner aspect of the distal skull surface, at right angles to the midline and across the widest diameter of the skull (Fig. 8.3A). This BPD measurement includes the thickness of only the proximal parietal bone and is commonly described as an 'outer-to-inner' measurement.

Growth of the 'outer-to-inner' BPD is illustrated in Appendix 7.

'Outer-to-outer' measurement

On the frozen image, place the intersection of the cross of the first linear calliper on the outer aspect of the proximal skull surface. Place the intersection of the cross of the second linear calliper on the outer aspect of the distal skull surface, at right angles to the midline and across the widest diameter of the skull (Fig. 8.4). This BPD measurement includes the thickness of both parietal bones and is commonly described as an 'outer-to-outer' measurement.

BPD measurements in breech and transverse presentations

In the second half of pregnancy, BPD measurements obtained from fetuses lying transversely or

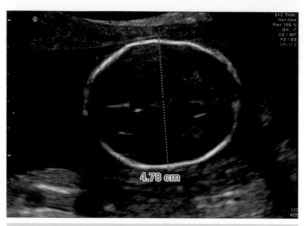

4.78 cm

Fig 8.4 • Measurement of the biparietal diameter using the 'outer-to-outer' placement of the callipers.

presenting by the breech may be unreliable. In these presentations the fetal head is often dolichocephalic (long and narrow) in shape. This produces a BPD measurement that is artefactually small for gestational age. The HC measurement, however, is unaltered by presentation. This is why the HC is a more reliable indicator of growth velocity and gestational age than the BPD.

Problems in Obtaining the Correct Sections for HC and BPD

Incorrect angle

If the angle of the probe on the maternal abdomen is incorrect, the midline echo does not lie centrally within the fetal skull and has a curved rather than a linear appearance. The echoes from the lateral ventricles will not be visualized symmetrically about the midline (Fig. 8.5A). In addition, there is dissimilarity in the appearance of the anterior and posterior skull bones, with one typically being smooth and regular and the other appearing broken and disrupted. To rectify this, the angle of the probe to the maternal abdomen should be altered, without sliding or rotating the probe.

Incorrect rotation

This is readily recognized because the shape of the fetal skull is not that of a rugby football and/or not all the required landmark features are seen. For example, visualizing the anterior horns together with the cerebellum indicates that your selected

level at the back of the head is too low (Fig. 8.5B). This is the suboccipito-bregmatic view section, which is the incorrect section for measurement of the HC and BPD but is required for measurement of the TCD (see later).

Visualizing the orbits together with the posterior horns of the lateral ventricles indicates that your selected level at the front of the head is too low (Fig. 8.5C). A slightly higher level at the front of the head, between the orbits and the anterior horns, may produce the false impression of a lemon-shaped skull (see Skull Shape later). Rotating the probe will correct the shape, but you must be careful to maintain the correct angle.

Incorrect level

Sliding movements of the probe will alter the level of section. A continuous midline indicates that your selected level is too high (Fig. 8.5D). Slide the probe inferiorly, towards the fetal body. A section demonstrating the orbits and the cerebellum is too low (Fig. 8.5E). Slide the probe superiorly, towards the top of the fetal head. Be careful not to rotate or change the angle of the probe as you slide.

Midline not horizontal

Having obtained the correct section in which the required landmarks are displayed, check that the midline is horizontal. If the midline is at an angle to the horizontal (Fig. 8.5F), dip one end of the probe gently into the maternal abdomen. This should bring the head into the required OT position, displaying the midline in the horizontal plane.

OA/OP position

Measurement of the HC and BPD should only be taken when the required landmarks are clearly visualized. This is normally when the fetal head is in the OT position, as the midline echo and the other landmarks will lie at 90° to the ultrasound beam. The HC and the BPD therefore should not be measured if the fetal head is directly OA, directly OP, or deep in the maternal pelvis, as in these situations the landmarks are poorly seen, making it difficult to obtain the correct section and therefore make the correct measurements.

When the position of the fetal head is OA or OP, ask the woman's permission first and then

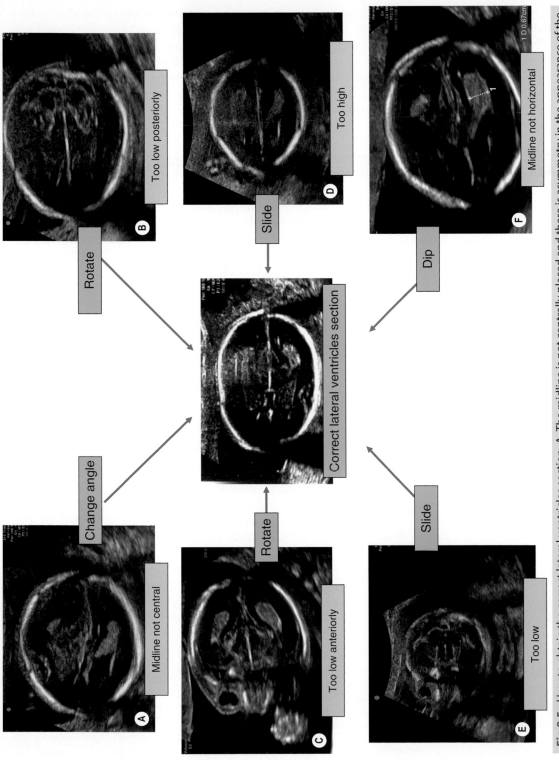

Fig 8.5 • How to obtain the correct lateral ventricles section. A. The midline is not centrally placed and there is asymmetry in the appearance of the parietal bones. Change the probe angle. B. The cerebellum is visible therefore the section is too low posteriorly. Rotate the probe away from the neck. C. The orbits are visible therefore the section is too low anteriorly. Rotate the probe away from the orbits. D. A continuous midline is visible therefore the section is too high. Slide the probe inferiorly. E. The orbits and the cerebellum are visible therefore the section is too low. Slide the probe superiorly. F. The section is correct but the midline is not horizontal. Dip the probe.

encourage the fetus to move by gently shaking the probe on the maternal abdomen. When the head is deep in the maternal pelvis, raising the foot of the scanning couch, so that the woman is in a 45° head-down position, may displace and rotate the fetal head such that it can be measured. Finally, imaging via the transvaginal route may be used but is not always successful in obtaining the correct section to assess. If these procedures are unsuccessful and it is still not possible to obtain the correct section, do not be tempted to take any measurements, as such measurements are likely to be inaccurate and potentially misleading.

THE VENTRICLES

The ventricular system consists of four irregularly shaped cavities the lateral, third and fourth ventricles as discussed in chapter 9. Fig. 8.6 illustrates a pathological specimen of a fetal head at approximately the same level as Fig. 8.2 and demonstrates that ultrasound produces a very good representation of the anatomy at this level. You will note that the pathological section of the fetal brain has the occiput on the left of the picture, whereas Fig. 8.2 has the occiput on the right. The ventricular cavities are filled with cerebrospinal fluid (CSF) which circulates through the ventricular system, around the brain and the spine and is then absorbed by specific areas of the arachnoid space.

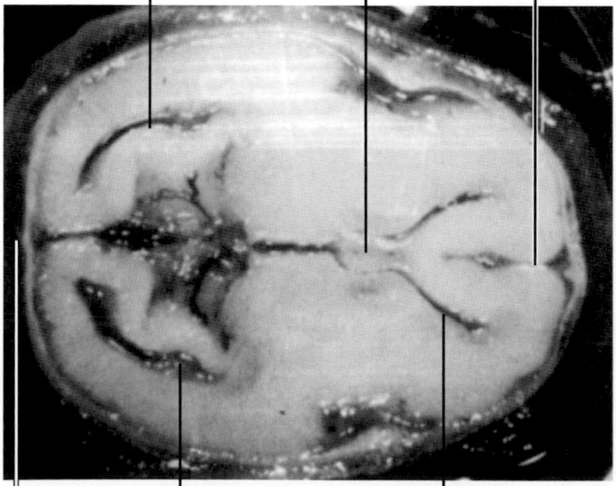

The anterior and posterior horns of the lateral ventricle in the upper hemisphere are obscured by artefacts generated as the acoustic beam passes through the fetal skull (Fig. 8.2). Reverberation artefact is rarely a problem in the distal hemisphere of the brain so the posterior horn of the lateral ventricle in the lower hemisphere should be assessed and measured. It is important that you make a subjective assessment of the lateral ventricle in both hemispheres of the brain to confirm they are of similar size and therefore to exclude possible unilateral dilation.

THE POSTERIOR HORN OF THE LATERAL VENTRICLE/ATRIUM

The posterior horn of the lateral ventricles are clearly visualized because of the presence of the hyperechoic choroid plexus within each ventricle. The posterior horn is a complex formed by the atrium that continues posteriorly into the occipital horn. *Atrium* describes the specific region of the posterior ventricle in which the glomus of the choroid plexus can be seen. The choroid plexus is normally hyperechoic and homogeneous in appearance. *Posterior horn* and *atrium* are terms that are interchangeable.

Posterior horn | Cavum septum pellucidum | Midline

Occiput | Choroid plexus | Anterior horn

Fig 8.6 • Pathological specimen of mid trimester fetal brain.

Measurement of the Posterior Horn of the Lateral Ventricle

In order to be able to measure the posterior horn of the lateral ventricle, the echoes generated by its medial and lateral walls, respectively, must be clearly defined. Once the two borders have been identified, the widest part of the atrium is measured. Usually this will be across the choroid plexus.

Current recommended practice is to measure the posterior horn according to the guideline published by the International Society of Ultrasound in Obstetrics and Gynaecology (ISUOG) in 2007 (Fig. 8.7).

The intersection of the cross of the callipers should be positioned on the inner edge of the echoes generated by medial and lateral borders of the ventricle to obtain an 'inner-to-inner' measurement of the posterior horn. This measurement must be at 90° to the axis of the posterior horn (Figs 8.7 and 8.8). The axis of the ventricle is not parallel to the midline but at a slight angle to it, so it is important that you position your callipers correctly, orthogonal to the long axis of the ventricle rather than to the midline (Fig. 8.9). Incorrect positioning of the callipers along and across the atrium alters the measurement as shown in Fig. 8.10. Measurements can be falsely increased with the use of an off-axis image plane, an improper

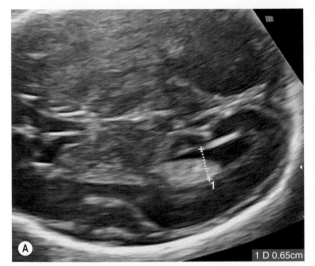

A

1 D 0.65cm

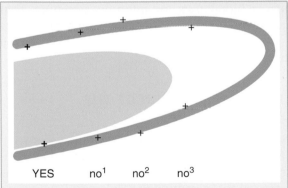

YES   no[1]   no[2]   no[3]

B

Fig 8.7 • Measurement of the posterior horn of the lateral ventricle i.e. inner to inner across the glomus. Current recommended practice is to measure the posterior horn according to the guideline published by the International Society of Ultrasound in Obstetrics and Gynecology in 2007. The caliper placement 'YES; is correct, being 'inner to inner'. THE 'no' caliper placements are incorrect, no[1] being 'mid to mid', no[2] being 'outer to outer' and no[3] is not placed across the widest part of the ventricle.

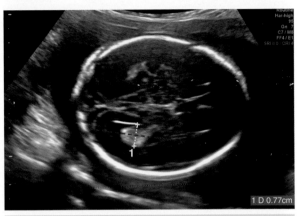

1 D 0.77cm

Fig 8.8 • Measurement of the posterior horn of the lateral ventricle. Correct placement of the callipers positioned on the inner edge of the echoes generated by the medial and lateral borders of the ventricle to obtain an 'inner-to-inner' measurement at 90' (dashed line) to the axis of the ventricle.

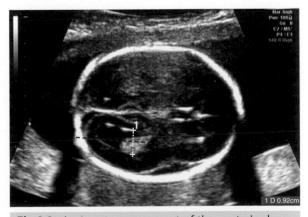

1 D 0.92cm

Fig 8.9 • Incorrect measurement of the posterior horn. The callipers have been positioned incorrectly at 90° to the midline echoes (dashed line) rather than orthogonal to the long axis of the ventricle.

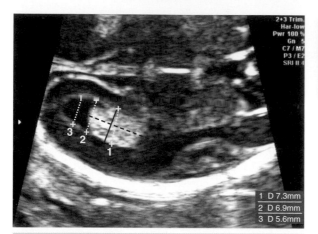

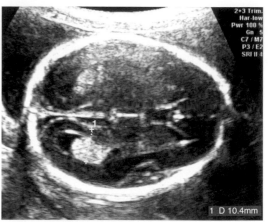

Fig 8.10 • Measurement of the posterior horn. Incorrect positioning of the callipers along and across the atrium alters the measurement significantly from 5.6 to 7.3 mm. The axis of the ventricle is shown by the dashed line. Measurement 1 is an overestimate because, although the callipers have been placed across the maximum diameter of the glomus, they are not orthogonal to the axis of the ventricle. The callipers for measurement 2 have been placed too far posteriorly, and only just include the glomus. Measurement 3 is an underestimate because the callipers have been placed across the tapering portion of the ventricle. The solid red line indicates the correct caliper placement.

Fig 8.11 • Incorrect identification of the ventricular boundaries when attempting to measure the posterior horn. The lower calliper has been positioned correctly onto the lateral wall of the ventricle but the upper calliper has been incorrectly positioned, above the medial border of the ventricle. The measurement obtained, of 10.4 mm, therefore suggests incorrectly that mild ventriculomegaly is present. When measured correctly, the size of this ventricle was within the normal range.

choice of ventricular boundary (Fig. 8.11) or poor cursor placement.

Occasionally the distal border of the lateral ventricle may not be clearly seen, so the posterior aspect of the choroid plexus may be used to determine where to position the distal calliper. Although the choroid plexus is normally homogeneous in appearance, one or more cystic areas may be seen within the choroid. These cystic areas are called choroid plexus cysts (CPCs) and are discussed in Chapter 9.

Irrespective of the precise method used to measure the posterior horn, it is accepted that the upper limit of the normal range for the posterior horn measurement at 18–22 weeks is 10.0 mm. Measurements larger than 10.0 mm warrant referral for detailed examination by a fetal medicine specialist. Consistency of the measurements is therefore critical when the ventricle is between 9.5 mm and 10.5 mm in order that the woman is referred appropriately. An overmeasurement could result in an unnecessary referral being made, which will increase the anxiety levels of the woman

concerned. An undermeasurement could result in the woman not being followed up appropriately. As a consequence, this woman would not be offered blood tests for infection screening, fetal karyotyping or the follow-up scans which are necessary to check for resolution or progression of the mild ventriculomegaly.

THE ANTERIOR HORN OF THE LATERAL VENTRICLE

The anterior horns of the lateral ventricles provide one of the landmarks used in the Chitty HC section and are therefore visualized in the same section as that used for measuring the HC and BPD.

Measurement of the Anterior Horn of the Lateral Ventricle

Historically, measurement of the anterior horn of the lateral ventricle was taken in the assessment of ventricular dilation, in preference to measurement of the posterior horn. 'Measurement' of the anterior horn was a misnomer as it was the distance between the lateral border of the anterior horn and

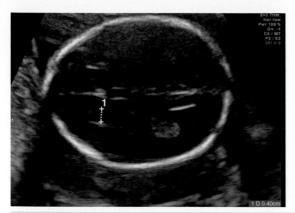

Fig 8.12 • Measurement of the anterior horn of the lateral ventricle.

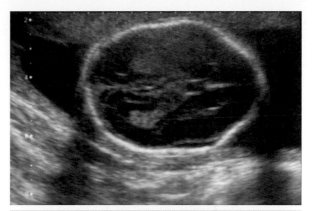

Fig 8.13 • Abnormal scalloping of the fetal skull may be obtained in a normal 18–22 week fetus from an incorrect HC/BPD section. This may be achieved when the probe is rotated slightly too far towards the fetal orbits at the front of the skull as in this case.

the midline directly anterior to it which was measured. In the normal fetus, this measurement was typically around 7.0 mm at 18–22 weeks.

The anterior horn is a fluid-filled cavity so it has both medial and lateral borders. With modern equipment and careful observation, the medial and lateral borders can be identified as separate echoes. The medial border is typically bowed, whereas the lateral border is more linear in appearance (Fig. 8.2). Measurement of the size of the anterior horn itself is therefore now possible. As with measurement of the posterior horn, the intersection of the cross of the callipers should be positioned on the inner edge of the echoes generated by medial and lateral borders, respectively, to obtain an 'inner-to-inner' measurement. This measurement should be at 90° to the axis of the anterior horn (Fig. 8.12).

Current practice

Measurement of the anterior horn is not a requirement of the routine 18–22 week examination. There is no normal range for the size of the anterior horn but we recommend further review if it appears unusually prominent and certainly if it measures more than 5.0 mm.

EVALUATING THE SKULL SHAPE FROM THE LATERAL VENTRICLES VIEW

As the fetal skull should have already been assessed at the 12-week scan, the acrania sequence as discussed in Chapter 7 will have been excluded.

It is important to observe the normal shape of the fetal skull and appreciate how this varies, albeit subtly, with increasing gestation. As discussed earlier, the shape of the normal skull after approximately 18 weeks is that of a rugby football.

Abnormal scalloping of the frontal bones produces a more angular appearance to the front of the skull in this view. It is known as the 'lemon' sign and is associated with spina bifida (see Chapter 12). However, a similar appearance is demonstrated by the skull of the normal fetus before 16 weeks. It can also be obtained in a normal 18–22 week fetus from an incorrect HC/BPD section, as described earlier, if the probe is rotated slightly too far towards the fetal orbits at the front of the skull (Fig. 8.13). Conversely fetuses with spina bifida rarely demonstrate a lemon-shaped skull after 24–26 weeks. These factors should be remembered if a lemon-shaped skull is suspected.

EVALUATING THE INTRACRANIAL ANATOMY FROM THE LATERAL VENTRICLES VIEW

Irrespective of which template you are using, it is important to observe the information presented in the sections selected for measurement and thus to familiarize yourself with the range of normal appearances of these sections at 18–22 weeks of gestation. Once you have this experience, you will hopefully identify a finding which is not normal even if you are unable to pinpoint the specific diagnosis. The skull and brain abnormalities introduced here are discussed in detail in Chapter 9.

Obtaining the correct sections, taking the required measurements properly and assessing the information demonstrated within the sections should allow you to answer the following questions correctly.

1a Does the overall appearance of the brain appear normal?

1b Is the surrounding skull present and/or normal in appearance?

If the answer to both of the above is 'yes', you are able to exclude anencephaly and an occipital encephalocele.

2 Is the CSP normal in size and position?

If the answer is 'yes', agenesis of the corpus callosum (ACC) is unlikely as it is associated with absence of the CSP.

3 Are the anterior horns of the lateral ventricles normal in position and appearance?

The answer 'yes' will exclude the sickle-shaped appearance of the monoventricle of alobar holoprosencephaly.

4a Is the posterior horn normal in appearance?

4b Is the choroid plexus homogeneous in its appearance?

4c Is the measurement of the posterior horn less than 10.0 mm?

4d Is the anterior horn normal in appearance?

If the answers to all of the above are 'yes', you are able to exclude CPCs and at least unilateral ventriculomegaly.

5a Is the echo pattern in both halves of the brain similar and symmetrical?

5b Are you able to exclude one or more unusual hypoechoic or hyperechoic areas in the brain?

If the answer to both is 'yes', you are able to exclude a porencephalic cyst, which is typically hypoechoic, or a recent intracranial bleed, which is typically hyperechoic. Both would produce an abnormally positioned mass within the brain.

6 Do the intracranial contents appear brighter than usual such that you may have reduced the gain slightly?

If the answer is 'no', you are able to exclude abnormalities of bone mineralization such as osteogenesis imperfecta type II or hypophosphatasia. This is because abnormally hyperechoic skull contents are usually not indicative of a brain abnormality but rather of skull hypomineralization (see Chapter 9).

THE CLINICAL IMPACT OF CORRECTLY EVALUATING THE CHITTY HC SECTION

Proper evaluation of the HC section has therefore excluded anencephaly, an encephalocele, possible ACC, alobar holoprosencephaly, choroid plexus cysts, ventriculomegaly, a large porencephalic cyst, a recent significant intracranial bleed and skull hypomineralization.

THE THALAMI VIEW/HADLOCK SECTION

The section described by Hadlock differs from that of Chitty in that it is slightly lower in the fetal head and includes the paired thalami as a landmark rather than the posterior horns of the lateral ventricles.

Finding the Thalami View

From the lateral ventricles view, make a *very* slight rotation of the probe towards the fetal neck (i.e. the back of the head) to image the W-shaped hippocampal gyrus in preference to the posterior horns of the lateral ventricles. This is followed by a *very* slight sliding movement of the probe downwards, towards the fetal body so that the lower border of the cavum is just visible together with the optimal view of the thalami. The third ventricle is centrally positioned between the two thalami and can be identified as a very small, pointlike structure between them.

The correct section is demonstrated in Fig. 8.14 and should include the following features:

- a rugby football-shaped skull, rounded at the back (occiput) and more pointed at the front (synciput)
- a short midline equidistant from the proximal and distal skull echoes

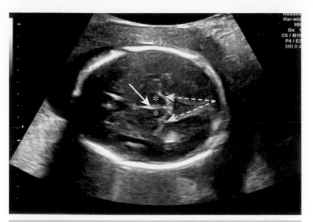

Fig 8.14 • The transthalamic level of the brain. The third ventricle (arrow) lies in the midline, between the two lobes of the thalamus (*). The hippocampal gyrus can be seen posterior to the thalamus (dashed arrows).

- the lower CSP bisecting the midline one third of the distance from the synciput to the occiput
- the paired thalami
- the third ventricle
- the hippocampal gyrus.

This is the correct section from which to measure the HC and BPD if using a Hadlock data set. A disadvantage of the thalami view is that you cannot measure the posterior horn from this section and you will therefore need to seek a higher section in the fetal head, by sliding the probe, in order to measure the posterior horn and assess the appearance of the lateral ventricles.

THE SUBOCCIPITO-BREGMATIC SECTION

FINDING THE SUBOCCIPITO-BREGMATIC PLANE

The required suboccipito-bregmatic plane is easily obtained from the lateral ventricles plane. Having obtained the correct HC section, rotate the probe slightly towards the fetal neck while keeping the CSP in view. Such rotation lowers the level of the section at the back of the brain away from the posterior horn of the lateral ventricle to the posterior fossa, within which you should see the cerebellum (Fig. 8.15).

THE CEREBELLUM

The cerebellum lies within the posterior fossa and is best visualized using the suboccipito-bregmatic plane. It is dumbbell-shaped and consists of two rounded lobes connected by the triangular-shaped vermis. The centrally positioned cerebellar vermis is hyperechoic compared with the cerebellar hemisphere on either side. The cerebellar hemispheres can be identified as discrete structures from 12–13 weeks of gestation with the vermis recognizable about 1 week later. Because the formation of the vermis is not complete until 19 weeks, care must be taken where vermian abnormalities are suspected prior to this gestation.

Measuring the TCD

The TCD is the measurement of the widest anteroposterior diameter of the cerebellum. The intersection of the cross of the callipers should be positioned on the outer edge of each hemisphere to obtain an 'outer-to-outer' measurement. This measurement should be taken at 90° to the midline as shown in Fig. 8.15.

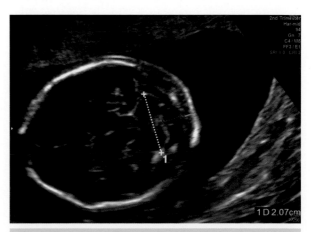

Fig 8.15 • Suboccipito-bregmatic plane of the fetal brain demonstrating the measurement of the TCD (dotted line), cisterna magna (red dotted line) and nuchal fold (blue line).

With advancing gestation, the cerebellum is less easy to see as the bones of the skull become progressively more ossified. It is often easier to see the cerebellum more clearly at later gestations if the probe is dipped so that the midline echo is at 30–45° to the horizontal, rather than perpendicular to the ultrasound beam. This angulation allows the ultrasound beam to be directed through the occipital suture of the skull.

In the normally developing fetus the TCD increases by approximately 1 mm per week of pregnancy between 14 and 22 weeks so that the TCD measured in millimetres equals the gestational age in weeks. After 24 weeks this numerical equivalence becomes unreliable as a result of the growth rate of the cerebellum. The normal TCD demonstrates a more than twofold increase in size during the second half of pregnancy.

In the majority of cases of open spina bifida the cerebellum is either banana-shaped or not visible in the posterior fossa because of the Arnold–Chiari type II malformation. Identifying the normal dumbbell shaped cerebellum is therefore important in excluding open spina bifida, together with other abnormalities as discussed in Chapter 9.

THE CISTERNA MAGNA

The cisterna magna (CM) lies in the posterior fossa, between the cerebellum and the occiput (Fig. 8.15). Although the CM is not routinely measured, you should always assess its size and be familiar with its normal appearance. This is because dilation of the CM is associated with a number of abnormalities including trisomies 13, 18, and 21 and Dandy Walker variant (see Chapter 9).

Measurement of the CM is made in the midline, at 90° to the TCD. The intersection of the cross of the callipers should be positioned on the outer edge of the cerebellar vermis and the inner border of the occipital bone to obtain an 'inner-to-inner' measurement as shown in Fig. 8.15. The normal range of the CM diameter in the second trimester is 4–10 mm. A measurement of less than 10.0 mm in the 18–22 week fetus should therefore be considered normal.

When obtaining the transcerebellar section used to measure the cisterna magna, it is important to make sure that you are not falsely elongating the posterior fossa by using either incorrect rotation or incorrect angle of the probe. Such elongation can result in a falsely increased CM measurement.

THE NUCHAL FOLD

The nuchal fold (NF) is the area of soft tissue at the back of the neck. An increased NF has a strong association with trisomy 21 and is also commonly associated with fetal hydrops (see Chapter 9). Although most women will already have had Down's screening before their anomaly scan, it is important that you do not overlook assessment of the fetal neck in this plane. Formal measurement of the NF is not normally performed unless the NF appears visually increased.

Measurement of the NF is made in the midline, at 90° to the TCD, and in the same plane as measurement of the CM. The section therefore should include the CSP, cerebellum, CM and NF with the midline echo of the brain ideally at 90° to the ultrasound beam. The intersection of the cross of the callipers should be positioned on the outer edge of the occipital bone and the outer edge of the skin to obtain an 'outer-to-outer' measurement of the NF as shown in Fig. 8.15. The normal NF should measure less than 6.0 mm in the second trimester.

Care must be taken when making this measurement as the range of sections demonstrating the ideal view is very small. It is very easy to obtain a falsely increased nuchal fold measurement if the skin over the upper neck is imaged rather than the skin over the base of the skull. The section can be corrected by rotating the probe cephalad away from the fetal neck.

THE CLINICAL IMPACT OF CORRECTLY EVALUATING THE SUBOCCIPITO-BREGMATIC SECTION

Proper evaluation of the suboccipito-bregmatic section has therefore excluded a range of abnormalities including the majority of cases of open spina bifida, Dandy Walker variant and increased nuchal fold.

MEASURING THE AC

Historically the AC has been used in the assessment of fetal growth, but its measurement was not always included in the fetal biometry performed at the time of the anomaly scan. The current national recommendation is that the AC is measured at 18–22 week scan. We consider measuring both the HC and the AC at every scan to be good clinical practice.

Because the AC is not used in pregnancy dating, the literature includes only AC size charts. As with the HC and BPD, the section that should be selected for measurement and assessment should be that described by the authors of the data set or 'chart' which you are using. Unlike the HC and BPD, the reference plane for AC described by most authors is the same. The national programme recommends the data set authored by Chitty.

FINDING THE AC

Obtain a longitudinal view of the fetus that demonstrates both the fetal heart and the fetal bladder. Make sure that the stomach is positioned below the diaphragm. This is important in the exclusion of a left-sided diaphragmatic hernia (see Chapter 11).

Slide the probe laterally until the fetal spine is visualized. Rotate the transducer through 90° at the level of the fetal stomach to obtain a cross-section of the fetal body.

The landmark features required to measure the AC are as follows:
- a circular section of the abdomen demonstrating an unbroken and short rib echo of equal size on each side
- a cross-section of *one* vertebra visualized as a triangle of three hyperechoic spots
- a short length of umbilical vein (UV). This length should be centrally placed between the lateral abdominal walls as opposed to at the cord insertion. It should be well within the fetal liver, ideally a third of the way along an imaginary line drawn from the anterior abdominal wall to the fetal spine

- the stomach, usually visualized as a circular or teardrop-shaped hypoechoic area, in the left side of the abdomen, positioned approximately halfway between the posterior and the anterior abdominal walls.

The outline of the section in which the above landmarks are seen should be circular (Fig. 8.16). If it is ovoid, make a small adjustment to the rotation of the probe or to the angle of the probe to the maternal abdomen, as discussed in the next section.

If the UV is not visualized as described here, make small sliding movements of the probe to change the level of the section.

MEASUREMENT OF THE AC

As with the HC, the AC can be calculated by one of three basic methods:
- the *ellipse method*
    This is the most commonly used method and the method we recommend.

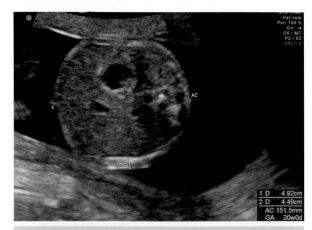

Fig 8.16 • Methods of measuring the AC. Cross section of a breech fetus showing the correct landmarks for the AC. The ellipse is placed around the outer edge of the abdomen, giving an AC measurement of 151.5 mm. The two diameter method shows the outer to outer placement of the two callipers to obtain an APAD diameter (1) of 49.2 mm and a TAD diameter (2) of 44.9 mm, giving a calculated AC of 147.7 mm.

As previously, the 'outer-to-outer' technique is used.

The intersection of the cross of the first ellipse calliper is placed on the outer border of the abdomen at the level of the vertebra. Place the intersection of the cross of the second ellipse calliper on the outer border of the anterior abdominal wall, following the axis of the UV. Using the appropriate control, a preformed ellipse of dots or crosses is moved out from between the two cursors until it matches the outline of the fetal abdomen (see Fig. 8.16). Adjustment of the position of both the cursors can be made after the ellipse is formed to achieve a more exact match.

- the *two-diameter method*

The transverse abdominal diameter (TAD) is measured in millimetres across the widest part of the AC section. The anteroposterior diameter (APAD) is measured in millimetres at 90° to the TAD, from the fetal spine to the anterior abdominal wall (Fig. 8.16). The short section of UV should lie along this axis.

Both diameters are measured using the 'outer-to-outer 'technique.

The mathematical formula for calculating the circumference of a circle is $2\pi r$ or a space 'πd' where r is the radius of the circle, d is the diameter of the circle and $\pi = 3.14$.

The ultrasound machine's software calculates the AC using the two diameters, TAD and APAD, as shown here:

$$AC\,(mm) = 3.14\,(TAD + APAD)/2$$

- the *plot method*

The intersection of the cross of the first calliper mark is placed, where it can be easily visualized, on the outer border of the abdomen. The correct position is then recorded in the machine's software by pressing the calliper 'enter' control.

Sequential marks are plotted and recorded around the whole circumference. In some equipment a continuous trace is produced rather than a series of dots or crosses.

On many machines adjustment of the last positions of the cursor can be made in case of error.

Growth of the AC is illustrated in Appendix 8.

PROBLEMS IN OBTAINING THE CORRECT SECTION FOR AC

Directly Anterior Fetal Spine

When the fetus is prone, its spine will be anterior. Thus, in transverse sections of the fetal abdomen and in the required AC section, the UV will not be seen as it lies in the acoustic shadow produced from the fetal spine. The fetal stomach will normally be seen when the spine is anterior but, as it has length as well as width, it will be seen over a number of sections of the fetal body of which only that in which the UV is also seen will give the correct measurement of the AC. Thus both landmarks should be seen to ensure the correct section is selected for measurement.

In the second trimester it is usually possible to slide the probe to a more lateral position on the maternal abdomen, or to dip one end of the probe gently into the maternal abdomen. This effectively rotates the image relative to the horizontal, thus repositioning the UV out of the acoustic shadow produced by the spine and thereby allowing it to be imaged.

Alternatively you can move on to another task within the examination and return to measuring the AC later, by which time the fetus may well have moved into a more favourable position.

Noncircular Outline

An oval outline indicates that you have obtained an oblique cross-section of the fetal body and therefore the AC. This can be rectified by a slight change in rotation or angle – the choice depends on the position of the fetal body relative to the horizontal plane. When the longitudinal fetal spine is in the horizontal plane, then rotation is required. When the longitudinal fetal spine is at an angle to the horizontal, angling of the probe is required.

Long Length of UV

The UV travels from the cord insertion up through the liver at an angle of approximately 45° to the horizontal. Thus if the section from which you intend to measure the AC demonstrates a long length of UV from, for example, the cord insertion through the fetal liver, you know you have an oblique section of the abdomen rather than the required cross-section. Where the longitudinal fetal spine is in the horizontal plane, angling the probe is required to obtain the required circular section in which only a small section of UV is demonstrated. When the longitudinal fetal spine is at an angle to the horizontal, rotation of the probe is required to obtain the required section.

EVALUATING THE FETAL ANATOMY FROM THE AC SECTION

As discussed earlier, irrespective of which template you are using, it is important to observe the information presented in the section selected for AC measurement and thus to familiarize yourself with the range of normal appearances of this section at 18–22 weeks of gestation.

Once you have this experience, you will hopefully identify a finding which is not normal even if you do not have the experience to pinpoint the specific diagnosis.

Is the stomach normal in position? It should be seen on the left side of the fetal abdomen and should be below the diaphragm. Seeing the stomach above the diaphragm would suggest a left-sided diaphragmatic hernia (see Chapter 10).

Is the stomach normal in size? A stomach 'bubble' may not be seen simply because the stomach has recently emptied. When this is the case, rescanning in 30–40 minutes should confirm the presence of a normal stomach. A persistently absent stomach is associated with oesophageal atresia, whereas a persistently very small stomach is associated with oesophageal atresia with fistula.

Two rounded areas at the level of the AC may represent the normal stomach together with the proximal duodenum, suggesting duodenal atresia. Although polyhydramnios normally accompanies upper gastrointestinal tract atresias in the third trimester fetus, the amniotic fluid volume in such atresias at 18–22 weeks is usually normal.

At 18–22 weeks, the echotexture of the normal fetal liver and bowel seen at the level of the AC section is homogeneous, and 'mid-grey'. An area of increased echogenicity, of similar 'whiteness' to the fetal iliac crests, indicates echogenic bowel (see Chapter 11).

The HC and AC should lie on approximately the same centile when plotted on their respective size charts. A significantly small AC relative to the HC may indicate early asymmetrical growth restriction, whereas a significantly small HC relative to the AC may indicate microcephaly.

THE CLINICAL IMPACT OF CORRECTLY EVALUATING THE AC SECTION

Proper evaluation of the AC section has therefore excluded left-sided diaphragmatic hernia, oesophageal atresia with and without a fistula, duodenal atresia and echogenic bowel. Comparison of the relative sizes of the HC and AC has excluded significant asymmetrical growth restriction and microcephaly.

MEASURING THE FL

Using measurement of the FL to assess gestational age was first suggested by O'Brien et al in 1981 and it describes measurement of the calcified portion of the femur, namely the diaphysis. Other authors describe the measurement as representing the metaphysis. Measurement of the FL is as accurate as the HC in the prediction of gestational age. As with the HC and BPD, the section that should be selected for measurement and assessment should be that described by the authors of the data set or 'chart' which you are using. The reference plane for FL shares similarities with the HC and BPD in that it varies between authors but, unlike the HC and BPD, the difference between authors relates principally to the angle of the bone relative to the horizontal rather than the content of the section.

As the FL can be used both for pregnancy dating and for size assessment, both dating (Appendix 9) and size charts (Appendix 10) for FL are available. The national programme recommends the data sets authored by Chitty.

From a practical point of view for the beginner, the accuracy of the FL measurement will be influenced by a combination of the speed with which the femur moves and your ability to anticipate this or activate the freeze control appropriately. Once you have the required expertise, you will find the FL is useful in confirming the gestational age estimated from HC measurements when dating a pregnancy in the second trimester and vice versa.

In addition, the FL can often be obtained when fetal position prevents accurate measurement of the HC. In such situations it is important that the intracranial anatomy has been assessed and is normal even if head measurements cannot be taken.

FINDING THE FL

Measuring the femur is ideally undertaken after the AC has been measured. Slide the probe caudally from the AC section until one or both of the iliac bones are visualized. At this point a part of one or both femurs is usually seen. Using this technique enables you to examine the abdominal wall, cord insertion, kidneys, bladder and spine and its skin covering en route to your search for the femur (see Chapters 11 and 12).

The upper femur should be selected for measurement. The lower femur is often difficult to image clearly because of acoustic shadowing from fetal structures above or anterior to it. Keeping the bright echo from the upper femur in view, rotate the probe slowly until the full length of the femur is obtained. Depending on whether you have rotated onto or away from the femur, you may need to make a *small* sliding movement after each rotational movement to bring the image of the femur back onto the screen.

MEASUREMENT OF THE FL

To ensure that you have obtained the full length of the femur and that your section is not oblique, soft

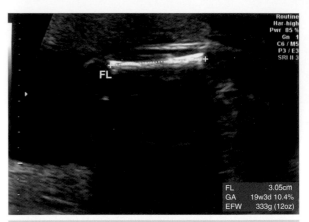

Fig 8.17 • Measurement of femur length (FL). Note the position of the callipers giving the correct measurement along the length and not diagonally across the femur.

tissue should be visible beyond both ends of the femur and the bone should not appear to merge with the skin of the thigh at any point (Fig. 8.17).

It should be noted that Chitty et al describe measurement of FL as being taken 'as close as possible to right angles to the ultrasound beam'. The end points of the femur are often difficult to define when the femur is imaged in the true horizontal plane but are much easier to define when the bone lies at a slight angle of 5–15° to the horizontal. There is therefore a decision to be made as to whether you are able to identify the end points of the femur better, and therefore your FL measurement is likely to be more accurate, if you image the femur as described by Chitty or at a slight angle.

The angle of the bone relative to the horizontal can be manipulated by dipping one end of the probe gently into the maternal abdomen. As your experience develops you will need to decide how best to measure the FL, relative to the horizontal, in order to obtain the most accurate FL measurement.

On the frozen image, place the intersection of the cross of the first linear calliper at one end of the FL. Place the intersection of the cross of the second linear calliper at the other end of the FL, therefore making sure that the callipers are placed in the centre at each end of the bone. This ensures that you measure the true length of the bone (Fig. 8.17) and are not falsely increasing its length by measuring diagonally across it.

It is good practice to obtain measurements from three separate images of the same femur. These should be within 1.0 mm of each other.

Growth of the FL is illustrated in Appendix 10.

PROBLEMS IN OBTAINING THE CORRECT SECTION FOR FL

Fetal Movements

Most problems arising with measuring the FL are due to a combination of fetal movements and slow use of the freeze button. The use of the cine-loop may be useful in such situations. However, reliance on the cine-loop rather than learning to obtain the correct section with timely use of the freeze button if the end points of the femur cannot be adequately visualized encourages what we consider to be a second-rate scanning technique. We recommend unfreezing the image and seeking another, better image. It is very easy to under- or overestimate the FL by 3–5 mm if a suboptimal image is measured.

One or Both End Points Are Difficult to Define

When one or both end points are difficult to define, dip one end of the probe gently into the maternal abdomen as described earlier.

The Upper Femur Appears Straight While the Lower Femur Appears Bowed

The slight bowing seen in the lower limb is a normal consequence of the imaging process. Unilateral femoral abnormalities are very rare but should always be considered as a possible, if unlikely, explanation for the dissimilarity, especially if the difference in the shape of the two femurs is marked. An experienced second opinion should be sought if necessary.

Gestational Age Equivalents of the HC and FL Disagree

The estimation of gestational age obtained from FL measurements should agree with that obtained from the measurement of the HC. If the FL is small (outside the normal range) compared with the HC (on the 50th centile), then all the long bones and the plantar view of the feet should be carefully measured to exclude skeletal dysplasia (see Chapter 12). A short femur can also be associated with trisomy 21. This discrepancy is discussed in greater length towards the end of this chapter.

EVALUATING THE FEMUR LENGTH VIEW

As discussed earlier, irrespective of which template you are using, it is important to observe the information presented in the section selected for FL measurement and thus to familiarize yourself with the range of normal appearances of this section at 18–22 weeks of gestation.

Once you have this experience, you will hopefully identify a finding which is not normal even if you do not have the experience to pinpoint the specific diagnosis.

Is the appearance of the femur normal, namely is its echogenicity normal and is its shape normal? Reduced echogenicity may be associated with a hypomineralization disorder such as osteogenesis imperfecta type II or hypophosphatasia.

If the shape is abnormal, does the femur appear abnormally broad, is it abnormally bent or bowed or does it appear fractured? An abnormally shaped or fractured femur may be associated with one or more of the skeletal dysplasias. Classification of skeletal dysplasias is discussed in Chapter 12.

EVALUATING THE ANATOMY BETWEEN THE AC AND FL SECTIONS

Although the main aim of this part of the exercise is to measure and assess the femur properly it is important that you make maximum use of the various sections of the fetal abdomen that you slide through between the AC section and the section demonstrating both iliac crests. Between these two planes lie a number of important parts of the fetal anatomy, namely both kidneys, the cord insertion, the fetal bladder and the lumbar and sacral vertebrae and their skin covering.

One of the reasons why we recommend that you find the femur by sliding down from the AC onto the femur is that this technique enables you to assess the fetal anatomy of the lower abdomen and pelvis while en route from the AC plane to the FL plane. There is no rush to move from the AC to the FL. Slide your probe slowly down the fetal abdomen, making sure the sections you obtain are true cross-sections – this is important for proper assessment of the vertebrae as discussed in Chapter 12 – rather than oblique sections of the fetal body. Assess all the fetal anatomical structures demonstrated in each section that you obtain.

THE CLINICAL IMPACT OF CORRECTLY EVALUATING THE FL SECTION

Proper evaluation of the FL section has therefore excluded a number of severe skeletal dysplasias and supported the low-risk result for Down's syndrome in those pregnancies in which Down's screening was undertaken.

Proper evaluation of the transverse sections between the AC and FL planes should have excluded major urinary tract abnormalities, omphalocele, gastroschisis and open lumbar or lumbosacral spinia bifida with meningocele/myelomeningocele involving – we would suggest – three or more vertebrae.

OBSERVATION OF THE FETUS FOR BODY AND LIMB MOVEMENTS

In the majority of situations movements of the fetal body and limbs will be only too apparent while attempting to obtain the required measurements. If the fetus appears to have remained uncharacteristically quiet during the examination, observe the fetus and ensure that flexion and extension of the limbs and some body movements have occurred. Conditions such as arthrogryposis and severe anaemia are associated with such loss of tone and movement.

EVALUATION OF AMNIOTIC FLUID VOLUME

From approximately 16 weeks of gestation the amniotic fluid is essentially fetal urine. Before this time, contributions to the amniotic fluid also come from the amniotic membranes, the umbilical cord, the fetal skin and the placenta. Thus, at 18–22 weeks, amniotic fluid is effectively produced solely by the fetal kidneys and removed by fetal swallowing and subsequent absorption by the fetal bowel. Disruption of this pathway will cause an abnormal reduction or increase in amniotic fluid volume. Abnormal amniotic fluid volume is therefore an important indicator of a range of varying fetal abnormalities. The amniotic fluid should be assessed for normality during every examination.

Normal amniotic fluid volume is shown in Figs 8.8, 8.9 and 8.16. Reduced fluid is described as *oligohydramnios*. As evident from Fig. 8.18, you must ensure that you have visually assessed the amniotic fluid throughout the entire uterus properly before making a diagnosis of oligohydramnios (Fig. 8.18). Anhydramnios describes absent amniotic fluid (Fig. 8.19). *Polyhydramnios* describes increased amniotic fluid (Fig. 8.20). As with oligohydramnios, and as shown in Fig. 8.20, you must evaluate the whole uterus before reaching a conclusion regarding a genuine increase in amniotic fluid.

Formal measurement of the amniotic fluid volume using the amniotic fluid index (AFI) is not normally undertaken before 24 weeks. The measurement techniques are described in Chapter 13. Before 24 weeks, visual assessment of the amount

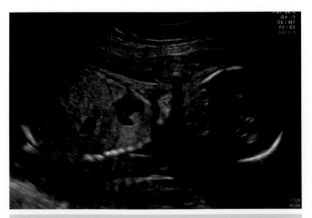

Fig 8.18 • Longitudinal section of a 20 week pregnancy. The amniotic fluid appears reduced in this section, suggesting possible oligohydramnios. This paucity of fluid however was confined to one area of the uterus only. When the uterus had been evaluated fully, it became apparent that the amniotic fluid volume overall was normal.

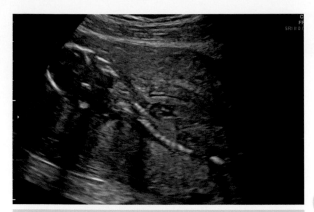

Fig 8.19 • A longitudinal section of a 16 weeks uterus following spontaneous rupture of membranes. No amniotic fluid is present. This is therefore a case of anhydramnios. The fetus is breech and the placenta appears to be posterior although the absence of amniotic fluid makes it difficult to distinguish placental tissue from uterine wall.

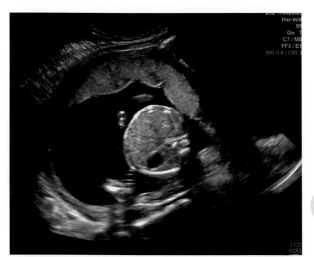

Fig 8.20 • Cross section of a 19 week uterus with a cross section of a breech fetus. The amount of amniotic fluid in this section appears visually increased, suggesting possible polyhydramnios. Having evaluated the uterus properly it was evident that the amniotic fluid volume overall was normal.

of amniotic fluid present, and its qualitative reporting, is acceptable.

VISUAL ASSESSMENT

Retaining a mental picture of the amount of amniotic fluid surrounding the normal fetus at each scan you undertake will soon provide you with the required experience to make an accurate visual assessment of the amniotic fluid volume.

In the normal pregnant uterus the fetal parts are surrounded by a number of clearly visible pockets of amniotic fluid. Some pockets will contain sections of the umbilical cord and others will not. Movements of the fetal body and limb are unrestricted. With the exception of Fig. 8.19, all the pregnancies in this chapter have a normal amniotic fluid volume.

OLIGOHYDRAMNIOS/ANHYDRAMNIOS

Diagnosis of oligohydramnios is made subjectively when only one or two small pockets of cord-free fluid either around the fetus or between its limbs can be identified within the uterus. *Anhydramnios* describes the absence of any such cord-free pools (Fig. 8.19). In both situations fetal limb and body movements are either absent or severely reduced. The fetal limbs are described as 'crowded' because of the lack of available space.

Severe oligohydramnios and anhydramnios are associated with lower urinary tract obstruction such as posterior urethral valves or urethral atresia or *bilateral* upper urinary tract abnormalities such as bilateral renal agenesis or bilateral multicystic renal dysplasia (see Chapter 11). Severe uteroplacental insufficiency and premature rupture of membranes are additional causes of oligo- or anhydramnios.

POLYHYDRAMNIOS

Polyhydramnios describes the presence of multiple large pools of amniotic fluid in which the fetus is normally moving freely with active limb movements. The need to increase the depth of view and/or reduce the gain, because the whole image appears unusually bright, are both useful indicators that increased fluid is present.

Polyhydramnios is associated with atresia or obstruction of the upper gastrointestinal tract, anencephaly, tumours of the face and neck (see Chapter 9) and conditions which cause pulmonary compression including congenital diaphragmatic hernia, congenital lung lesions and skeletal disorders presenting with a small chest (see Chapters 10–12). A quiescent fetus in the presence of polyhydramnios is a very unusual and often abnormal finding.

LOCALIZATION OF THE POSITION OF THE PLACENTA RELATIVE TO THE INTERNAL OS

The purpose of identifying the site of the placenta is to assess its position relative to the internal os. This is because of the important clinical implications associated with a placenta which encroaches on, or covers, the internal os both during the pregnancy and at the time of delivery.

The placenta is best identified by scanning the uterus longitudinally and is easily recognized by its more hyperechoic appearance compared with that of the underlying myometrium. Careful inspection will demonstrate the chorionic plate as a bright linear echo between the homogeneous echoes of the body of the placenta and the amniotic fluid (Fig. 8.21 and 8.22).

It is unnecessary to ask women to attend with a full bladder at the time of the 18–22 week scan as the majority will have a placenta which is obviously 'not low'. The cervical canal lies directly posterior to the bladder, typically at about 30–45° to the horizontal (Fig. 8.22). It is best imaged by placing the probe in the midline with its lower end just above the symphysis; slight dextrorotation may be necessary.

The actual internal os may be difficult to identify transabdominally, but its position can be assumed by visualizing the slight dimple at the upper end of the cervical canal below the maternal bladder. Therefore, providing you are able to visualize the lower placental edge and the assumed internal os, making the diagnosis of a low-lying placenta is possible even with a partially filled bladder.

The placenta may be positioned at the fundus of the uterus, on the anterior wall of the uterus, on the posterior wall of the uterus, on the left lateral wall or the right lateral wall or centrally over the internal os. Its position relates to the original site of implantation of the blastocyst at the beginning of the pregnancy. This is the position you will include in your reporting of placental site.

You must then decide where the leading edge of the placenta lies relative to the internal os. A pregnancy in which the placenta is correctly reported as 'upper' or 'not low' at 18–22 weeks is not at risk of later placenta praevia.

The term placenta praevia should not be used in the second trimester. *Placenta praevia* is a term relating placental position to the lower segment of the uterus. The uterus does not have a true lower segment in the second trimester. Thus it is preferable to retain the term *placenta praevia* until after

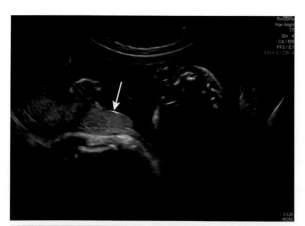

Fig 8.21 • A longitudinal section of the uterus showing a posterior placenta. The placental tissue is more hyperechoic compared with that of the underlying myometrium. The chorionic plate (arrow) is visible as a bright linear echo between the homogeneous echoes of the body of the placenta and the amniotic fluid.

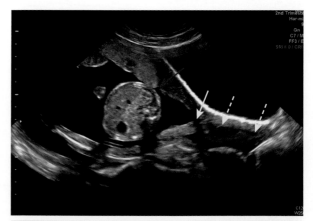

Fig 8.22 • A longitudinal section of the uterus showing an anterior placenta. The plaenta is not low lying as its leading edge (red arrow) is well clear of the assumed internal os (yellow arrow). The dashed yellow arrows show the cervical canal. The cervical canal lies directly posterior to the bladder typically at 30° to 45° to the horizontal (solid lines).

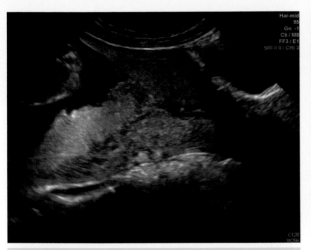

Fig 8.23 • A longitudinal section of the lower uterus and cervix of a 21 week pregnancy showing a low-lying placenta extending to and covering the internal os.

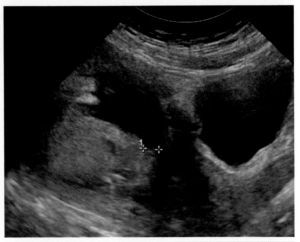

Fig 8.24 • A longitudinal section of the lower uterus and cervical canal at 21 weeks, demonstrating a low lying posterior placenta. The crosses demonstrate the distance (7.4 mm) between the leading edge of the placenta and the assumed internal os. Note the moderately full maternal bladder on the right of the image. Posterior placenta reaching the internal os but not covering the cervix.

36 weeks of gestation, when the formation of the lower segment is complete.

A pregnancy is at high risk of later placenta praevia if the placenta completely covers the assumed internal os at 18–22 weeks (Fig. 8.23). Such pregnancies should always be rescanned in the third trimester in order that appropriate plans for delivery can be made. We recommend that such a placenta at 18–22 weeks is reported as follows: 'The anterior/posterior placenta is centrally positioned over the internal os, as assessed by transabdominal imaging. A further scan has been arranged at 32 weeks to review placental site to exclude a major degree of placenta praevia'.

The risk of later placenta praevia is less easy to quantify if only the leading edge of the placenta extends to and/or covers the assumed internal os. What is important is that you are able to accurately determine and report the relationship between the leading edge of the placenta and the assumed internal os at this gestation (Fig. 8.24). We recommend that only pregnancies in which the leading edge of the placenta extends to or covers the assumed internal os at 18–22 weeks are reassessed in the third trimester for placental site. Thus the pregnancy shown in Fig. 8.23 has a high risk of having placenta praevia while this is unlikely in the pregnancy shown in Fig. 8.24.

We recommend that such a placenta at 18–22 weeks is reported as follows: 'The anterior/posterior,

right lateral, left lateral placenta is low lying, with its leading edge extending to but not covering the internal os, as assessed by transabdominal imaging. A further scan has been arranged at 36 weeks to review placental site and exclude a minor degree of placenta praevia'.

A transvaginal scan should always be performed when accurate assessment of the relative positions of the placental edge and the internal os is needed, irrespective of the gestational age, or if views are suboptimal and a low-lying placenta is suspected. The distance between the leading edge of the placenta and the internal os should be measured using linear callipers and this measurement included in the report. Such quantitative information allows comparison of the placental position with later scans and for optimal clinical management regarding delivery (see Chapter 14).

It is important that you are able to exclude the less common features associated with the placenta, including a succenturiate lobe and vasa praevia. These, together with other anomalies associated with the placenta, are discussed in Chapter 14.

Filling the maternal bladder and then rescanning with the transabdominal probe is an inferior imaging choice compared with emptying the maternal bladder and scanning with the transvaginal probe and is one which we do not recommend.

PROBLEMS OF PLACENTAL LOCALISATION

Overdistension of the Maternal Bladder

Where the maternal bladder is overfull it compresses the uterus, causing the low anterior and low posterior walls to abut each other, simulating a low-lying placenta. This provides a further good reason for not requiring women to attend with full bladders

Braxton Hicks Contractions

Fig. 8.25 demonstrates how the Braxton Hicks contraction may be a trap for the unwary. These contractions cause a 'bunching' of the myometrium, particularly on the low posterior wall of the uterus, and are easily mistaken for a low posterior placenta (or a fibroid). To avoid making this mistake, first examine the entire uterus. Identifying the placenta elsewhere indicates that what you initially thought was a posterior placenta was indeed a Braxton Hicks contraction.

Second, you should always look for strong linear echo resulting from the interface between the chorionic plate of the placenta and the amniotic fluid

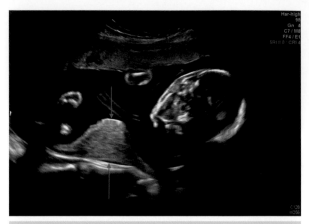

Fig 8.25 • A longitudinal section of the uterus of a 21 week pregnancy showing a Braxton Hicks contraction (arrows) on the posterior wall of the uterus. Note that there is absence of a strong linear echo representing the chorionic plate and therefore this is uterine wall not placental tissue.

adjacent to it. A Braxton Hicks contraction does not produce this strong echo as the interface is between the uterine wall, rather than the chorionic plate, and the amniotic fluid.

Finally, if you are still in real doubt, you should rescan the woman after a 20 minute period, during which time the Braxton Hicks contraction will have either disappeared or changed in appearance or position.

ASSESSMENT OF FETAL BIOMETRY

Interpretation of the measurements taken at the time of the routine 18–22 week ultrasound examination will depend on whether measurements have been taken at an earlier examination, but one which was performed after 10 weeks of pregnancy. When reliable measurements were taken at the earlier examination, the gestational age should have been calculated and the EDD assigned at that examination. The second trimester measurements you have just taken are thus used to assess fetal growth velocity.

Establishing gestational age requires the assumption that the fetus is of average size – that is, its measurements lie on the 50th centile for its gestational age. Having made this assumption, the gestational age of the pregnancy is then calculated by using the 50th centile gestational age equivalent of the fetal measurements taken, using the appropriate dating algorithm or chart. It follows therefore that the subsequent measurements of a fetus that is growing normally will also plot onto the 50th centile of the relevant size charts.

It is likely that you are using a computer program into which you enter the measurements of HC, BPD, AC and FL. As the EDD of the pregnancy was assigned at the earlier dating scan, the program calculates the current gestational age based on this previously assigned EDD. Having calculated the gestational age at the time of your scan, it then plots the measurements you have just obtained on the relevant size charts, at the appropriate gestational age. If you do not have access to such software, you should plot the measurements by hand on the appropriate size charts.

Confirmation of 'normal' growth velocity should, in theory, only be reported if the HC, AC and FL measurements plot onto the 50th centile. In practice it is reasonable to use 'normal growth' to describe measurements that plot between, we suggest, the 40th and 60th centiles. We suggest that growth velocity is best described as 'within normal limits' if the measurements plot between either the 60th and 97th centiles or 40th and 3rd centiles using the Chitty size charts.

Where one of the HC, AC or FL measurements plots onto a significantly different centile from the other two, you must consider what this combination of measurements may indicate. The first thing you should do is review the measured sections of all three parameters. This is to ensure, first, that the sections selected for all three measurements were correct and, second, that the sections for all three parameters were measured correctly. You should not assume that the measurement that disagrees with the other two was incorrect because only it was over- or under measured. Poor section selection or poor measurement of one, two or all of the parameters may influence, incorrectly, the conclusions reached.

It is unusual for growth-related problems to manifest themselves at 18–22 weeks, but a significant centile discrepancy between one or more measurements can be associated with a range of abnormalities as shown in Table 8.1. Having reviewed the measured sections and confirmed that the combination of measurements obtained cannot be considered to be consistent with normal fetal growth, such pregnancies should be reviewed in a timely fashion by a more senior sonographer colleague or referred to a fetal medicine specialist.

Fetal growth is discussed in more detail in Chapter 13.

DATING THE PREGNANCY

If the examination you have just performed is the first of the pregnancy or if the pregnancy was scanned previously but only before 10 weeks of pregnancy, the gestational age should be calculated, and the EDD assigned, from the HC.

Although you will use the HC, with support from the FL, to calculate the gestational age assessment, the measurement of the AC should also be used to provide confirmation that fetal growth, as indicated by the AC, is normal.

It is important to confirm that the data sets used by the ultrasound equipment software manufacturers, and therefore the gestational age equivalents displayed on the ultrasound monitor, conform to national guidance. As discussed earlier, the data sets should be those from Chitty et al.

As discussed in Chapter 7, it is important that you understand the differences between dating and growth charts, the specific role each has in the correct application of the measurements you take and therefore their correct clinical applications.

In cases such as those which we are discussing here, where the gestational age is unknown, estimation of gestational age and assignment of the

HC CENTILE	AC CENTILE	FL CENTILE	POSSIBLE ASSOCIATION
50th	50th	3rd or below	Skeletal dysplasia, trisomy 21
3rd or below	50th	50th	Microcephaly
50th	3rd	50th	Early asymmetrical growth restriction
3rd or below	3rd or below	3rd or below	Early symmetrical growth restriction, trisomy 13, trisomy 18, triploidy

Table 8.1 Possible complications associated with disparities of the three measurements taken to assess fetal size at 18–22 weeks, following accurate dating performed after 10 weeks of gestation

AC, abdominal circumference; FL, femur length, HC, head circumference.

EDD should be made from a *dating* chart in which the HC is plotted on the *x*-axis (independent variable) and the gestational age is plotted on the *y*-axis (dependent variable), or from tables derived in the same manner (see Appendix 3). In practical terms this means that, having measured the HC, you estimate the gestational age by use of the relevant dating table. The measurement can then be plotted on the growth chart according to the gestational age assigned from the dating table by the ultrasound measurements. The electronic package that you use for reporting should go through the same process for you when you select the 'calculating gestational age' tab combined with the HC 'option'.

We recommend that dating charts are used in look-up table format and, having calculated the gestational age and assigned the EDD, that all measurements are then graphically represented on the relevant Chitty size charts.

DATING A TWIN PREGNANCY

The HC measurement from the larger fetus should be used to determine the gestational age of a twin pregnancy.

REPORTING THE SCAN FINDINGS

Having successfully completed the first steps of your scan, you must now record your findings in the report. The woman should have a copy of this to place in her own handheld record and a further copy should be filed in the hospital medical record. The latter may be either a paper or an electronic copy.

As this chapter deals with the first steps of the 18–22 week scan, our recommendations here only include the reporting of what has been discussed in this chapter. Reporting of abnormal or unusual anatomical findings is discussed elsewhere in this text.

REPORTING THE FINDINGS WHEN THE EDD HAS ALREADY BEEN ACCURATELY ASSIGNED

We suggest the following template of information that should be included in a scan report when the EDD has already been accurately assigned:
- the date of the examination
- the reason for the examination
- the machine used for the examination
- the approach used, whether transabdominal, transvaginal or both
- recording of latex allergy and documentation of appropriate management if the transvaginal probe was used
- number of fetuses present (for twin pregnancy, see Chapter 15)
- the ultrasound-assigned EDD

- gestational age as calculated from either the CRL or HC at the earlier scan
- confirmation that the fetus was alive
- measurement of HC, BPD, FL and AC
- measurement of PH and TCD
- assessment of amniotic fluid volume
- position of placenta relative to the internal os
- position and size of fibroids and description and size of any ovarian pathological conditions
- interpretation of fetal size relative to gestational age
- interpretation of the fetal anatomy
- documentation of relevant management after the scan, such as referral if indicated and arrangements for further scans, together with the gestational age at which these scans are to be performed
- the name and professional role of the operator/supervisor
- the name and status of the trainee if performing any aspect of the examination.

REPORTING THE FINDINGS WHEN THE GESTATIONAL AGE AND THE EDD ARE TO BE ASSIGNED

We suggest the following template of information that should be included in a scan report when the gestational age and the EDD are to be assigned:

- the date of the examination
- the reason for the examination
- the machine used for the examination
- the approach used, whether transabdominal, transvaginal or both
- recording of latex allergy and documentation of appropriate management if the transvaginal probe was used
- number of fetuses present (for twin pregnancy, see Chapter 15)
- confirmation that the fetus was alive
- measurement of HC, BPD, FL and AC
- measurement of PH and TCD
- assessment of amniotic fluid volume
- position of placenta relative to the internal os
- gestational age as calculated from the HC

- the ultrasound-assigned EDD
- interpretation of size of AC and FL relative to HC, based on assigned gestational age
- interpretation of the fetal anatomy
- position and size of fibroids and description and size of any ovarian pathological conditions
- documentation of relevant management after the scan, such as referral if indicated and arrangements for further scans, together with the gestational age at which these scans are to be performed
- the name and professional role of the operator/supervisor
- the name and status of the trainee if performing any aspect of the examination.

SCREENING FOR DOWN'S SYNDROME WITH THE QUADRUPLE TEST

Those women attending for their first scan in the second trimester and who are requesting screening for Down's syndrome should be offered the quadruple test. This is because combined screening for Down's syndrome is not possible after 14^{+1} weeks of gestation.

The Down's syndrome risk can be calculated from the quadruple test from 14^{+0} weeks to 22^{+0} weeks, although the national recommendation is that this test should be offered from 14^{+2} weeks to 20^{+0} weeks only. As the sensitivity of the test is greatest at around 16 weeks, this is the optimal time at which to perform the test.

As its name suggests, the quadruple test measures the levels of four analytes or markers in the maternal blood, namely alpha-fetoprotein (AFP), unconjugated oestriol (uE_3), total human chorionic gonadotropin (hCG) and inhibin-A.

In pregnancies affected with Down's syndrome, AFP and uE_3 levels tend to be about 25% lower than in unaffected pregnancies. Conversely, levels of total hCG and inhibin-A tend to be higher in cases of Down's syndrome, with levels on average about double those of unaffected pregnancies (Table 8.2). The measured levels of the markers will vary between different laboratories so the concentration of each marker is expressed as a multiple of the median (MoM) for pregnancies of the same gestational age.

The concentrations of the markers vary with gestational age. Concentrations of AFP and uE_3 increase

ANALYTE	PATTERN	MEDIAN MoM*
AFP	Low	0.74
Total hCG	High	2.05
uE_3	Low	0.70
Inhibin-A	high	2.54

Table 8.2 The pattern and average MoM of the four analytes of the quadruple test in pregnancies affected with Down's syndrome compared with unaffected pregnancies where the MoM for each analyte in a normal pregnancy is 1.0 MoM

*Wald N et al. First and second trimester antenatal screening for Down's syndrome; the results of the Serum, Urine and Ultrasound Screening Study (SURUSS) Health Technology Assessment 2003; 7(11): 1288.

AFP, alpha-fetoprotein; hCG, human chorionic gonadotropin; MoM, multiple of the median; uE_3, oestriol.

189

DOWN'S SYNDROME	HEAVIER WOMEN		LIGHTER WOMEN	
	LEVEL	SCREENING EFFECT	LEVEL	SCREENING EFFECT
AFP	Lower	Increase FPR	Higher	Decrease DTR
Total hCG	Lower	Decrease DTR	Higher	Increase FPR
uE$_3$	Lower	Increase FPR	Higher	Decrease DTR
Inhibin-A	Lower	Decrease DTR	Higher	Increase FPR

Table 8.3 The effect of maternal weight on levels of AFP, total hCG, uE3 and inhibin-A in the detection rate and false-positive rate of Down's syndrome

AFP, alphafetoprotein; DTR detection rate; FPR, false-positive rate; hCG, human chorionic gonadotropin; uE$_3$, oestriol.

with gestational age, that of total hCG decreases with gestational age and that of inhibin-A decreases up to 17 weeks of gestation and then increases.

As with the serum analytes used in combined screening, the quadruple test markers are affected by a number of factors.

MATERNAL WEIGHT

Serum dilution effects will falsely decrease levels of all four markers in heavier women and produce falsely increased levels of all four markers in lighter women unless the risk calculation is adjusted for maternal weight. The impact of maternal weight on the detection rate and false-positive rate for Down's syndrome is shown in Table 8.3.

ETHNICITY

Levels of AFP tend to be about 20% higher and total hCG levels about 10% higher in Afro-Caribbean women than in Caucasian women. Inhibin-A levels tend to be about 5% higher in South Asian women than in Caucasian women. Failure to adjust for ethnic group will therefore lead to a decrease in the detection rate and an increase in the false-positive rate for Down's syndrome in Afro-Caribbean women and in South Asian women to a lesser degree.

SMOKING STATUS

Total hCG levels tend to be about 20% lower in women who smoke or have smoked at any time since conception or embryo transfer compared with women who have not. Inhibin-A levels are about 60% higher in these women. Failure to adjust for smoking will therefore lead to an increase in the false-positive rate for Down's syndrome in these women.

METHOD OF CONCEPTION

Total hCG levels tend to be 10% higher and uE$_3$ levels about 10% lower in women who conceive after in vitro fertilization, compared with pregnancies conceived naturally. Both these markers will contribute to an increase in the false-positive rate for Down's syndrome in in vitro fertilization pregnancies.

INSULIN-DEPENDENT DIABETES MELLITUS

Insulin-dependent diabetes mellitus (IDDM) has a small but important effect on AFP and uE$_3$ levels. Levels of AFP tend to be about 8% lower and uE$_3$ about 6% lower in women with IDDM, leading to an increase in the false-positive rate for Down's syndrome in these women.

SCREENING FOR EDWARDS' AND PATAU'S SYNDROMES WITH THE QUADRUPLE TEST

Quadruple screen testing can also be performed for Edwards' and Patau's syndromes but its performance is poor.

Levels of AFP, oestriol and hCG tend to be reduced in Edwards' syndrome, but there is no significant difference in the level of inhibin-A compared with karyotypically normal pregnancies. By contrast, levels of inhibin-A are increased in Patau's syndrome and there is no significant difference in levels of the other three analytes compared with karyotypically normal pregnancies.

Ultrasound examination is the nationally recommended screening test for Edwards' and Patau's syndromes in the second trimester; thus second trimester serum testing is not normally offered to screen for trisomy 18 and trisomy 13.

Further reading

Altman D G, Chitty L S 1997 New charts for ultrasound dating of pregnancy. Ultrasound Obstet Gynecol 10:174–179

International Society of Ultrasound in Obstetrics and Gynaecology 2007 Sonographic examination of the fetal central nervous system guidelines for performing the 'basic examination' and the 'fetal neurosonogram'. Ultrasound Obstet Gynecol 29:109–116

Loughna P, Chitty L, Evans T, Chudleigh T 2009 Fetal size and dating; charts recommended for clinical obstetric practice. Ultrasound 17:161–167

National Health Service 2010 18+0 to 20+6 weeks fetal anomaly scan – national standards and guidance for England 2010. http://fetalanomaly.screening.nhs.uk/standardsandpolicy

Wolfson Institute of Preventive Medicine 2011 Antenatal screening for Down's syndrome and open neural tube defects; the quadruple test. Information for health professionals. Wolfson Institute of Preventive Medicine, London

Assessing the fetal head, brain, neck and face

9

CONTENTS

This chapter addresses the ultrasound examination of the fetal head, face and neck with particular reference to the second trimester of pregnancy. The aims of this chapter are to describe the correct techniques used in order to assess the:

- shape of the head
- integrity of the bones of the skull
- echogenicity of the brain and bones of the skull
- size of the head
- appearances of the intracranial anatomy
- appearances of the posterior fossa of the brain

- appearances of the neck
- appearances of the face.

The examination of the skull and intracranial anatomy should follow on naturally after measuring the head circumference (HC), biparietal diameter (BPD), posterior horn (PH) of the lateral ventricle and the transcerebellar diameter (TCD) (see Chapter 8). You are already aware of the benefits of a systematic approach in order to maximize the likelihood of your exclusion or detection of the various abnormalities associated with the fetal head, neck and face.

The descriptions of the various abnormalities included in this chapter have been arranged to link with the scanning sequence recommended in Chapter 8.

THE SHAPE OF THE SKULL

The shape of the normal skull in the lateral ventricles plane is that of a rugby football, being rounded at the back (occiput) or posteriorly and more pointed at the front (sinciput) or anteriorly (see Fig. 8.2). Remember that the shape of the skull is altered by the orientation of the probe relative to the position of the fetus.

DOLICOCEPHALY AND BRACHYCEPHALY

The skull can appear elongated in the axial plane when a fetus is in a breech presentation or in transverse lie. This results in a skull shape that is longer and thinner than the more usual shape and is termed dolicocephaly. The BPD measurement in such situations is therefore smaller than in a cephalic presentation. The HC is unaffected by presentation or lie, so dolicocephaly will result in a BPD measurement that lies on a lower centile than the HC. Dolicocephaly is considered to be a normal variation in skull shape providing the HC is a normal size for the gestational age (Fig. 9.1). The effect on the BPD measurement of a non-cephalic presentation becomes more marked with increasing gestation.

A skull shape that is more rounded in appearance than the more usual rugby football shape is termed brachycephaly. The BPD measurement in such situations is therefore larger than in the more usual head shape. The HC is unaffected by brachycephaly, which will result in a BPD measurement that lies on a higher centile than the HC. Brachycephaly is considered to be a normal variant providing the HC is a normal size for the gestational age.

LEMON-SHAPED SKULL

A normal-shaped head can appear abnormal if an incorrect section is used to measure the HC. Where the orientation of the probe at the front of the fetal head is too low – that is, between the correct level demonstrating the anterior horns and the incorrect level demonstrating the fetal orbits – the frontal bones of the head may appear scalloped. This produces a skull which is lemon-shaped (see Fig. 8.13). If the rotation of the probe is adjusted to obtain the correct section but the skull still appears 'lemon-shaped', this should be considered abnormal.

Open spina bifida is associated with a lemon-shaped skull in approximately 90% of cases

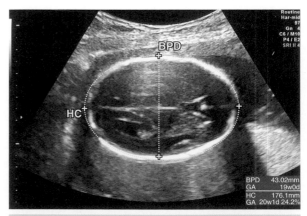

Fig 9.1 • A dolicocephalic-shaped skull of a fetus in a breech presentation at 20 weeks of gestation. The biparietal diameter measurement is equivalent to only 19 weeks, whereas the head circumference measurement is equivalent to 20 weeks and 1 day. BPD, biparietal diameter; HC, head circumference.

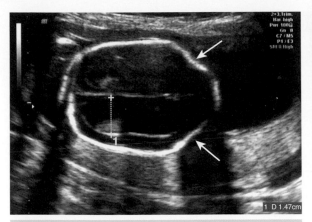

Fig 9.2 • A lemon-shaped skull in a case of spina bifida at 16⁺⁴ weeks. Note the significant scalloping of the frontal bones (arrows). Severe ventriculomegaly is also present with a posterior horn measurement of 14.7 mm.

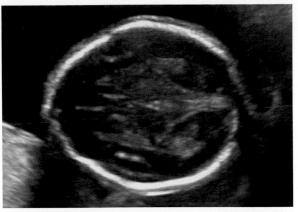

Fig 9.3 • A strawberry-shaped skull in a fetus with trisomy 18 at 20 weeks of gestation. The frontal bones appear pointed, the occiput is flattened and the shape is brachycephalic.

examined at 18–22 weeks. The 'lemon sign' describes the abnormal scalloping of the frontal bones, which produces a more angular appearance to the front of the skull (Fig. 9.2). This is thought to be as a result of the caudal displacement of the cranial contents within the skull, which is pliable at this stage of development. This abnormal appearance of the skull should only be used as a marker for spina bifida between 16 and 24 weeks. The lemon-shaped skull is not a reliable feature of open spina bifida after this gestation, thus a normally shaped skull should not be used to exclude spina bifida after 24 weeks of gestation.

STRAWBERRY-SHAPED SKULL

The skull is considered to be abnormal when it resembles the shape of a strawberry in the lateral ventricles plane. In a strawberry-shaped skull, the occiput is flattened and there is a pointed appearance to the frontal bones and the head appears brachycephalic (Fig. 9.3). This appearance is associated with trisomy 18 and with abnormalities of suture development such as craniosynostosis.

CLOVER-LEAF-SHAPED SKULL

A clover-leaf-shaped skull describes a skull that has a diamond-shaped appearance in the lateral ventricles plane, with marked bulging of the parietal bones. This skull shape is associated with the most

common of the lethal skeletal dysplasias, namely thanatophoric dysplasia. A clover-leaf-shaped skull should prompt a thorough examination of the length and appearance of all the fetal limbs (see Chapter 12) and an assessment of the shape and size of the fetal chest (see Chapter 10).

Craniosynostosis describes the premature fusing of the sutures between the bones that form the cranium and the clover-leaf-shaped skull is a result of this process. There are various types of craniosynostosis that relate to the specific sutures involved.

PRACTICAL MANAGEMENT OF AN ABNORMALLY SHAPED SKULL

The classic appearances of lemon-, strawberry- and clover-leaf-shaped skulls are easily distinguished from each other, as can be seen by comparing Figs. 8.2 with Figs 9.2 and 9.3. In some situations it may be difficult to decide whether the skull is more strawberry- than lemon-shaped or clover-leaf- rather than strawberry-shaped. These skull shapes are associated with structural abnormalities elsewhere in the fetus which differ significantly from each other. Identifying an abnormal skull shape should therefore prompt a detailed assessment of specific parts of the fetal anatomy as it is the combination of abnormalities which will enable the correct diagnosis to be made. It is very unlikely that abnormal skull shape is the only detectable feature of the structural abnormality which is present.

THE INTEGRITY OF THE SKULL BONES

The individual bones that make up the cranium appear as hyperechoic, curved lines surrounding the brain tissue. The spaces between the bones of the cranium represent the sutures that separate the frontal, parietal and occipital bones and, with careful examination, can be seen from the late first trimester onward.

Ossification of the fetal skull is normally completed by 12 weeks of gestation and therefore the bony structures of the skull above the orbits should be visible after this time. The vault of the skull should therefore be assessed at the first scan performed at or after 12 weeks to ensure that it is normal in shape and echogenicity and completely surrounds the fetal brain (see Fig. 7.5). As discussed in Chapter 7, when examining and measuring the fetus between 12 and 14 weeks of gestation, the skull should be assessed not only in the sagittal plane used to measure the crown–rump length but also in the plane used to measure the HC.

ACRANIA, EXENCEPHALY AND ANENCEPHALY

Absence of the cranium should be identified from 12 weeks of gestation onward (see Chapter 7). Acrania describes the condition in which the bones that make up the cranial vault are absent. The brain tissue is commonly disorganized and may be incompletely formed. As the brain tissue is not protected by the skull, it is exposed to the amniotic fluid and becomes progressively eroded with increasing gestation. Its appearance will therefore change as the pregnancy advances.

Some authors use the term 'exencephaly' to describe the appearances just outlined, whereas others assign exencephaly to the condition where the brain is still visible but is abnormal in shape. Anencephaly correctly describes the appearance when the brain has been effectively destroyed. This results in no skull and brain above the fetal orbits. It produces the characteristic ultrasound appearance of anencephaly described as the 'frog's eyes' appearance (Fig. 9.4).

Acrania and exencephaly are typically seen in the late first and early second trimester fetus,

whereas anencephaly is more typically seen in the later second trimester and third trimester.

The progressive conditions of acrania, exencephaly and anencephaly are commonly grouped together and all referred to, incorrectly, as 'anencephaly'. In accordance with common usage, this term is therefore used here to encompass the ultrasound appearances of the three phases of the condition.

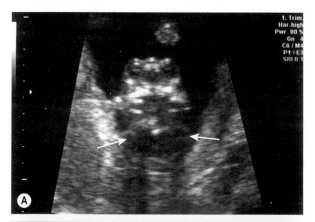

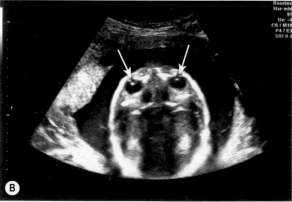

Fig 9.4 • A. Transverse section of a fetal head with acrania and exencephaly at 14^{+1} weeks of gestation demonstrating the presence of brain tissue (arrows), which is an abnormal shape. Note the prominent orbits resulting in a 'frog eyes' appearance. B. Coronal view of the fetal face demonstrating the two orbits and lenses (arrows) with the fetal nose towards 12 o'clock. Note the appearance of the normal, intact skull vault of this 20 week fetus, included for comparison.

Anencephaly is the most severe form of neural tube defect (NTD) and is a lethal condition. It is unreasonable to expect every anomaly that is amenable to ultrasound detection to be identified by ultrasound screening, but anencephaly is a diagnosis that should not be overlooked after 12 weeks of gestation. In the majority of cases, failure to identify an anencephalic fetus after this gestation would be considered substandard care and therefore potentially negligent.

The diagnosis of anencephaly may be missed in the first trimester because the brain may appear normal (as in acrania) and it is the absence of the bones of the cranial vault that has been overlooked. The most common reason for missing the diagnosis in the second or third trimesters is due to the position of the fetal head deep in the maternal pelvis. The assumption is made that the head and intracranial anatomy cannot be assessed because of the fetal position but are assumed to be normal. Thus, when the fetal head is so low in the pelvis that the intracranial anatomy cannot be visualized, a transvaginal scan should be offered. When this is refused, the woman should be reexamined with a full bladder and scanned with the foot of the couch raised in order to encourage the fetus to move up out of the pelvis. If the fetal position is still not favourable, a further scan should be performed no more than 1 week later in order to check the integrity of the skull and brain.

ENCEPHALOCELE

As discussed earlier, the complete integrity of the bones of the cranial vault should be checked in order to exclude absence of any part of the skull. An encephalocele is a meningeal sac containing brain tissue which herniates through a defect in part of the skull. The majority of encephaloceles are skin-covered. The defect most commonly involves the occipital bone (Fig. 9.5), with less common sites being the frontal, nasal (Fig. 9.6) or parietal bones. Such a mass which contains cerebrospinal fluid (CSF) only is more correctly described as a meningocele rather than an encephalocele.

The prognosis will depend on the size, position and content of the encephalocele and the presence of associated abnormalities including karyotypic abnormalities. Structural abnormalities are

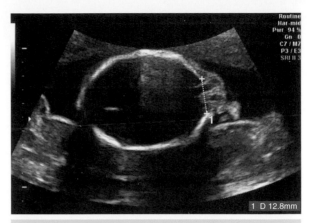

Fig 9.5 • Transverse section of the head of a 20 week fetus with an occipital encephalocele. There is a 12.8 mm defect (identified by the two crosses) in the skull with herniation of the brain tissue into the amniotic fluid.

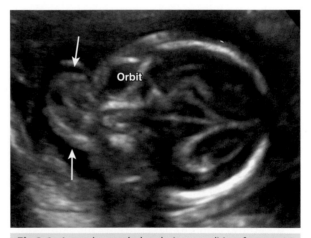

Fig 9.6 • A nasal encephalocele (arrowed) in a fetus at 14 weeks of gestation.

described in 60–80% of antenatal series and in approximately 50% of postnatal series. The risk of associated chromosomal abnormalities is reported in the literature as between 10% and 45%, indicating that the offer of karyotyping should form part of the subsequent discussion with the parents.

Encephalocele may be one component of genetic conditions, the most common of which are Meckel-Gruber syndrome and Walker-Warburg syndrome. Meckel-Gruber syndrome is a rare condition which is characterized by occipital encephalocele, bilaterally enlarged, dysplastic kidneys; and postaxial polydactyly. It is an autosomal recessive condition and therefore has a 1 in 4 recurrence risk.

Bilateral renal dysplasia is often associated with oligohydramnios. Thus, a marked reduction in amniotic fluid volume should always initiate careful examination of not only the urinary tract but also the skull for its integrity and the intracranial contents to exclude Meckel-Gruber syndrome (see Chapter 11).

Walker-Warburg syndrome is also an autosomal recessive condition. It is characterized by ventriculomegaly, cerebellar abnormalities and agyria.

Identifying this lack of ridges or gyri in the surface of the brain is beyond the capabilities of routine screening. An occipital encephalocele may be present, but renal or digital involvement are not features of this condition.

When an encephalocele is detected, therefore, the appearances of the kidneys are particularly important when considering the differential diagnoses of Meckel-Gruber and Walker-Warburg syndromes and discussing the appropriate information with the parents.

THE ECHOGENICITY OF THE BONES OF THE SKULL AND OF THE BRAIN

Normal ossification of the skull produces acoustic shadowing posterior to the skull (see Fig. 8.2). The normally ossified cranium is slightly more echogenic than the cerebral falx or midline. With normal mineralization of the skull, the anterior and posterior horns of the lateral ventricle in the proximal hemisphere of the brain are generally obscured by reverberation artifacts generated as the acoustic beam passes through the fetal skull.

HYPOMINERALIZATION OF THE SKULL

A poorly ossified skull permits a higher proportion of the sound beam to pass through the skull bones to the brain, rather than be reflected back to the probe at the skull surface. This results in a brain which appears much brighter than normal and a skin + skull outline, which, instead of being thin and white, is thicker and much less echogenic than normal. The skull appears thickened because the sound beam is able to resolve interfaces within the skull bone. By contrast, in the normally mineralized skull, the skull echo primarily represents information returning to the probe from the amniotic fluid/skin + skull interface, with the thickness and brightness of this echo being determined largely by the machine's controls.

The net effect of poor ossification therefore is a thicker and less echogenic skin + skull outline surrounding a brain which is noticeably more echogenic or hyperechoic than normal. When imaging

the majority of normal skulls and their intracranial contents, the amount of gain required to image the brain varies little at 18–22 weeks. You should be suspicious of a potential mineralization problem if you find yourself turning down the gain in order to assess the fetal brain because it appears unusually bright.

A poorly ossified skull is softer than a normal skull. Thus the ability to flatten the skull by applying pressure with the probe is another indicator of hypomineralization.

The most common conditions in which deficient mineralization of the skull bones is sufficiently severe to be detected routinely are the skeletal dysplasias of hypophosphatasia and osteogenesis imperfecta type II. As with all skeletal dysplasias, both these conditions are rare. Table 9.1 illustrates the differential diagnoses of abnormal skull appearances.

INCREASED ECHOGENICITY OF THE BRAIN

In the presence of a normally mineralized skull, increased brightness of the noncystic areas of the brain is associated with maternal infections in which the fetus itself is affected. Such infections are cytomegalovirus (CMV), parvovirus and toxoplasmosis and are identified through a maternal blood test for TORCH screening. The TORCH blood test includes screening for TOxoplasmosis, Rubella, Cytomegalovirus, and Herpes simplex.

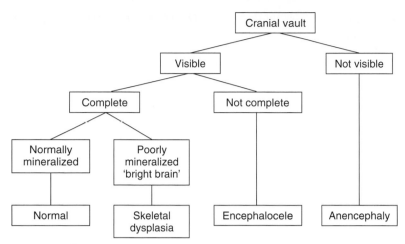

Table 9.1 The more common differential diagnoses of abnormal skull appearances

The intracranial appearances most commonly associated with an affected fetus are ventriculomegaly and areas of calcification within the brain. Infection can also cause haemorrhage. When haemorrhage occurs into the ventricles, it may produce inflammation of the walls of the ventricles or chemical ventriculitis. The ultrasound appearances of ventriculitis include increased echogenicity and/or increased thickness of the ventricular walls.

Table 9.1 illustrates the more common differential diagnoses of abnormal skull appearances.

THE SIZE OF THE HEAD

As discussed in Chapter 8, the HC and abdominal circumference (AC) measurements may not necessarily both lie on the same centile in a normal fetus. However, the HC and AC should remain on approximately their same centiles when these measurements are made sequentially in a normally growing fetus.

MICROCEPHALY

Microcephaly describes an abnormally small head and brain. It is not a structural abnormality but rather an abnormally slow growth velocity of the fetal head. The time of onset of this condition and its progression are variable, with only the most severe being amenable to detection between 18 and 22 weeks. 'Primary microcephaly' is the term used when the condition is identified prior to 36 weeks of pregnancy. Other cases of microcephaly are mild and some, termed 'secondary microcephaly', only develop after birth. Many infants with the severe condition die soon after birth, and those who survive are not only severely mentally compromised but are also dwarfed.

Microcephaly should be suspected where there is an abnormally large difference in the comparative sizes of the fetal head and abdomen – for example, where the AC lies on the 50th centile but the HC lies on or below the 3rd centile. The diagnosis of microcephaly should only be made after serial measurements of the HC, AC and femur length (FL) demonstrate abnormally poor head growth in association with normal growth of the AC and femur. Where microcephaly is suspected, using the head/abdomen (H/A) ratio for assessing the comparative growth of the HC and AC is useful.

Microcephaly is caused by a heterogeneous group of conditions including viral infections, in particular rubella, irradiation, some drugs exposure, including maternal heroin addiction, and excessive alcohol intake during pregnancy.

Antenatal screening of a pregnancy after a pregnancy affected with microcephaly should include early and accurate assessment of growth velocity by measurement of the crown rump length twice, once between 8 and 10 weeks and again at around 12 weeks. Serial measurements of the HC and AC, together with the FL and BPD, should be performed by the same operator using the same machine on a 2 or 3 weekly basis between 15–16 weeks and 24 weeks of gestation. The diagnosis is not normally made until the H/A ratio has fallen below the normal range.

HEAD SIZE AND SPINA BIFIDA

The BPD and HC are commonly reduced compared with the femur and AC in cases of spina bifida in the second trimester. Indeed, if the BPD and HC are found to be small compared with the femur, this should prompt a careful search for both spina bifida and microcephaly.

THE H/A RATIO

The head/abdomen ratio is obtained by dividing the HC measurement by the AC measurement and can be plotted on the H/A ratio chart. It is often easier to assess whether or not the comparative growth rates of the head and abdomen are normal by using one value derived from both of them than by trying to compare the growth velocity of both circumferences separately from their respective size charts.

The H/A ratio falls during normal pregnancy. This is because the HC is larger than the AC in earlier pregnancy, with the comparative difference decreasing until 38 weeks, when both circumferences are the same size. After 38 weeks the AC is larger than the HC. Thus the normal H/A ratio is >1.0 before 38 weeks, 1.0 at 38 weeks and <1.0 after 38 weeks. The abnormally poor head growth in microcephaly produces an H/A ratio which decreases abnormally.

THE APPEARANCES OF THE INTRACRANIAL ANATOMY

THE CEREBRAL FALX AND THE MIDLINE

The cerebral falx is a double fold of dura mater lying in the interhemispheric fissure that separates the right and left cerebral hemispheres. The 'midline' is a constant feature of all transverse sections of the fetal brain from 12 weeks of gestation. It is linear and hyperechoic and arises from the differences in acoustic impedance between the two boundaries of the interhemispheric fissure and the falx lying within it (see Fig. 8.6 and Fig. 9.1).

As some severe brain abnormalities are associated with absence of the midline, confirming the presence of a normal midline echo is important in the exclusion of hydranencephaly and holoprosencephaly.

THE CAVUM SEPTUM PELLUCIDUM

The septum pellucidum is a thin triangular vertical membrane, composed of two leaflets or laminae, that separates the anterior horns of the left and right lateral ventricles of the brain. It runs as a sheet from the corpus callosum above to the fornix below. At around 12 weeks of gestation a space develops between the two lamina. This is the cavum septum pellucidum (CSP). A normal CSP is a strong indicator of normal development of the forebrain. The CSP should always be seen in fetuses between 18 and 37 weeks of gestation and in approximately 50% of fetuses at term. The laminae slowly start to close from mid-gestation with the process normally being completed by 6 months after birth.

In the lateral ventricles section of the brain, the normal CSP is seen as two thin hyperechoic parallel lines that interrupt the midline, between the frontal horns, in the anterior third of the brain. These lines that represent the cavum make a rectangular, three-sided box which appears open anteriorly and has a characteristic anchor shape (see Figs. 8.2 and 9.1).

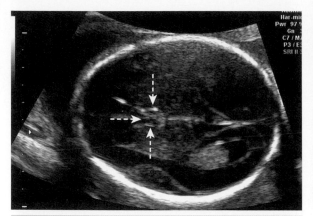

Fig 9.7 • A section of a fetal brain at 20 weeks of gestation which is very slightly too low anteriorly because the three parallel lines of the fornix (arrows) can be seen rather than the three sided box of the CSP in which no central echo is present. The red dot demonstrates the Sylvian fissure. CSP, cavum septum pellucidum.

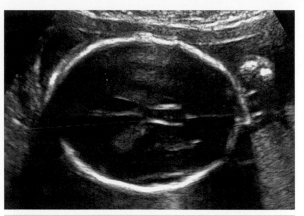

Fig 9.8 • Transverse section of the brain demonstrating elongation of a normal cavum septum showing the cavum vergae (red dot).

The paired nerve columns of the fornix lie directly below, or inferior to, the CSP. They can be identified as three lines which display a similar echogenicity to the CSP but are slightly thinner than the 'sides' of the CSP. A very slight sliding movement caudally, towards the bottom of the fetal head, will allow you to distinguish between the relative positions and appearances of the fornix and the CSP (Fig. 9.7). Making this distinction is very important as there are several conditions in which an absent CSP is a critical diagnostic feature. Mistaking the three lines of the fornix for the CSP when the latter is absent is an example of poor technique.

The normal width and length of the CSP can vary. The cavum can sometimes appear prominent and wider than usual or elongated, extending towards the thalamus. This posterior continuation of the cavum is due to the presence of a second cavity within the septum pellucidum, the cavum vergae (Fig. 9.8). The two cava normally communicate with each other, although they may appear as separate structures in the lateral ventricles view. Unlike the CSP, the cavum vergae is not present in all fetuses.

Because of its position in the centre of the midline, the cavum vergae can be confused with a dilated third ventricle or an arachnoid cyst, so care must be taken when considering the differential diagnosis.

Absent Cavum Septum Pellucidum

An absent CSP is associated with holoprosencephaly and agenesis of the corpus callosum. As discussed later, these conditions demonstrate characteristic and differing ultrasound features. Septo-optic dysplasia is also associated with absence of the CSP. Approximately half of cases of septo-optic dysplasia have moderate or severe developmental delay, but the subtlety of its ultrasound features in the fetus mean that its diagnosis is difficult to make in the antenatal period and certainly beyond the expectations of routine screening.

THE THALAMUS/THALAMI

The thalamus is composed of two lobes which are positioned symmetrically on either side of the midline, immediately posterior to the CSP (see Fig. 8.14). The two hypoechogenic thalami form the side walls of the third ventricle and are therefore useful when trying to locate the third ventricle. They become fused in alobar holoprosencephaly but are otherwise of limited significance in assessment of the fetal brain.

THE SYLVIAN FISSURE/INSULA

The Sylvian fissure or lateral sulcus separates the frontal and parietal lobes of the brain from the temporal lobe. The middle cerebral artery lies within it. The tissue adjacent to the fissure is the insula. Early in development the insula lies on the surface of the brain but, as the brain grows and the complex patterns of sulci and gyri develop and the frontal and temporal lobes grow towards each other, the insula and Sylvian fissure become buried deeper into the brain. This process of invagination is called 'opercularization' and continues with advancing gestation.

Opercularization normally starts between the 20th and the 22nd weeks of pregnancy, until by 32–34 weeks the insula is completely covered and internalized within the brain. It is clear, therefore, that the ultrasound appearances of the insula/Sylvian fissure complex will change with gestation. The complex is commonly referred to simply as the 'Sylvian fissure' and this is the term used in this text to describe the complex.

The Sylvian fissure can be recognized on ultrasound from around 18 weeks when it appears as a thin, curved line, immediately adjacent to the skull and lateral to the thalami. The changes in appearance of the Sylvian fissure complex are highly gestational age specific, such that some authors use these changes of appearance as an aid in assessing the gestational age.

The Sylvian fissure is of importance as the unobservant sonographer might confuse its appearance with the lateral wall of the lateral ventricle, which is medial to the fissure in the normal brain (Fig. 9.7). A useful way of distinguishing between the Sylvian fissure and the lateral wall of the ventricle is to look for the pulsations from the middle cerebral artery, which lies within the fissure.

THE VENTRICULAR SYSTEM

The ventricular system consists of four irregularly shaped cavities, namely the two lateral ventricles, the third ventricle and the fourth ventricle (Fig. 9.9). The lateral ventricles each communicate with the third ventricle via the foramen of Munro. The third and fourth ventricles communicate via the aqueduct of Sylvius or the cerebral aqueduct, whereas the fourth ventricle communicates with the subarachnoid space via the foramina of Luschka and Magendie. The CSF is produced by the choroid plexus present in each of the ventricular cavities and circulates through the ventricular system. After circulating through the subarachnoid cisterns, it is reabsorbed by the arachnoid villi or granulations of Pacchioni, which are distributed primarily along

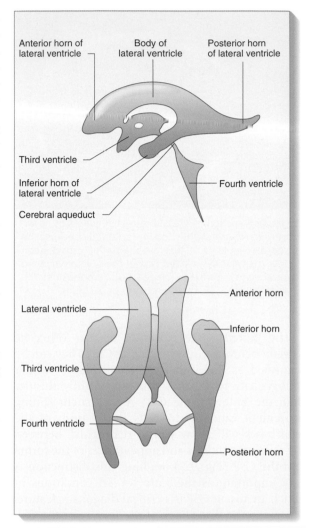

Fig 9.9 • The ventricular system of the fetal brain consists of four irregularly shaped cavities.

the superior sagittal sinus. The system is normally in equilibrium, with production of CSF equalling absorption. Dilatation of all or part of the ventricular system usually arises from a blockage or obstruction in this pathway (Fig. 9.10).

The Lateral Ventricles

As stated in Chapter 8, the part of the ventricular system which is best visualized with ultrasound is the lateral ventricles. The lateral ventricles each have three components, namely the frontal or anterior horn, the posterior horn and the inferior horn (Fig. 9.9). The anterior and posterior horns

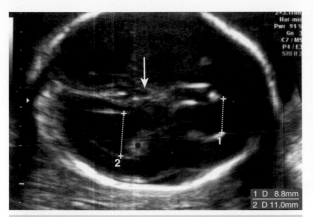

Fig 9.10 • Moderate ventriculomegaly at 20 weeks gestation. Both the anterior and posterior horns of the lateral ventricle are dilated. The measurement of the anterior horn is 8.8 mm. Note the lateral border is clearly demonstrated but the medial border is indistinct in this image. The posterior horn measures 11.0 mm. Note the 'dangling choroid' sign (red dot). The 3rd ventricle is prominent (arrow).

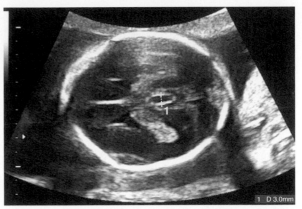

Fig 9.11 • The third ventricle appears prominent in this image of a 19 week fetus. Its measurement of 3.0 mm is at the upper limit of the normal range.

can be routinely imaged with ultrasound, whereas the inferior horn cannot. It is obviously important to be familiar with the appearances of the anterior and posterior horns at 18–22 weeks and, equally as important, the way in which these appearances change as the fetal brain grows and matures.

The Third Ventricle

The third ventricle is a small, slit or 'pin prick'-shaped structure that lies in the midline, between the two triangular-shaped thalami. The 'inner-to-inner' anteroposterior (AP) diameter of the normal third ventricle should be less than 3.0 mm at 18–22 weeks. A prominent 3rd ventricle should always be reassessed. It is most likely to be of no clinical significance if the rest of the ventricular system is normal (Fig. 9.11).

The Fourth Ventricle (See Later in Text)

Measurement of the Posterior and Anterior Horns of the Lateral Ventricles

These measurements are described in Chapter 8.

VENTRICULOMEGALY/HYDROCEPHALUS

'Ventriculomegaly' is the term used to describe enlargement of part or all of the intracranial ventricular system and is the most common cranial abnormality. Hydrocephalus describes a pathological increase in the size of the cerebral ventricles. Ventriculomegaly is found in approximately 1 in 100 or 1% of fetuses at 18–22 weeks, whereas hydrocephalus is present in approximately 2 per 1000 or 0.2% of births. Thus most fetuses with ventriculomegaly do not develop hydrocephalus.

The most common cause of congenital ventriculomegaly is aqueduct stenosis, caused by a narrowing of the aqueduct of Sylvius between the third and fourth ventricles. Aqueduct stenosis is more common in males than females because up to 25% of this obstruction in males is due to the result of an X-linked recessive disorder termed 'X-linked hydrocephalus'.

The second most common cause of ventriculomegaly is due either to obstruction to CSF flow outside the ventricular system or its impaired reabsorption. This type of ventriculomegaly is usually, and incorrectly termed, 'communicating hydrocephalus' and leads to dilatation of the third and fourth ventricles in addition to dilatation of the lateral ventricles. Dilatation of the fourth ventricle is often minimal, which makes the differential diagnosis from aqueduct stenosis difficult.

Ventriculomegaly is frequently described as mild, moderate or severe, depending on the size of the posterior horn, as shown in Table 9.2.

Ventriculomegaly is associated with a range of structural abnormalities, the most well known of which is spina bifida. It is associated with chromosomal abnormalities in approximately 10% of cases, most commonly trisomy 21 and trisomy 18,

DEGREE OF VENTRICULOMEGALY	POSTERIOR HORN MEASUREMENT (mm)
Mild	10.0–12.0
Moderate	12.1–15.0
Severe	>15.0

Table 9.2 The degree of ventriculomegaly as defined by the anteroposterior measurement of the posterior horn of the lateral ventricle

>, greater than.

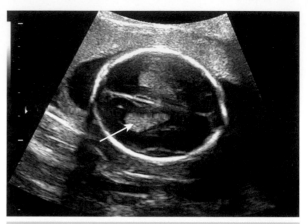

Fig 9.12 • Transverse section of the brain at 20 weeks demonstrating the normal choroid plexus (arrow) within the posterior horn of the lateral ventricle.

and also with fetal infection. It is clear, therefore, that the identification of ventriculomegaly warrants a careful assessment of the whole fetus.

Ventriculomegaly is often the first clue to the presence of spina bifida as the head is usually the first part of the fetus to be examined. Identification of ventriculomegaly should therefore prompt careful assessment of the shape of the skull, the shape and size of the cerebellum and the spine and its skin covering – using sagittal, coronal and transverse planes (see Chapter 12). Ventriculomegaly occurs in about 80% of fetuses with spina bifida. Its presence makes the prognosis for the spina bifida much worse as neurodevelopmental delay is more common if both conditions are present.

In severe ventriculomegaly, the ventricular system can be so dilated that it can be very difficult to identify the normal landmarks such as the CSP and even the midline. This can make it very difficult to distinguish between severe ventriculomegaly, hydranencephaly and holoprosencephaly.

The initial management of ventriculomegaly, after detailed anatomical assessment for the presence or otherwise of associated structural abnormalities, is usually the offer of a maternal blood test for TORCH screening followed by discussion of fetal karyotyping.

THE CHOROID PLEXUS

Choroid tissue is present in all of the ventricular cavities but is only seen on ultrasound in the lateral ventricles, where it is identified as a tear-shaped, homogeneous, hyperechoic structure within each of the posterior horns (Fig. 9.12).

In the normal fetus, the choroid plexus lies snugly within the ventricle, with minimal CSF

between it and the medial wall of the posterior horn. A posterior horn in which the choroid plexus is surrounded by fluid is therefore unusual and should be measured with extreme care to determine whether or not ventriculomegaly is present. As the choroid plexus is gravity-dependent, the extra fluid within the ventricle causes the choroid to hang down close to the medial border of the upper/proximal posterior horn and to the lateral border of the lower/distal posterior horn (Fig. 9.10). This is known as the 'dangling or hanging choroid' sign and is a characteristic feature associated with ventriculomegaly.

Choroid Plexus Cysts

A choroid plexus cyst (CPC) is a hypoechoic cystic structure within the body of the choroid plexus. It is poorly named as it is a collection of CSF and cellular debris within the choroid rather than a true 'cyst' as defined in histological terms. These fluid-filled areas can vary in size but are typically small (mean diameter ~5.0 mm). They can be unilateral (Fig. 9.13A) or bilateral (Fig. 9.13B) and typically occur as a single 'cyst' within one or both choroids. Occasionally, very small, less than 3.0 mm, multiple CPCs are present in the same choroid plexus (Fig. 9.13C). The mean diameter of the CPC should be calculated from two measurements orthogonal to each other using 'inner-to-inner' calliper placement (Fig. 9.13A).

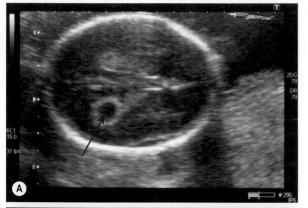

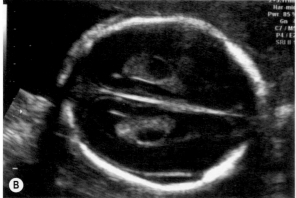

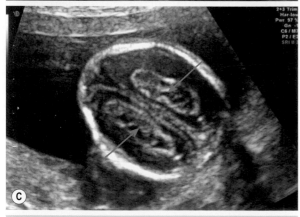

Fig 9.13 • Transverse sections of three fetal brains. A. A single, unilateral CPC (red arrow) in a 20 week fetus. B. Single bilateral CPCs in a 20 week fetus. C. Multiple small bilateral CPCs (green arrows) in a 17 week fetus. CPC, choroid plexus cyst.

Choroid plexus cysts have no pathological significance in the developing fetus, but there is an association reported in the literature between CPCs and trisomy 18. This association is weak in populations at low risk of chromosomal abnormalities and when the CPCs are an isolated finding. Thus when CPCs are seen it is important to confirm whether screening for trisomy 18 was performed earlier in gestation and that the resulting risk was low. As with every fetus, a fetus with CPCs should be examined thoroughly to exclude other anomalies associated with trisomy 18 (see Appendix 11).

The natural history of CPCs is to resolve by 24–26 weeks of gestation, and they are therefore very rarely seen in the third trimester fetus. The current recommendation for the management of isolated CPCs in a pregnancy which is known to be at low risk for trisomy 18 is to treat them as a normal variant.

The circular hypoechoic appearance of CPCs within the choroid plexus means they are often readily noticed by the woman during the examination. It is therefore important that you are able to discuss and report the implications of this ultrasound finding with the woman appropriately and according to departmental guidelines. Although they are an innocuous finding in the majority of cases, the finding of CPCs generates significant anxiety for women. As with the detection of most 'not normal' findings, parents' fears can be allayed by a sensitive and honest approach to their discussion. Such fears will almost certainly be fuelled by a defensive, dismissive and/or uninformed approach.

PORENCEPHALIC CYST

Porencephaly is a destructive cerebral condition that results from the liquefaction of an intracranial haemorrhage in one of the cerebral hemispheres. The most common cause is hypoxic rupture of the small vessels of the germinal matrix that surround the ventricles of the brain. These cysts usually communicate with the ventricular system, the subarachnoid space or both. Porencephalic cysts are usually single and unilateral. The mean diameter of the cyst should be calculated from two measurements orthogonal to each other using 'inner to inner' calliper placement.

Porencephalic cysts are distinguishable from choroid plexus cysts because of their position close to, but separate from, the lateral ventricle. The prognosis depends on the size and the location of the cyst. There is an increased risk of neurodevelopmental delay, although in some cases development may be normal, making prognosis difficult.

HYDRANENCEPHALY

Hydranencephaly is another rare destructive cerebral condition, which is thought to occur because of an early occlusion or developmental defect of both internal carotid or cerebral arteries, prolonged and severe ventriculomegaly/hydrocephalus or an overwhelming infection such as CMV or toxoplasmosis. In hydranencephaly the cerebral hemispheres are destroyed and effectively reduced to a sac of CSF. The midline, CSP, lateral ventricles and cortex are absent. The ultrasound appearance of the lateral ventricles views is therefore of a skull filled primarily with fluid. The parts of the brain, such as the cerebellum and midbrain, which receive their blood supply from other blood vessels are unaffected.

The differential diagnosis is of severe ventriculomegaly or alobar holoprosencephaly. A thin rim of cortex is present in hydrocephalus and alobar holoprosencephaly but absent in hydranencephaly. Pulsations of the middle cerebral artery in the Sylvian fissure are present in hydrocephalus but will be absent in hydranencephaly, allowing, in theory, the two conditions to be distinguished. In practice, distinguishing between the hydranencephaly and severe ventriculomegaly is likely to be academic as both have a very poor prognosis.

HOLOPROSENCEPHALY

Holoprosencephaly is a severe brain abnormality arising from incomplete division of the prosencephalon or early forebrain. The prosencephalon is the embryological structure which gives rise to the cerebral hemispheres, the thalami, the third ventricle and the median facial structures, namely the forehead, nose, interorbital area and upper lip.

As the prosencephalon gives rise to the midline structures of the face, it is not surprising that alobar and semilobar holoprosencephaly are associated with midline facial defects including cyclopia, proboscis and midline clefts. Holoprosencephaly has a strong association with chromosomal abnormalities, principally trisomy 13.

There are three types of holoprosencephaly, based on the degree of incomplete division of the prosencephalon:

- alobar
- semilobar
- lobar.

Alobar holoprosencephaly is the most severe of the three types and is characterized by absence of the interhemispheric fissure, falx and third ventricle (see Fig. 7.11). The thalami are fused and there is a single primitive ventricle. It is the single ventricle which provides the characteristic ultrasound appearance of alobar holoprosencephaly. The normal features of the lateral ventricles section are replaced by a sickle-shaped monoventricle anteriorly. The midline echo and CSP are absent. A small rim of cortex should be present. The fused thalami appear bulb-shaped with no discernible third ventricle in their centre. This condition is lethal.

Semilobar holoprosencephaly is also characterized by a monoventricle anteriorly but, as some division of the forebrain takes place, the two cerebral hemispheres are partially separated posteriorly. There is incomplete fusion of the thalami. In practice it is often difficult to distinguish between the alobar and semilobar conditions with ultrasound imaging.

Lobar holoprosencephaly is the least severe condition. The interhemispheric fissure is well developed but a certain degree of fusion of structures is present. There is typically normal separation of the ventricles and thalami but the CSP is absent. Owing to the subtle features of this type, lobar holoprosencephaly is rarely detected prenatally. However, it should be considered as a differential diagnosis if the CSP cannot be demonstrated.

THE CORPUS CALLOSUM

The corpus callosum (CC) is a bundle of nerve fibres which lies immediately anterior to the CSP and connects the two cerebral hemispheres together. The corpus callosum is closely related both embryologically and anatomically to the CSP. It is, however, possible to have a normal corpus callosum without a normal CSP.

The CC is not visualized from the standard transverse views used in assessment of the intracranial anatomy. It is best identified from the sagittal section of the fetal head used to visualize the profile of the face. In this view, the CC is seen as a thin, comma-shaped hypoechoic strip clearly delineated by its hyperechoic edges (Fig. 9.14).

Agenesis of the Corpus Callosum

The ultrasound features of agenesis of the corpus callosum (ACC) are often subtle but can be

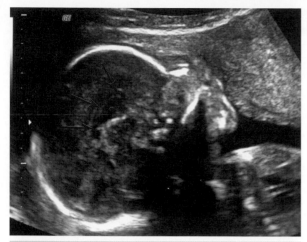

Fig 9.14 • Midsagittal view of the fetal brain demonstrating the cavum septum pellucidum (red dot) and corpus callosum (red arrows) at 20 weeks.

Fetal magnetic resonance imaging (MRI) is helpful in confirming the diagnosis of ACC and generally provides more specific and detailed information regarding the structures in the brain than ultrasound examination.

ARACHNOID CYST

The brain is covered by three membranes or meninges (singular meninx), namely the dura mater, which is the most external and lines the skull; the arachnoid; and the pia mater; which is the most internal and is in direct contact with the brain. The arachnoid is composed of two layers. The space between the pia mater and the inner layer of the arachnoid is filled with CSF and is called the subarachnoid space. Arachnoid cysts can be found anywhere in the central nervous system, but they are most commonly found on the surface of the cerebral hemispheres and in the sites of the major fissures of the brain, namely the interhemispheric and the Sylvian fissures. They are avascular. Interhemispheric arachnoid cysts will obviously be seen in the midline. An arachnoid cyst of the Sylvian fissure is likely to be unilateral and will be seen close to the fetal skull. Arachnoid cysts can vary in size but can grow rapidly, displacing the normal contours of the brain tissue around the cyst, and can lead to the development of ventriculomegaly and hydrocephalus. The mean diameter of the cyst should be calculated from two measurements orthogonal to each other using 'inner to inner' calliper placement (Fig. 9.15).

excluded in most cases with careful examination of the landmarks of the lateral ventricles section. Agenesis of the corpus callosum should be suspected if the CSP cannot be identified in this plane, the anterior horns of the lateral ventricles are displaced laterally and the posterior horns are 'teardrop' in shape. Enlargement of the posterior horns may be present. Another hallmark feature of ACC is the cystic structure, which is often present in the midline, in the centre of the brain. This is not the CSP but is the upwardly displaced third ventricle, filling the void left by the absent CSP and CC.

Ventriculomegaly and ACC have several features in common, so it is important that you make an informed attempt to distinguish between the two conditions when you identify mild dilatation of the posterior horns of the lateral ventricles.

Agenesis of the corpus callosum is one of the most common brain malformations found in children and is found in about 5 per 1000 births. In apparently isolated cases of ACC postnatal development is normal in about 85% of children. The association of ACC with other structural abnormalities, most commonly of the brain and including neuronal migration disorders, with chromosome abnormalities, principally trisomies 8, 13 and 18, and with genetic syndromes, makes prognosis difficult. Chromosomal abnormalities can be excluded by diagnostic testing, but there may be no other ultrasound features associated with the neuronal migration disorders or genetic syndromes, which may have serious prognostic implications.

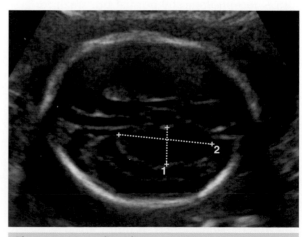

Fig 9.15 • An arachnoid cyst measuring 10.3 × 27.1 mm at 21^{+3} weeks of gestation.

THE APPEARANCES OF THE POSTERIOR FOSSA

The posterior fossa contains the cerebellum, the medulla and pons (the brainstem) and the cisterna magna. The posterior fossa lies between the tentorium cerebelli superiorly and the occiput and foramen magnum inferiorly. The tentorium is a posterior extension of the falx that splits over the cerebellum to form a tentlike covering that separates the cerebellum and the other contents of the posterior fossa from the occipital lobes. The foramen magnum is the large opening in the occipital bone through which the spinal cord enters the skull vault.

The posterior fossa is best visualized using the suboccipito-bregmatic plane as described in Chapter 8. The transcerebellar section should demonstrate the midline echo perpendicular to the ultrasound beam, with the CSP, the cerebellum, cisterna magna and nuchal fold clearly identified (see Fig. 8.15).

THE CEREBELLUM

Finding and assessing the cerebellum are described in Chapter 8.

Abnormal Size

As stated in Chapter 8, the TCD, measured in millimetres, is equivalent to the gestational age, assessed in weeks, up to approximately 24 weeks of gestation. In cerebellar hypoplasia, the cerebellum is morphologically normal but small for gestational age (Fig. 9.16). Cerebellar hypoplasia is associated with cytomegalovirus and karyotypic abnormalities and may only manifest itself in the third trimester of pregnancy. As the cerebellum controls balance, co-ordination and ocular movement, the prognosis is dependent on underlying aetiology.

Abnormal Shape: The Banana Sign

The normal cerebellum is dumbbell-shaped. The 'banana sign' describes a crescent- or banana-shaped cerebellum, the diameter of which is abnormally small. These features are due to the downward displacement of the cerebellum towards

the foramen magnum and result in a partially or totally obliterated cisterna magna. A small, banana-shaped cerebellum is abnormal and has a very strong association with open spina bifida (Fig. 9.17).

In some cases of open spina bifida the cerebellum cannot be visualized within the posterior fossa

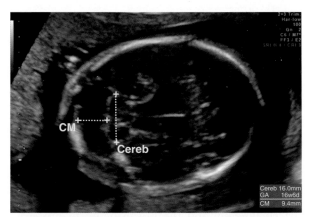

Fig 9.16 • Cerebellar hypoplasia. The cerebellum is visibly small at 20^{+5} weeks of gestation with the TCD measuring 16.0 mm, equivalent to only 16 weeks and 6 days. The cisterna magna appears enlarged due to the small size of the cerebellum, but its measurement, of 9.4 mm, is within normal limits. Cereb, cerebellum; CM, cisterna magna; TCD, transcerebellar diameter.

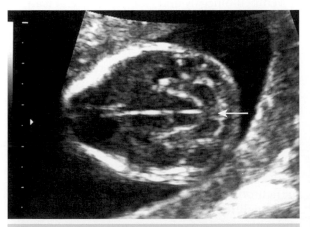

Fig 9.17 • Suboccipito-bregmatic view of the head of a fetus at 16 weeks and 4 days. The size and shape of the cerebellum are abnormal, demonstrating the 'banana sign' (arrow) typical of fetuses with open spina bifida. Note the lemon shaped skull.

ARNOLD CHIARI TYPE	PRESENTATION
I	Minor downward displacement of the cerebellar tonsils through the FM. Usually asymptomatic during childhood
II	Significant displacement of cerebellar vermis, tonsils and medulla through the FM, usually associated with lumbar or lumbosacral myelomeningocele
III	Displacement of the cerebellum through the FM in association with occipital encephalocele
IV	Equivalent to primary cerebellar agenesis

Table 9.3 Classification of Arnold Chiari malformations based on severity of downward displacement of the cerebellum

FM, foramen magnum.

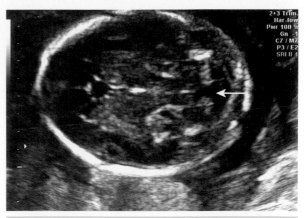

Fig 9.18 • The suboccipito-bregmatic view of a 21 week fetus showing absence of the vermis (arrow). Only the inferior part of the vermis was missing as normal vermis was present when slightly more superior sections of the cerebellum were imaged. A similar appearance is also shown in Fig. 9.20.

and is described as 'absent'. This is a misnomer as the cerebellum is present but is displaced downward into the foramen magnum. This is known as the Arnold Chiari malformation type II.

The sensitivity of the banana sign is greater than that of the lemon-shaped skull in the detection of spina bifida in the second trimester. Both these intracranial signs of spina bifida and the Arnold Chiari malformation are thought to result from traction on the brainstem and/or tethering of the cord at the site of the spinal defect.

Arnold Chiari malformation

Arnold Chiari malformations are a group of related abnormalities of the hind brain and in particular the downward displacement of the cerebellum. The cerebellar tonsils are the rounded lobules situated on the undersurface of each cerebellar hemisphere and are therefore the part of the cerebellum which is in the closest proximity to the foramen magnum.

Four categories of Arnold Chiari malformation are described, as shown in Table 9.3. The severity of the condition increases, with type IV being the most severe. Type II is the type you are most likely to detect owing to its strong association with spina bifida.

Agenesis of the cerebellar vermis

Agenesis of the cerebellar vermis may be either complete or partial (Fig. 9.18). In complete vermian agenesis, as the term suggests, the whole of the cerebellar vermis is absent. In partial vermian agenesis, the inferior portion of the vermis is absent and the superior portion is anatomically normal. It is therefore important to examine the cerebellum thoroughly, to check that the two cerebellar hemispheres are connected by the vermis both superiorly and inferiorly. It is important to remember that an absent vermis will increase the diameter of the cisterna magna (CM) at that level. In such cases the measurement of the CM may be outside the normal range because of the CM occupying the space normally filled by the vermis rather than 'enlargement' of the CM.

Vermian agenesis can be an isolated finding but can also be associated with many syndromes, including Joubert syndrome, Walker-Warburg syndrome and the CHARGE association. CHARGE is a combination of anomalies including **C**oloboma, **H**eart defect, **A**tresia choanae, **R**etarded growth and/or CNS abnormalities, **G**enital anomalies and **E**ar anomalies and/or deafness, of which only the heart defect, CNS abnormality and growth restriction are potentially amenable to ultrasound detection.

THE FOURTH VENTRICLE

The fourth ventricle is best appreciated in the suboccipito-bregmatic plane. The thalami lie on either side of the midline, in the centre of this brain section. Immediately posterior to the thalami, towards the occiput, lie the cerebral peduncles. The fourth ventricle lies in the midline as a small, hypoechoic, box-shaped structure between the cerebral peduncles (anteriorly) and the cerebellar vermis (posteriorly). The normal fourth ventricle is not usually visible.

THE CISTERNA MAGNA

The CM is a fluid-filled cavity lying between the cerebellum and the occiput within the posterior fossa. It is part of the subarachnoid space and is a reservoir for the CSF produced by the fourth ventricle, which drains into the CM via the median foramen of Magendie and the lateral foramina of Luschka. The CM is typically completely anechoic. However, it is not uncommon to visualize two fine, linear and parallel or slightly curved echoes extending posteriorly across the CM from the cerebellum to the occiput (Fig. 9.19A). These septa are thin strands of tissue which are thought to represent remnants of the walls of Blake's pouch and can be seen in many second and third trimester fetuses. They are a normal finding and should not be misinterpreted as a cyst in the posterior fossa. Blake's pouch is important in the early embryological development of the fourth ventricle.

Visual assessment, rather than measurement, of the CM is an important component of the routine 18–22 week anomaly scan. The CM should be measured if it appears prominent (Fig. 9.19B) or abnormal in size, its normal size range being 4–10 mm. Measurement of the CM is described in Chapter 8.

Dandy-Walker complex

Cystic abnormalities of the posterior fossa have traditionally been divided into four conditions, namely Dandy-Walker malformation (Fig. 9.20), Dandy-Walker variant, mega cisterna magna and posterior fossa arachnoid cyst. Current thinking is that Dandy-Walker malformation, Dandy-Walker variant and mega cisterna magna are all part of

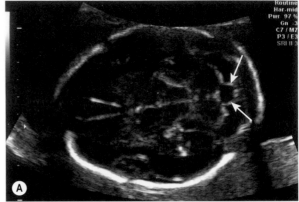

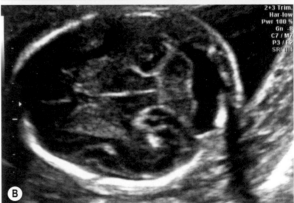

Fig 9.19 • Suboccipito-bregmatic views demonstrating the posterior fossa. A. The transcerebellar diameter demonstrating normal remnants of the Blake's pouch (arrows) within the cisterna magna at 20^{+1} weeks. The cerebellum, including the vermis, is normal. B. The cisterna magna is completely anechoic in this fetus of 20+ weeks. No remnants of Blake's pouch are therefore present. Although the cisterna magna appears prominent, it measured 9.0 mm and was therefore normal.

a continuum of abnormalities that is termed the 'Dandy-Walker complex'. Some authors also include Blake's pouch cyst in this spectrum of disorders. Differentiating between these conditions is often beyond the scope of antenatal ultrasound imaging.

Dandy-Walker malformation (DWM) is characterized by the presence of three specific features:
- cystic dilatation of the fourth ventricle
- enlargement of the posterior fossa
- hypoplasia or aplasia of the cerebellar vermis.

The posterior fossa is enlarged due to the cystic dilatation of the fourth ventricle, which balloons out into the posterior fossa and into the foramen

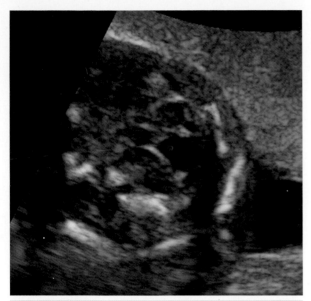

Fig 9.20 • Dandy-Walker malformation at 21 weeks of gestation. Note the cerebellar vermis is absent (red dot).

magnum. This dilatation causes upward displacement and lateral separation of the cerebellar hemispheres, and the tentorium above, together with subsequent abnormal development of the cerebellar vermis. Obstruction to the normal flow of CSF may also occur, resulting in ventriculomegaly or hydrocephalus.

It has been suggested that the dilatation of the fourth ventricle may be associated with atresia of the foramen of Magendie and also possibly of the foramina of Luschka.

Dandy-Walker malformation is associated with chromosomal problems, in particular trisomies 13, 18 and 21, and therefore karyotyping should be discussed and offered.

Dandy-Walker variant (DWV) describes the cystic dilatation of the fourth ventricle and hypoplasia or aplasia of the cerebellar vermis but with no enlargement of the cisterna magna.

Mega cisterna magna describes a posterior fossa in which the cisterna magna is enlarged (i.e., measuring more than 10.0 mm) but the fourth ventricle and cerebellar vermis are normal.

Blake's pouch cyst

'Blake's pouch' refers to an evagination of the posterior membranous area of the roof of the rhombencephalon, or future fourth ventricle. This thin membrane is called Blake's pouch. It develops at around 9 weeks of gestation, grows and then perforates by the end of the 10th week of gestation, forming the foramen of Magendie. The remnants of the walls of Blake's pouch form the thin strands of tissue commonly seen in the cistern a magna as described previously.

Blake's pouch cyst arises when perforation of the Blake's pouch membrane fails to occur. The cyst-like structure protrudes into the cisterna magna and acts as a wedge under the developing cerebellum causing upward displacement of the cerebellar vermis.

A small number of cases of Blake's pouch cyst are reported in the literature and indicate that Blake's pouch cysts often resolve spontaneously during pregnancy, typically at around 26 weeks. This is possibly related to the foramina of Luschka becoming patent at this gestation.

An association between Blake's pouch cyst and cardiac abnormalities and with trisomy 21 have been reported, although these findings should be interpreted with caution because of the small numbers in the various studies.

THE NUCHAL FOLD

Finding and measuring the nuchal fold are described in Chapter 8.

Increased Nuchal Fold/Skin Fold Thickness

Thickening of the back of the neck identified in the second or third trimester fetus is called increased nuchal fold (NF) or increased skinfold thickness (IST). Although the nuchal fold of the second and third trimester fetus and the nuchal translucency of the first trimester fetus both relate to the fetal neck, it is important to appreciate that they are different entities. These terms should therefore *not* be used interchangeably. 'Increased nuchal fold' or skin fold thickness is not a term that is used in the first trimester, unlike 'nuchal translucency', which is *only* used in the first trimester.

The NF measurement is the most sensitive and specific marker for the mid-trimester detection of Down's syndrome. The upper limit of the normal range for nuchal fold thickness at 18–22 weeks is 6.0 mm (Fig. 9.21). Increased NF thickness is

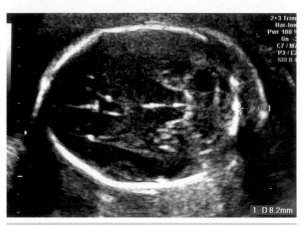

Fig 9.21 • Sub occipito-bregmatic section of the brain demonstrating an increased nuchal fold of 8.2 mm at 20+ weeks.

associated with chromosomal abnormalities, in particular with trisomy 21, hydrops and other conditions including genetic syndromes. Thus an NF thickness greater than 6.0 mm should be considered abnormal irrespective of whether or not earlier screening for Down's syndrome has been accepted or declined.

Table 9.4 provides an algorithm to guide you towards the more likely diagnosis if you have identified or are suspicious of an abnormality of the brain.

THE APPEARANCES OF THE NECK

The neck should be evaluated from the occiput to the cervical spine in order to check its shape, the normal alignment of the vertebral bodies and the integrity of the skin covering the back of the neck (see Chapter 12).

The most common abnormality of the fetal neck is cystic hygroma (see Fig. 7.13). Other abnormalities are rare and include goitre, cervical teratoma and cervical meningomyelocele (see Chapter 12).

CYSTIC HYGROMA

Cystic hygroma is an abnormality of the lymphatic system which arises during early embryonic development from a failure in communication between the lymphatic and venous systems. This results in excess fluid collecting under the skin of the posterior aspect of the fetal neck. The fluid can extend anteriorly, effectively encompassing the whole neck. Cystic hygromata are septated and it is the single central septum, or multiple septa radiating from the cervical spine to the skin, which produce the characteristic appearance of the cystic hygroma (see Fig. 7.13). This feature is useful in distinguishing between a cystic hygroma and an occipital encephalocele. The latter condition is also associated with a defect in the skull, whereas cystic hygroma is associated with an intact skull.

Cystic hygroma are often associated with chromosomal abnormalities, principally Turner's syndrome (45XO) and therefore fetal karyotyping should be discussed. Because of its strong association with aneuploidy, other abnormalities, particularly fetal hydrops, are often present with cystic hygroma. The prognosis is dependent on the accompanying abnormalities but is poor in the presence of hydrops.

NECK MASS

The differential diagnosis of a subcutaneous mass presenting within the neck (more commonly anteriorly) includes goitre and teratoma. The echo pattern of either may be mainly cystic, mainly solid or mixed. A large mass which demonstrates significant vascularity (Fig. 9.22) is more likely to be a teratoma than a small mass with minimal vascularity.

A large mass situated anteriorly may cause hyperextension of the fetal neck and may also obstruct swallowing, causing polyhydramnios and a smaller stomach than normal. Anticipation of respiratory difficulties at birth in such cases is important, although the likelihood and/or degree of this is difficult to predict before delivery.

Table 9.4 provides an algorthim to guide you towards the more likely diagnoses if you have identified or are suspicious of an abnormality of the fetal neck.

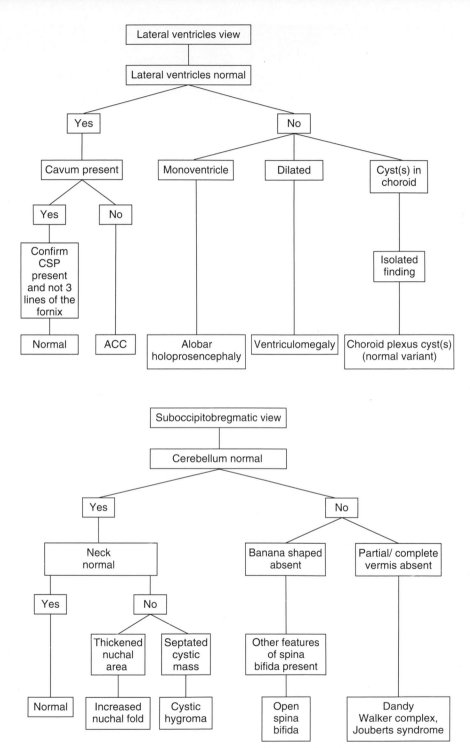

Table 9.4 The more common differential diagnoses of abnormal brain and neck appearances.
ACC, agenesis of the corpus callosum; CSP, cavum septum pellucidum.

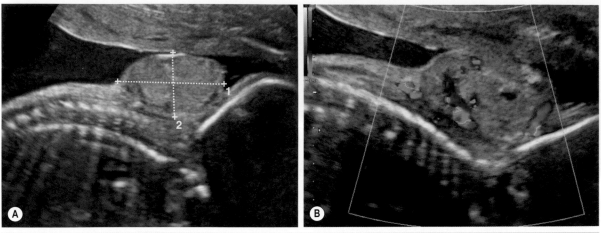

Fig 9.22 • Sagittal sections of the head and upper body of a 22 week fetus. A. A posterior heterogeneous cervical teratoma located within the occipital region and measuring 40.1 × 23.7 mm. B. Vascularity of the neck mass is demonstrated with colour flow Doppler.

THE APPEARANCES OF THE FETAL FACE

The face should be examined in the coronal plane to confirm normality of the upper lip, in the transverse plane to assess the normality of the alveolar ridge and in the sagittal plane to confirm normality of the fetal profile.

DEVELOPMENT OF THE FACE

The development of the face is a complex embryological process that involves the fusion, between the 4th and 10th weeks of gestation, of five different tissue masses, the frontonasal process, the paired maxillary swellings and the paired mandibular swellings.

The frontonasal process will form the nose, including the nostrils, the philtrum and the central portion of the alveolar ridge of the upper jaw. The philtrum is the central portion of the upper lip together with the soft tissue in the depression between the upper lip and the nose.

Part of the maxillary swellings will each fuse with the frontonasal process to form the philtrum, the central portion of the alveolus and the primary palate. Part of the maxillary swellings will fuse with each other to form the outer portion of the alveolus on each side and the secondary palate.

The hard palate is composed of the primary palate and the secondary palate. The primary palate is the small triangular area at the front of the roof of the mouth, directly behind the four incisors. The remaining part of the hard palate is formed from the secondary palate.

The mandibular swellings will fuse to form the lower jaw.

The fact that the upper lip, alveolar ridge and palate derive from two different tissue masses which fuse in various planes is important in understanding how clefting of the upper lip, alveolus, primary palate and secondary palate occur.

Failure of fusion between various of these structures results in clefting of either the upper lip, upper lip and alveolus, palate or upper lip, alveolus and palate as described later.

OBTAINING A CORONAL VIEW OF THE FACE

Assessing the soft tissues of the face in the coronal plane follows on naturally from measurement of the HC (and BPD), measurement of the PH and assessment of the rest of the intracranial anatomy presented in the lateral ventricles view.

To view the face in coronal section(s), ensure that the midline is as close to the horizontal as possible before leaving the HC section. Slide the probe down the fetal head, towards the body until you see the orbits anteriorly and the cerebellum posteriorly. Rotate the probe through 45°, towards the front of the face. You should now have obtained a coronal section of the face. Sliding movements will now allow you to examine the orbits, confirm the presence of the lens in both orbits and examine the upper lip. The upper lip is best assessed with the fetus in the occipito transverse position while assessment of the orbits is much easier when the fetus is in the occipito posterior (OP) position.

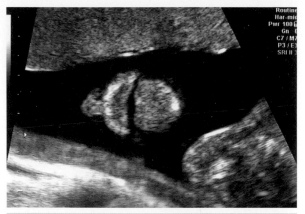

Fig 9.23 • Coronal section of the fetal face at 20 weeks of gestation demonstrating the nasal tip, the nostrils and the lips with the mouth slightly open. Note that this is the section required to exclude a cleft in the upper lip.

THE ORBITS AND EYES

The fetal orbits should appear as two symmetrical hypoechoic circles on either sides of the fetal nose in the coronal section of the face. Orbital diameter and interorbital diameter charts exist, but assessment of the size of the orbits is usually made subjectively. However, the orbits should appear equal in size and separated by a distance that is roughly equal to the diameter of each orbit. Hypotelorism describes the condition in which the orbits are abnormally close to each other. Hypertelorism is the converse condition in which the distance between orbits is abnormally large.

The lens has a characteristic appearance of a hyperechoic ring within the orbit (Fig. 9.4B). The lenses can be seen to move within their respective orbits; you will note that their movement is not always synchronous – this is a normal finding in the developing fetus. The lens itself should be hypoechoic with only its rim appearing hyperechoic. Cataracts have been described in the fetus and produce an opaque appearance of the lens.

THE NOSE AND UPPER LIP

Having obtained a coronal section of the face, you need to slide the probe forward towards the front of the face. If you have obtained a section that is too far back into the face, slide the probe, minimally, towards the front of the face until you are imaging the fetal lips. The correct section (Fig. 9.23) for assessment of the lips should include the lips, nostrils and nasal tip only. If the section contains the orbits and the chin, your probe is angled too far into the fetal face. Correct this by rotating the probe slightly to either side to obtain the correct section.

The nostrils should appear as two small hypoechoic circles just below the rather triangular-shaped nasal tip. The nostrils should be symmetrical, with no deviation of either one or the nasal tip to either side of the midline of the face. It is more important to image the upper lip in detail rather than the lower lip because of the upper lip's association with facial clefting.

The upper lip has 'thickness', so you must ensure that you have imaged the whole lip properly in the coronal plane. Assessing the upper lip from only one section is unlikely to result in its adequate examination, so use small sliding movements to ensure you have examined the upper lip properly from front to back. Also ensure that you have imaged the full extent of the upper lip to either side of the nose. Both sides of the upper lip should look symmetrical about the nose; if they do not, make very small adjustment to the angle of the probe on the maternal abdomen to rectify the problem. We recommend assessing the upper lip with the axis of the coronal section between 2 and 4 o'clock or between 8 and 10 o'clock (Fig. 9.23). It is much more difficult to obtain the correct angle to the face in order to image the upper lip properly if the fetus is OP or occipito anterior (OA).

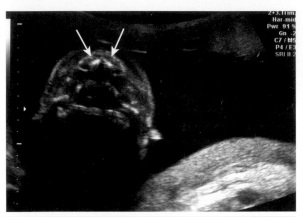

Fig 9.24 • Transverse section of the face at 20 weeks demonstrating the alveolus (arrows). Note that this view is required to exclude a cleft of the alveolar ridge. Both sides of the alveolus can be clearly visualized with the nose upward to 12 o'clock.

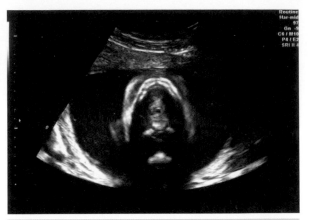

Fig 9.25 • Transverse section of the face at 20 weeks demonstrating the shape of the lower jaw. Note the different shape compared with the alveolar ridge.

THE ALVEOLAR RIDGE OR ALVEOLUS

A transverse section of the head is required to image the alveolar ridge or alveolus. From the HC section, slide the probe down the fetal head, towards the body, until you see the orbits anteriorly and the cerebellum posteriorly. A further minimal sliding movement towards the fetal body should result in the transverse section demonstrating the alveolus. As the alveolus is best examined with the fetus in the OP position, with the occiput between 4 and 8 o'clock, you may need to dip one end of the probe into the maternal abdomen to bring the head from an OT position to the required OP position.

The ultrasound appearance of the normal alveolus is of a hyperechoic horseshoe, which is slightly pointed in the centre (Fig. 9.24).

Care must be taken to distinguish the alveolus and maxilla anteriorly from the mandible posteriorly. Their shapes are similar but the mandible is slightly broader, more rounded in shape and surrounds the tongue, movements of which can be identified from the mandibular section (Fig. 9.25).

THE PALATE

The normal palate is not routinely visualized using two-dimensional (2D) imaging. The tongue should not be confused with the palate. The tongue's median lingual sulcus produces a very 'palate-like' appearance. This tends to excite the inexperienced operator until a tongue movement confirms that this structure is indeed the tongue and not the palate.

Facial Clefting

Facial clefting is a common abnormality both as an isolated condition and in association with other abnormalities. It has a birth incidence in the UK of approximately 1 in 700. Thus a relatively large number of fetuses that you scan will have a facial cleft. It is therefore important that you understand how to examine the face properly to exclude facial clefts, are aware of the different types of facial clefting and can differentiate between their ultrasound appearances.

Failure of fusion between the maxillary swelling and the frontonasal process on one side will result in unilateral clefting of the upper lip only, clefting of the upper lip and alveolus or clefting of the upper lip, alveolus and primary palate. Failure of fusion on both sides will result in a bilateral cleft.

The line of fusion of each side of the upper lip is demarcated by the borders of the philtrum or, when assessing the ultrasound image, at a position slightly lateral to the centre of the lip. The cleft of the 'cleft lip' will always occur at this site. Other types of cleft of the lips can occur but are very rare and their description is beyond the scope of this text.

A cleft of the lip that extends into the nose is termed a 'complete cleft'; a cleft of the lip in which the nose is not affected is termed an 'incomplete cleft'.

The four incisors, or 'front teeth' will arise from the central portion of the alveolus. The canine, premolar and molar teeth will arise from the outer portion of the alveolus on each side. The line of fusion, and therefore potential clefting, of the alveolus lies between the incisors and the canine teeth.

Failure of fusion between the maxillary swellings will result in clefting of the secondary palate. It is this defect which is commonly referred to as 'cleft palate'. As the maxillary swellings fuse in the midline, clefting of the secondary palate will always result in a central, linear defect.

As stated previously, facial clefting is a common abnormality. Cleft lip, with or without cleft palate, is found in approximately 1 in 700 to 1 in 1000 births. Cleft palate is found in approximately 1 in 2,500 births. There is a racial variation with a higher incidence of facial clefting in Asian populations of approximately 1 in 500–600 births. This can be compared with Caucasian populations where the incidence is approximately 1 in 800 births and black populations where the incidence is approximately 1 in 2000 births.

Clefting of the lip and alveolar ridge is twice as common in males than females, except in black populations, where the incidence in males is very low.

Approximately 80% of unilateral clefts are left-sided and 20% right-sided.

The most common combinations of facial clefting are:

- unilateral cleft lip
- unilateral cleft lip and alveolus
- unilateral cleft lip, alveolus and palate (primary and secondary)
- bilateral cleft lip, alveolus and palate (primary and secondary)
- isolated cleft palate (secondary).

Cleft lip is associated with chromosomal abnormalities, principally trisomy 13 and 18, exposure to teratogens, including antiepileptic drugs, and a large number of genetic syndromes.

As the embryological basis for cleft lip and for cleft palate differs, the recurrence risks for these conditions vary. The risks also vary between published series. The literature rarely differentiates between cleft lip alone and cleft lip and alveolar ridge when addressing recurrence rates. These two conditions therefore tend to be grouped together as 'cleft lip' when compared with cleft palate alone.

Having had a pregnancy affected with an isolated cleft, the risk of a second child having a cleft is quoted as 2–5%. This risk increases to 10–12% if more than one member of the immediate family has a cleft. The risk of an unaffected sibling of an individual with a cleft having a child with a cleft is in the order of 1%, rising to 5–6% if more than one close family member has a cleft.

The recurrence risk for isolated cleft palate is around 3% where a sibling has an isolated cleft palate and around 5% when one parent has an isolated cleft palate. Screening for clefting of the palate is beyond the scope of this text.

Cleft lip

Imaging the upper lip, nostrils and nasal tip in the coronal plane and imaging the alveolus in the transverse plane are required to exclude a cleft of the upper lip and alveolus or gum, respectively. The ultrasound appearance of the normal upper lip is of a crescent shape of homogeneous echoes. A cleft of the lip appears as a vertical hypoechoic area on one side of the lip, usually just to the left of the midline. This area may involve the lip only (i.e., an incomplete cleft), or may extend up into the nose (i.e., a complete cleft). The symmetry of the nostrils is often affected by a complete unilateral cleft, with distortion of the ipsilateral nostril (Fig. 9.26). A bilateral cleft lip will demonstrate these features on both sides of the midline (Fig. 9.27A).

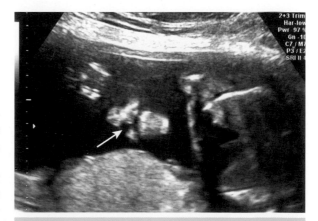

Fig 9.26 • A coronal section of the face demonstrating a unilateral right sided cleft lip (arrow) with slight distortion of the nasal tip toward the side of the defect.

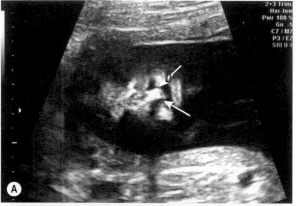

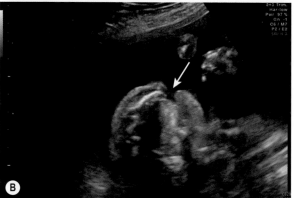

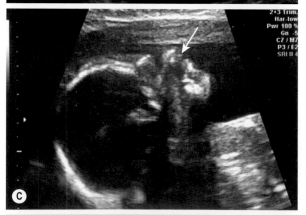

Fig 9.27 • A. Bilateral complete cleft of the lip. The coronal view of the face demonstrating the defect in the upper lip on both sides (arrows) extending up into each nostril. B. The transverse view of the alveolus demonstrating interruption of the alveolus (arrow) on one side. C. Midsagittal section of the fetal face demonstrating the prominent premaxilla (arrow).

Clefting of the alveolus

A cleft may involve only the lip or may also include the alveolus. As the management for the two conditions after birth and into early adulthood varies considerably, it is important that the alveolus is examined carefully when a cleft lip is suspected.

The ultrasound appearance of the normal alveolus is of a hyperechoic horseshoe which is slightly pointed in the centre. As with the cleft lip, a cleft in the alveolus appears as a vertical hypoechoic area on one side of the ridge, usually just to one side of the midline (Fig. 9.27B).

The premaxilla

Where a bilateral cleft lip and alveolus is present, the tissues of the philtrum and mid-alveolus are disrupted and present as a mass, which protrudes forward from the face. This mass is called the premaxilla and may be of such a size that it obscures the clefts present on either side. The premaxilla is best identified when examining the fetal face in the sagittal plane and is often the first indication that a bilateral cleft lip is present (Fig. 9.27C).

Midline cleft

A midline cleft describes a defect in which the philtrum and central part of the alveolus have failed to form. It is part of the spectrum of midline defects that includes holoposencephaly and, as such, is associated with trisomy 13.

Table 9.5 provides an algorithm to guide you to the most likely diagnosis if you have identified or are suspicious of an abnormality of the upper lip.

THE PROFILE

The profile of the fetal face requires a sagittal section, obtained by rotating the probe through 90° from the coronal view of the face (Fig. 9.28A). Small sliding movements are then required until the frontal bones of the forehead, nasal tip, nasal bone, upper and lower lips and chin are all clearly delineated. If the orbit of one eye is seen but the nasal tip is not, the section is parasagittal (Fig. 9.28B). Slide the probe towards the centre of the face to obtain the correct, sagittal section. If you have obtained a section in which the chin and an orbit can be seen, the section is oblique. Rotate the probe away from the orbit to obtain the correct

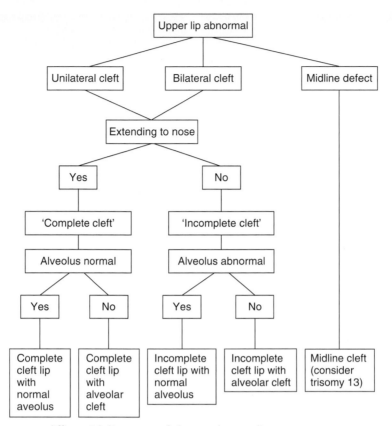

Table 9.5 The more common differential diagnoses of abnormal upper lip appearances

sagittal section. If you have rotated the wrong way, you will need to slide from the side of the face to the centre of the face.

The ease with which this view can be obtained varies with fetal position. If the fetus is OP, with the face looking upward towards the probe, the profile is easily obtained.

When the fetus is lying OT, you need to position the probe so that it is virtually parallel to the scanning couch in order to obtain the correct fetal profile view. It is not possible to obtain a profile view when the fetus is OA, as the face is towards the maternal spine. It may be necessary to turn the woman onto her side to encourage the fetus to change its position in order that the profile view can be obtained.

Once a correct section is obtained, draw an imaginary line along the length of the forehead to the lower protrusion of the chin. In the normal fetus the forehead and chin are in line with each

other while the nose and the lips lie anterior to, or in front of, this line (see Fig. 9.28A).

The profile view of the face is useful in excluding a number of the more subtle features associated with various chromosome abnormalities and in refining the differential diagnosis of a number of the skeletal dysplasias.

THE FOREHEAD

Although normal values of facial angles have been published, normal practice at the 18–22 week routine scan is to make a subjective assessment of the angle of the forehead relative to the rest of the profile.

Flat Forehead

A forehead which slopes acutely towards the face is abnormal and is described as 'flat'. A flattened

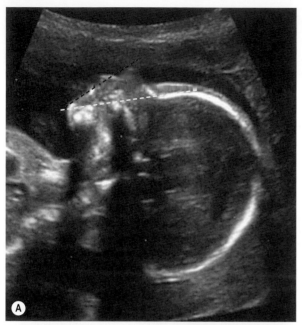

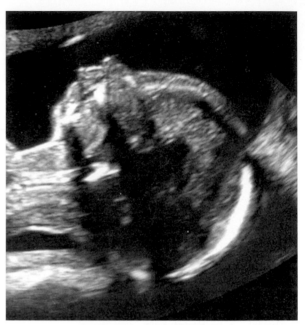

Fig 9.29 • Midsagittal section of the fetal face at 20^{+2} weeks demonstrating a slightly small receding chin. Compare this to the size of the chin in Fig. 9.28A.

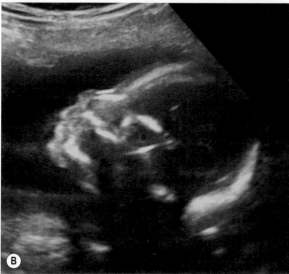

Fig 9.28 • A. Midsagittal view of the fetal face demonstrating the normal profile with the tip of the nose, lips and chin along the same line (red dashed line). The yellow dashed line demonstrates the forehead and chin in line with each other, confirming a normal profile. Note in particular the presence of the nasal bone, normal contours of the nose, lips and normal size and angle of the chin. B. A parasagittal section of the fetal face demonstrating one orbit (red dot).

forehead is associated with trisomy 21 and a range of conditions, the most common of these being Apert's syndrome.

THE NOSE

The features of importance when assessing the nose are the nasal bone and the nasal bridge (see Chapter 12, p. 303).

Nasal Bone

Measuring the length of the nasal bone is not a requirement of the routine 18–22 week scan, but you should make yourself familiar with the echogenicity, shape and length of the nasal bone at this gestation (Fig. 9.28A). An absent or hypoplastic nasal bone in the second trimester fetus can be associated with Down's syndrome. The significance of this finding should be interpreted against the background of previous Down's screening results.

Proboscis

The normal nose may be absent and replaced by an abnormal structure called a proboscis, which typically is positioned above the eyes or single midline eye. This severely abnormal profile is part of the spectrum of midline abnormalities associated with trisomy 13.

THE CHIN

The protrusion of the normal chin lies directly underneath the lower lip (Fig. 9.28A) and, as described earlier, is in line with the normal forehead. As with the other features of the profile, the angle made by the chin to the lips is assessed subjectively.

It is difficult to assess the size of the chin when the fetus is in a flexed position and the chin is down onto the fetal chest. You should also be aware that the chin may appear small and/or receding if an oblique, rather than a sagittal, section of the face is obtained. Dip the probe slightly until you have obtained a section whereby the facial profile is perpendicular to the beam before making your final assessment.

Micrognathia

A chin that forms an acute angle with the lips is abnormal and is described as receding (Fig. 9.29). 'Micrognathia' is the term used to describe an abnormally small or receding chin. Micrognathia is associated with trisomy 18, triploidy and various genetic syndromes such as the Pierre Robin sequence and Roberts syndrome.

THE TONGUE

In the normal fetus, the tongue is accommodated within the mouth. The tongue is often seen moving during swallowing and other activities.

Macroglossia

An abnormally large tongue may protrude beyond the lips and remain outside the mouth for long periods. An abnormally large tongue is termed 'macroglossia'. It can be associated with Down's syndrome and is a feature of Beckwith-Wiedemann syndrome. Other features of Beckwith-Wiedemann syndrome include macrosomia, exomphalos and large dysplastic kidneys.

Having completed your assessment of the head, brain, neck and face you will have decided whether or not the anatomy you have examined is normal.

Further reading

CLAPA 2001 Cleft lip & palate: a guide for sonographers. The Cleft Lip and Palate Association (CLAPA)

Gandolfi Colleoni G et al 2012 Prenatal diagnosis and outcome of fetal posterior fossa fluid collections. Ultrasound Obstet Gynecol 39:625–631

Guibaud L, des Portes V 2006 Plea for an anatomical approach to abnormalities of the posterior fossa in prenatal diagnosis. Ultrasound Obstet Gynecol 27:477–481

Malinger G, Lev D, Lerman-Sagie T 2009 The fetal cerebellum. Pitfalls in diagnosis and management. Prenat Diag 10:2196

Paladini D et al 2012 Abnormal or delayed development of the posterior membranous area of the brain: anatomy, ultrasound diagnosis, natural history and outcome of Blake's pouch cyst in the fetus. Ultrasound Obstet Gynecol 39:279–287

Robinson A J, Goldstein R 2007 The cisterna magna septa: vestigial remnants of Blake's pouch and a potential new marker for normal development of the rhombencephalon. JUM 26:83–95

Sepulveda W Dezerga V, Be C 2004 First-trimester sonographic diagnosis of holoprosencephaly. American Institute of Ultrasound in Medicine 23:761–765

Sonographic examination of the fetal central nervous system guidelines for performing the 'basic examination' and the 'fetal neurosonogram'. 2007 Ultrasound Obstet Gynecol 29:109–116

Winter T C, Kennedy A M, Bryne J, Woodward P J 2010 The cavum septi pellucidi. Why is it important? JUM 29:427–444

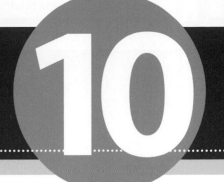

Assessing the chest and heart

This chapter addresses the ultrasound examination of the thorax with particular reference to the second trimester of pregnancy. The aims of this chapter are to describe the correct techniques to be used to assess the following:

- the chest and ribs
- the diaphragm
- the lungs
- the heart.

THE CHEST AND RIBS

THE CHEST

The bony thorax is the skeleton of the chest within which the heart, lungs and other organs are situated and which is delineated inferiorly by the diaphragm. From an ultrasound point of view, the chest and the ribs should be evaluated separately as the abnormalities associated with them, although rare, differ.

The shape of the chest is best assessed in transverse section, whereas the size of chest, relative to the abdomen, is best assessed in longitudinal section. The ribs are readily recognized in both longitudinal and transverse sections of the thorax.

In the normal fetus there is no visual difference in the circumference of the chest above the diaphragm compared with that of the abdomen immediately below the diaphragm. Thus a smooth outline

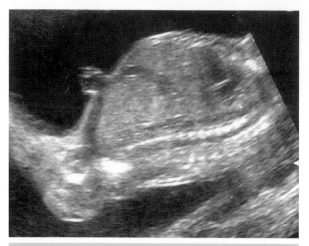

Fig 10.1 • A sagittal view of the chest and abdomen showing a normal sized chest and thorax in relation to the abdomen.

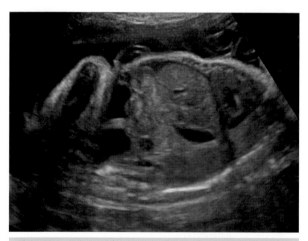

Fig 10.2 • A sagittal section of the chest and abdomen showing a small chest and enlarged abdomen. This champagne-cork-shaped small chest cavity was seen in a fetus with osteogenesis imperfecta type II.

of the fetal chest and abdomen is seen when the fetus is imaged in sagittal section (Fig. 10.1).

A disproportion in size between the chest and abdomen causes protuberance of the abdomen below the diaphragm and thus a disruption in the smooth outline of the fetal body. This may be due to either a small chest with an abdomen of normal size or a chest of normal size with an abdomen of increased size (Fig. 10.2). When the chest cavity is abnormally small, the normal sized heart will appear abnormally large within the chest.

Champagne Cork Chest

The most common abnormality of chest shape is the so-called champagne cork or bell-shaped chest. The chest is abnormally small compared with the abdomen, causing the normally sized abdomen to bulge below the diaphragm producing an appearance similar to the shape of a champagne cork (Fig. 10.2). This is part of the spectrum of abnormalities seen in lethal skeletal dysplasias such as achondrogenesis, asphyxiating thoracic dystrophy and thanatophoric dysplasia. The small chest in these conditions affects the development and growth of the lungs. The reduced lung volume results in pulmonary hypoplasia and therefore is the primary cause of the lethal outcome in the majority of cases.

THE RIBS

The shape and curvature of each rib should be regular and its echogenicity consistent along its length.

Abnormalities of the ribs are rare, although pathological variations in size, shape and ossification are associated with a number of skeletal dysplasias, including the group of self-explanatory short rib–polydactyly syndromes.

Rib Fractures

Fractures can be identified if they result in abnormal angulation of the ribs, whereas those which contain healed or healing fractures may display localized areas of thickening and/or hyperechoic at the site of the fractures. Such rib fractures are characteristic of osteogenesis imperfecta type II. This condition is divided into three subgroups. Type IIA has short and fractured long bones and 'beaded' ribs because of multiple fractures. Type IIB has short and fractured long bones but no rib fractures, whereas type IIC has thin and fractured long bones and thin ribs. Should you suspect that a fetus has osteogenesis imperfecta, you will impress your fetal medicine and genetics colleagues greatly if, based on your careful and thorough examination, you are able to suggest not only the condition but also the subgroup correctly.

In practice it is much more likely that you will be alerted to a potential diagnosis by the significant abnormalities in size and/or appearance of the limbs or skull rather than those of the ribs.

DIFFERENTIAL DIAGNOSIS OF CHEST MASSES

With the obvious exception of the heart, single or multiple hypo- or hyperechoic areas within the thorax are abnormal. Their differential diagnoses include diaphragmatic hernia, pleural effusions, pericardial effusions, cystic lung lesions and tracheal occlusion.

THE DIAPHRAGM

It is important to appreciate the spatial relationship between the various organs that are normally located in the chest and those organs usually within the abdomen. The diaphragm can be identified in both longitudinal and coronal sections as a thin, echo-poor, concave line that separates the lungs and heart in the thorax from the stomach, liver and bowel in the abdomen (Fig. 10.3).

The diaphragm is formed by the fusion of four structures, namely the anterior *septum transversum*, the dorsal oesophageal mesentery, the lateral pleuroperitoneal membranes and the body wall. This process of fusion takes place between the sixth and ninth weeks of gestation.

CONGENITAL DIAPHRAGMATIC HERNIA

Congenital diaphragmatic hernia (CDH) occurs in approximately 1 in 4000 births and arises from the defective development and/or fusion of the

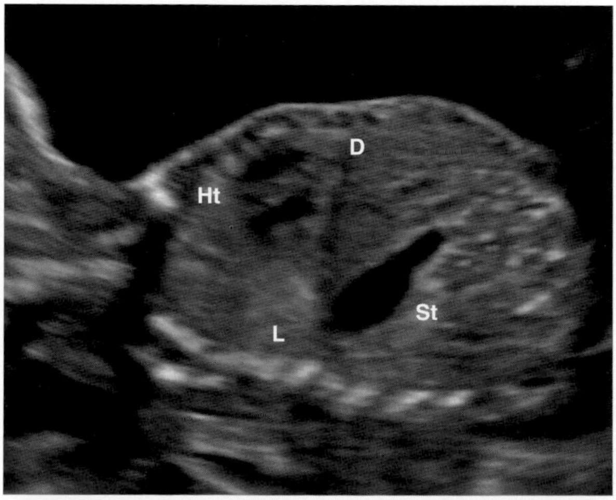

Fig 10.3 • A sagittal section of the fetal body illustrating the diaphragm (D), lung fields (L) and heart (Ht). Note the concave shape of the diaphragm and the normal position of the stomach (St) below the diaphragm.

pleuroperitoneal membranes. This results in an opening, called the foramen of Bochdalek, in the posterolateral part of the newly formed diaphragm. In the normal fetus the physiological herniation of the bowel into the base of the umbilical cord takes place between approximately 8 and 10 weeks of gestation. In the presence of an incomplete diaphragm, some of the abdominal contents will herniate into the chest following the return of the intestines into the abdomen, indicating that in theory CDH could be suspected on ultrasound examination from 12 weeks of gestation.

Defects in the diaphragm are themselves rarely identified on ultrasound but are inferred by the abnormal position in the chest of one or more of the organs which are normally located in the fetal abdomen. Diaphragmatic hernia is normally unilateral and occurs four times more often on the left side than on the right; thus 80% of cases of CDH are left-sided.

A left-sided diaphragmatic hernia should be suspected if a cystic mass is seen in the left side of the fetal chest with no stomach bubble visible in its normal position, below the diaphragm and on the left side of the abdomen (Fig. 10.4A and B). These appearances suggest that the stomach has entered the fetal chest through a defect in the diaphragm. Bowel loops may also move into the chest through the defect. The ultrasound appearances of bowel and lung are similar, but you should suspect bowel in the chest if you can see peristaltic movements within the mass in addition to the cystic mass of the stomach. With a left-sided CDH, the heart is often pushed into the right side of the chest. This itself is another suspicious finding of left-sided CDH and should prompt careful evaluation of the contents of the chest to exclude bowel in the chest, even if the stomach is correctly situated below the diaphragm.

In right-sided CDH the fetal liver is the organ most likely to herniate through the defect in the diaphragm into the chest. Right-sided cases are

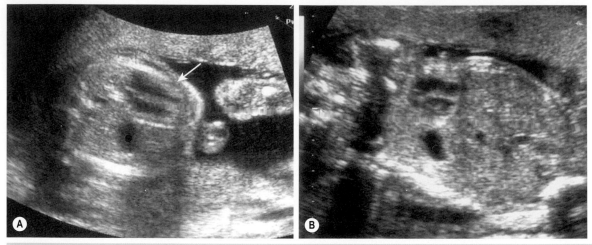

Fig 10.4 • A. A transverse section of the chest demonstrating a left-sided congenital diaphragmatic hernia. The stomach (red dot) is visible within the chest cavity. Note the deviation of the heart to the right side (arrow) of the chest. B. The sagittal section of the same fetus demonstrating the stomach (red dot) above the diaphragm within the chest cavity.

thus less amenable to prenatal ultrasound detection because of the normally positioned stomach and the relative similarity of the echotexture of the liver and lung. Abnormal positioning of the heart in the left side of the chest may provide the only diagnostic clue in such cases.

The ultrasound appearances of CDH are known to vary over time as a result of the mobility of the abdominal organs through the defect in the diaphragm. It is probable, therefore, that there are times when neither the stomach nor the bowel is in the fetal chest, meaning that the effects of the left-sided CDH may not be apparent. This fact restricts the sensitivity of ultrasound in the detection of CDH and may explain why cases with obvious findings in the third trimester were not suspected in the second trimester.

Pregnancies with isolated CDH are usually not complicated, although impaired absorption of amniotic fluid by the fetal gut may cause polyhydramnios in the late second and third trimesters. A significant amount of the bowel in the fetal chest may result in a reduced abdominal circumference (AC) measurement, giving the impression of asymmetrical growth restriction. Serial measurements, however, usually demonstrate normal growth velocity. It should be remembered, however, that fetal weight estimations in such cases are likely to be underestimated because of the inaccurate contribution made by the AC.

Approximately half of cases of CDH are associated with chromosomal abnormalities, principally trisomies 13 and 18. Diagnosis of CDH should therefore always prompt discussion with the parents regarding invasive testing in order to obtain a fetal karyotype.

Although the defect in the diaphragm is readily amenable to surgery, up to 50% of neonates will die of associated pulmonary hypoplasia or associated abnormalities. Poor prognostic indicators in cases of isolated CDH include evidence of early (i.e. at or before 20 weeks) herniation of abdominal organs into the chest, early left ventricular compression of the heart and polyhydramnios.

THE LUNGS

The most prominent structure in the chest is the fetal heart. The remainder of the chest cavity is filled with the lungs, which produce homogeneous low level echoes. Thus single or multiple hyperechoic or hypoechoic areas within either or both lung fields are an abnormal finding. You should be able to recognize and differentiate between the appearances of fluid around one or both lungs, namely pleural effusion, a cystic mass in the chest, a solid mass in the chest and a mass in the chest which contains both solid and cystic elements. Your aim is to be able to identify the different ultrasound appearances of a diaphragmatic hernia, pleural or pericardial effusion and a congenital lung lesion.

HYDROPS FETALIS

The strict definition of hydrops fetalis is the presence of excess fluid in more than one body cavity with a combination of at least two of the following: subcutaneous oedema, pericardial effusion, pleural effusion or abdominal or urinary ascites. This is discussed in more detail in Chapter 11.

Pleural Effusion

A collection of fluid surrounding the lung is called a pleural effusion or chylothorax. It can be unilateral or bilateral (Fig. 10.5). The fluid, or chyle, can result from an overproduction or impaired reabsorption of lymph. Pleural effusion may be an isolated finding but is more commonly present as part of the spectrum of features of hydrops fetalis.

Pleural effusion is also associated with other conditions involving lymphatic abnormalities, including Down's syndrome and Turner's syndrome or 45XO. Diagnosis of pleural effusion should therefore always prompt discussion with the parents regarding invasive testing in order to obtain a fetal karyotype.

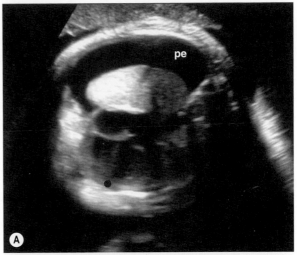

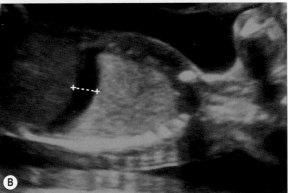

Fig 10.5 • A. A transverse section of the fetal chest demonstrating a unilateral pleural effusion, (pe), affecting the left lung. Note the deviation of the heart (red dot) from its normal axis within the chest cavity. B. A sagittal section of the fetal chest. The fluid can be seen at the base of the lung and measures 3.6 mm.

Pericardial Effusion

Pericardial effusion is the abnormal collection of fluid surrounding the heart.

CONGENITAL LUNG LESIONS

Congenital lung lesions occur in approximately 1 in 4000 births and include bronchopulmonary sequestration (BPS) and a condition previously described, in all but the most modern literature, as congenital cystic adenomatoid malformation (CCAM). The latter has recently been reclassified and is now correctly described as cystic pulmonary airways malformation (CPAM). The reclassification took place on the basis that not all lesions are cystic and the majority of the types are not adenomatoid on pathological examination.

Bronchopulmonary Sequestration

Bronchopulmonary sequestration describes a mass of lung tissue that is separated, or sequestrated, from the normal lung. The most common site for a BPS is between the lower lobe of either lung and the diaphragm. It does not usually communicate with the rest of the bronchial tree and usually receives

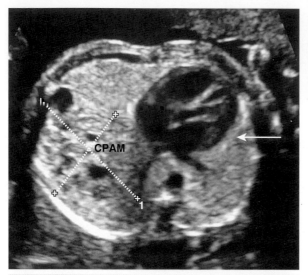

Fig 10.6 • Large type II CPAM at 20 weeks of gestation. The mass measures 33 × 24 mm and consists of numerous small cysts less than 10.0 mm in diameter. It has deviated the heart towards the left side of the chest (arrow). CPAM, cystic pulmonary airways malformation.

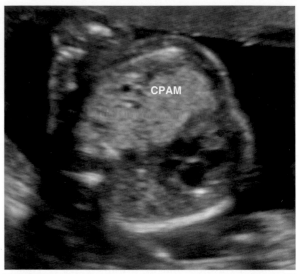

Fig 10.7 • Microcystic CPAM at 20 weeks of gestation showing a large area of uniformly bright tissue in the left lung with deviation of the heart (red dot) to the right of the chest cavity. CPAM, cystic pulmonary airways malformation.

its blood supply from arteries arising from the descending aorta rather than from a pulmonary artery. The ultrasound appearance of BPS is of a discrete mass of homogeneous, bright echoes, typically just above the diaphragm. Identifying such a mass should prompt you to apply the colour Doppler in an attempt to identify a blood vessel leading from the aorta to the mass. This will support the diagnosis of BPS as opposed to other conditions such as tracheal occlusion, which results in part of or a whole lung being abnormally bright as described later.

Cystic Pulmonary Airways Malformation

These lesions are usually unilateral and confined to a single lobe of the lung. Three types are described:

Type I (macrocystic). This type consists of a small number of large cysts, usually more than 10 mm in diameter, and is usually confined to a single lobe (Fig. 10.6).

Type II (mixed). This type consists of numerous smaller cysts, usually less than 10 mm in diameter, and again may be confined to a single lobe.

Type III (microcystic). This type consists of numerous microcysts that cannot be resolved as individual cysts on ultrasound examination. In the same way as the appearances of the kidneys in infantile polycystic disease, the multiple interfaces within this type of CPAM result in a uniformly bright appearance of the affected tissue (Fig. 10.7).

A wide spectrum of outcomes from CPAM has been reported, ranging from fetal hydrops, intrauterine death and postnatal surgical intervention to resolution during pregnancy and postnatal regression. This makes counselling at the time of diagnosis difficult in many cases. The prognosis is dependent on the degree of involvement of the lung tissue and is worst in the presence of the associated findings such as mediastinal shift and hydrops. Polyhydramnios is a common finding and is thought to be due either to oesophageal compression causing a reduction in fetal swallowing or excess fluid production from the abnormal lung tissue.

It is unclear whether those cases which resolve antenatally are true cases of CPAM or whether the identical appearances are due to a different

ULTRASOUND FINDING IN THE CHEST	ADDITIONAL ULTRASOUND APPEARANCES	MOST LIKELY DIAGNOSIS
Single left sided cystic mass	Stomach not visible below the diaphragm, heart deviated to right	Left sided CDH
Single right sided cystic mass	Stomach normally positioned below the diaphragm	CPAM type 1
Echobright mass	Blood vessel to mass from aorta, position of mass relative to diaphragm	BPS – typically in the lower chest, with feeder vessel from aorta
Echobright mass	No feeder vessel	CPAM type 3 – site non-specific. Tracheal occlusion
Mass with mixed echo pattern	Stomach normally positioned below the diaphragm; no peristaltic movements within mass	CPAM type 2
Heart deviated to left	Stomach normally positioned below the diaphragm; peristaltic movements of tissue in left side of chest	Right sided CDH

Table 10.1 Abnormal findings in the fetal chest and additional ultrasound appearances used to aid in the most likely diagnosis

BPS, bronchopulmonary sequestration; CDH, congenital diaphragmatic hernia; CPAM, cystic pulmonary airways malformation.

underlying cause, namely transient or intermittent tracheal occlusion.

TRACHEAL OCCLUSION

Tracheal occlusion describes the condition in which the lumen of the trachea is obliterated. This may be due to part of the trachea being atretic or obstructed, and the latter may be partial and/or intermittent. In the presence of occlusion or obstruction, the fluid secreted by the lungs cannot be expelled and the lung fields appear abnormally hyperechoic. Although intermittent tracheal occlusion has a far better prognosis than true CPAM, its intermittent appearance and similarity of appearance only contribute further to the difficulty in providing an accurate prognosis at the time of differential diagnosis.

Once you are familiar with the normal appearances of the chest, it should be relatively easy to differentiate among the more common abnormalities discussed here and summarized in Table 10.1.

THE FETAL CIRCULATION

The embryonic structure that will become the heart first appears early in the fifth week of gestation as a pair of endothelial tubes which fuse to form a single tube. Differential growth occurs within the tube causing bending into, first, a U-shaped and then, an S-shaped structure. The heart becomes partitioned into four chambers between the sixth and ninth weeks of gestational age.

Contractions of the heart begin in the fifth week of gestation, initially as an ebb and flow motion. Coordinated contractions resulting in unidirectional flow supersede this by the end of the sixth week of gestation.

The normal heart has four chambers, namely two atria and two ventricles. The postnatal circulation is as follows: oxygenated blood enters the left atrium from the lungs via two left and two right pulmonary veins. The oxygenated blood is pushed into the left ventricle through the mitral valve. Ventricular contraction (systole) forces the aortic valve to open, pushing the oxygenated blood from the left ventricle into the ascending aorta, through the aortic arch and isthmus into the descending aorta aorta and then round the body. Deoxygenated blood returns from the body to the right atrium via the inferior vena cava (IVC) and from the head via the superior vena cava (SVC). The deoxygenated blood is pushed into the right ventricle through the tricuspid valve. Ventricular systole forces the pulmonary valve to open, pushing the deoxygenated blood from right ventricle into the main pulmonary artery. This divides into the left and right pulmonary arteries, which carry the deoxygenated blood to the left and right lung, respectively, where it is oxygenated. The oxygenated blood leaves the left and right lungs via the left and right pulmonary

veins, which carry it to the left atrium to begin the cycle again.

The fetal circulation differs from the adult circulation because the lungs do not perform the function of oxygenating the blood before birth. The fetal circulation is designed to oxygenate the blood at the placenta, from where it is circulated round the fetal body, thus effectively bypassing the fetal lungs.

The modifications in the fetal circulation compared with the circulation after birth are the presence of the foramen ovale, the ductus arteriosus, the ductus venosus and the umbilical vessels. These modifications result in a fetal circulation in which the pulmonary and systemic circulations are in parallel rather than in series (Fig. 10.8.).

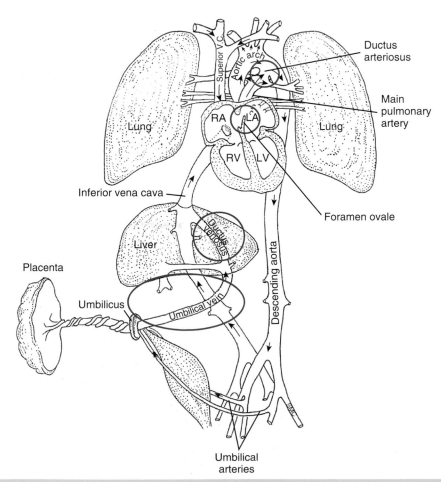

Fig 10.8 • Diagramatic representation of the fetal circulation. This differs from the circulation after birth due to the presence of the ductus arteriosus, foramen ovale, ductus venosus, umbilical vein and the umbilical arteries (red circles). LA, left atrium; LV, left ventricle; RA, right atrium; RV, right ventricle.

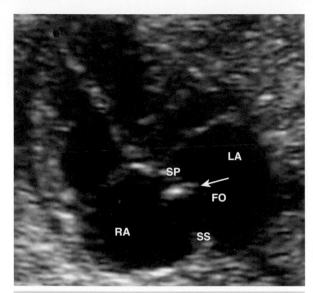

Fig 10.9 • The four chamber view with the apex (red dot) towards 11 o'clock, demonstrating that the left atrium (LA) and right atrium (RA) are equal in size, the flap of the foramen ovale (FO) can be seen in the left atrium, and the septum primum (SP) and septum secundum (SS) comprising the atrial septum.

THE FORAMEN OVALE

The interatrial septum between the left and right atria is formed from two septa, the smaller septum primum, at the crux of the heart, and the larger septum secundum, which extends to the roof of the atria (Fig. 10.9). The foramen ovale (FO) is a perforation in the septum secundum and lies in the centre of the interatrial septum. The FO is covered by a flap or leaflet, the foramen ovale leaflet, which lies within the left atrium. This leaflet allows blood to flow from the right atrium into the left atrium during diastole but not vice versa.

THE DUCTUS ARTERIOSUS

The ductus arteriosus or ductal arch (DA) is the vessel which connects the main pulmonary artery (MPA) to the descending aorta. Its function is to allow blood to bypass the lungs, thus producing two effectively parallel systemic circulations round the body and brain which result in the pressure between the left and right sides of the heart being essentially equal. The majority of the blood from the right ventricle is received by the DA, with only a small portion, approximately 10%, going to the lungs. It is commonly referred to simply as 'the duct', and this is the terminology that will be used here. It is important that you remember there is a second duct, the ductus venosus so you must be careful that you are not introducing confusion when referring to the DA as 'the duct'.

The DA is one of the largest blood vessels in the fetus, being approximately the same diameter as the aorta. Shortly after leaving the heart, the MPA divides into left and right branches. The DA arises at the anatomical origin of the left pulmonary artery (PA).

THE DUCTUS VENOSUS

The ductus venosus (DV) is the vessel which connects the umbilical vein (UV) to the inferior vena cava (IVC), shortly before the IVC enters the right atrium. The function of the DV is to allow oxygenated blood from the umbilical vein to bypass the lungs and to enter the right atrium, from where it crosses the foramen ovale into the left atrium and then into the ascending aorta via the left ventricle. The UV contains well oxygenated blood from the placenta, whereas the IVC contains deoxygenated blood from the lower limbs and body. Thus the blood entering the right atrium has a somewhat lower oxygen concentration than that of the UV because of the mixing of the blood from the DV and the IVC. This system means that the blood vessels to the heart, head, neck and upper limbs receive as well oxygenated blood as possible.

THE UMBILICAL VESSELS

The umbilical cord contains three blood vessels, namely the umbilical vein and two umbilical arteries. The umbilical vein carries oxygenated blood from the placenta to the right atrium via the ductus venosus, whereas the right and left umbilical arteries carry deoxygenated blood from the fetus back to the placenta.

As in postnatal life, the fetal aorta bifurcates into the right and left iliac arteries, which in turn divide into the right and left internal and external iliac arteries. The umbilical arteries arise from their respective internal iliac arteries and course round the fetal bladder before joining the umbilical vein at the site of the cord insertion.

CHANGES AT DELIVERY

During fetal life the pressures in both sides of the heart are essentially the same because oxygen transfer is provided through the placenta rather than via the lungs as in postnatal life. At delivery, changes to the circulation are necessary so that sufficient and immediate perfusion of the lungs can take place. In the fetus the vascular resistance in the lungs is very high as they are nonfunctioning and therefore require minimal blood supply. The first breath of air after birth causes a dramatic fall in the vascular resistance of the lungs, which results in a marked increase in pulmonary blood flow. Separation from the placental circulation causes an immediate fall in blood pressure in the IVC and right atrium of the infant. This increase in pulmonary blood flow causes the pressure in the left atrium to increase above that of the right atrium. The increase in pressure in the left atrium causes the foramen ovale flap to be pressed against the atrial septum, resulting in its closure (Fig. 10.10).

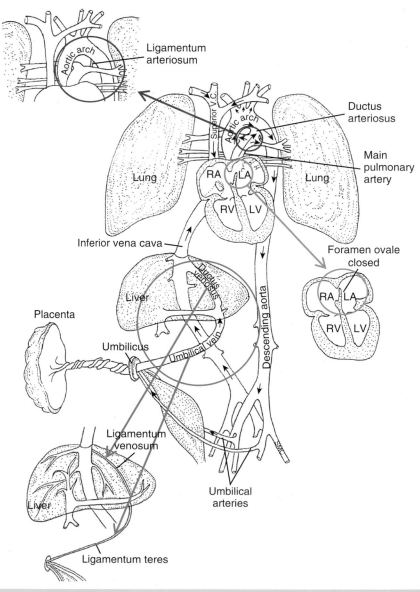

Fig 10.10 • Diagramatic representation of the fetal circulation demonstrating the postnatal fate of the ductus arteriosus (in red), the foramen ovale (in blue), the ductus venosus and umbilical vein (in green). LA, left atrium; LV, left ventricle; RA, right atrium; RV, right ventricle.

The ductus arteriosus begins to close immediately after birth, in response, it is thought, to a decrease in prostaglandins resulting from the increase in oxygen tension occurring at birth. The ductus arteriosus is normally closed within 24–48 hours of life in the term infant. It eventually becomes the ligamentum arteriosus, which passes from the left pulmonary artery to the arch of the aorta (Fig. 10.10).

Once separation from the placenta has taken place after birth, the ductus venosus has no further role to play. It becomes the ligamentum venosum, which passes through the liver from the left branch of the portal vein to the IVC, to which it is attached (Fig. 10.10). The umbilical vein similarly as no further role to play and becomes the ligamentum teres (Fig. 10.10).

The umbilical arteries constrict at birth to prevent blood loss from the infant. If the cord is not cut immediately after birth, for a short time blood will continue to flow through the umbilical vein, continuing to transfer blood from the placenta to the infant. Most of the intra-abdominal portions of the two umbilical arteries form the medial umbilical ligaments, and the proximal parts persist as the right and left superior vesical arteries.

THE FETAL HEART

Evaluation of the fetal heart is an essential component of the 18–22 week anomaly scan. The heart is complex both in terms of its structure and its function and thus provides a potentially daunting challenge to the beginner. It is important, first, to ignore the mystery which has built up, historically, over examination of the fetal heart. Second remember that a clear understanding of the anatomy of the heart, together with keen attention to your scanning technique, will ensure that you are able to assess the heart properly. With time and experience you will be able to exclude or identify those abnormalities which are amenable to detection during routine examination.

To examine the heart properly requires a systematic approach which incorporates assessment of the following six views:

- situs
- four chamber view
- left ventricular outflow tract (LVOT)
- right ventricular outflow tract (RVOT)
- three vessel view (3vv)
- three vessel trachea view (3vt).

In addition to being able to obtain the various sections that include these views, you also need to remember that the heart is a moving organ and that assessing the movements of its various constituent parts is as important a part of your examination as assessing the parts themselves. You should therefore think of your examination as a sweep through the heart that incorporates the required views rather than a set of static views that, when added together, equate to the full examination. We recommend that you learn to image the heart properly using grey scale imaging in the first instance. Once you are able to obtain the correct views relatively easily, you should then apply colour and/or power Doppler imaging. When used properly, the use of colour and/or power Doppler will provide you with additional, useful information in your examination of the heart.

We recommend that you approach the six views in the following sequence:

- obtain the AC section, and use this to assess normality of abdominal situs
- slide up to the four chamber view. Confirm cardiac situs and laterality. Assess the four chamber view
- slide the probe up towards the fetal head to obtain the 3vt
- slide back to the four chamber view, rotate the probe towards the right should to obtain the LVOT
- slide the probe very slightly up towards the fetal head, and then rotate it slightly towards the left shoulder to obtain the RVOT
- confirm a normal crossover of the LVOT and RVOT before sliding from the RVOT up towards the fetal head to obtain the 3vv.

COLOUR DOPPLER SETTINGS

Examining the fetal heart using colour requires a rapid frame rate combined with an acceptable 233

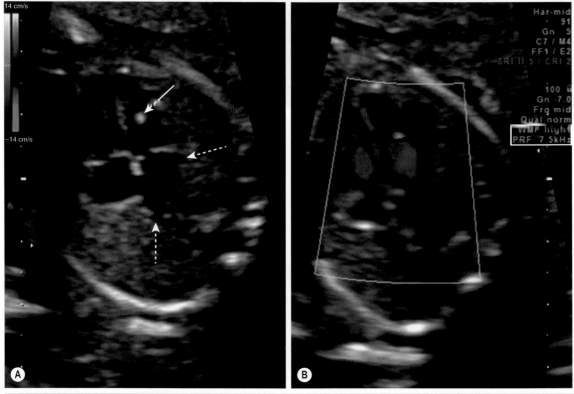

Fig 10.11 • A four chamber view of the heart with the apex (red dot) at 11 o'clock. A. The grey scale image demonstrates normal anatomy. Note the hyperechoic 'echogenic cardiac focus' (arrow) in the left ventricle. Two pulmonary veins can be seen entering the left atrium (dashed arrows). B. Colour Doppler has been applied to the grey scale image using a small colour box and a high frame rate, with a PRF of 7.5 kHz (white box).

image quality. Frame rate can be increased by manipulation of depth, magnification, zoom box and sector width. The frame rate is influenced by the size of the colour box. You should therefore apply as small a colour box as possible over the area of interest in order to maintain as high a frame rate as possible (Fig. 10.11).

The velocity scale or pulse repetition frequency (PRF) determines the range of mean velocities demonstrated within the colour box. A higher velocity range is required for the colour Doppler assessment of the atrioventricular (AV) valves, the filling of the atria and ventricles, and the aortic valve, pulmonary valve and great vessels than that required to assess the pulmonary veins as flow in the latter is slower than elsewhere in the heart.

Applying a velocity range that is too low for the valve, chamber or vessel being interrogated will result in aliasing. This gives the artefactual impression of turbulent flow across that valve or within

the chamber or vessel. As aliasing can occur in pathological situations, mitral or tricuspid valve regurgitation being typical examples, it is important that you adjust the PRF correctly after applying colour. This is because in the normal heart the blood flow should be clearly demonstrated as only red or only blue flashes rather than a mixture of colours.

Similarly, the colour gain setting must be set correctly. This control works in the same way as the gain setting control for grey scale imaging – that is, in this case, by altering the amount of colour shown on the screen. Thus, if the colour gain is set too high, the colour information will 'bleed' over into structures adjacent to the one you are trying to interrogate. This will reduce the quality of the information you obtain and, importantly, can also lead to diagnostic errors. This is important when examining the AV valves, as too high a colour gain setting can produce a false impression of a septal defect. You should therefore start your examination with the colour gain turned to a minimum, increasing it until the optimum colour information is obtained.

M MODE

We do not consider the use of M mode is required in the routine assessment of the fetal heart.

AIM OF THE EXAMINATION

You are examining the heart to exclude a range of abnormal appearances, the implications of which will vary depending on the specific cardiac abnormality and whether it is an isolated condition or associated with other structural and/or chromosomal abnormalities. Unfortunately, for the screening sonographer, most cardiac conditions that are amenable to detection at the 18–22 week anomaly scan present with varying degrees of severity. This means that although the 'typical' appearances of a condition may be well described, your ability to identify the abnormal features of the condition will depend on the degree of severity of that condition in that fetus at the time of your examination. The ultrasound appearances of a number of cardiac conditions may not be present at the 18–22 week examination. Some cardiac conditions may not be present in the views examined at the 18–22 week examination. Others may be present but have appearances which are too subtle to be suspected or detected at the 18–22 week examination. It is also important to remember that some abnormalities can only be detected after birth because of the differences between the antenatal and postnatal circulations.

We suggest that correct examination of the fetal heart as described in this text provides a screening examination for the conditions listed in Table 10.2 and described in the following text. You will note that the characteristic ultrasound appearances of some features and conditions may be too subtle to be identified at 18–22 weeks, although incorporation of the 3vt into the routine screening examination should now make a positive and significant contribution to the likelihood of their detection.

The development of the heart is complex and cardiac abnormalities in the fetus are relatively common. The prognosis for a cardiac abnormality will vary depending on whether the abnormality is isolated or is associated with other structural anomalies and whether the fetal chromosomes are normal. As with all abnormal findings, should you suspect a cardiac abnormality, the woman should be referred for a specialist cardiac evaluation. As there is a strong association between cardiac abnormalities, other structural abnormalities and chromosomal abnormalities, the fetus should also be examined by a fetal medicine specialist if the cardiac abnormality is confirmed. The cardiac and fetal medicine specialists may be the same individual; if not, separate referrals to the two different specialists should be made.

THE FOUR CHAMBER VIEW

The four chamber view was the first cardiac view to be incorporated into the routine assessment of the fetal heart and it remains, arguably, the most important of the views that you need to be able to assess at the 18–22 week examination.

The key to obtaining the correct section for the four-chamber view is first to obtain a correct abdominal circumference section, and then slide the probe up to the thorax. When you have arrived at the heart, make sure your image displays a complete rib on both sides of the chest. If the rib on one or both sides appears incomplete, you are not imaging a true cross-section of the chest or, as the heart lies horizontally in the chest, of the heart.

As discussed in Chapter 7, the axis of the fetus relative to the horizontal within the uterus will influence whether a slight rotation of the probe or a small change of angle of the probe is required to produce the correct four chamber view (Fig. 10.12).

It is generally easier to start examining the heart if it is 'apex-up' – that is, with the apex pointing to 11, 12 or 1 o'clock – than if the apex is 'transverse' – that is, pointing between 2 and 4 o'clock or between 8 and 10 o'clock. This is because it is easier to assess the relative positions and movement of the valves from the apex-up view, as these structures lie at roughly 90° to the insonant sound beam in this view (Fig. 10.12).

By definition, therefore, apex-up is not the best position from which to assess the integrity of the interventricular septum or the interatrial septum. When the apex is up, the two septa will lie parallel to the insonant sound beam. As discussed later, the

CARDIAC ABNORMALITY	VIEWS REQUIRED	MAIN ULTRASOUND FEATURES	CHANGES IN ULTRASOUND APPEARANCE WITH INCREASING GESTATION
Dextrocardia	Situs	Heart in right side of chest	Consistent
Common arterial trunk	1 LVOT & RVOT 2 3vt	1 Only one vessel arising from heart, so no crossover 2 Single large vessel (aortic arch) & SVC; arch right sided in 30%	1 Consistent 2 Consistent
HLHS	1 4ch 2 3vv/3vt	1 LV significantly smaller than RV 2 Aortic arch very small or not visible	1 & 2. May be too subtle to identify at 18–22 weeks. Appearances of all views typically become more abnormal with increasing gestation
Significant (moderate or large) AVSD	4ch	No offset cross at crux	Consistent
Significant (moderate or large) VSD	4ch with septum horizontal	Lack of continuity of IVS. Jet of colour flow across septum at site of defect	Consistent
TGA	1 LVOT & RVOT 2 3vv/3vt	1 No crossover 2 Single large vessel (aortic arch) & SVC (PA/DA present but not seen in this view)	1 Consistent 2 Consistent
Tetralogy of Fallot (VSD, overriding aorta, pulmonary stenosis & enlarged RV)	1 4ch with septum horizontal 2 4ch 3 LVOT 4 RVOT 5 3vv/3vt	1 VSD 2 Hypertrophy of RV wall 3 Aortic valve straddles VSD 4 Post valvular dilatation of PA 5 DA larger than aortic arch	1 Consistent 2 May be too subtle to identify at 18–22 weeks; disparity typically increases in severity with increasing gestation 3 Consistent 4 May be too subtle to identify at 18–22 weeks; appearance typically becomes more abnormal with increasing gestation 5 Consistent
Coarctation	3vv/3vt	Aortic arch significantly smaller than DA	Consistent
Pulmonary stenosis	1 RVOT 2 3vv/3vt	1 Post valvular dilatation of PA 2 DA larger than aortic arch	1 May be too subtle to identify at 18–22 weeks; appearance typically becomes more abnormal with increasing gestation 2 Consistent
Right aortic arch (v sign)	3vt	Arches form a normal V, but to the right of the trachea	Consistent
Right aortic arch (U shape)	3vt	Arches form a wide U, with the trachea in the 'bend' of the U	Consistent
Double aortic arch	3vt	Arches form a wide U, with the trachea in the 'bend' of the U, and surrounded by a vascular ring.	Consistent

Table 10.2 Cardiac abnormalities which can be detected at the 18–22 week routine screening examination, the principal views required to suspect or exclude them and the change in the ultrasound appearances of the abnormality with increasing gestation

ARSA, aberrant right subclavian artery; AVSD, atrioventricular septal defect; DA, ductal arch; HLHS, hypoplastic left heart syndrome; LV, left ventricle; LVOT, left ventricular outflow tract; PA, pulmonary artery; RV, right ventricle; RVOT, right ventricular outflow tract; TGA, transposition of the great arteries; VSD, ventricular septal defect; 3vt, three vessel trachea view; 3vv, three vessel view; 4ch, four chamber view.

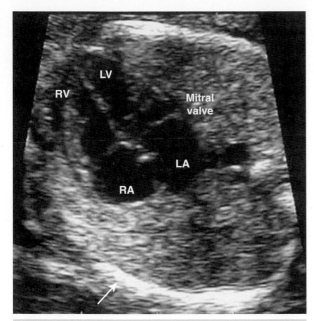

Fig 10.12 • A transverse section of the chest demonstrating the normal four chamber view of the heart. Note the apex is pointing towards 11 o'clock. The normal offsetting of the atrioventricular valves can be seen together with a single rib (arrow) on the right side. LA, left atrium; LV, left ventricle; RA, right atrium; RV, right ventricle.

- the angle of the cardiac axis is noted
- there are two atria of approximately equal size
- the leaflet of the foramen ovale is seen flickering in the left atrium in the moving image
- the interatrial septum appears intact below and above the foramen ovale
- there are two ventricles of approximately equal size and with walls of approximately equal thickness
- the ventricles show equal contraction in the moving image
- the moderator band can be seen in the right ventricle, towards its apex
- the left ventricle extends to the apex of the heart
- the two AV valves are seen to open equally in the moving image
- the atrial and ventricular septa meet the two AV valves at the centre or crux of the heart, forming an offset cross. The valve on the right side, the tricuspid valve, inserts slightly lower in the ventricular septum – that is, closer to the apex of the heart – than the valve on the left side, the mitral valve
- the interventricular septum (IVS) is intact.

The normal appearances of the various components of the four chamber view are described next. Those cardiac abnormalities described in this text that often produce abnormal appearances in more than one of the five views are described at the end of this chapter, after the five cardiac views have been described. Those abnormalities that are most commonly specific to one of the five views only are described in situ.

Situs Solitus

Assessing situs should be the starting point of your cardiac examination. Confirming that the stomach and the apex of the heart are both on the same side of the fetal body does not constitute adequate assessment of situs solitus. Determining where the left and right sides of the fetus are on the ultrasound monitor must be your first task before assessing the relative positions of the stomach and heart.

Assessing situs and confirming *situs solitus* are discussed in Chapters 3 and 8, respectively. *Situs solitus* describes the normal arrangement of the

presence of the foramen ovale in the interatrial septum results in difficulties in assessing the integrity of the rest of the interatrial septum. Assessment of the interventricular septum, however, is a crucial part of your examination. Although the interventricular septum can be assessed from the apex-up view, and ventricular septal defects (VSD) certainly can be detected from this view, complete assessment of the interventricular septum should always include the apex-horizontal view. This ensures that optimal visualization of the septum takes place, that is when it is positioned at roughly 90° to the insonant sound beam.

The relative sizes and appearances of the heart chambers can be assessed equally effectively from either apex-up or apex-horizontal views.

There are 14 components that must be evaluated in order for the four chamber view of the heart to be reported as normal. These are as follows:

- situs solitus is present
- the size of the heart is noted
- the apex of the heart is noted

stomach, cardiac apex and aortic arch on the left side of the body and the IVC on the right. *Situs inversus* is a mirror image of this arrangement, whereas *situs ambiguous* (heterotaxy or isomerism) describes the condition in which some, but not necessarily all, of the organs are incorrectly positioned. Bilateral left sidedness is termed *left isomerism* and bilateral right-sidedness *right isomerism*. *Solitus* is the Latin term for 'common', *ambiguous* for 'unknown' and *inversus* for 'inverted'.

Situs inversus is associated with a slight increase (0.3–0.5%) in complex heart disease. *Situs ambiguous* is commonly associated with complex heart disease, an irregular arrangement of the nonpaired abdominal organs together with bowel, spleen, biliary and bronchial abnormalities and abnormalities in venous drainage. *Situs ambiguous* occurs in 2–4% of infants with congenital heart disease.

Situs abnormalities

In situs solitus the intrahepatic portion of the umbilical vein curves towards the right side of the fetus, the descending aorta lies to the left of the spine and the IVC lies to the right of the spine and is more anterior than the aorta (Fig. 10.13).

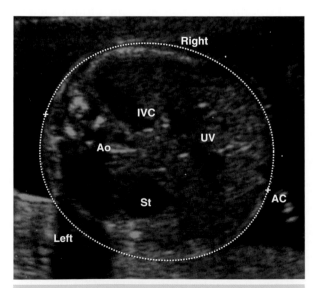

Fig 10.13 • A measured abdominal circumference section of a breech fetus at 21 weeks of gestation, showing the correct positions of the organs required to confirm situs solitus. AC, abdominal circumference; Ao, aorta; IVC, inferior vena cava; St, stomach; UV, umbilical vein.

Situs abnormalities should be suspected if the following are identified:

- the heart and/or stomach is not found on the left side of the fetus
- the intrahepatic portion of the umbilical vein curves towards the left side of the fetus
- the aorta and the 'IVC' or the azygous vein (see below) lie beside each other and on the same side of the abdomen.

Left atrial isomerism

In left atrial isomerism both atria have the morphological characteristics of the left atrium and the IVC is interrupted in its course through the abdomen to the right atrium and connects with the azygous circulation via an azygous vein. The azygous vein is an important component of a complex vascular system called the azygous system. This runs parallel to the vena cava system and serves as an alternative venous pathway. It is not normally visible in the fetus. In left atrial isomerism the azygous vein, which drains into the SVC, is dilated and therefore visible. This is termed *interruption of the IVC with azygous continuation*. The azygous vein, which you may understandably assume is the IVC, is adjacent to, rather than in front of, the aorta in cross-section of the abdomen and produces what is called 'the double vessel sign'.

Left isomerism is more common than right isomerism in the fetus and is associated with complete heart block and hydrops and therefore an increased rate of intrauterine demise.

Right atrial isomerism

In right atrial isomerism both atria have the morphological characteristics of the right atrium. Complex cardiac abnormalities are associated with this condition. The IVC is normally positioned anterior to the aorta but both lie on either the left or the right of the spine.

Right isomerism is less common than left isomerism in the fetus but is more common in the neonate because of the increased rate of fetal demise in left isomerism.

Size of the Heart

The heart should occupy approximately one third of the chest cavity. As discussed earlier, it is important to be able to distinguish between a normal-sized heart in a small chest and an enlarged heart in a normal sized chest. Calculation of the thoracic/abdominal circumference ratio can be made by measuring the circumferences of the thorax and abdomen and using the appropriate charts for the gestation but this is not a requirement of the routine screening examination.

Enlarged heart

An abnormally large heart, or cardiomegaly, typically is due to cardiac overload, or increased cardiac output, for which a number of causes need to be considered. Certain fetal tumours which are highly vascular can cause high cardiac output, which can result in cardiomegaly and eventual heart failure. Sacrococcygeal teratoma is one such tumour.

Other causes of high cardiac output leading to cardiomegaly and which are within the remit of a routine screening examination include placental chorioangioma (see Chapter 14), recipient twin-to-twin transfusion and cardiac abnormalities including tricuspid atresia, atrioventricular septal defect (AVSD), Ebstein's anomaly and heart block.

Severe anaemia is another important cause of cardiomegaly and is usually identified from velocity measurements of the middle cerebral artery. Such measurements are beyond the remit of the routine assessment of the fetus.

In the third trimester of pregnancy a normal heart can appear abnormally large (Fig. 10.14).

The Apex of the Heart

In mid-gestation, the heart lies horizontally within the left chest, at the level of the fourth rib, with the apex of the heart pointing towards the left anterior chest wall.

The normal position of the heart within the left chest is termed *levocardia*. *Dextrocardia* describes a heart located in the right chest and *mesocardia* describes a heart with a central position in the chest.

Dextrocardia

Dextrocardia describes the condition where the heart is located in the right chest. As discussed earlier in this chapter, displacement of the heart from its normal anterior left position can be caused by diaphragmatic hernia and lung lesions. The apex of the heart in these cases is normally to the

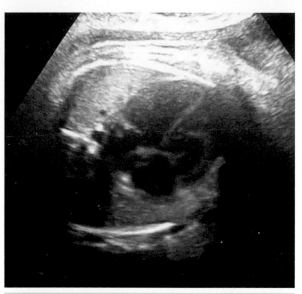

Fig 10.14 • A normal sized heart in the third trimester. Note the heart appears abnormally large when compared with its size relative to the fetal chest in the second trimester.

left. This type of dextrocardia, also referred to as *dextroposition*, is usually transitory, the heart assuming its correct position within the chest once the extracardiac condition has been treated.

Dextrocardia can also be secondary to situs inversus, situs ambiguous and conditions in which there is discordance between the atrioventricular connections, as in transposition. In these cases the apex of the heart is typically to the **right**. This type of dextrocardia is also referred to as *dextroversion*.

Angle of the Cardiac Axis

The *angle of the cardiac axis* describes the angle of the interventricular septum to a line drawn from the fetal spine to the anterior chest wall at the level of the four chamber view. The normal angle of the cardiac axis is 45° to the left of this line, with the normal range being between 25° and 65° (Fig. 10.15).

Abnormal axis

A heart in which the axis is less than 25° or more than 65° is abnormal. An abnormal axis increases the risk of cardiac abnormalities, especially those including the outflow tracts, and is also reported

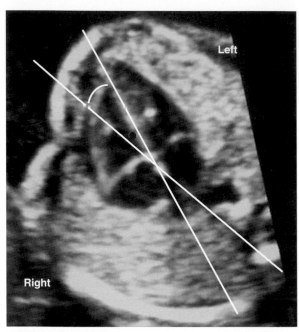

Fig 10.15 • A four chamber view of the heart demonstrating a normal cardiac axis (red dot).

in association with omphalocele and gastroschisis (see Chapter 11).

The Atria

The right and left atria are of approximately equal size in the normal heart (Fig. 10.9). At first glance the ultrasound appearance of both atria is similar. However, on closer examination you will be able to recognize that the inner wall of the left atrium appears less smooth than that of the right atrium (Fig. 10.11). This is because two of the four pulmonary veins, the right and left inferior pulmonary veins, enter the left atrium at the level of the four-chamber view, enabling you to distinguish between the two atria. Confirmation that these vessels are pulmonary veins can be made using colour flow.

As discussed earlier, blood flow in the pulmonary veins is much slower than in adjacent vessels, so you will need to select a lower velocity setting than normally used in the heart for your colour mapping of the pulmonary veins. Lowering the velocity will naturally result in oversaturation of the colour map of the blood vessels other than the pulmonary veins. You must make sure that the direction of flow, or the colour, of these vessels

indicates that they are going into rather than coming out of the left atrium. Remember that the pulmonary arteries, which lie in close proximity to the pulmonary veins, will demonstrate blood flow in the opposite direction.

Failing to identify the pulmonary veins entering the left atrium is associated with the rare condition of total anomalous pulmonary venous drainage.

The Foramen Ovale

As discussed earlier, the foramen ovale (FO) is a perforation in the septum secundum and lies in the centre of the interatrial septum. It is covered by a flap or leaflet which lies within the left atrium, and this leaflet allows blood to flow from the right atrium into the left atrium during diastole but not vice versa.

The Atrial Septum

As discussed earlier, the septum between the left and right atria is formed from two septa, the smaller septum primum, at the crux of the heart, and the larger septum secundum, which extends to the roof of the atria. The atrial septum is interrupted in its mid-portion by the foramen ovale (Fig. 10.9).

Atrial septal defect

Atrial septal defect (ASD) describes an abnormal opening in the atrial septum allowing an additional communication between the left and right atria, over and above that of the foramen ovale.

Atrial septal defects are classified according to the position of the defect, in either the septum primum or in the septum secundum. The septum primum is very short, but you should still learn to recognize its appearance, as it is an important component of the crux of the heart and therefore in the exclusion of AVSDs.

The more common site for an ASD is adjacent to the FO in the septum secundum, with about 80% of all ASDs occurring along this part of the septum. Due to the proximity of the majority of secundum ASDs to the foramen ovale, it is very difficult to identify this type of ASD.

Although detecting an isolated ASD is not an expectation of a routine 18–22 week examination of the fetal heart, this should not preclude you from examining the atrial septum to familiarize yourself with its normal appearance and thus to increase the possibility of your identification or exclusion of an ASD.

If you are suspicious of an ASD, applying colour flow over the septum to determine whether there is shunting of blood across the septum, other than through the foramen ovale, will be helpful. Remember that in the normal fetus blood should flow through the foramen ovale from the right atrium to the left atrium.

The Ventricles

As discussed earlier, the axis of the heart points towards the left chest. This results in the right ventricle lying closer to the anterior chest wall than the left ventricle in the normal heart (Fig. 10.12). In the first, second and early third trimester fetus, the two ventricular chambers should be of a similar size, although the left ventricle is anatomically slightly narrower and longer than the right ventricle (Fig. 10.16). The thickness of the two ventricular walls should also be similar. In later gestations, the right side of the heart may appear slightly larger than the left side; this is a normal finding.

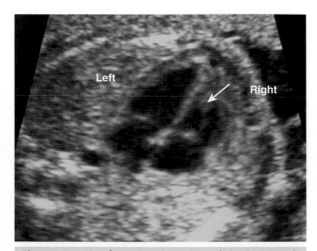

Fig 10.16 • The four chamber view of the heart with apex (red dot) to 1 o'clock showing the apical insertion of the chordae tendineae of the tricuspid valve to the right ventricular wall and apex of the heart. Note that the morphological left ventricle extends to and effectively occupies the apex of the heart. The moderator band is visible within the right ventricle (arrow).

The right and left ventricles both have their own characteristic features, and it is these appearances which you must learn to recognize. This is to enable you to determine whether it is the morphological right ventricle or the morphological left ventricle which is nearer the anterior chest wall.

Difference in size of the ventricles

A difference in size between the two ventricles is an abnormal finding. Having identified a size discrepancy between the two ventricles, you must decide whether this is a result of one ventricle being larger than normal or the other ventricle being smaller than normal.

One ventricle may appear enlarged because its cavity is enlarged or because its walls are thickened. These appearances will look very different. An enlarged ventricular cavity will present with a hypoechoic ventricular chamber that is larger than normal, surrounded by a wall of normal thickness and echogenicity. By contrast, a ventricle with abnormally thickened walls will usually present with a ventricular cavity which is normal, or more commonly reduced, in size, and which is surrounded by a wall of increased thickness or echogenicity and which typically demonstrates poor contractility.

You must then decide whether it is the left or the right ventricle which is abnormal. Remember to confirm that the right ventricle is nearer to the chest wall by identifying the moderator band within it, as described later.

Enlarged ventricle

An enlarged ventricle suggests obstruction to forward flow across the outlet valve. Thus if the left ventricle is enlarged, you should consider the possibility of aortic (valve) stenosis. If the right ventricle is enlarged because the walls are thickened but the size of the ventricular cavity is reduced, you should consider the possibility of pulmonary (valve) stenosis.

Small ventricle

A small ventricle is the likely result from underdevelopment of that ventricle and its outflow tract. The condition most likely to present with a small left ventricle is hypoplastic left heart syndrome (HLHS), whereas the condition most likely to present with a small right ventricle is pulmonary atresia with intact ventricular septum.

The Moderator Band

The distinguishing feature of the morphological right ventricle is the presence of a large muscle bundle, the septoparietal muscle bundle or moderator band, which crosses the cavity of the ventricle obliquely towards the ventricular apex (Fig. 10.16). The presence of the moderator band may give you the initial impression that the morphological right ventricle is significantly shorter than the morphological left ventricle. You should always confirm that you have visualized the moderator band and that you have seen it in the ventricle lying nearer to the chest wall.

Moderator band in the 'wrong' ventricle

The moderator band lying within the ventricle further from the anterior chest wall is an abnormal finding because this indicates that the left ventricle is nearer the chest wall rather than the right ventricle. This arrangement is associated with congenitally corrected transposition of the great arteries (ccTGA) but not complete transposition of the great arteries (TGA). These conditions are both discussed later in this chapter.

The Left Ventricle

The distinguishing feature of the morphological left ventricle is its length (Fig. 10.16). The morphological left ventricle is longer than the morphological right ventricle because of, first, the mitral valve inserting into the interventricular septum closer to the crux of the heart than the tricuspid valve and, second, because the morphological left ventricle extends to, and effectively occupies, the apex of the heart. There is a close relationship between the inlet (mitral) and outlet (aortic) valves of the morphological left ventricle. This is not a feature of the inlet (tricuspid) and outlet (pulmonary) valves of the morphological right ventricle.

The AV Valves

Examination of the two AV valves includes assessing the position of their relative insertions into the interventricular septum, the differing appearance of both valves and confirmation that both valves open and close freely.

The valve 'belongs' to its ventricle rather than its atrium; thus the tricuspid valve is associated with the right ventricle and the mitral valve with the left ventricle. Appreciating these relationships is important in the recognition of a possible ccTGA or TGA.

The tricuspid valve

The tricuspid valve is situated between the right atrium and the right ventricle and prevents backflow of blood into the right atrium during ventricular systole. The valve, as its name suggests, has three leaflets – anterior, posterior and septal. These are attached to thin muscle strands, the chordae tendinae. The chordae tendinae insert into three papillary muscles and also directly into the wall of the interventricular septum. The insertion of some of the leaflet's chordae tendinae directly into the wall of the septum is a distinguishing feature of the tricuspid valve, although assessment of this level of detail is not a requirement of the routine 18–22 week examination.

The insertion of the tricuspid valve into the interventricular septum is closer to the apex and further from the crux of the heart than that of the mitral valve. This contributes to the right ventricle being smaller than the left ventricle. In Ebstein's anomaly the tricuspid valve is positioned more apically than normal, resulting in a smaller right ventricle and a larger right atrium than in the normal heart.

The tricuspid (inlet) valve and the pulmonary (outlet) valve are separated by an area of tissue (the subpulmonic conus). The inlet and outlet valves of the right ventricle therefore do not have the same close anatomical relationship as found between the inlet and outlet valves of the left ventricle.

The mitral valve

The mitral valve is situated between the left atrium and the left ventricle and prevents backflow of blood into the left atrium during ventricular systole. The valve has two leaflets, anterior and posterior, which attach to chordae tendinae. As with the tricuspid valve, the chordae tendinae of the mitral valve insert into papillary muscles, of which there are two, and which attach to the free wall of the left ventricle. Unlike the tricuspid valve, there is no direct insertion of the mitral valve's chordae tendinae into the wall of the interventricular septum, with the attachment of both papillary muscles being to the free ventricular wall rather than the septum. As with the tricuspid valve, assessment of this level of detail of the mitral valve is not a requirement of the routine 18–22 week examination.

The insertion of the mitral valve into the interventricular septum is farther from the apex and closer to the crux of the heart than that of the tricuspid valve. This contributes to the left ventricle being slightly longer than the right ventricle (Fig. 10.16).

There is a close anatomical relationship between the mitral (inlet) valve and the aortic (outlet) valve such that the anterior leaflet of the mitral valve is in fibrous continuity with the aortic valve. This is an important component of the left ventricular outflow tract view and important in the exclusion of a VSD.

The Crux of the Heart

The crux of the heart describes the area of the heart where the atrial and ventricular septa meet the two atrioventricular valves. Due to the more apical insertion of the tricuspid valve compared with that of the mitral valve, this junction has the appearance of an offset cross (Fig. 10.12 and Fig. 10.17). The differential insertion of the AV valves into the ventricular septum is important in the identification of the right and left ventricles in the normal fetus and in recognizing AVSDs.

AVSD

Atrioventricular septal defect describes the combination of an ASD, a VSD and a common AV valve. The crux therefore is absent. The resulting ultrasound appearances are as follows. The crux is replaced by a black void resulting from the two septal defects (Fig. 10.17). The common AV valve has a characteristic linear appearance when closed, and its motion can be likened to the flapping of 'seagull wings'.

As AVSD has a strong association with Down's syndrome, the importance of, not only, achieving a correct four chamber view, but also of evaluating its component parts rigorously, cannot be emphasised enough.

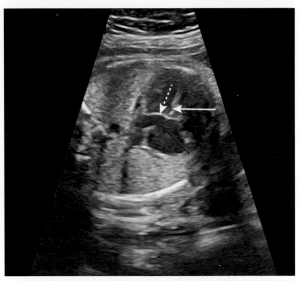

Fig 10.17 • A four chamber view at 20 weeks, with an AVSD. The atrial component (red arrow) can be seen above the (closed) common valve which has the appearance of flapping 'seagull wings' (dashed arrow). The ventricular component of the defect is seen below the common valve (white arrow). AVSD, atrioventricular septal defect.

The Ventricular Septum

The right and left ventricles are separated by a septum, the interventricular or ventricular septum (IVS). The septum consists of four component parts:

- inlet septum
- outlet septum
- membranous septum
- muscular or trabecular septum.

When imaging the heart in two-dimensional (2D) imaging, the ventricular septum appears as a bright and relatively thin linear structure. It is helpful to remember that the ventricles are separated by a sheet of tissue which has both depth and width outside the plane in which you are imaging it. The inlet septum separates the two AV valves. The outlet septum lies beneath the pulmonary valve. The membranous septum is the small, thin area of the left ventricular outflow tract which lies just beneath the aortic valve, whereas the muscular or trabecular septum is the largest part of the septum which extends from the apex of the heart to the insertion of the tricuspid valve.

The purpose of imaging the ventricular septum is to confirm its continuity from the crux of the

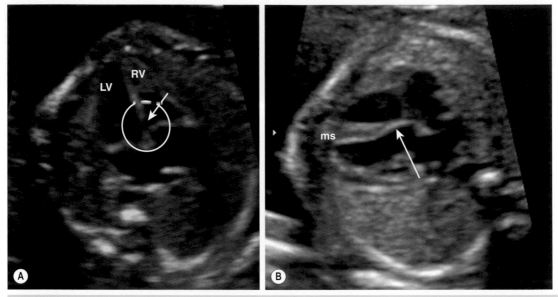

Fig 10.18 • A. Four chamber view with apex up (red dot) demonstrating a thinner appearance of the ventricular septum and dropout artefact (arrow) within the membranous portion of the septum (the area within the circle). B. A normal four chamber view with the apex (red dot) at 9 o'clock. The ultrasound beam is perpendicular to the ventricular septum. This image clearly shows the thickened appearance of the muscular ventricular septum (ms) and the thinner membranous (arrow) portion of the septum indicating that the ventricular septum is intact in this view. LV, left ventricle; RV, right ventricle.

heart to its apex, thus hopefully excluding the larger of one of the most common cardiac abnormalities, namely a defect in the septum or a VSD.

Imaging the heart using the apex-up view will demonstrate the muscular portion of the septum but will often fail to image the membranous part of the septum. This is because the angle of insonation, of approximately 0° to the vertical often is unable to resolve the membranous part of the septum as it is so thin (Fig. 10.18). This results in an apparent lack of continuity of the septum, thus mimicking a VSD. This lack of visualization is called acoustic dropout. As discussed earlier, the correct way to image the ventricular septum is to apply an angle of insonation of 90°. You should manipulate the probe, therefore, so that the apex of the heart is between 2 and 4 o'clock or between 8 and 10 o'clock. Colour flow Doppler is useful to check for ventricular septal defects by demonstrating that there is no blood flow across the septum at any point (Fig. 10.19).

You may mistake acoustic dropout for a VSD using the apex-up view but must then determine whether or not the appearance is artefactual by using the correct orientation for assessing the

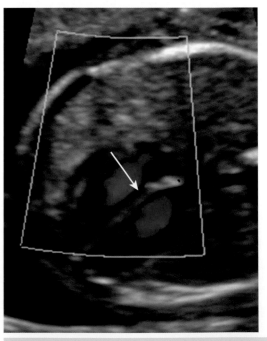

Fig 10.19 • A four chamber view with the apex at 7 o'clock (red dot). Colour Doppler shows that there is no flow across the ventricular septum, excluding a VSD in this view. Note particularly the intact membranous portion of the septum (arrow). VSD, ventricular septal defect.

septum, namely with the septum horizontal (compare Figs. 10.18A and 10.18B). You must never assume that the defect in the septum using the apex-up view is dropout and thus fail to proceed to the horizontal septum view. This is poor practice and is very likely to result in your failing to identify a true VSD.

Although many of the significant cardiac defects can be detected from the four chamber view, it is important to remember that this view will typically be normal in a number of other severe cardiac abnormalities. In tetralogy of Fallot for example, the four chamber view may appear normal unless the ventricular septal defect is large and therefore obvious in this view. In TGA, the four chamber view is likely to appear normal, with the defect only being suspected from the outflow tract views.

Conversely, it is important to be aware that an incorrect section of the four chamber view can give the false impression of disproportion either between the two atria, between the two ventricles or between the two sides of the heart (Fig. 10.20).

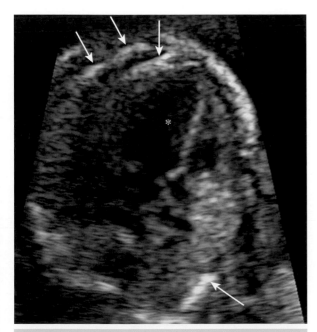

Fig 10.20 • Oblique view of the chest demonstrating multiple segments of ribs (arrows) at each lateral chest wall falsely demonstrating ventricular disproportion resulting in a non-diagnostic attempt at a four chamber view of the heart. The apparent ventricular disproportion, with the left ventricle (*) appearing much larger than the right ventricle, is artefactual due to poor technique.

THE LEFT OUTFLOW TRACT VIEW

The *left ventricular outflow tract view (LVOT)*, or left ventricle long-axis view, describes the section of the heart in which the aorta is seen arising from the left ventricle. The aims of obtaining this view are to confirm the following:

- the normal size of the left ventricle
- continuity between the interventricular septum and the anterior wall of the ascending aorta
- the direction of the ascending aorta towards the right shoulder
- the presence of the aortic valve, lying completely within the aorta
- the normal diameter of the ascending aorta
- forward, laminar flow from the ventricle across the aortic valve into the ascending aorta.

To image the LVOT, obtain the four-chamber view and identify the left ventricle. Slide the transducer minimally towards the fetal head. Rotate the probe slightly towards the right shoulder to demonstrate the blood vessel leaving the left ventricle. This should be the first vessel you see leaving the heart and should be the aorta. The direction of the aorta is across the chest towards the right shoulder of the fetus (Fig. 10.21). Due to the close proximity of the inlet (mitral) and outlet (aortic) valves in this view, you are likely also to observe the mitral valve opening and closing, adjacent to the ascending aorta.

One diagnostic feature of the aorta is that, unlike the main pulmonary artery, it does not divide. The second diagnostic feature of the aorta is that three vessels, the head and neck vessels, arise from the arch of the aorta – although a different view of the vessel is required to demonstrate their presence, thereby confirming this vessel is the aorta. This is discussed towards the end of this chapter.

The bright white echo flicking at the junction of the left ventricle and the aorta is the aortic valve. The flicking confirms that the valve is opening and closing. The valve is closed when this white echo is seen and open when the echo cannot be seen (Fig. 10.21). The purpose of visualizing the aortic valve lying completely within the aorta is to exclude an overriding aorta as described later.

Make sure you have rotated the probe sufficiently to image the full length of the left ventricle and as

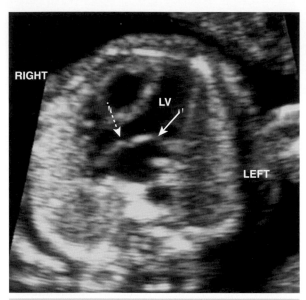

Fig 10.21 • The LVOT view demonstrating the origin of the ascending aorta as it leaves the left ventricle (LV). As no white echo can be seen within the aorta, this suggests that the aortic valve (dashed arrow) is open. Part of the mitral valve (arrow) can be seen directly adjacent to the origin of the ascending aorta. LVOT, left ventricular outflow tract.

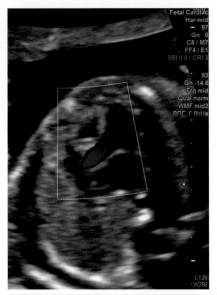

Fig 10.22 • The left outflow tract with the apex (red dot) at 12 o'clock, demonstrating continuity of the ventricular septum, suggesting that the septum is intact in this view. Compare the similar appearances of Fig. 10.21.

much of the ascending aorta as possible. The aim of ensuring there is continuity between the septum and the anterior wall of the aorta is to exclude a VSD and conotruncal abnormalities as discussed later. Although the purpose of your grey scale image is to demonstrate continuity of the posterior wall of the aorta with the anterior leaflet of the mitral valve, and the continuity of the anterior wall of the ascending aorta with the ventricular septum, you should now confirm these normal appearances by applying colour Doppler (Fig. 10.22). The role of colour in identifying VSDs is discussed in more detail later in this chapter. The heart is a three-dimensional structure and so it is important to remember that the LVOT should be assessed from more than one ultrasound slice. Having assessed your first LVOT slice, make very small sliding movements to each side of the original section to examine as much of the septum as you can.

Confirm again that the aortic valve lies completely within the aorta. The diameter of the aorta should remain constant along its length in this view. Both a narrow and a dilated ascending aorta are abnormal findings and result from an abnormality above, below or at the level of the aortic valve. The diameters of the aorta and pulmonary artery as they leave the heart should be approximately the same size – you will use the three vessel (3vv) and three vessel trachea (3vt) views to confirm this later in your examination. If you suspect that the size of the aorta is abnormal in the LVOT view, remember that it is likely also to be abnormal in the 3vv and 3vt views.

Colour flow Doppler is useful to demonstrate continuity of laminar flow from the left ventricle through the aortic valve and into the ascending aorta. A jet of blood crossing the IVS is an abnormal finding and suggestive of a VSD. You must take care to ensure that the jet results from a defect in the septum and is not an artefact caused by the close proximity, and often rather confusing blood flow patterns, of other structures. Remember that you will achieve the best Doppler signal and therefore the most informative colour mapping when the vessel(s) you are insonating lie parallel – that is, at 0° – to the ultrasound beam. This means that flow in the LVOT is best imaged with the apex towards 12 o'clock. A VSD, however, is best excluded when the LVOT is imaged with the apex at 3 or 9 o'clock. In this orientation, the abnormal jet will be crossing the defect in the septum at around 0° to the ultrasound beam.

The inability to obtain a normal LVOT is most commonly the result of poor technique. Visualizing the continuity of the aorta with the ventricular septum is important in the exclusion of abnormalities that may not be evident from the four-chamber view, namely outlet VSDs, aortic override and conotruncal abnormalities.

THE 3VT VIEW

The *3vt view* describes the section of the heart in which the pulmonary artery/ductal arch and transverse arch of the aorta meet as they join the descending aorta and in which both the SVC and trachea are seen.

The aims of obtaining this view are to confirm the following:

- three vessels and the trachea are present
- from left to right, these vessels are the pulmonary artery/duct or ductal arch, the transverse arch of the aorta and the SVC
- the diameters of the ductal and aortic arches should appear approximately the same size, which should be greater than that of the SVC
- the two arches merge in a tight V shape
- both arches lie to the left of the spine and the trachea
- the trachea lies posterior to the SVC
- forward, laminar flow is present in the three vessels.

The 3vt view includes the longitudinal view of the aortic arch, the longitudinal view of the ductal arch and a cross section of the SVC. The 3vt view is most easily obtained as follows. Manipulate the probe so that the ventricular septum in the 4 chamber view is as horizontal as possible. Make sure that you have 'opened out' the ventricles as much as possible so that the LV is imaged in its maximum length. You may need to rotate the probe slightly to maximize its length. Now slide the probe towards the fetal head from this 4 chamber view. A very slight rotation towards the left side of the fetus may also be required. We do not recommend trying to obtain the 3vt view using the 3vv as your starting point as you are unlikely to be successful. This is due to the spatial arrangement of the two arches.

The spatial relationship between the three vessels and their relative sizes are as follows. The ductal arch lies to the left of the aortic arch which lies to the left of the SVC. Both the ductal arch and the aortic arch are seen in longitudinal section. The SVC is seen in cross section. The ductal and aortic arches form an acute V, to the left of the spine, as they merge into the descending aorta. The SVC and the trachea are seen in cross-section, to the right of the aortic arch and the spine. The trachea appears as a small hyperechoic ring surrounding a fluid-filled space (Fig. 10.23).

In the normal fetus no cardiovascular vessels lie to the right of the trachea in the 3vt view (Fig. 10.23). This gives rise to the descriptor of the aortic arch in the normal fetus as being 'left-sided'– that is, lying to the left of the trachea.

The 3vt view is best imaged with apex of the heart at 1 or 11 o'clock. In this position, blood flow in both arches, the descending aorta and the SVC should be in an anteroposterior direction. Colour flow Doppler is useful in confirming the sizes of and relative flow patterns within the two arches and the SVC. It should also ensure that the flow in all three vessels is away from the transducer and should therefore result in a blue signal in all three vessels if standard colour flow mapping is applied (Fig. 10.23). Remember that the colour presented by each of the three vessels will depend on the orientation of that vessel relative to the horizontal.

Note that this view differs from the 3vv in that the middle vessel, the aortic arch, is seen in longitudinal section in the 3vt view, whereas in the 3vv the arch is seen in cross-section.

The cardiac conditions that should be suspected either when the 3vt view is abnormal or cannot be obtained, include tetralogy of Fallot, TGA, coarctation and aortic arch abnormalities. These are discussed in more detail later in this chapter.

THE RIGHT OUTFLOW TRACT VIEW

Authors differ in their definitions of the right ventricular outflow tract view (RVOT). This text describes the RVOT as the section of the heart in which the main pulmonary artery is seen arising from the right ventricle and bifurcating into right and left branch pulmonary arteries (Fig. 10.24). The pulmonary valve should be seen within the MPA.

247

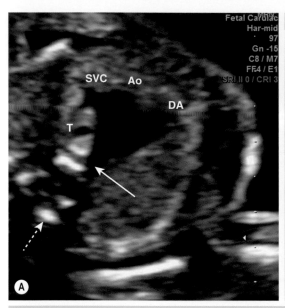
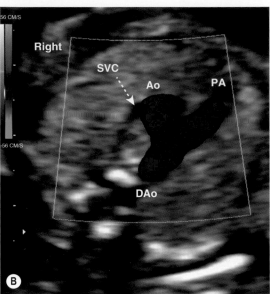

Fig 10.23 • A. A grey scale image of a normal 3vt view without colour Doppler. The ductal arch (DA) can be seen merging with the descending aorta (arrow), to the left of the spine (dashed arrow) and trachea (T). The superior vena cava (SVC) is seen in cross section and to the right of the aortic arch. B. The same 3vt view with colour Doppler superimposed, confirming that the two arches (Ao and PA) meet in a tight V shape (DAo, descending aorta), to the left of the spine, SVC (dashed arrow) and trachea (red dot).

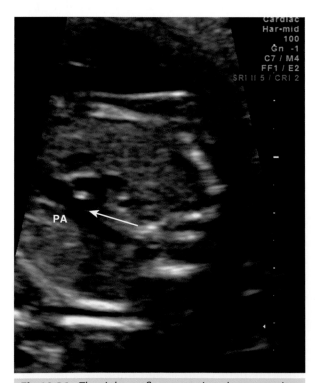

Fig 10.24 • The right outflow tract view demonstrating the bifurcation (arrow) of the pulmonary artery (PA) leaving the right atrium towards the fetal spine.

The aims of obtaining this view are to confirm the following:

- the right ventricle is of normal size
- the direction of the MPA is towards the spine
- the diameter of the MPA is normal
- the MPA bifurcates
- forward, laminar flow is present from the ventricle into the MPA and its branches.

To obtain the RVOT from the LVOT, slide the probe very slightly towards the fetal head and then rotate it slightly away from the right shoulder. The main aim of this view is to visualize the bifurcation of the great vessel originating from the right ventricle, thus confirming that this vessel is the MPA, as the aorta does not divide in the fetal chest.

The direction of the MPA is towards and slightly to the left of the spine. You must make sure you visualize the pulmonary valve within the MPA and that it is moving freely – seen as flicking – within the vessel and does not appear to be thickened. The MPA divides after a short course into the right and the left pulmonary arteries which are sometimes referred to as the branch pulmonary arteries. The right PA crosses the fetal chest towards the right side, but it is often difficult to image any length of this vessel. You must, however, make sure you have identified origin of the right PA at the bifurcation, as this ensures that the vessel arising from the right ventricle is the MPA and not the aorta (Fig. 10.24).

Colour flow Doppler is useful to demonstrate continuity of laminar flow from the right ventricle through the pulmonary valve into the main pulmonary artery, the bifurcation and continuing forward flow through the left pulmonary artery and the arterial duct towards the descending aorta.

The cardiac conditions that should be considered when the RVOT cannot be obtained or is abnormal should include TGA, tetralogy of Fallot and pulmonary atresia/stenosis. These conditions are discussed in more detail later in this chapter.

THE CROSS OVER OF THE GREAT VESSELS

You now will appreciate that the directions of the two outflow tracts differ as they leave the heart. In the normal heart the aorta leaves the left ventricle towards the right shoulder and the pulmonary artery leaves the right ventricle towards the spine.

The aims of obtaining the cross over view are to confirm the following:

- the direction of the aorta is towards the right shoulder
- the direction of the main pulmonary artery is towards the spine
- in a caudal to cephalad sweep, the first vessel to leave the heart is the aorta
- the main pulmonary artery crosses over the aorta as it leaves the heart
- forward, laminar flow is present in both outflow tracts.

The plane in which the aorta leaves the heart is lower, or more caudal, than the comparative plane for the main pulmonary artery. Thus when you are scanning the heart and performing your sweep up from the four chamber view towards the fetal head, you will image the LVOT first, then the RVOT. Note that the pulmonary artery crosses over the aorta as you sweep cephalad.

Colour flow Doppler is useful to demonstrate forward laminar flow in both outflow tracts.

Identifying a normal crossover of the great arteries is an important adjunct to your assessment of the LVOT and RVOT views. A normal crossover excludes the majority of transpositions of the great vessels and double-outlet right ventricle.

THE 3VV

The *3vv* describes the section of the heart in which the MPA/DA, ascending aorta and SVC are seen.

The aims of obtaining this view are to confirm the following:

- three vessels are present
- from left to right, these vessels are the pulmonary artery/DA, the ascending aorta and the SVC
- the pulmonary artery/DA is the most anterior vessel, and the SVC is the most posterior
- the diameter of the pulmonary artery/DA is similar to that of the aorta and larger than that of the SVC
- forward, laminar flow is present in the three vessels.

The 3vv is obtained by sliding the probe up slightly cephalad from the RVOT. The 3vv is best imaged with the apex of the heart at 1 or 11 o'clock and the spine therefore at 7 or 5 o'clock.

This view demonstrates a longitudinal section of the pulmonary artery/DA, whereas the descending aorta and SVC are imaged in cross-section (Figs. 10.25 and 10.26). The spatial relationship between the three vessels and their relative sizes are as follows. The pulmonary artery/DA is the most anterior of the three vessels and lies to the left of the aortic arch, which lies to the left of the SVC. The pulmonary artery/DA is seen in longitudinal section. The aortic arch and SVC are seen in cross-section. The pulmonary artery/DA is the largest in diameter of the three vessels, although this difference in size in the normal heart is subtle. The SVC is the smallest in diameter of the three vessels, lies to the right of the aortic and pulmonary/ductal arches and is the most posterior of the three vessels (Fig. 10.25).

Although the trachea is not a component part of this view, you may identify it lying directly posterior to the aorta (Fig. 10.25). You may also identify the oesophagus, which lies posterior and to the right of the tachea. The lumen of the trachea and of the oesophagus present as small hypoechoic linear and circular structures, respectively, each surrounded by a thicker hyperechoic ring.

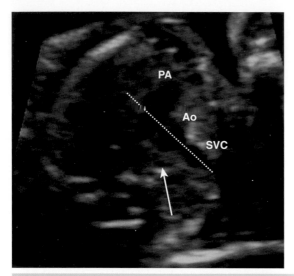

Fig 10.25 • The 3vv demonstrating the pulmonary artery (PA), the ascending aorta (Ao) and the superior vena cava (SVC) in the upper chest arranged in an oblique line, as shown by the dotted line. Although not a component part of this view, the trachea (arrow) can be seen posterior to the aorta. This fetus is cephalic.

Colour flow Doppler is useful in confirming the location, sizes of and relative flow patterns within the three vessels. Flow in all three vessels should be in an anteroposterior direction. Thus, if you are imaging the 3vv using the apex-up view, blood flow in all three vessels should be away from the transducer and should therefore result in a blue signal in all three vessels if standard colour flow mapping is applied (Fig. 10.26). Remember that the colour presented by each of the three vessels will depend on the orientation of that vessel relative to the horizontal. Make sure you have correctly determined the direction of flow in each vessel, relative to the horizontal, before applying colour. This will ensure that you do not falsely identify reverse flow in one or more of the vessels, which would be an abnormal finding.

An inability to identify three vessels in this view or disproportion in size of one or more of the three vessels are abnormal findings and may be associated with transposition, tetralogy of Fallot, coactation or pulmonary atresia/stenosis (Table 10.2).

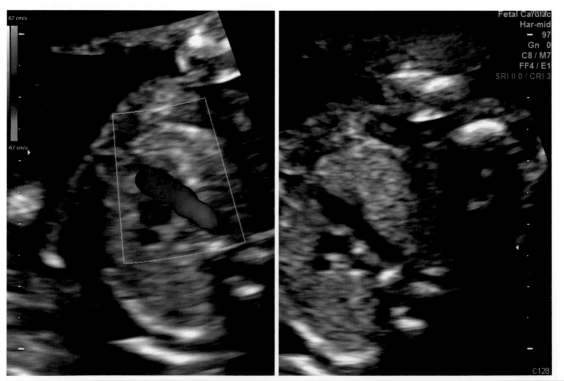

Fig 10.26 • The 3vv view with (left image) and without (right image) colour Doppler. The left image demonstrates the direction of blood flow within the pulmonary artery/DA and the aorta. Note the direction of flow is the same in each vessel, as demonstrated by the blue signal in both.

Note that the 3vv differs from the 3vt view in that the middle vessel, the aortic arch, is seen in cross-section in the 3vv, whereas in the 3vt view the aortic arch is seen in longitudinal section.

OTHER CARDIAC ABNORMALITIES

The purpose of examining the fetal heart during routine screening is to distinguish between normal appearances and abnormal appearances, rather than make a specific diagnosis when abnormal findings are identified.

The reason why you should be able to obtain and interpret correctly the six views is to exclude the following seven serious cardiac conditions:

- common arterial trunk
- HLHS
- AVSD
- moderate VSD
- TGA
- tetralogy of Fallot
- coarctation.

Described next in more detail are the conditions that are most commonly diagnosed when one or more of the standard views are abnormal.

Aortic Stenosis

Aortic stenosis describes the condition where there is narrowing at (valvular), just below (subvalvular) or just above (supravalvular) the level of the aortic valve which results in obstruction to forward flow into the ascending aorta. The most common type is valvular stenosis where one or more leaflets of the valve are dysplastic. The condition varies in its severity, from mild to critical, with critical aortic stenosis being the severe expression of the condition.

The features of mild aortic stenosis are unlikely to be amenable to detection at the 18–22 week examination.

Critical Aortic Stenosis

Critical aortic stenosis is the severe expression of the condition and is associated with a left ventricle which is enlarged, rather globular in shape and has hyperechoic walls with reduced contractility. The left atrium may also be dilated as a result of a poorly functioning and regurgitant mitral valve. In severe cases reduced filling of the left ventricle is seen with reversed, and therefore abnormal, left-to-right shunting through the foramen ovale. Critical aortic stenosis therefore can develop into hypoplastic left heart syndrome. The ascending aorta is often narrowed at its root, close to the aortic valve, but then balloons out past the stenosis. This may result in abnormal appearances in the 3v and 3vt views, as the size of the aorta may be greater than that of the pulmonary artery.

Pulmonary Stenosis

Pulmonary stenosis (PS) describes obstruction to the right ventricular outflow tract as a result of an abnormality of the pulmonary valve or narrowing above or below the valve. As with aortic stenosis, the severity of PS varies from mild cases, which are typically not identified in the fetus, to severe cases in which hypertrophy of the right ventricle is present and which are amenable to detection at 18–22 weeks. The condition is also progressive, meaning that appearances that are abnormal in later gestation may not necessarily be abnormal at 18–22 weeks.

In PS the walls of the right ventricle are thickened, making the chamber of the ventricle appear small. The tricuspid valve opens and closes normally. Assessing the deficiency of the pulmonary valve requires the RVOT view which will typically demonstrate postvalvular dilation of the pulmonary artery. In the normal fetus the pulmonary valve can be seen flicking in the pulmonary artery as the valve opens and closes. In pulmonary stenosis, the deficient valve can be seen within the artery throughout the cardiac cycle. The dilation of the pulmonary artery will also be evident in the 3v and 3vt views.

Pulmonary stenosis is one of the components of tetralogy of Fallot.

Hypoplastic Left Heart Syndrome

Hypoplastic left heart syndrome (HLHS) is an abnormality that involves significant underdevelopment of the left ventricle and its outflow tract (Fig. 10.27). There are two types of HLHS. One involves atresia of both the mitral and aortic valves. This results in no communication between the left

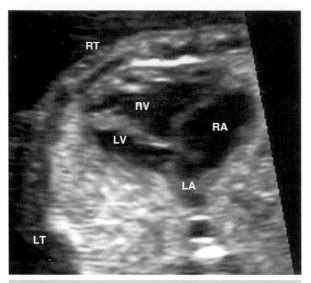

Fig 10.27 • A four chamber view of the heart showing marked disproportion of the chambers in a case of HLHS at 20 weeks of gestation. The left ventricle (LV) is significantly smaller in diameter than the right ventricle (RV). The left atrium (LA) is significantly smaller than the right atrium (RA). It is not possible to determine the type of HLHS from this image.

from the SVC in both the 3v and 3vt views will be the same – all will either be red or all will be blue. In a fetus with HLHS, the colour map from the SVC and pulmonary artery/ductal arch will be the same but will differ from that of the transverse aortic arch because of flow reversal in this vessel. This colour difference is a typical finding in HLHS.

Hypoplastic left heart syndrome has been described in the first trimester but is more commonly a second trimester diagnosis. It is also recognized that, although features of HLHS may be present at 18–22 weeks, their appearances at this gestation may be too subtle to be detected during a routine screening examination. Thus HLHS is one of the relatively small number of conditions that can present with normal appearances at mid-trimester screening but abnormal appearances in later gestations.

Hypoplastic left heart syndrome is often fatal without early intervention and therefore a number of operations over several years are necessary to correct this complex heart condition. A series of reconstructive operations are necessary to repair the HLHS using the Norwood, Glenn and Fontan procedures known as a 'staged reconstruction'.

atrium and ventricle, which in turn results in a tiny left ventricle. The second type involves a patent, often dysplastic mitral valve with aortic atresia and a globular, hyperechoic and poorly contracting left ventricle.

The normal circulatory patterns within the heart are disrupted in HLHS, leading to compensatory dilation of the pulmonary artery and abnormal left-to-right shunting across the foramen ovale because of the increased pressure in the left atrium resulting from the mitral atresia. In addition to the abnormal appearance of the four chamber view, the 3v and 3vt views will be abnormal.

In the grey scale 3v and 3vt views only two vessels – the SVC and enlarged pulmonary artery/ductal arch – may be seen. This is because the aortic atresia results in a transverse aortic arch which is either not visible or extremely small. Blood must reach the descending aorta in order to maintain a fetal circulation and does this by flow reversal across the aortic isthmus and aortic arch. In the normal fetus, the flow in the pulmonary artery/ductal arch and the ascending aorta/transverse arch is in the same direction. Thus the colour map obtained from these two vessels and

Pulmonary Atresia

Pulmonary atresia with intact ventricular septum (PA-IVS) describes a rare condition in which there is no communication between the right ventricle and the pulmonary artery and in which the interventricular septum is intact. In the majority of cases the cavity of the right ventricle is very small and the walls are thickened and contract poorly. In some cases, however, the appearance is very different with both the right ventricle and right atrium being dilated, the latter because of significant tricuspid regurgitation.

The features of PA-IVS have many similarities with those of HLHS. In addition to the abnormal appearance of the four-chamber view, the 3vv and 3vt view will also be abnormal. The pulmonary artery/ductal arch will appear small compared with the ascending aorta/transverse arch and there is typically reverse flow in the pulmonary artery/ductal arch.

Pulmonary atresia is also similar to HLHS in its spectrum of appearances and its progression in severity with advancing gestation.

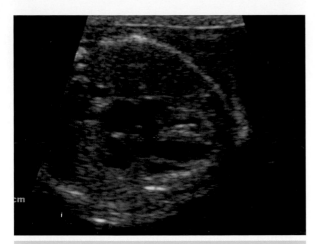

Fig 10.28 • Four chamber view of the heart, with the apex pointing towards 4 o'clock. The callipers identify a moderate, perimembranous VSD, measuring 3.6 mm.

Ventricular Septal Defect

Ventricular septal defect describes a defect in the septum that separates the right and left ventricles (Fig. 10.28), allowing haemodynamic communication between the two ventricles. As stated earlier, VSD is a common abnormality. Approximately 30% of children born with congenital heart disease have an isolated VSD, although the incidence in the fetus is much lower, on the order of 5–10%. Ventricular septal defect is found in association with other cardiac abnormalities in a further 30% of postnatal cases.

As described earlier, both the four chamber and the LVOT views should be used to confirm an intact ventricular septum and therefore to exclude significant defects in the septum. Although an expectation of the cardiac examination is that VSDs of significant size will be detected, their position must be within part of the septum that is assessed in the standard views. Detecting those cases in which the VSD does not lie in the part of the septum assessed in the standard views is beyond the remit of the 18–22 week examination.

It is likely that you will first be suspicious of a VSD because you have identified a black or hypoechoic gap somewhere along the hyperechoic ventricular septum on grey scale imaging of the four chamber view. Alternatively, you may suspect a VSD in the LVOT because there is a break or gap in the hyperechoic, linear echo representing the continuity between the ventricular septum and the anterior wall of the aorta. Where a true VSD is present the borders of the defect in either view may appear slightly more hyperechoic than the normal septum. Although this is a subtle feature it can be helpful in differentiating a true VSD from artefact.

The most common type of VSD is the perimembranous type, which involves the small thin region of the septum just beneath the aortic valve. Perimembranous VSDs account for about 80% of VSDs. The importance of differentiating between this type of VSD and acoustic fallout cannot be over emphasised. Muscular VSDs involve the larger thicker, muscular part of the septum which extends from the attachments of the atrioventricular valves to the apex of the heart.

Debate remains as to what size of VSD should be detectable at 18–20 weeks. In paediatric surgical terms, a VSD would be described as *moderate* if it was of a similar size to the diameter of the aorta. As measuring the 'inner-to-inner' diameter of the aorta at, for example, the level of the aortic valve is feasible in the 18–22 week fetus, comparing this with the size of the VSD in either the four chamber view or the LVOT view would provide a useful comparator in terms of size when a VSD was suspected.

As a VSD results in an abnormal communication between the left and right ventricles, interrogating the septum with colour flow Doppler should demonstrate the abnormal jet of blood flow across the defect. Remember that maximum sensitivity will be achieved when the presumed defect within the ventricular septum is aligned at 90° to the Doppler beam. The jet of blood flow through the septum where the defect is located may not be visible if the velocity of the colour Doppler signal is set too high. Alternatively, if it is set too low the image will be saturated with colour, making identification of anything impossible.

The treatment of a VSD depends on the size of the defect and whether it is an isolated defect or part of a more complex heart abnormality. Some will require surgery to correct the defect; however, smaller VSDs often close spontaneously within the first 2 years of life.

Overriding Aorta

Overriding aorta describes the incorrect alignment of the aorta in the presence of a VSD where the aorta straddles, or overrides, the defect in the inter-ventricular septum. Overriding aorta is a component of tetralogy of Fallot.

Conotruncal Abnormalities/Truncus Arteriosus

Conotruncal abnormalities arise from the unequal or defective partitioning of an important structure in the embryological heart called the truncus conus. Internal segmentation of the truncus conus is essential for the separation of the great vessels and the formation of the outflow tracts. Defective segmentation may result in a common outflow tract, rather than a separate aorta and pulmonary artery, and the abnormal origin of the aorta.

Truncus arteriosus is a life-threatening congenital heart defect and therefore most babies will not live for more than a few months without treatment. Several operations are required to correct this heart abnormality, and usually take place within the first 2 months of life.

Tetralogy of Fallot

Tetralogy of Fallot describes a spectrum of four (hence 'tetralogy') abnormalities, namely an overriding aorta, pulmonary stenosis, VSD and right ventricular hypertrophy. As the right ventricular hypertrophy is not typically seen antenatally, there are only three features of the condition that you need to exclude. The four chamber view with the apex up (apex to 11, 12 or 1 o'clock) will typically demonstrate the aorta overriding a perimembranous VSD. In the normal fetus the ascending aorta points to the right fetal shoulder with a wide angle between the direction of the ventricular septum and the anterior wall of the ascending aorta. In tetralogy of Fallot the aorta arises astride the crest of the ventricular septum and therefore the course of the ascending aorta is parallel to the ventricular septum rather than following a wide angle.

This defect can be corrected with surgery being performed typically in the first few months of life to close the VSD and widen the pulmonary valve or artery. In some cases a temporary repair is performed initially until a complete repair is possible. Most children born with tetralogy of Fallot go on to lead healthy lives as adults; however, some experience heart problems later in life, including leaking of the pulmonary valve or arrhythmias.

TGA

Transposition of the great arteries (TGA) describes the condition where the great arteries are 'transposed' or switched. It is also called complete transposition, simple transposition or transposition. The connections between the atria and ventricles are normal. Thus the right atrium is connected to the right ventricle by the tricuspid valve and the left atrium is connected to the left ventricle by the mitral valve. Remember therefore that the moderator band will be visible in the right ventricle which is correctly situated closer to the chest wall. The connections of the great vessels, however, are switched. The aorta therefore arises from the right ventricle, the pulmonary artery arises from the left ventricle and they leave the heart in a parallel arrangement, with no crossover (Fig. 10.29).

This results in an abnormal 3vv where only two vessels are visible. The larger vessel is the transverse aortic arch and the smaller is the superior vena cava, which is located to its right (Fig. 10.30).

This is an important diagnosis to make prenatally as it is one of the few cardiac conditions where prior knowledge before delivery enables immediate postnatal intervention. All babies born

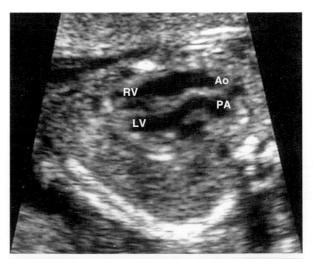

Fig 10.29 • A cross-over view of the fetal heart. The view is abnormal because the two great vessels leave the heart in a parallel arrangement, rather than crossing over each other. This is a typical feature of TGA. The two vessels are transposed with the pulmonary artery (PA) arising from the left ventricle (LV) and the aorta (Ao) arising from the right ventricle (RV). TGA, transposition of the great arteries.

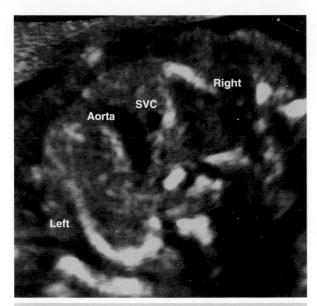

Fig 10.30 • The 3vv demonstrating the two vessels seen in TGA. The larger vessel is the transverse aortic arch (Aorta) with the smaller SVC to its right. In TGA the duct is present but usually not visible in this view, as in this case. SVC, superior vena cava; TGA, transposition of the great arteries; 3vv, three vessel view.

with transposition of the great vessels will require an arterial switch operation to correct this serious defect. Several operations are necessary to reconstruct the heart so that the aorta is attached to the left ventricle and the pulmonary artery is attached to the right ventricle. It is anticipated that the overwhelming majority of children born with TGA will go on to lead healthy, lives. Confusingly 'transposition' or TGA is normally used to refer to complete transposition, as opposed to corrected transposition.

Corrected Transposition

Corrected transposition describes the condition in which the morphological right atrium is connected to the morphological left ventricle by the mitral valve and the morphological left atrium is connected to the morphological right ventricle by the tricuspid valve. The great vessels are also transposed as in TGA. Thus the aorta arises from the morphological right ventricle, the pulmonary artery arises from the morphological left ventricle and they leave the heart in a parallel arrangement with no crossover. The ventricle closer to the chest wall is the morphological left ventricle. In corrected

transposition therefore the moderator band is seen in the more medial ventricle, the right ventricle. This provides the most obvious feature to distinguish corrected transposition from TGA.

The relationships between the chambers of the heart, the AV valves and the great arteries in TGA and corrected transposition, compared to the arrangement in the normal fetus are shown in Table 10.3.

Double Outlet Right Ventricle

Double outlet right ventricle (DORV) describes a group of cardiac abnormalities in which the aorta and pulmonary artery arise primarily from the morphological right ventricle. This condition is commonly associated with a VSD. Pulmonary and, less commonly, aortic outflow obstruction may also be present. The aorta and pulmonary artery leave the heart in a parallel arrangement with no crossover, although this is unlikely to be the only abnormality you should identify in this condition.

Coarctation

This condition is characterised by a narrowing of the aorta in the region of the isthmus. The isthmus describes the segment of the aorta adjacent to the entry point of the ductus arteriosus into the aortic arch. This narrowing can result in disproportion of the ventricles although this feature is frequently too subtle to be identified at the routine anomaly scan. However, the narrowing results in disproportion of the aorta and duct in the 3vv and 3vt view.

As with TGA, coarctation is an important diagnosis to make prenatally as it is one of the few cardiac conditions where prior knowledge before delivery enables appropriate postnatal management plans to be put in place.

Right Aortic Arch (V Sign)

A right aortic arch (V sign) is identified in the 3vt view. Although the two arches merge normally, into a tight V, they lie to the right of the spine, trachea and SVC.

Right Aortic Arch (U Sign)

A right aortic arch (U sign) is also identified in the 3vt view. The ductal arch is in the normal position

NORMAL HEART			
	DIRECTION OF FLOW THROUGH THE HEART		
	RIGHT SIDE	↓	**LEFT SIDE**
Anterior chest wall	RA	↓	LA
	Tricuspid valve	↓	Mitral valve
	RV (moderator band)	↓	LV
	MPA	↓	Aorta
TGA			
	DIRECTION OF FLOW THROUGH THE HEART		
	RIGHT SIDE	↓	**LEFT SIDE**
Anterior chest wall	RA	↓	LA
	Tricuspid valve	↓	Mitral valve
	RV (moderator band)	↓	LV
	Aorta	↓	MPA
CORRECTED TGA			
	DIRECTION OF FLOW THROUGH THE HEART		
	RIGHT SIDE	↓	**LEFT SIDE**
Anterior chest wall	RA	↓	LA
	Mitral valve	↓	Tricuspid valve
	LV	↓	RV (moderator band)
	MPA	↓	Aorta

Table 10.3 Relationships between the left and right atria, the left and right ventricles and their respective AV valves, the moderator band, the great vessels and the anterior chest wall in the normal heart, in TGA and in corrected TGA

LA, left atrium; LV, left ventricle; MPA, main pulmonary artery; RA, right atrium; RV, right ventricle; TGA, transposition of the great arteries.

but the aortic arch lies to the right of the trachea. This results in the two arches meeting to form a wide U shape, rather than a tight V, with the trachea in the 'bend' of the U (Fig. 10.31).

Double Aortic Arch

The U shape described above is also associated with a condition called 'double aortic arch' which can therefore also be identified in the 3vt view. In this condition the trachea lies in the 'bend' of the U but is surrounded by a circle of blood vessels, known as a vascular ring. There is therefore a subtle difference in the ultrasound appearance of a double aortic arch compared to that of a right aortic arch (U sign).

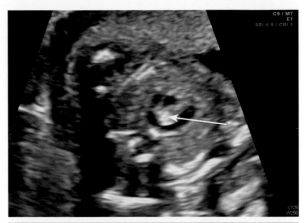

Fig 10.31 • Cross section of the fetal chest showing an abnormal 3vt view. The two vessels form a wide U, with the trachea (arrow) lying between them, rather than a tight V to the left of the trachea, as seen in Fig. 10.23.

ADDITIONAL VIEWS OF THE HEART

There are two other views which can be used to examine the fetal heart:

- ductal arch view
- aortic arch view.

These two sagittal views do not tend to form part of the routine screening of the heart at the anomaly scan. Their value lies in confirming the relative positions, sizes and appearances of the duct and the aorta.

THE DUCTAL ARCH VIEW

This view is obtained from a sagittal section of the fetus and is most easily achieved when the spine is posterior (Fig. 10.32). The purpose of this view is to demonstrate that the vessel arising from the more anterior chamber of the heart is the duct and not the aorta. Thus no vessels should be visualised arising from its arch. This is important in the exclusion of TGA and corrected TGA. The shape of the arch should be a broad 'hockey stick' shape.

THE AORTIC ARCH VIEW

This view is obtained from a sagittal section of the fetus and is most easily achieved when the spine is posterior but can be obtained when the spine in

anterior (Fig. 10.33). The purpose of this view is to demonstrate that the vessel arising from the more posterior chamber of the heart is the aorta and not the duct. The aortic arch forms a tight 'shepherd's crook' that appears to arise from the centre of the heart. Head and neck vessels (the brachiocephalic, left common carotid and left subclavian arteries) arise from the aortic arch and at least two should be identified, thus confirming that this is the aortic arch and not the ductal arch (Fig. 10.33). When a

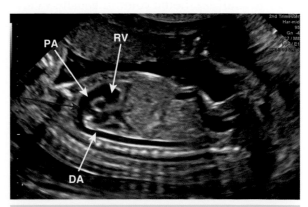

Fig 10.32 • Sagittal section of the fetal body demonstrating the ductal arch (arrow). DA, descending aorta; PA, main pulmonary artery; RV, right ventricle.

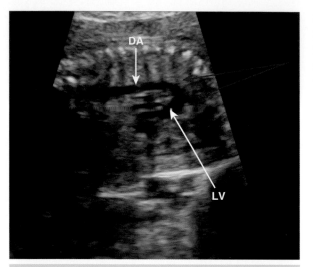

DA

LV

Fig 10.33 • Sagittal section of the fetal chest demonstrating the aortic arch. The aorta arises from the left ventricle (LV) in the centre of the heart, and produces the tight 'shepherd's crook' shape of the aortic arch. This can be compared with the ductal arch which arises from the outer chamber of the heart and produces the wider 'hockey stick' shape. The head and neck vessels (arrows) arising from the arch are distinguishing features of the aortic arch; two can be seen in this image. DA, descending aorta.

coarctation is suspected from the 3vt view, the narrowing at the isthmus should, in theory, be visible in the aortic arch view. However, in practice the narrowing produces an appearance which is often too subtle to be detected in this view.

FETAL HEART RATE AND RHYTHM

The function of the heart, heart rate and heart rhythm should be observed as part of the examination of the fetal heart. As discussed earlier, the right and left ventricles should contract equally. Colour flow Doppler provides a rapid assessment of blood flow to identify normal contractility, turbulent, reversed or even absent flow within a chamber. Backflow across a valve is termed regurgitation and is characterised by turbulent flow across a valve, vessel, or chamber that is narrowed. Mild regurgitation, identified as a small flash of red colour in the blue (or vice versa) jet of bloodflow through the open valve, is a relatively common finding in the second trimester fetus. It is usually of no clinical significance if the rest of the heart is normal. However it is always wise to refer an unusual finding for a more experienced assessment to confirm that your initial assumption of likely normality was correct.

The heart should be observed to confirm symmetry of movement between the atria and ventricles and between the left and right sides of the heart. In HLHS, for example, there is either minimal or absent filling of the left ventricle, which can be demonstrated using colour flow Doppler.

The heart should have a regular beat and rate of between 110 and 160 beats per minute (bpm). During the anomaly scan it is not uncommon to observe short periods of fetal bradycardia, where the fetal heart rate is less than 110 bpm, lasting several seconds. This is considered normal providing the bradycardia is not persistent. In the third trimester a persistent bradycardia or repeated decelerations of the fetal heart rate can be caused by fetal hypoxia and requires immediate attention.

An increase in the fetal heart rate of more than 160 bpm (tachycardia) is also common during periods of fetal movement. A persistent tachycardia requires further evaluation or possibly early delivery, as it can be associated with fetal hypoxia or serious tachydysrhythmias.

Occasional ectopic or skipped beats are often benign and resolve spontaneously with advancing gestation. Ectopic beats are usually not associated with an increased risk of structural heart disease.

Further reading

International Society of Ultrasound in Obstetrics and Gynaecology 2013 Guidelines (updated): sonographic screening examination of the fetal heart. Ultrasound Obstet Gynecol 41:348–359

Assessing the abdomen

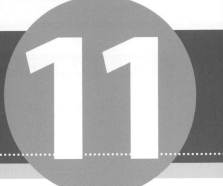

11

CONTENTS

This chapter addresses the ultrasound examination of the fetal abdomen with particular reference to the second trimester of pregnancy.

The aims of this chapter are to describe the correct techniques used to assess the following:

- abdominal size
- the gall bladder, liver and spleen
- the stomach
- the bowel
- the anterior abdominal wall
- the umbilical cord and cord insertion
- the kidneys
- the bladder
- genitalia.

As discussed in Chapter 8, the examination of the fetal abdomen should follow on naturally after you have measured the abdominal circumference (AC). You are already aware of the benefits of a systematic approach to maximize the likelihood of your exclusion or detection of the various abnormalities identified within the fetal abdomen.

The descriptions of the various abnormalities included in this chapter have been arranged to link with the scanning sequence recommended in Chapter 8.

ABDOMINAL SIZE

Measurement and evaluation of the AC has already been described in Chapter 8. An AC measurement that is outside the normal range is, by definition, abnormal. The association of an isolated small AC is with growth restriction rather than a fetal abnormality, providing of course you have excluded an abdominal wall defect.

Similarly a large AC is more likely to be associated with a normal, large fetus than an abnormality that is not apparent in the AC cross-section but is increasing the girth of the fetus. Diabetes in the mother may be associated with a large AC, although this is usually a finding of the later second and third trimester fetus, rather than at 18-22 weeks. You should, however, consider Beckwith–Wiedemann syndrome, which is characterized by generalized overgrowth of the fetus, in particular the abdominal organs.

THE GALL BLADDER

In the normal fetus the gall bladder, being fluid filled, appears as a hypoechoic sausage-shaped or pear-shaped structure in the right side of the abdomen (Fig. 11.1). Part of it is often seen in the AC section and mistaken, by the uninitiated, for the umbilical vein, which lies medially to it. The full length of the gall bladder is best imaged in a transverse section very slightly below the AC section. It can be distinguished from the stomach by its elongated pear shape, its more anterior position and the fact that it lies in the right abdomen rather than the left.

The gall bladder is visible in most fetuses at 18–22 weeks but is much more variable in size than the stomach. Do not be tempted to misdiagnose a normal gall bladder for an enlarged loop of bowel.

ABSENT GALL BLADDER

Although the size of the gall bladder is very variable, an absent gall bladder is an abnormal finding which is associated with left atrial isomerism and biliary atresia.

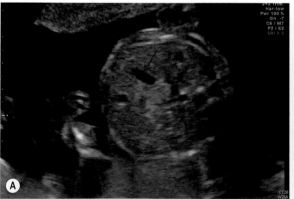
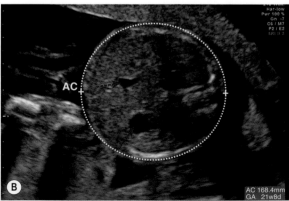

Fig 11.1 • A. Transverse section of the abdomen, at 21⁺ weeks of gestation, demonstrating the gall bladder (solid arrow) lying to the right of the umbilical vein (dashed arrow). This can be compared with the transverse section of the same fetus shown in B. B. This is the correct section for measuring the abdominal circumference (AC), in which the stomach (arrow) and umbilical vein (dashed arrow) are shown.

THE LIVER

The fetal liver lies in the right side of the abdomen inferior to the diaphragm and has a similar echogenicity to the lungs, spleen and bowel. The similarity in its echogenicity to the organs adjacent to it makes it difficult to define the limits of the fetal liver. Fortunately, this is of limited significance as structural abnormalities of the fetal liver are rare. The most common abnormal findings within the liver are pinpoint hyperechoic areas or echogenic foci and choledocal cysts. Echogenic foci have a known association with infection, most commonly varicella or chickenpox and cytomegalovirus (Fig. 11.2).

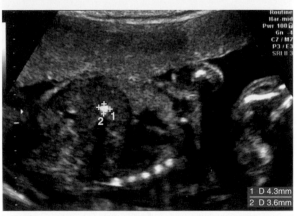

Fig 11.2 • Sagittal section of the fetal body showing an echogenic focus within the liver measuring 4.3 × 3.6 mm at 20 weeks of gestation.

THE SPLEEN

The fetal spleen is located on the left side of the abdomen inferior to the diaphragm. As with the liver, the spleen has a similar echogenicity to the lungs and the bowel. The similarity in its echogenicity to the organs adjacent to it makes it difficult to define the limits of the fetal spleen. Fortunately, this is of limited significance because, as with the liver, structural abnormalities of the spleen are rare. Also as with the liver, echogenic foci may be seen within the spleen, although they are less common than in the liver, with infection being suspected as the most likely cause.

Cysts of the spleen can occur, are usually isolated findings and normally have a good prognosis.

THE STOMACH

In the normal fetus the stomach, being fluid-filled, is seen as a typically circular hypoechoic area in the left side of the abdomen, approximately halfway between the posterior and the anterior abdominal walls (Fig. 11.1B). The stomach communicates with the duodenum at the pylorus, and, although the pyloric sphincter itself is not visible on ultrasound, the communication can be assumed when the full length of the stomach is imaged. To obtain the full length of the stomach, which is teardrop-shaped, from the AC section, rotate the probe to obtain an oblique longitudinal section of the body, while keeping the stomach in view. The point of the teardrop represents the communication between the stomach and the proximal duodenum at the pylorus.

The fetus swallows amniotic fluid, and the stomach fills and empties into the duodenum in a cyclical fashion. The size of the stomach therefore varies over time. If you are unable to visualize the stomach, or it is unusually small, rescan in 30–40 minutes. This should allow sufficient time for the stomach to fill and achieve a normal size. With experience you will learn how to determine when the stomach is a normal size and when it is abnormally small (Fig. 11.3).

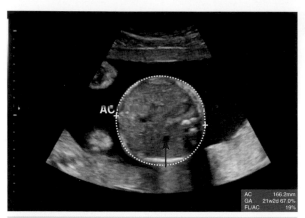

Fig 11.3 • A transverse section of the abdomen of a 21 week fetus showing an abnormally small stomach (arrowed). Compare these appearances with those shown in Fig. 8.1 and Fig. 11.1B. Note also the amount of amniotic fluid which appears subjectively increased in this section. AC, abdominal circumference.

The stomach is often visible in the first trimester fetus but should always be seen at the 18–22 week examination. A persistently absent or a very small stomach are both abnormal findings.

RIGHT SIDED STOMACH

As confirming situs is one of the first actions you undertake during the 18–22 week scan, you should not fail to identify a stomach that is located on the right side of the fetal abdomen. This is an abnormal finding and suggestive of situs inversus or heterotaxy, as discussed in Chapter 10.

ABSENT OR SMALL STOMACH

The stomach may not be visible in the abdomen for two reasons. First, it is abnormally positioned in the fetal chest because of the presence of a left-sided diaphragmatic hernia (see Chapter 10). Alternatively the stomach is normally positioned but is not filling with the amniotic fluid swallowed by the fetus because of obstruction or compression of the oesophagus.

An absent or a very small stomach, in the absence of a left-sided diaphragmatic hernia, is associated with a spectrum of abnormalities but as an isolated finding is most commonly associated with oesophageal atresia.

OESOPHAGEAL ATRESIA AND TRACHEO-OESOPHAGEAL FISTULA

Oesophageal atresia describes a condition in which there is a blind-ending oesophagus which results in no direct communication with the stomach. *Tracheo-oesophageal fistula (TOF)* describes the condition in which there is communication between the blind-ending oesophagus and the trachea. The oesophagus and trachea arise from the primitive foregut. They are separated by the development of a longitudinal septum within the primitive foregut during the sixth and seventh weeks of gestation. Oesphageal atresia results from this division being deficient. The incomplete formation of the dividing septum results, most commonly, in a blind-ending upper oesophagus with the lower oesophagus communicating with the trachea through a fistula. This arrangement allows fluid to pass into the trachea, through the fistula to the lower oesophagus and into the stomach. The majority – around 90% – of cases of oesophageal atresia are associated with a TOF.

Oesophageal atresia should be suspected if there is persistent absence of the stomach and a TOF should be suspected in the persistent presence of an abnormally small stomach (see Fig. 11.3). Polyhydramnios often accompanies both of these conditions in the third trimester but is not a commonly associated finding at 18–22 weeks.

VATER AND VACTERL

Associated abnormalities are common with oesophageal atresia and TOF, including what are described as the VATER or VACTERL complexes. The two complexes are essentially the same, differentiated by cardiac defects being included in VACTERL but not in VATER.

VATER complex is a synonym for the following cluster of abnormalities:

V	vertebral anomalies
A	anorectal anomalies
TE	tracheo-oesophageal anomalies and duodenal atresia
R	renal anomalies
	radial anomalies

VACTERL complex is a synonym for the following cluster of abnormalities:

V	vertebral anomalies
A	anorectal anomalies
C	cardiac anomalies
TE	tracheo-oesophageal anomalies and duodenal atresia
R	renal anomalies
L	radial limb anomalies

Although oesophageal atresia is the congenital anomaly most often associated with an absent or very small stomach, there are a number of conditions that compress the fetal oesophagus or affect the central nervous or musculoskeletal systems and which may therefore impair swallowing. They commonly, therefore, result in no stomach being seen. As with other conditions that affect the gastrointestinal tract, polyhydramnios is often present in the late second and third trimester pregnancy.

'DOUBLE BUBBLE'

This is described in the following section.

THE BOWEL

In anatomical terms the *bowel* describes the small and the large bowel. The small bowel comprises the duodenum, jejunum and ileum. The large bowel comprises the caecum, ascending-, transverse- and descending colon, sigmoid colon, rectum and anal canal.

In the normal second trimester fetus the echogenicity of the liver, spleen and bowel is very similar, making their identification and separation difficult. However, with modern machines the loops of the small bowel now can be identified and therefore distinguished from the adjacent liver and spleen. Should your equipment allow you to visualize the small bowel, it is important that you can distinguish between the normal ultrasound appearance of small bowel and 'bright' or 'echogenic' bowel, which is not normal.

The large bowel is not routinely visible in the 18–22 week fetus but becomes progressively more visible with increasing gestation and is a normal appearance in the third trimester fetus. Haustrations within the large bowel can be seen from about 30 weeks, and peristalsis can be often observed. These are important features in distinguishing the large bowel from other structures within the fetal abdomen. The normal internal diameter of the large bowel should be no greater than 10.0 mm at 28 weeks, 15.0 mm at 32 weeks and 20.0 mm towards term.

From approximately 16 weeks of gestation, the majority of amniotic fluid is fetal urine. The fetus swallows (and inhales) amniotic fluid, which passes down the oesophagus into the stomach, through the pylorus into the small bowel and into the large bowel where it is absorbed.

As the large bowel is the site of fluid absorption within the gut, impaired swallowing and obstruction of the gastrointestinal tract above the level of the large bowel are commonly associated with polyhydramnios. Thus the lower the obstruction in the gastrointestinal tract (GIT), the more likely it is that the amniotic fluid volume will be normal. Conversely, the higher the obstruction, the more likely is the presence of polyhydramnios, although you must remember that this is gestational age related. Polyhydramnios is an infrequent finding at 18–22 weeks but a common finding in the third trimester. Therefore, when polyhydramnios is identified, the ultrasound features of GIT abnormalities should always be sought and excluded, or otherwise.

BRIGHT OR ECHOGENIC BOWEL

A localized area of increased echogenicity within the small bowel, commonly described as bright or echogenic bowel, is an abnormal finding (Fig. 11.4). Increased echogenicity is defined as

265

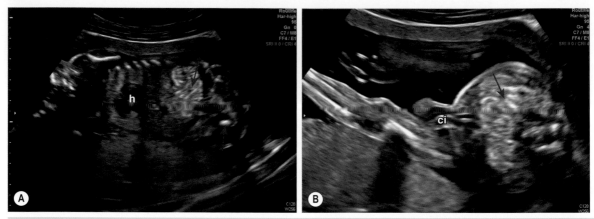

Fig 11.4 • Longitudinal section of the fetal abdomen (A) and transverse section (B) of the fetal abdomen, at the level of the cord insertion, demonstrating echogenic bowel (solid arrow) at 20⁺ weeks. The echogenicity of the bowel loops can be compared with that of the iliac crest (dashed arrow). ci, cord insertion; h, heart.

echogenicity that is as bright as bone. You will soon discover that the echogenicity of the bones of the fetus varies and thus a specific bone needs to be used as a reference comparator to ensure consistency in defining echogenic bowel. We recommend that you use the iliac crest as your reference bone.

Should you suspect echogenic bowel, turn down the overall gain of the ultrasound machine until you can no longer visualize the bowel you are interrogating. If you are still able to visualize the iliac crests but can no longer see the bowel, then the bowel is not echogenic. Where it 'disappears' at the same, or at an even lower, level of gain as the iliac crest, then the bowel can be described as echogenic (Fig. 11.5).

Intra-amniotic bleeding is the most common cause of echogenic bowel. The fetus swallows blood-stained amniotic fluid, which causes a local inflammatory response within the wall of the small bowel. Echogenic bowel is also described in association with cystic fibrosis (CF), congenital infection and chromosomal abnormalities, particularly Down's syndrome. It is a useful marker where there is a family history of CF but is of no value in screening for CF. When echogenic bowel is present in association with a small or growth-restricted fetus, congenital infection should always be considered. Maternal blood should therefore be taken for CF and TORCH screening.

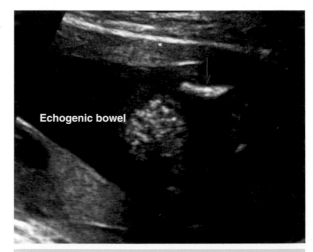

Fig 11.5 • Transverse section of the fetal abdomen demonstrating echogenic bowel, of similar 'brightness' as the iliac crest (arrowed).

The association with echogenic bowel and an increased risk of Down's syndrome is historical, with the majority of the literature relating to populations at high risk of, or unscreened for, Down's syndrome. This is problematic, therefore, when attempting to extrapolate the risk increase to the low-risk population. A body of literature suggests that echogenic bowel confers a threefold increase in the Down's risk. This means that, in practice, echogenic bowel in a fetus with an *a priori* risk of less than 1 in 450 for Down's syndrome can be treated as a normal variant. Where the *a priori* risk is greater than 1:450, for example, 1:300, identifying echogenic bowel would increase the Down's risk to 1:100 (300/3 = 100), thereby placing the pregnancy into the higher-risk group as the adjusted risk is now greater than the threshold risk of 1:150.

The majority of cases of echogenic bowel will be TORCH- and CF-negative and the Down's risk will remain low. Thus in the majority of cases, echogenic bowel will be of no pathological significance. You should, however, be aware of the anxiety you may generate with the mother when you initiate discussion of your finding of echogenic bowel at the 18–22 week scan, irrespective of whether or not the forthcoming results are normal.

BOWEL OBSTRUCTION

In the normal fetus, the stomach is the only part of the GIT that should be visible at 18–22 weeks. The presence of one or more hypoechoic areas within the abdomen, other than the stomach and the gall bladder, is an abnormal finding. The differential diagnosis for cystic masses within the abdomen includes bowel obstruction at various levels within the GIT. Other causes are discussed later in this chapter.

'Double Bubble' or Duodenal Atresia

The clinical term for 'double bubble' is *duodenal atresia*. This describes a blockage in the upper duodenum formed by an atretic segment of the duodenum (Fig. 11.6A). The normal passage of fluid from the stomach through the duodenum, via the pylorus, is interrupted by the atretic segment. The proximal duodenum thus becomes dilated between the pylorus and the site of the obstruction.

As the stomach is the only part of the gastrointestinal tract that is visualized in the normal fetus at 18–22 weeks, identifying a second hypoechoic structure, of a similar size to the stomach and lying medial to it in the AC section, is an abnormal finding. This is suggestive of either duodenal atresia or an abdominal cyst.

To make the presumed diagnosis of duodenal atresia you must be able to join stomach and presumed proximal duodenum at the pylorus as described earlier (Fig. 11.6B). A connection between the stomach and duodenum indicates duodenal atresia and effectively excludes an abdominal cyst.

The double bubble sign is usually not apparent at 18–22 weeks. This is a finding that is more typical of the late second or third trimester pregnancy. Polyhydramnios develops in around 50% of pregnancies with duodenal atresia and is the most common precursor to its diagnosis in later

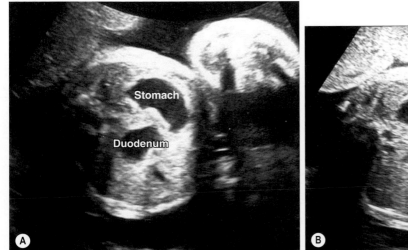

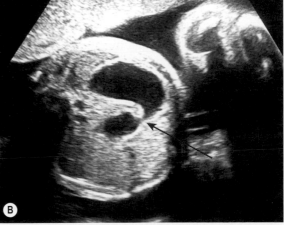

Fig 11.6 • Cross sections of the fetal abdomen at 26 weeks of gestation. A. Two hypoechoic structures can be seen, representing the stomach and the dilated proximal duodenum. B. The two 'bubbles' communicate with each other, at the pylorus (arrow). Note the amniotic fluid is generous but within normal limits.

pregnancy. The onset or severity of polyhydramnios is dependent on the degree of duodenal obstruction and the presence or absence of other gastrointestinal abnormalities that may affect amniotic fluid resorption.

Isolated duodenal atresia is surgically correctable. However, approximately 50% of fetuses with duodenal atresia have other abnormalities, including the VATER or VACTERL complexes. Historically there has been a strong association between duodenal atresia and trisomy 21, with approximately 30% of cases of duodenal atresia being associated with Down's syndrome. As a significant proportion of fetuses with Down's syndrome are now detected through combined screening, this association is likely to reduce, although data supporting this fact are not currently available. However, where duodenal atresia is detected, a discussion that includes the offer of karyotyping should still take place irrespective of whether or not the pregnancy has already been screened for Down's syndrome.

Lower Bowel Atresia or Obstruction

Identifying multiple cystic masses in the fetal abdomen is an abnormal finding. The presence of multiple fluid-filled bowel loops is suggestive of bowel obstruction or atresia distal to the duodenum. A 'triple' bubble is characteristic of jejunal atresia. In general, the more 'bubbles' that are present, the lower in the bowel is the atretic segment or the obstruction likely to be.

The normal appearances of the large bowel in the later second and third trimesters of pregnancy are varied owing to the motility of its fluid- and meconium-filled loops. Obstruction should be suspected if the internal transverse diameter, as measured using the 'inner-to-inner' technique, of the large bowel loops exceeds 10.0 mm before 28 weeks, 15.0 mm at 32 weeks or 20.0 mm towards term.

The differential diagnosis of multiple cystic masses in the fetal abdomen includes multicystic kidney.

THE ANTERIOR ABDOMINAL WALL

The anterior abdominal wall forms during the fourth week of gestation, from the fusion of four embryonic body folds – the cephalic, caudal and two lateral folds. Incomplete fusion of these folds results in ectopic cordis, omphalocele or bladder extrophy, also known as *ectopia vesicae*. Confirming the integrity of the anterior body wall therefore should be part of the cross-sectional assessment of the fetal chest and abdomen when sliding the probe from the chest through the abdomen to the pelvis.

PHYSIOLOGICAL HERNIATION OF THE BOWEL

Before 8 weeks of gestation the bowel grows exclusively within the abdominal cavity but, because there is insufficient room within the abdomen for the rapidly growing midgut, it also occupies the base of the umbilical cord for approximately 2 weeks. The shortage of space primarily is due to the relatively large liver and kidneys. Thus between 8 and 10 weeks of gestation the bowel develops both within the abdominal cavity and within the base of the umbilical cord. The latter is termed the physiological herniation of the gut and is a normal finding in all embryos across this gestational age range. The herniation appears as a hyperechoic mass in the base of the umbilical cord (see Fig. 7.13). The bowel should always have returned completely into the abdominal cavity by the end of the 11th week of gestation. Failure of the bowel to return to the abdominal cavity results in the abnormality of omphalcele or exomphalos. It is clear therefore that this diagnosis cannot be made or excluded until 12 weeks of gestation at the earliest.

THE UMBILICAL CORD

The normal umbilical cord contains three blood vessels, namely a central umbilical vein and two umbilical arteries that spiral around it (Fig. 11.7A). The umbilical vein carries oxygenated blood from the placenta to the fetus and the two arteries carry deoxygenated blood from the fetus back to the placenta. The cord vessels are surrounded by Wharton's jelly, which protects them from compression.

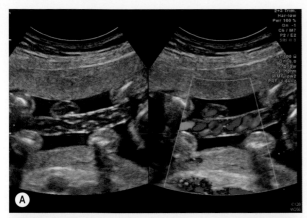

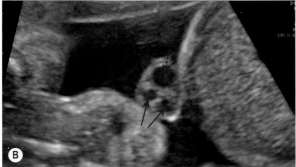

Fig 11.7 • A. A longitudinal section of a segment of umbilical cord at 19⁺ weeks demonstrating the two arteries spiralling around a single vein with B mode imaging (left panel) and colour flow mapping (right panel). The two arteries are blue and the vein is red. B. The Mickey Mouse sign. A transverse section of the normal umbilical cord at 28 weeks of gestation, demonstrating the two arteries (solid arrows) and one vein (dashed arrow).

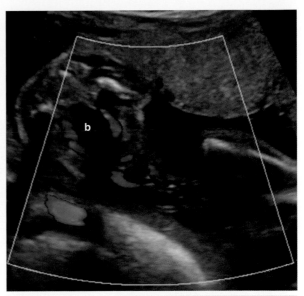

Fig 11.8 • A transverse section of the fetal pelvis at 20 weeks of gestation using colour flow mapping to demonstrate the two umbilical arteries, shown in blue, on either side of the bladder (b). The blue colour confirms that blood in both umbilical arteries flows from the fetus to the umbilical cord.

Vessel number can be evaluated from a transverse section of the cord within the amniotic fluid. The technique you require is very straightforward. Select a long length of cord lying horizontally within the amniotic fluid. Rotate your probe through 90° to obtain a cross-section of the cord. The three vessels produce what is often described as the 'Mickey Mouse' sign with the umbilical vein representing Mickey's face and the two umbilical arteries his ear on either side (Fig. 11.7B). The small size of the umbilical vessels often makes it difficult to obtain a cross-section of the cord at 18–22 weeks because of the tight spiralling of the blood vessels and the relative speed at which the cord moves in the amniotic fluid. However, it is usually a straightforward exercise in the later second and third trimesters of pregnancy.

The umbilical cord inserts into the fetal abdomen at a level slightly below, or inferior to, the AC section and above the bladder. The umbilical arteries branch off from their respective internal iliac artery and course around each side of the fetal bladder before leaving the fetal abdomen in the umbilical cord. Colour Doppler can be used to confirm arterial flow in, and the presence of, both umbilical arteries as they pass on either side of the fetal bladder (Fig. 11.8). Identifying the presence of both umbilical arteries confirms a three-vessel cord and is a far easier method of confirming a normal cord at the routine anomaly scan than trying to image the cord in cross-section in the amniotic fluid.

Two-Vessel Cord or Single Umbilical Artery

The normal umbilical cord consists of a vein and two arteries. *Two-vessel cord* or *single umbilical artery (SUA)* describe an umbilical cord in which only one artery and one vein are present (Fig. 11.9). This is a relatively common event, occurring in approximately 1% of live births.

Two-vessel cord can be an isolated finding or, because it occurs relatively commonly, in association with a wide range of structural abnormalities including cardiac and urinary tract abnormalities and chromosomal anomalies. The increased risk of a chromosomal abnormality in association

isolated SUA remains debatable, but most authors consider it to be low. Thus isolated SUA in the presence of a low-risk Down's, Edwards' and Patau's screening result can be considered a normal variant in terms of aneuploidy risk.

There is good evidence that the risk of growth restriction is increased in the presence of isolated SUA. Thus a third trimester growth scan should be considered when an SUA is identified.

THE CORD INSERTION

The *cord insertion* describes the area of the anterior abdominal wall where the two umbilical arteries leave, and the single umbilical vein enters, the fetal abdomen within the umbilical cord (Fig. 11.10).

The cord insertion can be identified from around 8 weeks of gestation and is best assessed from a transverse section of the abdomen. Obtain an AC section of the embryo or fetus and slide the probe caudally from the AC section to the site of the cord insertion. As discussed earlier, bowel will be seen within the base of the umbilical cord between 8 and 10 weeks of gestation. Before and after this gestational window only the three blood vessels should be visible within the cord.

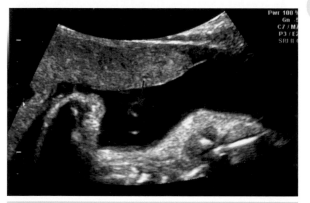

Fig 11.9 • A two-vessel cord with a single umbilical artery (arrowed). This can be compared with the normal cord as seen in Fig. 11.7B.

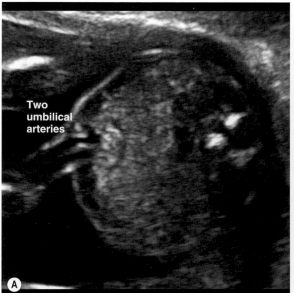
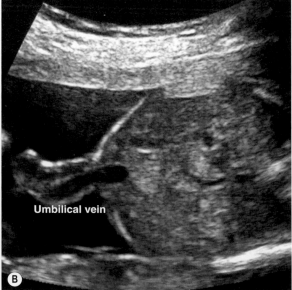

Fig 11.10 • Normal insertion of the umbilical cord into the fetal abdomen showing (A) the two umbilical arteries and (B) the single umbilical vein.

Confirming the normal appearance of the cord insertion and the abdominal wall, particularly below and to the right of the cord insertion, are component parts of the routine 18–22 week anatomical assessment. Confirming these appearances are normal excludes omphalocele, or exomphalos, and gastroschisis, as discussed later.

It may be of interest to consider that, after delivery, the position of the umbilicus is at waist level, which is roughly equivalent to the level of the AC. In the 18–22 week fetus, however, the cord insertion is not at the level of the AC, but is more inferior, roughly halfway between the level of the AC and the fetal bladder.

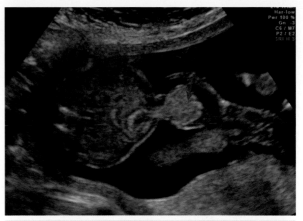

Fig 11.11 • A cross section of 21 week fetal abdomen at the level of the cord insertion. An exomphalos (arrowed) demonstrating a small quantity of bowel within the base of the umbilical cord can be seen.

CHEST WALL AND ABDOMINAL WALL DEFECTS

Ectopia Cordis

Where the cranial fold fails to fuse in very early gestation, the resulting midline defect involves the chest with the fetal heart being fully or partially outside the body cavity. This is termed *ectopia cordis* and is extremely rare.

Bladder Extrophy or Ectopia Vesicae

Where the caudal fold fails to fuse in very early gestation, the defect may extend down into the pelvis, resulting in extrophy of the bladder, or *ectopia vesicae*, and separation of the pubic bones. Bladder extrophy affects the anterior wall of both the bladder and the abdomen. The muscle in the abdominal wall anterior to the bladder fails to form, resulting in the anterior wall of the bladder being covered only by a thin membrane. This membrane is easily ruptured, causing the bladder to open into the amniotic fluid. Bladder extrophy is a very rare condition, being estimated to occur once in 40 000–50 000 births and occurs primarily in males.

Omphalocele

Omphalocele or *exomphalos* describes a midline defect in the anterior abdominal wall through which a sac protrudes which contains some contents of the abdominal cavity. It is thought to arise because the two lateral folds of the early embryo fail to fuse during the formation of the abdominal wall. The bowel therefore remains within the base of the umbilical cord after the period of physiological herniation of the gut. For this reason diagnosis of omphalocele should not be attempted before 12 weeks of gestation. The contents of the sac vary, with liver and bowel being most commonly described.

As the abdominal contents lie within the base of the cord, a distinguishing feature of an omphalocele is the insertion of the umbilical cord into the apex of the defect. Thus the diagnosis should be straightforward providing the site of the cord insertion is examined properly (Fig. 11.11).

The contents of the sac are normally covered by a layer of peritoneum, amnion and skin. This means that the typical second trimester maternal serum alpha-fetoprotein (AFP) level of, for example, the quadruple Down's screening test will be unaffected by the presence of an omphalocele. This contrasts with the level of AFP in gastroschisis, which will be raised.

Monitoring fetal growth and estimating fetal weight in the presence of an omphalocele is problematic because a significant proportion of the abdominal contents may lie outside the abdomen. This results in difficulties in deciding how to measure the AC, in a falsely reduced AC measurement and therefore in a falsely reduced estimated fetal weight.

Omphalocele is surgically repairable after birth, with the survival rate depending largely on the presence of other abnormalities. The literature indicates that, before the introduction of Down's sceening, up to 50% of cases were associated with chromosomal abnormalities, principally trisomies 18 or 13, or cardiac lesions. There is currently insufficient post routine Down's screening data available to determine whether these figures remain correct or whether they are overestimated. As an association between omphalocele and abnormal karytoype undoubtedly exists, it is likely that discussions relating to the prognosis for the pregnancy will include the offer of karyotyping.

A detailed cardiac scan should also be offered. If the pregnancy continues, vaginal delivery may be considered because the omphalocele rarely causes dystocia and the toughened peritoneal sac is rarely ruptured during delivery. When the condition is isolated, postoperative survival rates of 90% can be expected.

Gastroschisis

Gastroschisis is a condition in which the body folds develop and fuse normally but a small defect arises in the abdominal wall, usually below and to the right of the cord insertion. This is thought to be due to vascular compromise of either the right umbilical vein or the omphalomesenteric artery. The umbilical cord therefore inserts normally into the abdominal wall, making the differentiation of gastroschisis from omphalocele relatively easy.

The abdominal wall defect is small and allows only the small bowel to escape into the amniotic cavity. The bowel is not usually covered by peritoneum so it floats freely within the amniotic fluid. This produces the characteristic cauliflower-like appearance of free-floating bowel and aids further in the differentiation of gastroschisis from omphalocele (Fig. 11.12).

The presence of gastroschisis has implications in the typical second trimester maternal serum AFP level of, for example, the quadruple Down's screening test. The maternal serum AFP level will be raised in the presence of gastroschisis because the fetal bowel is exposed to the amniotic fluid. This contrasts with the AFP level in the presence of omphalocele, which will be normal because the defect is skin-covered.

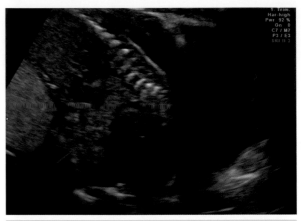

Fig 11.12 • A sagittal section of the fetal abdomen, at 20 weeks, demonstrating a gastroschisis. The bowel (arrowed) is floating freely within the amniotic fluid. Note the normal amount of amniotic fluid.

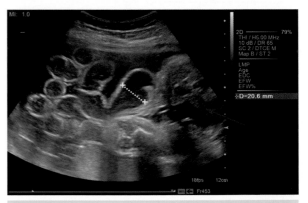

Fig. 11.13 • An oblique cross section of the lower abdomen (arrow) of a fetus with gastroschisis at 28 weeks of gestation. Dilated loops of bowel can be seen floating within the amniotic fluid. The diameter of the most dilated loop measures 20.6 mm.

Gastroschisis is usually an isolated abnormality, and its association with chromosomal anomalies is rare. About 25% of cases are associated with other abnormalities of the gut such as malrotation and atresia caused by vascular impairment. Obstruction of the bowel can cause dilation of bowel loops both inside and outside the abdomen as the pregnancy progresses (Fig. 11.13).

Gastroschisis is surgically repairable after birth, and postoperative survival rates of 90% can be expected. Postnatal morbidity is dependent on the quantity of nonfunctioning bowel which is removed and the problems resulting from short gut syndrome.

THE KIDNEYS

The development of the urinary system is complex and it is therefore not surprising that abnormalities of the urinary system are relatively common. Assessing the presence, position and appearance of both kidneys and the bladder is an important component of the 18–22 week anomaly scan.

The kidneys can be identified from the end of the first trimester and, as you are aware, must always be sought and identified at the anomaly scan. It is a matter of preference as to whether they are sought and assessed from cross-sections of the abdomen in the first instance or from sagittal or coronal sections. As discussed in Chapter 8, we recommend that, as you locate the femur by sliding the probe in a caudal direction from the AC section, you learn to recognize the kidneys in cross-section in the first instance. It is important that you also learn to recognize and assess both kidneys from the coronal and sagittal planes because different information can be obtained from the various planes.

TRANSVERSE SECTION OF THE KIDNEY

By sliding caudally from the transverse section required for measurement of the AC towards the femur, the two kidneys should appear, as circular areas, on either side of the ossification centres of the lumbar spine (Fig. 11.14). They are most easily imaged when the fetal spine is directly anterior. If the spine is lateral, at 3 or 9 o'clock, then the lower kidney is usually hidden in the acoustic shadow from the spine. In order to see the lower kidney, the probe should be rotated around the maternal abdomen to bring the spine to the top of the screen.

The echogenicity of the renal cortex is similar to that of the surrounding tissues, and this can make its identification a challenge for the beginner. The interface between the renal tissue and the surrounding tissue produces a brighter, hyperechoic rim surrounding the renal cortex, and searching for this, together with the hypoechoic renal pelvis which is also delineated by a hyperechoic bright border, often provides a useful clue as to the position and size of each kidney (Fig. 11.14). The kidneys do not both lie at exactly the same level in the fetal abdomen. This means you will not obtain the optimal image of them both in transverse section in the same cross section of the abdomen. You will therefore need to make small sliding movements of the probe up or down the abdomen to assess each kidney properly.

SAGITTAL SECTION OF THE KIDNEY

Having located the kidneys in the transverse plane, bring one kidney into the centre of the screen by sliding the probe across the maternal abdomen. Rotate the probe through 90°, keeping the kidney in view until a longitudinal, sagittal section of that kidney is obtained (Fig. 11.15). The kidneys are bean-shaped structures in this plane. Now angle the probe, if necessary, so that the spine is anterior. You are now imaging the fetal body in sagittal view. Because the kidneys are essentially parasagittal, you will now need to slide the probe to either side of the spine to image each kidney in its sagittal section. Remember that the kidneys do not normally lie in a true parasagittal plane but at a slight angle to the fetal spine, with the upper pole of the kidney lying closer to the spine that the lower pole. You are therefore now likely to have to rotate the probe very slightly towards the fetal spine to obtain

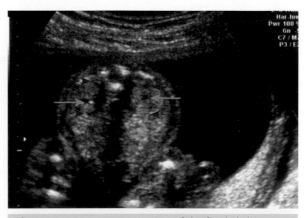

Fig 11.14 • A transverse section of the fetal abdomen at 19 weeks, with the spine anterior demonstrating both kidneys. The renal pelves (solid arrows) are visualized and are not dilated. The anterior and posterior margins of both kidneys are delineated (dashed arrows).

273

the full length of each kidney in sagittal section. If the upper and lower limits of the kidney are difficult to see, make tiny lateral sliding movements of the probe, or change the degree of rotation very slightly. Because the kidneys move up and down the abdomen during fetal breathing, you will find this activity will help you in the identification of the renal endpoints. Unfortunately, we are unable to provide guidance as to how best to encourage fetal breathing during your examination of the kidneys.

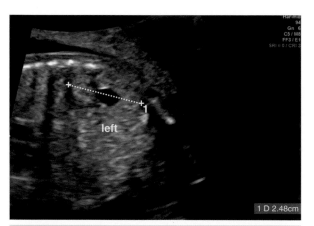

Fig 11.15 • The left kidney, measured in sagittal section, of a 20 week fetus. Note the prominent appearance of the renal pelvis, which, in AP diameter, measured 7.2 mm (see Fig. 11.26). AP, antero-posterior.

CORONAL SECTION OF THE KIDNEY

From the sagittal section of the abdomen, angle the probe by 90° away from the sagittal plane to obtain a coronal section of the abdomen. This view enables you to image both kidneys in longitudinal section. You will notice that they lie on either side of the aorta, immediately cephalad to its bifurcation (Fig. 11.16). Not only can you image both kidneys together from the coronal section but you can also use colour flow Doppler to demonstrate the renal artery which branches off the aorta on each side, at an angle of 90° to the aorta, before entering the kidney. Orientating the fetal aorta in the horizontal plane and applying colour Doppler will thus reveal the renal artery of the more anterior kidney in red and of the more posterior kidney in blue. If you are having difficulty in identifying one or both kidneys, using colour Doppler to image the renal arteries will help you 'see' where the kidney is positioned. Reducing the velocity of

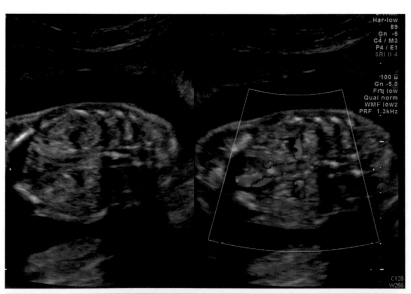

Fig 11.16 • A longitudinal section of a 20 week fetus demonstrating both kidneys in coronal section (left panel). Colour flow mapping of the renal arteries (red anterior, blue posterior) confirms the position of the kidneys above the bifurcation of the aorta (right panel).

the colour flow may help you to pick up the flow in the renal arteries if you are having difficulty in imaging them.

MEASUREMENT OF THE KIDNEYS

Renal size can be assessed from longitudinal, anteroposterior and transverse diameter measurements. The maximum longitudinal renal diameter should be measured from a longitudinal, sagittal section of the fetus, rather than a longitudinal, coronal section (Fig. 11.15). As discussed earlier, slight rotation of the probe away from the long axis of the fetus may be necessary to obtain the maximum length of each kidney. Care should be taken to make sure the adrenal gland, lying immediately superior to the upper pole of the kidney, is not included in the renal measurement. As mentioned previously, fetal breathing movements aid in the delineation of the end points of the kidneys, and therefore their measurement, when imaged in sagittal section.

To obtain a view of the kidney in transverse section from the sagittal section, rotate the probe through 90°. Make small sliding movements of the probe up and down the renal axis to obtain the optimal transverse section of each kidney separately. The maximum transverse and anteroposterior (AP) diameters of one kidney should be taken from the same image (Fig. 11.17).

All three renal diameters are measured using the same method of placing the intersection of the two arms of the on-screen callipers on the outer aspects of the renal outline using the 'outer-to-outer' technique (Figs. 11.15 and 11.17).

Charts showing normal values for these renal parameters are available.

THE RENAL PELVIS AND URETER

As the renal pelvis contains urine, it appears as a hypoechoic area within the kidney. In the normal kidney the pelvis lies equidistant between the upper and lower poles of the kidney and, because of the position of the ureter medial to the kidney, lies towards the medial rather than the lateral aspect of the kidney.

The extrarenal pelvis lies immediately medial to the intrarenal pelvis and varies in its size and therefore prominence. The extrarenal pelvis joins the ureter at the pelviureteric junction. The ureter inserts into the posterior and inferior aspect of the bladder.

The undilated ureter is not readily visible on ultrasound, although you may be able to image a short length of the proximal ureter immediately distal to the pelviureteric junction. The proximal ureter is best imaged from a sagittal view of the kidney and pelvis. The diameter of the ureter, as measured using the 'inner-to-inner' technique, should be less than 3.0 mm.

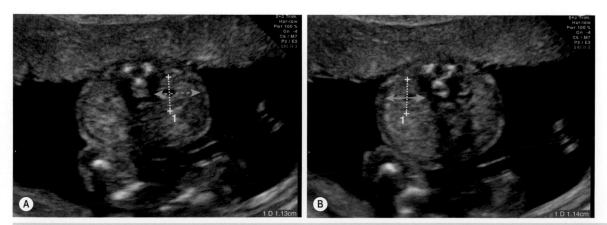

Fig 11.17 • A transverse section of the right kidney (A) and left (B) kidney at 19⁺ weeks demonstrating measurement of the AP (yellow, dashed arrows, with the respective measurements displayed) and transverse diameters blue arrows of the kidney. The measurements are 'outer to outer' and orthogonal to each other. The pelvis is of normal size in both kidneys.

MEASUREMENT OF THE RENAL PELVIS

Assessment of the size of both renal pelves is an important component of your assessment of the fetal kidneys and is undertaken from transverse sections of the kidneys in the first instance.

Renal pelvic size is typically reported using the AP pelvis diameter only and is best assessed and measured with the spine uppermost. The AP pelvis diameter is measured by placing the intersection of the two arms of the on-screen callipers on the inner aspects of the renal pelvis outline to obtain an 'inner-to-inner' measurement (Fig. 11.18). Make sure you are imaging the kidney in true cross-section before you start your assessment of the renal pelvis, as oblique sections of the kidney are likely to produce oblique sections of the renal pelvis which, if measured, will give a false estimation of the AP pelvis diameter.

The renal pelvis fluctuates in size, although this does not appear to correlate simply with fetal bladder volume. Controversy remains as to what constitutes normal renal pelvic size in the fetus. At the current time, in England, an AP diameter of 7.0 mm is taken as the upper limit of normal renal pelvis in the second trimester. The definition of mild renal pelvic dilation (RPD) also varies between authors. Some use quantitative criteria to distinguish between mild, moderate and severe RPD, whereas others use qualitative criteria such as calyceal dilation. The quantitative definition of moderate second trimester RPD is commonly described as an AP pelvis of 10.0 mm.

There is no agreed recommendation of normal renal pelvic size in the third trimester, but an AP diameter of 10.0 mm is commonly taken as the upper limit of normal in the third trimester fetus.

DUPLEX KIDNEY

A duplex kidney is one in which two pelvicalyceal systems are present. You are unlikely to suspect this condition prenatally unless one or both moieties are full or pelvic dilation in one or both moieties is present. Pelvic dilation more commonly affects the upper pole moiety, and this will be evident because the renal pelvis will not lie centrally within the length of the kidney but more towards its upper pole (Fig. 11.19). If you suspect a duplex kidney, you should always examine the fetal bladder carefully, as RPD may be secondary to a ureterocele in the bladder.

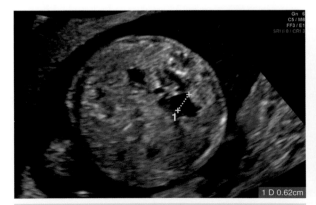

Fig 11.18 • Measurement of the AP diameter of the renal pelvis at 20 weeks. The inner-to-inner measurement of 6.2 mm is within the normal range for the gestation. AP, antero-posterior.

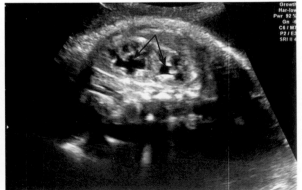

Fig 11.19 • A sagittal section of a duplex kidney showing the two collecting systems (arrowed). They are not connected. The lower moiety is more prominent than the upper moiety in this 28 week fetus.

THE BLADDER

The fetal bladder can be identified in approximately 80% of fetuses at 11 weeks of gestation and more than 90% at 13 weeks of gestation. As the bladder empties and fills over a 30–40 minute period, it may not be visible in a small proportion of fetuses because it may just have emptied. The bladder is visible as a circular, hypoechoic, structure lying between the iliac crests of the pelvis when the fetus is imaged in transverse section (Fig. 11.20). In longitudinal section the bladder is more oval in appearance, depending on its degree of fullness. In the transverse plane, the rectum may also be visible adjacent and posterior to the fetal bladder, just in front of the spine (Fig. 11.20).

Demonstration of fetal bladder filling implies that renal function from at least one kidney is present, whereas demonstration of bladder emptying confirms a patent outlet for the urine to be released into the amniotic cavity.

URETEROCELE

A ureterocele appears as a thin-walled circular cystic mass within the bladder and is associated with duplex kidney (Fig. 11.21). It looks rather like an ovarian follicle or a yolk sac within the fetal bladder. Identifying or excluding the presence of a ureterocele is important, as its presence is likely to affect the postnatal management of a fetus in which other abnormalities of the urinary tract have been detected. In such situations, your report should state whether or not a ureterocele was present.

Ureteroceles can be unilateral or bilateral and can be large enough to cause obstruction to the contralateral kidney.

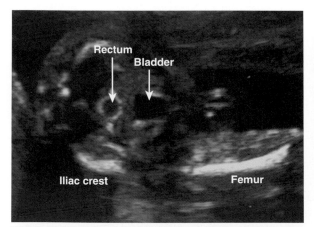

Fig 11.20 • A transverse section of the fetal pelvis, at 22 weeks, demonstrating the normal bladder and rectum.

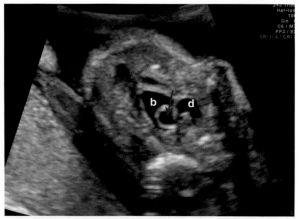

Fig 11.21 • An oblique section of the pelvis of a 26 week fetus demonstrating a ureterocele (arrowed) within the partially full fetal bladder (b). The dilated distal ureter (d) can be seen adjacent to the bladder.

URINARY TRACT ABNORMALITIES

RENAL AGENESIS

Renal agenesis describes the condition in which one or both kidneys are absent, together with the corresponding ureter and renal artery. It can therefore be either unilateral (Fig. 11.22) or bilateral renal agenesis. The adrenals are present in renal agenesis, may be enlarged and thus may be mistaken for normal renal tissue. Unlike the kidney, the adrenal gland does not have a collecting system and thus will not demonstrate 'pelvic' echoes.

Because the majority of amniotic fluid consists of fetal urine after the 16th week, a normal amount of amniotic fluid implies the presence of at least one functioning kidney and a patent urethra to allow the urine produced to be passed into the amniotic cavity. In bilateral renal agenesis, no urine is produced at all, so the bladder never fills and therefore is not visible. Bilateral renal agenesis is invariably associated with anhydramnios. When anhydramnios is present, the differential diagnosis includes bilateral renal agenesis, severe intrauterine growth restriction and premature rupture of membranes. The fetus is often severely flexed when

anhydramnios is present, and this further compounds the difficulties of making the correct differential diagnosis. If the fetal bladder is seen to fill, this effectively excludes the diagnosis of bilateral renal agenesis.

Irrespective of the underlying cause of the anhydramnios or severe oligohydramnios, when the condition is longstanding, the prognosis is poor because of the pulmonary hypoplasia resulting from the ongoing lack of amniotic fluid.

Unilateral renal agenesis has a very different prognosis. This is because, first, adequate postnatal renal function can be provided by one kidney only and, second, as the amniotic fluid is normal, pulmonary hypoplasia will not be a compounding prognostic factor.

As identifying the normal appearance of both kidneys is a component of the 18–22 week scan, and as unilateral renal agenesis is a relatively common condition, it would seem reasonable to assume that unilateral renal agenesis would be a condition that was identified relatively commonly during routine screening. In reality, identifying unilateral renal agenesis is reported relatively rarely in the fetus, suggesting that correct assessment of both kidneys at the 18–22 week scan leaves something to be desired.

Failing to identify both kidneys in their normal positions in the presence of a normal amniotic fluid volume does not automatically imply unilateral renal agenesis. You should also consider a horseshoe or pelvic kidney as a differential diagnosis. Neither is an easy condition to diagnose because of the similarity in echotexture of the renal cortex and surrounding tissues, as discussed earlier, but nevertheless you should try to define the outline of the single kidney to determine whether it is normal or not.

CONGENITAL CYSTIC DISEASE OF THE KIDNEY

Classifications

Enid Potter made the original pathological classification of cystic diseases of the kidney in 1972. She described four types of disease: Type I described the kidneys seen in infantile polycystic kidney

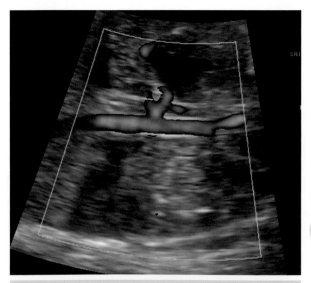

Fig 11.22 • Coronal section of a 29 week fetus. Imaging with power Dopper demonstrates the presence of only one renal artery. The lower kidney is absent, therefore suggesting the diagnosis of unilateral renal agenesis.

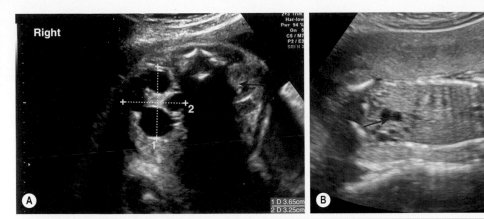

Fig 11.23 • A. A transverse section of a 33 week fetus with a unilateral Potter type IIA multicystic kidney. Note that the contralateral kidney, which is partially obscured by the acoustic shadow from the spine (arrowed), is normal. The amniotic fluid volume is also normal, consistent with a unilateral condition. B. A coronal section of a 22 week fetus with Potter type IIB multicystic dysplasia (arrow). Multiple small cysts are present. The contralateral kidney is not visualized in this section but was also abnormal. Note the complete absence of amniotic fluid, consistent with a severe bilateral condition.

disease (IPCK). Types II and III described multicystic disease and type IV described obstructive disease. Type II involved the nephrons, whereas type III involved the collecting tubules in addition to the nephrons. Potter subdivided type II into IIA (multicystic and large) (Fig. 11.23A) and IIB (multicystic and small) (Fig. 11.23B).

The Potter classification is still used by many authors, although variations of these criteria are also commonly used. Type II disease is also now commonly described as multicystic renal dysplasia or multicystic dysplastic kidney disease (MCDK).

Type III disease is also now commonly described as renal dysplasia or type III renal dysplasia. Type III kidneys are found in autosomal dominant or adult polycystic kidney disease (APK), Meckel–Gruber syndrome (autosomal recessive) and tuberous sclerosis (autosomal dominant). Confusingly, the ultrasound appearances of the kidneys in IPCK and in Meckel–Gruber syndrome can look very similar, in that both conditions are characterized by kidneys which are enlarged and 'bright'.

It is important to be aware that inconsistencies of definition are occasionally apparent in the literature, which can cause confusion to the reader. It should also be remembered that the terms *polycystic* and *multicystic* describe specific and different ultrasound appearances and they should therefore

not be used interchangeably. Unfortunately, the ultrasound literature has not always adopted this rigorous approach.

Many centres have adopted a classification based on ultrasound findings of laterality, cyst number, cyst size, appearance of the cortex, bladder size, thickness of the bladder wall and amniotic fluid volume.

Infantile Polycystic Kidney Disease

Infantile polycystic disease is a rare condition with an incidence of about 1 in 30 000 births which affects both the kidney and the liver. It has an autosomal recessive inheritance pattern. The condition is amenable to prenatal diagnosis, as the gene responsible lies on chromosome 6.

Four types of the disease are described (prenatal, neonatal, infantile and juvenile) based on the age at presentation and the degree of renal involvement. The prenatal type is the most common and it is this type which is most amenable to prenatal detection, but not always with ease. This condition is always bilateral, with cysts that may vary in size from microscopic to several millimetres. The appearance of the renal cortex is dependent on the size of the cysts. The microcysts which typify the condition cannot be resolved by ultrasound. The multiple interfaces caused by the cysts return multiple echoes producing the hyper-echoic appearance which characterises IPCK (Fig. 11.24). Slightly larger cysts can be resolved by ultrasound, producing the second characteristic 'spongy' appearance of this condition. The differential diagnosis of enlarged hyperechoic kidneys includes APK and Meckel–Gruber syndrome.

As IPCK is an abnormality of tubular development, the calyceal system and renal pelvis are present and can be identified. Oligohydramnios is often present but not invariably so, suggesting some degree of renal function is retained in some cases.

The gestational age at which these findings become apparent vary and therefore not all are amenable to second trimester diagnosis. It is possible to identify, and record, normal renal appearances at 20–22 weeks, with subsequent examination in the third trimester demonstrating the typical features of IPCK. Women carrying a fetus at risk of IPCK should therefore be offered serial ultrasound examinations through pregnancy.

Multicystic Dysplastic Kidney Disease

Multicystic dysplastic kidney disease encompasses a spectrum of renal appearances that reflect the size of the cysts and the degree of renal involvement. The condition is thought to arise either as a consequence of early obstruction to the ureter or bladder or as a failure in the development of the nephrons. It may be bilateral, unilateral or segmental, affecting only part of one kidney. Presence of the renal artery or ureter is variable. The unilateral condition may be accompanied by agenesis of the contralateral kidney.

The affected renal tissue is replaced by noncommunicating cysts of varying size (Fig. 11.23). The kidney may therefore be enlarged or small. In cases where the kidney is enlarged, it is important to differentiate between MCDK and severe renal pelvic dilation. In the latter condition the cystic areas, representing dilated calyces, intercommunicate. Other abnormalities including chromosomal abnormalities, particularly trisomy 18, and cardiac abnormalities are associated with approximately 50% of cases of MCDK.

Bilateral MCDK is always associated with severe oligohydramnios and has a poor prognosis irrespective of the presence of other abnormalities. Conversely, isolated unilateral MCDK carries a normal prognosis.

Multicystic dysplastic kidneys tend to involute or shrink over time. This may occur prenatally or in infanthood. Nephrectomy may be indicated if the affected kidney remains grossly enlarged.

The recurrence risk of MCDK is low, as the condition is generally sporadic. As the renal ultrasound appearances of MCDK and renal dysplasia may be very similar, it is important to be aware of the association of the latter with Mendelian disorders, which therefore have recurrence risks of 1 in 2 or 1 in 4.

Renal Dysplasia

The ultrasound appearances of renal dysplasia cover a wide spectrum of conditions and include findings that may be indistinguishable from IPCK or bilateral MCDK. Renal dysplasia is characterized by enlarged kidneys that contain cysts of varying size. Microcysts will therefore produce an appearance indistinguishable from IPCK, whereas larger or more variably sized cysts will produce appearances similar to those of MCDK. The condition tends to be bilateral, with both kidneys being equally enlarged. As discussed earlier, MCDK has

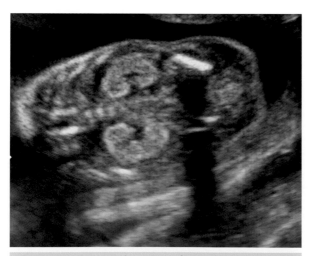

Fig 11.24 • A coronal section of a 20 week fetus with bilateral hyperechoic kidneys. Note the renal pelvis can be identified in each kidney and that the amniotic fluid is normal, suggesting some functioning renal tissue is present.

a low recurrence risk. A number of the conditions amenable to prenatal diagnosis and which are associated with renal dysplasia are autosomal dominant (APK) or autosomal recessive conditions (Meckel–Gruber syndrome) with recurrence risks of 1 in 2 or 1 in 4, respectively. The characteristic association with other abnormal findings in some of these conditions provides an important aid in the differential diagnosis of enlarged cystic kidneys and thus the recurrence risk of this condition for future pregnancies.

Adult Polycystic Kidney Disease

The finding of large cysts in the fetal kidney, especially in the presence of a normal amniotic fluid volume, should raise the possibility of the antenatal expression of APK. The prenatal diagnosis of APK has been reported sporadically, and it is associated with a spectrum of appearances. No, single and multiple cysts are described in association with either normally sized and enlarged kidneys which are of normal or increased echogenicity. The differential diagnosis of enlarged, hyperechoic kidneys includes IPCK (see earlier).

Adult polycystic kidney disease is an autosomal dominant condition that is usually asymptomatic until the third or fourth decades of life. The condition is amenable to prenatal diagnosis, as the gene responsible lies on chromosome 16. Due to the inheritance pattern of this condition, scanning the kidneys of the parents should be considered after suitable discussion has taken place.

Meckel–Gruber Syndrome

Meckel–Gruber syndrome is an autosomal recessive condition characterized by Potter type III renal dysplasia, encephalocele and polydactyly. An occipital encephalocele is the most common neural tube defect found in this condition, although anencephaly, hydrocephalus and microcephaly are also reported associations. Detection of enlarged kidneys should therefore always prompt the search for the other abnormal findings characterized by Meckel–Gruber syndrome. As bilateral renal disease is often associated with oligohydramnios, such an examination may be difficult.

Although both bilateral renal dysplasia and Meckel–Gruber syndrome carry a poor prognosis

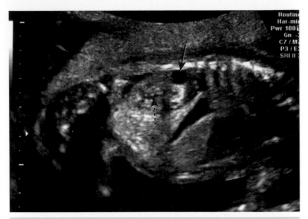

Fig 11.25 • A sagittal section of a 28 week fetus demonstrating a unilateral, simple cyst (arrowed) in the upper pole of the left kidney. Note that the renal pelvis (dashed arrow) is separate from the cyst.

for the index pregnancy, it is important that the parents are made aware of the difficulties that arise regarding counselling for future pregnancies from a suboptimal examination.

Renal Cysts

Unilateral isolated cysts of the fetal kidney are a relatively common finding and are found more often than other types of abdominal cyst. Isolated renal cysts arise from the renal cortex and should be distinguished from dilation of the renal pelvis (Fig. 11.25). Cases of isolated renal cyst should be reviewed in the third trimester to ensure that the AC is not so large as to prevent safe vaginal delivery. This is an unusual occurrence, as the majority of renal cysts are of no clinical significance.

OBSTRUCTIVE UROPATHY

Obstructive uropathy is the name given to a range of conditions in which there is dilation of some or all of the urinary tract as a result of an obstruction. The obstruction may be intermittent, partial or complete. The ultrasound appearances produced are dependent on the site and severity of the obstruction. The prognosis is dependent on the degree of renal compromise and the pulmonary hypoplasia associated with prolonged anhydramnios or oligohydramnios.

Urethral Obstruction

In this condition, flow of urine from the bladder to the amniotic fluid via the urethra is blocked. The most common cause of urethral obstruction is posterior urethral valves (PUV), although urethral atresia is another, less likely cause. Posterior urethral valves are folds of mucosa at the bladder neck that act as a one-way valve and prevent urine from leaving the bladder. They occur in male fetuses exclusively. In both PUV and urethral atresia renal function is initially preserved, producing the features characteristic of urethral obstruction, namely a markedly distended bladder and severe oligohydramnios. Back pressure from the site of the obstruction causes dilation of the upper urinary tract and progressive renal dysplasia. It is difficult to determine the degree of dysplasia, although increased cortical echogenicity is taken as indicative by some authors. The longer or the more severe the obstruction is, therefore, the greater is the likelihood of renal dysplasia and thus the poorer the prognosis. In the most severe cases the only organ that can be identified below the diaphragm is the fetal bladder. Intrauterine death is common and, for those fetuses that survive, the prognosis is poor because of pulmonary hypoplasia in addition to the severe renal compromise.

Urethral valves may also be associated with other anomalies such as chromosomal abnormalities, bowel atresias and craniospinal defects. Although the postnatal management of PUV is a straightforward procedure, the prenatal challenge is to identify those fetuses that have sufficient renal function and that may therefore benefit from vesicoamniotic shunting. Such shunting involves insertion of a suprapubic catheter into the fetal bladder under ultrasound control to bypass the obstruction caused by the urethral valves. Even with careful selection of fetuses thought to be suitable for such treatment, only about one quarter will survive. However, such treatment is now rarely performed because of the long-term morbidity associated with these cases.

Renal Pelvic Dilation

Renal pelvic dilation is a relatively common finding and may be unilateral or bilateral (Fig. 11.26). Mild RPD has been reported in association with Down's

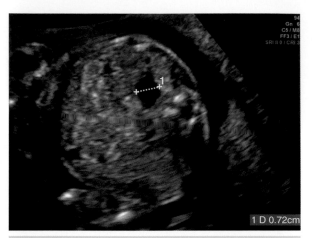

Fig 11.26 • A transverse section of a 20 week fetus demonstrating unilateral mild renal pelvic dilation of 7.2 mm.

syndrome, but the strength of this association in the pregnancy at low risk of Down's syndrome has been a subject of controversy for many years. At the current time, in England, mild RPD is considered to confer no additional risk of Down's syndrome to a pregnancy that is at low risk of this condition. It is therefore considered to be a 'normal variant' in terms of karyotypic risk in the pregnancy at low risk of Down's syndrome. However, this does not mean that mild RPD should be considered a 'normal variant' in terms of the fetal renal tract.

In a small number of cases mild RPD is the first sign of progressive renal tract dilation. This may result in postnatal uropathies, including pelviureteric junction obstruction and reflux, which may require postnatal investigations and treatment, including surgery. Mild RPD is also associated with duplex kidney and may be a precursor for a multicystic kidney.

Mild renal pelvic dilation can either progress, resolve or remain unchanged. The majority of cases of mild second trimester RPD will either 'resolve' – that is, the AP pelvis diameter will be less than 7.0 mm – or will remain unchanged. A small number, however, will progress in size (Fig. 11.27), whereas others develop calyceal (Fig. 11.28) or ureteric dilation. For this reason it is recommended that all cases of mild RPD are rescanned in the third trimester, commonly around 32 weeks, to exclude worsening dilation of the renal pelvis and ureteric dilation.

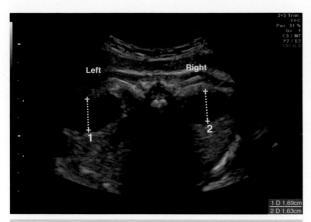

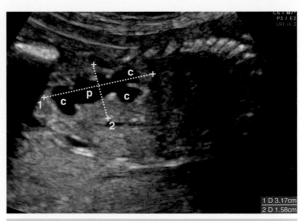

Fig 11.27 • A transverse section of a 34 week fetus with bilateral renal pelvic dilation. The AP diameter of the left and right renal pelves measures 16.9 mm and 16.3 mm, respectively. No calyceal dilation is evident. AP, antero-posterior.

Fig 11.28 • An oblique sagittal section of a 22 week fetus showing the dilated renal pelvis (p) and calyceal dilation (c) in the kidney. The callipers indicate the outline of the kidney. The longitudinal diameter (31.7 mm) can be taken as an accurate assessment of the renal length. However the second measurement (15.8 mm) should not be used as the AP diameter, for reasons discussed in the text. AP, antero-posterior.

Second trimester RPD will resolve before delivery in up to 80% of cases and in the majority of cases has no postnatal sequelae. However, a postnatal urinary tract pathological condition is present in approximately 10% of fetuses with mild second trimester RPD, and approximately 4% of fetuses with mild second trimester RPD will require postnatal surgery.

The postnatal management of prenatal mild RPD varies, with some units scanning the kidneys of all babies in whom antenatal mild RPD was reported, irrespective of the subsequent findings at 32 weeks, whereas other units will only scan those babies in whom dilation, however it is defined locally, was still present at 32 weeks. Postnatal ultrasound investigations should always be arranged for those fetuses demonstrating progressive dilation – that is, when the AP pelvis diameter in the third trimester is greater than 10.0 mm – as this group demonstrates the highest association with postnatal uropathies and subsequent surgery.

ABDOMINAL CYSTS

Abdominal cysts are a relatively common finding in the second trimester fetus. The normal fetal abdomen will contain a number of cystic areas, namely the stomach, gall bladder and bladder. Where you suspect an abdominal cyst is present, it is important that you have seen, and confirmed the normal appearances of, the stomach, gall bladder, kidneys, bladder and as much of the bowel as you are able to identify before deciding you have indeed found an abdominal cyst. As described earlier, the most common types of abdominal cyst are renal, whereas cysts within the liver, the adrenals or the spleen are rare.

Excluding cysts of the renal tract, ovarian cysts are the most common cause of abdominal cysts in the female fetus. Determining the fetal gender therefore is also helpful, as an ovarian cyst will be your most likely differential diagnosis in a female fetus. Ovarian cysts are typically unilocular and tend to occur towards the end of the second trimester or during the third trimester and are hormone-sensitive to human chorionic gonadotropin produced from the placenta. They may reach 10.0 cm in diameter, although the majority are smaller and asymptomatic. As you will have asked the parents whether or not they wish to know the

283

gender of their fetus at the start of your examination, you will already know whether or not you must ask them to shut their eyes or look away when you examine the genital area in such cases.

The second most common type of non renal abdominal cyst is a duplication cyst. This is a typically unilocular cystic malformation associated with the bowel, which may be seen in the second and third trimester fetus and may be several centimetres in diameter.

Other types of abdominal cyst are choledocal and mesenteric cysts. Choledocal cysts are associated with the common bile duct, and therefore will be seen in the upper right side of the fetal abdomen, and are typically unilocular. They can cause obstructive jaundice and so may require removal after birth. Mesenteric cysts can be distinguished from ovarian or duplication cysts, as they are typically multilocular.

Remember that abdominal cysts are not associated with polyhydramnios and are rarely associated with chromosome abnormalities. Thus if you have found what you consider to be an abdominal cyst in the presence of increased amniotic fluid, you should seek advice, as the diagnosis may not be as straightforward as you initially thought.

FETAL HYDROPS OR HYDROPS FETALIS

As outlined briefly in Chapter 10, the strict definition of fetal hydrops is the presence of excess fluid in more than one body cavity with a combination of at least two of the following being required: subcutaneous oedema, pericardial effusion, pleural effusion, abdominal ascites (Fig. 11.29A).

Subcutaneous oedema is the accumulation of fluid in the skin. Abdominal ascites is accumulation of fluid within the peritoneal cavity of the abdomen (Fig. 11.29B). The normal fetal skin is barely resolved with ultrasound, appearing simply as a thin bright edge to the underlying organs. Distension of the skin tissue in oedema produces a characteristically thicker and less bright ultrasound appearance that can be readily recognized.

Abnormal collections of fluid within the fetal body are also readily recognized, as they produce a characteristic hypoechoic rim of varying depth which surrounds the heart, lung and/or abdominal organs.

Hydrops is traditionally divided into two groups: immune (because of maternal antibodies) and nonimmune. The majority of cases are now due to nonimmune causes, which are many and varied. These include conditions that cause alterations in cardiac output, venous and lymphatic drainage and membrane permeability. Structural abnormalities involving mediastinal compression such as some skeletal dysplasias, cystic adenomatoid malformation, diaphragmatic hernia and

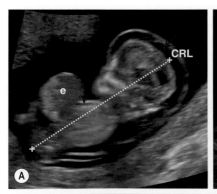
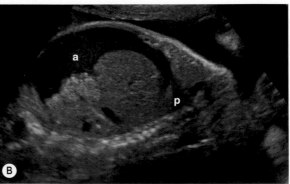

Fig 11.29 • A. A sagittal section of a 12+ week fetus with generalized skin oedema (solid arrow) and a small pleural effusion (dashed arrow). An exomphalos (e) is also present. B. A sagittal section of a 29 week fetus with severe abdominal ascites (a). Although the diaphragm cannot be clearly seen in this image, a pleural effusion (p) is present. Note the absence of skin oedema. CRL, crown rump length.

abnormalities causing cardiac compromise, including tachyarrhythmias, are associated with hydrops. Hydrops is associated with trisomies 13, 18 and 21, Turner's syndrome (45XO) and triploidy. Fetal infections and anemia are also important causes of hydrops, with parvovirus, cytomegalovirus and toxoplasmosis being the most common infectious causes.

It is important to exclude a structural abnormality such as those listed earlier as the underlying cause when hydrops is present. Maternal antibody and infection status can be evaluated from maternal blood sampling and the fetal status from fetal blood sampling. Despite the range of diagnostic tools currently available, the cause of many cases of hydrops remains unproven.

THE GENITALIA

Parents seem to be equally divided as to whether they wish to know the sex of their fetus. We recommend that you ascertain whether or not the parents want to be given this information during your discussion with them, before you start scanning. Many parents will assume, often incorrectly, that their fetus must be male if you ask them this question once you have started scanning.

It is possible to identify male genitalia in fetuses from 12 weeks onwards using the abdominal route, but it is often difficult to make a definitive diagnosis until several weeks later. The diagnosis depends on the fetus having its legs apart and on recognizing the echo patterns characteristic of the male and female, respectively. Both the scrotum and penis should be identified in the male fetus (Fig. 11.30A).

The testes may be visualized in the scrotum in the third trimester. The female labia are smaller than the male scrotum and have an appearance similar to two lips lying between the fetal legs (Fig. 11.30B).

You should not make the diagnosis unless the views you have obtained are unequivocal, and do not be tempted to diagnose a female by an apparent lack of male parts.

In clinical conditions in which identifying fetal gender is important, such as in women who are carriers of sex-linked conditions, identifying gender using ultrasound should not be attempted. Such pregnancies require accurate diagnostic testing rather than a potentially inconclusive screening test.

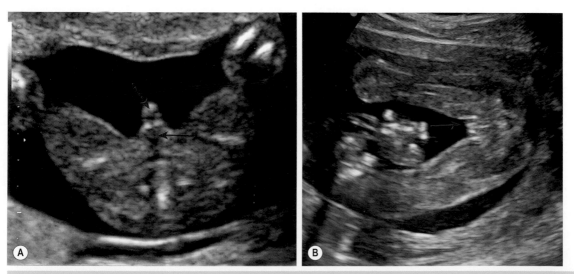

Fig 11.30 • A. A cross section of the fetal pelvis at 19 weeks showing the penis (dashed arrow) and scrotum (solid arrow) of the male genitalia. B. A cross section of the fetal pelvis at 20 weeks showing the labia (arrow) of the female genitalia.

Further reading

Public Health England 2015 Fetal Anomaly Screening Programme. Programme Handbook. NHS Screening Programmes; London

Salomon L J, Alfirevic Z, Berghella V, et al; ISUOG Clinical Standards Committee 2011 Practice guidelines for performance of the routine mid-trimester fetal ultrasound scan. Ultrasound Obstet Gynecol 37(1):116–26

Ultrasound assessment of the spine and limbs

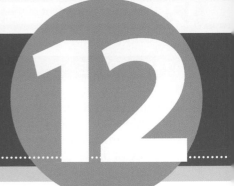

CONTENTS

This chapter addresses the ultrasound examination of the fetal spine and limbs with particular reference to the second trimester of pregnancy.

The aims of this chapter are to describe the correct techniques used to assess the following:
- the spine and its skin covering
- the long bones, hands and feet.

Examination of the spine and its skin covering has been an integral part of the second trimester examination since screening for fetal anomalies was first introduced, with detection of open spina bifida contributing to the earliest series of abnormalities detected with ultrasound being published.

You are already aware, from your reading of Chapter 8, that assessing the full length of the spine, including the sacrum and its skin covering, in sagittal section is an essential requirement of the 18–22 week scan. Having examined the spine and its skin covering in this plane, you should then evaluate the fetal spine in coronal view. Finally, you should assess the spine and its skin covering in transverse sections from the neck to the sacrum. Assessment of the spine and skin covering in transverse view can be done simultaneously with that of the chest, stomach, kidneys, bladder and abdominal wall, providing you are able to image each vertebra correctly. Alternatively, you may prefer to assess the individual vertebrae with one sweep and the abdominal organs and cord insertion with another.

THE SPINE

The normal fetal spine is easily visualized because of the high-level echoes produced by the three ossification centres within each vertebra. These are in the body of the vertebra and one from the lamina–pedicle junction on each side. The spine and skin covering should be examined using the sagittal, transverse and coronal views. Your aim should be to examine the neural arch of every vertebra in all three views before reporting the spine as normal.

SAGITTAL VIEW OF THE SPINE

First locate a portion of the spine. Keeping this part of the spine in view rotate the probe until you have obtained the full length of the spine. You now need to decide whether you are viewing the spine in coronal section or sagittal section. Your aim is to obtain a sagittal view of the fetal body with the spine and its skin covering lying anteriorly on the screen. If the fetus is lying prone in the uterus, this will be straightforward; if it is lying on its side, then you will need to change the angle of the probe on the maternal abdomen to bring the spine and its skin covering into the anterior position on the screen. You will be able to manipulate the spine into the correct position by changing the angle of the probe on the maternal abdomen, providing the fetus is lying with its spine between 9 o'clock through 12 o'clock to 3 o'clock, but not if it is between 3 o'clock through 6 o'clock to 9 o'clock. Thus, if the fetus is supine, you will not be able to manipulate the probe around the maternal abdomen sufficiently to bring the spine and its skin covering into the correct anterior position. In this situation the best use of your time is to move on to examining another part of the fetal anatomy, returning to the spine later with the hope that the fetal position will be more favourable for you. If the fetus remains with its spine persistently in the lower half of the clock, then your only option is to rebook the woman at a later date. What you must not do is report the spine as being normal when you have not been able to assess it and its skin covering properly.

Assuming the fetus is cooperating, you should now have an image which demonstrates the normal curve of the spine in its thoracic region, the upsweep of the sacrum and the integrity of the overlying skin (Fig. 12.1). If you cannot see the entire spine, rotate and/or make small sliding movements of the probe to obtain the entire spine and its skin covering in sagittal section. In this section the spine appears as two parallel lines of small hyperechoic dots that gradually taper towards and meet at the base of the sacrum. The echo immediately under the skin surface is produced by the vertebral body, whereas the echo lying more posteriorly (within the image, but more anteriorly within the fetus) is produced by one of the lamina–pedicle junctions. You will appreciate that the ossification centre from the junction lies very slightly lateral to that from the vertebral body, so this view does not demonstrate a true sagittal section of the spine. A true sagittal section of the spine would demonstrate the echoes from the verbal bodies only. However, the view you are seeking is that in which the two rows of echoes tapering to the sacrum can be seen. Note the small distance between the spine and the fetal skin. This distance should be consistent along the length of the spine; if it is not, then you have obtained an oblique view of the spine and skin covering. This can be rectified by a small change in the angle of the probe to the maternal abdomen, a very small rotational movement or a combination of both. When the spine is anterior but lying

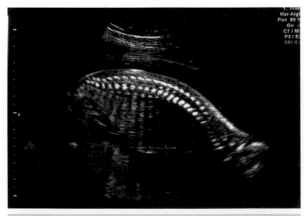

Fig 12.1 • A sagittal section of the fetal body at 20 weeks. The normal curve of the spine in its thoracic region, the upsweep of the sacrum and the integrity of the overlying skin can be seen.

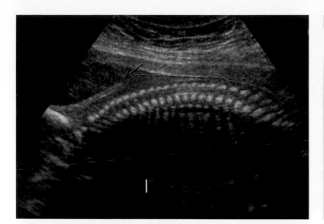

Fig 12.2 • The spine is too close to the uterine wall at the level of the dashed line to assess the continuity of the skin. The skin overlying the cervical vertebrae can be seen sufficiently well to be assessed, but that overlying the lumbar and sacral vertebrae cannot.

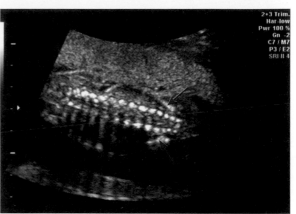

Fig 12.3 • The lumbar and sacral spine in coronal section demonstrating the three echoes representing the ossification centres of each vertebra. In this fetus the ossification centres from the lamina/pedical junctions are seen more clearly than the ossification centres from the vertebral bodies lying between them. These will be optimally visualised by a very slight sliding movement of the probe towards the fetal skin. The iliac crests (arrows) can be seen on either side of the sacrum.

very close to the uterine wall, or an anterior placenta, it is difficult to examine the continuity of the skin covering in the sagittal plane (Fig. 12.2). Reducing the pressure of the probe on the maternal abdomen may produce more space between the fetal skin and the uterine wall or placenta. Alternatively, the fetus can be encouraged to move away by applying and then releasing gentle pressure to the surface of the mother's abdomen with the ultrasound probe.

The sagittal view is used to confirm the integrity of the skin directly overlying the spine, thereby excluding the abnormal appearances caused by the meningocele or myelomenigocele, which are commonly associated with open spina bifida. Remember that this view is not the view to exclude or identify the actual vertebral defect of spina bifida. This view is also used to confirm the presence of a normal sacrum, thus excluding caudal regression syndrome or sacral agenesis.

CORONAL VIEW OF THE SPINE

To obtain a coronal view of the spine, return to the longitudinal view of the fetal body. The ease with which this view can be obtained varies with fetal position. If the fetus is lying on its side, the coronal view of the spine is easily obtained by sliding the probe towards the fetal back, until the spine is

visualised. As the fetal body has very little 'depth' at this gestation, only very small sliding movements of the probe are required to move from a coronal section of the front of the fetus to its back. If the fetus is lying with its spine directly anterior or posterior, then the coronal view is much more difficult to obtain. Begin with the longitudinal section of the fetal spine and then angle the probe through 90°. The angle of the probe to the maternal abdomen must be such that it produces a section that is virtually parallel to the scanning couch in order for a coronal spine view to be obtained. Owing to the anteroposterior curvature of the spine, you are unlikely to be able to view the whole spine in one coronal section. Small sliding movements through this plane are therefore needed to visualize all the vertebrae adequately in this view (Fig. 12.3).

In the coronal section, the spine has a characteristic rail-track appearance with the three echoes from each vertebra derived from the ossification centre of the vertebral body centrally and that of each lamina on either side. The coronal view is used to identify abnormal splaying of the ossification centres from the laminae, which characterizes the ultrasound appearance of open spina bifida.

TRANSVERSE VIEW OF THE SPINE

Rotate the probe through 90° from either the coronal or sagittal view to demonstrate the spine in transverse section. In this view each vertebra appears as three echoes which form an inverted triangular shape (Fig. 12.4). The side arms of this triangle immediately underneath the fetal skin surface represent the ossification centres from the two lamina, with that from the vertebral body, lying more anteriorly, producing the apex of the triangle. Note the small distance between each vertebra and the skin overlying it. Your aim is to slide down the spine from the neck to the sacrum, examining each vertebra and its skin covering in turn.

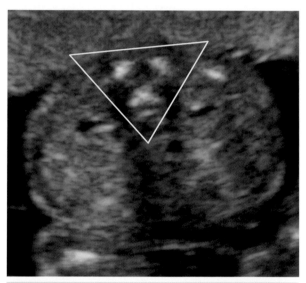

Fig 12.4 • A transverse section of the fetal abdomen demonstrating the inverted triangle of a normal lumbar vertebra. This appearance is produced by the three ossification centres of the vertebra.

You must therefore take care to keep the probe at right angles to the long axis of the spine when examining the spine transversely. This ensures that the inverted triangle for each vertebra and the slight curve of the overlying skin are maintained – this is especially important when examining the sacrum. The anteroposterior curvature of the spine means that you will need to make subtle adjustments to the angle of the probe on the maternal abdomen as you slide down the spine in transverse section. In addition, as the fetal position is not always directly occipito-anterior (OA), you will often need to rotate the probe slightly to allow for the lateral flexion of the fetal body, and therefore the spine, within the maternal abdomen.

Incorrect angling and/or rotation of the probe will result in an image that demonstrates oblique sections of two or more vertebrae. This is an appearance that it is important for you to recognize so that you can adjust your technique accordingly. Remember that the majority of spina bifidas are lumbar or lumbosacral, so it is particularly important to make sure you are examining a single vertebra only in each image. If you have examined the spine correctly, your sliding technique should result in your demonstrating both iliac crests in the same image when you arrive at the sacrum.

The spine and its skin covering are best examined in transverse section with the vertebrae positioned at about 1 or 2 o'clock or 10 or 11 o'clock and not at 12 o'clock. For the same reasons outlined earlier when obtaining sagittal views of the spine, you will be able to manipulate the spine into the correct position by changing the angle of the probe on the maternal abdomen, providing the fetus is lying with its spine between 9 o'clock through 12 o'clock to 3 o'clock, but not if it is between 3 o'clock through 6 o'clock to 9 o'clock.

NEURAL TUBE DEFECTS

More than 90% of infants born with neural tube defects (NTDs) are born to women who have not had a previously affected child. Before the widespread use of periconceptual folate therapy, a woman who had had one child or fetus with an NTD was advised that the risk of recurrence in a subsequent pregnancy was 1 in 20. If she had had two affected infants, the chances would be increased to 1 in 10. Periconceptual folate therapy reduces these recurrence risks by approximately one half. Therefore women are now advised to take a folic acid supplement daily 3 months before conception and until 12 weeks of gestation to reduce the risk of an NTD.

The two most common forms of NTD are spina bifida and anencephaly, and they are equal in occurrence. Acrania with anencephaly (see Chapter 9) is incompatible with life, so prenatal diagnosis is desirable and, as discussed previously, should be an expectation of all dating scans performed after 12 weeks of gestation. Prenatal diagnosis is also desirable in cases of spina bifida because only about half of the infants with open spina bifida will survive 5 years and the vast majority of the survivors have major degrees of handicap.

ALPHA-FETOPROTEIN

Alpha-fetoprotein (AFP) is virtually undetectable in the adult but is easily detectable in embryonic and fetal life. It is a glycoprotein produced first from the yolk sac and later by the fetal liver and gastrointestinal tract. In the normal fetus AFP is excreted into the amniotic fluid via the fetal urine and crosses the placenta to enter the mother's blood. The level of AFP reaches a peak in the fetal blood at 10–13 weeks and in the amniotic fluid at 12–15 weeks. In maternal blood AFP continues to increase in concentration until 32 weeks, probably because of increasing placental permeability. Any defect that exposes fetal tissue to the amniotic fluid will result in increased levels of AFP in the amniotic fluid and in the maternal blood. Thus raised serum or amniotic AFP levels are associated with open spina bifida and gastroschisis.

In the past screening for NTD was performed by measuring the level of AFP in the maternal serum at around 16 weeks of gestation. This was originally offered as a stand-alone test and, more latterly, as part of the 'double' and then the 'triple' and now the 'quadruple' screening test for Down's syndrome.

As with other serum analytes, maternal serum AFP (MSAFP) levels are reported in multiples of the median (MoM). The upper limit of normal MSAFP is generally taken as 2.5 MoM. About 2 per 100 women (2%) will have an MSAFP value greater than this level. In areas where the incidence of NTDs is 2–3 per 1000 births, the chances of a woman with an MSAFP greater than 2.5 MoM having a fetus with an NTD are about 1 in 20. The MSAFP level in normal pregnancies is higher in obese women and Afro-Caribbean women and lower in women with insulin-dependent diabetes.

The combined screening test for Down's syndrome is now offered to all women in England in the first trimester of pregnancy. With first trimester combined screening the AFP level is not measured and therefore only those women having second trimester screening for Down's syndrome using the quadruple test will have their AFP level measured. Even though the AFP is measured, the examination of choice for the detection of spina bifida should be a detailed ultrasound examination of the fetal spine in the second trimester.

Having a normal MSAFP result is not a guarantee that the fetus does not have an NTD, as an MSAFP greater than 2.5 MoM will only detect about 85% of cases of open spina bifida. Therefore a normal MSAFP result should not be taken as a guarantee that the fetus does not have spina bifida.

Conversely, women who have the second trimester quadruple screening test and have an elevated AFP level should be offered an early anomaly scan to assess the normality of the spine, brain anatomy and abdominal wall to exclude open spina bifida and gastroschisis. In skilled hands, such as yours in time, it should be possible to decide from the ultrasound examination if the fetus is abnormal, to specify the type of anomaly and to say how extensive it appears in order that a prognosis may be given.

SPINA BIFIDA

Spina bifida describes a defect in the fusion of the two halves of the vertebral arch of one or more vertebrae. It results in external protrusion of the meninges or the spinal cord and the meninges through this dorsal defect. It is the most common malformation of the central nervous system. Its incidence varies because of a range of factors including geographical location, ethnicity, maternal obesity and seasonal variation. Thus historically spina bifida was a relatively common condition in the British Isles but uncommon in Far Eastern countries such as Japan. It was more commonly found in Caucasian populations and less commonly in Oriental or black populations.

Women with diabetes have an increased risk of fetal malformations compared with the general population, with the risk of NTD in the former being quoted at around 2% although the incidence of anencephaly in these women is higher than that of spina bifida. Women with diabetes also have an increased risk of fetal caudal regression syndrome. Taking the antiepileptic drug sodium valproate in the first trimester of pregnancy (i.e. when the spine is forming) is associated with an increased risk of spina bifida.

There are two types of spina bifida, namely spina bifida occulta (closed spina bifida) and spina bifida aperta (open spina bifida). Spina bifida occulta represents approximately 15% of cases and is characterized by a small vertebral defect which is completely covered by skin. The intracranial signs associated with spina bifida are absent and MSAFP levels, if performed, are normal. This condition is usually completely asymptomatic and is often only diagnosed incidentally from an x-ray examination or suspected by the presence of a small dimple on the spine or a subcutaneous lipoma. Screening for spina bifida occulta is not an expectation of the 18–22 week examination.

The majority of cases of open spina bifida present with the open neural canal covered by a cystic mass (spina bifida cystica) which contains meninges only and is termed a meningocele or which contains meninges and neural tissue and is termed a myelomeningocele. In a minority of cases the defect will be covered by a thin meningeal membrane only, with no associated cystic mass. This latter group therefore poses the greater diagnostic challenge to the sonographer.

The vertebral defect of spina bifida can occur anywhere along the spine, although the majority, around 75%, are lumbosacral in origin. The location, size and type of the spinal defect should be determined, as this will influence the prognosis. As discussed earlier, extreme care must be taken to ensure the correct sections of the vertebrae are obtained for evaluation. It is easy to miss a small or subtle defect through a technique that is less than rigorous.

The ultrasound appearances of open spina bifida cystica are characteristic. When examined in transverse section, the splaying of the abnormal vertebral arch produces a wider V (Fig. 12.5A) or a U-shaped (Fig. 12.5B) appearance compared with the inverted triangular shape of the normal vertebra (Fig. 12.4). The virtually flat appearance of the skin overlying the normal vertebra is lost, being replaced by the bulging, rounded cystic mass of the

meningocele or myelomeningocele of varying size and appearance (Fig. 12.5B).

When examined in coronal section, the abnormal vertebrae will cause a bowing of the two outer parallel lines of the spine (Fig. 12.5C). With practice and the use of very subtle probe movements, the cystic mass of the meningocele or myelomeningocele can also be seen in the coronal plane (Fig. 12.5D). Very small sliding movements between the section demonstrating the vertebrae and that showing the disrupted skin overlying it are required to achieve this view.

The sagittal view is of limited value in identifying the *spinal* defect of spina bifida unless kyphoscoliosis is present, which is unusual. It will, however, demonstrate the disruption of the normal skin line because of the presence of the meningocele or myelomeningocele (Fig. 12.5E).

Thus examination of the spine in transverse section will demonstrate or exclude both the vertebral defect and the skin defect, whereas the standard coronal and sagittal sections will demonstrate the vertebral defect and skin defect, respectively.

It is the disruption of the nervous tissue of the spinal cord accompanying the vertebral defect of spina bifida that causes the paralysis associated with the condition. This disturbance of the nerves is not fully developed until the nerves are exposed to air (i.e. not until after delivery). This means that the fetus with spina bifida (or anencephaly) will empty its bladder and kick. It is therefore incorrect to report a fetus 'at risk' of an NTD as being 'normal' because it is moving its legs. In 40% of open spina bifida cases there will be additional anomalies, including ventriculomegaly, which can progress during the pregnancy, and abnormalities of the lower limbs such as talipes or rockerbottom feet.

The 'Lemon' and 'Banana' Signs

As discussed in Chapter 9, open spina bifida is strongly associated with a lemon-shaped skull, but this appearance is unreliable before 16 weeks and after 24 weeks of gestation. Thus a normally shaped skull should not be used to exclude spina bifida after 24 weeks of gestation. Also remember that the lemon-shaped skull can be produced in a second trimester fetus from an incorrect BPD section that is rotated slightly too far towards the fetal orbits

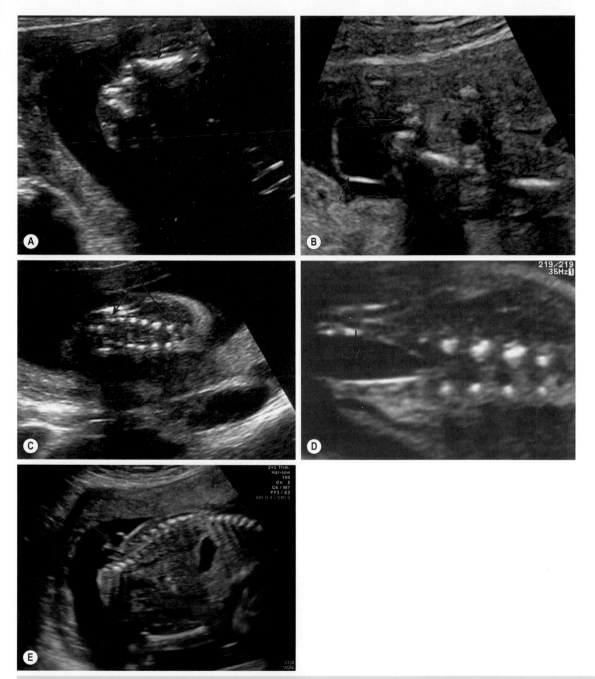

Fig 12.5 • A. Transverse section of a sacral spina bifida in a 21 week fetus showing splaying of the abnormal vertebral arch, which produces a typical wide V-shaped appearance (arrow). The iliac crest (dashed arrows) can be seen on either side of the defect. No obvious saclike protrusion of an accompanying meningocele is seen. This appearance can be compared with that of Fig. 12.5B. B. Transverse section of a sacral spina bifida in a 23 week fetus showing splaying of the abnormal vertebral arch, which produces a typical U-shaped appearance (arrow). The large sac like structure (dashed arrow) appears to contain fluid only, suggesting this is a meningocele rather than a myelomeningocele. C. Coronal view of a lumbosacral spinal bifida involving five or six vertebrae in a fetus of 19^+ weeks. Note the bowing of the normally parallel lines and the non visualisation of the ossification centres from the bodies of the abnormal vertebrae. D. Coronal view of the meningocele (arrow) associated with the lumbosacral spinal bifida shown in Fig. 12.5C. E. Sagittal section of a 22 week fetus with spina bifida, demonstrating the disruption of the normal skin covering by the rather complex cystic mass (arrow). This therefore is more suggestive of a myelomeningocele than a meningocele.

(see Chapter 8). If the rotation of the probe is adjusted to obtain the correct section but the skull still appears 'lemon-shaped', this should be considered abnormal.

The 'banana sign' describes a crescent or banana-shaped cerebellum that consequently produces an abnormally small transcerebellar diameter measurement (see Fig. 9.17). In some cases of open spina bifida the banana sign will be present, whereas in others the cerebellum cannot be identified within the posterior fossa because it has herniated into the foramen magnum. This is known as the Arnold–Chiari malformation type II.

Both these intracranial signs of open spina bifida and the Arnold–Chiari malformation are thought to result from traction on the brainstem and/or tethering of the cord at the site of the spinal defect. It is very unusual for a fetus with open spina bifida to have normal head appearances. One or both of the intracranial signs are reported as being present in at least 90% of fetuses with open spina bifida.

OTHER ABNORMALITIES ASSOCIATED WITH THE SPINE

SACRAL AGENESIS (CAUDAL REGRESSION SYNDROME)

Sacral agenesis is an extremely rare abnormality that is almost exclusively seen in infants born to mothers who have insulin-dependent diabetes mellitus. It ranges in severity from absence of the sacrum with short femora to complete fusion of the lower limbs – the mermaid syndrome (sirenomelia). Thus when checking the spine, it is particularly important to assess the sacral vertebrae to ensure that they are both present and normal in appearance. Fig. 12.3 demonstrates the normal sacrum seen in coronal section at the level of the sacral alar.

SACROCOCCYGEAL TERATOMA

Sacrococcygeal teratoma, although rare, is the most common type of congenital tumour with a live birth incidence of 1 in 40 000. It is found three times more commonly in female babies than in male babies.

There are four types of sacrococcygeal teratoma, the classification depending on the amount of the tumour that is intra-abdominal. Type I is predominantly extra-abdominal, whereas type IV is totally intra-abdominal. The majority (more than 80%) of these teratomas are benign, but malignancy rates are highest, approaching 40%, in the type IV tumours. One of the reasons why you should always examine the spine and its skin covering in sagittal section is to exclude a sacrococcygeal teratoma with an extra-abdominal component.

The ultrasound appearances of sacrococcygeal teratoma are varied. The mass arises from the sacral area and can appear completely solid or, more commonly, contains both cystic and solid components (Fig. 12.6). These tumours are usually highly vascular (Fig. 12.6B), can grow rapidly and are often associated with polyhydramnios. This may be due to excessive urine production (polyuria) or direct transudation of fluid from the tumour into the amniotic cavity. Hydrops may also be present, as a consequence of the hyperdynamic fetal circulation caused by the rapidly growing, highly vascular tumour. Preterm delivery is often required because of polyhydramnios. The delivery of a preterm, often hydropic, fetus requiring major surgery results in the high perinatal mortality rate of around 50%.

HEMIVERTEBRA, SCOLIOSIS, LORDOSIS AND KYPHOSIS

Hemivertebra is a rare congenital spinal deformity in which only one side of the vertebral body develops. It most commonly affects the thoracic and lumbar regions of the spine and affects one or more vertebrae. This results in a disruption of the normal vertebral alignment producing an abnormal lateral (scoliosis) or anteroposterior curvature of the spine. The abnormal anteroposterior curvature is described as lordosis when present in the lumbar region and kyphosis when present in the thoracic region. The abnormal shape of the vertebra produces a subtle change in the appearance of

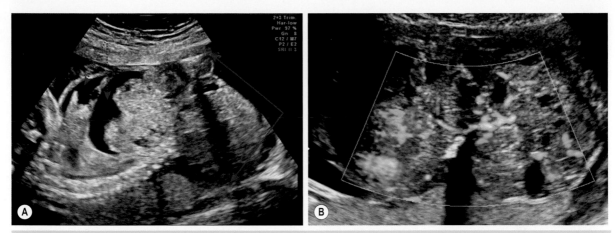

Fig 12.6 • A. A sagittal section of a 29⁺ week fetus with a large sacrococcygeal teratoma (arrows). The complex mass is composed of both cystic and solid components and extends into the pelvis and abdomen. Note the presence of abdominal ascites and fluid in the chest (dashed arrows). B. A coronal section of the tumour seen in Fig. 12.6A using colour flow mapping which demonstrates the presence of significant vascularity within the mass.

the spine which can be best identified using the coronal view of the spine (Fig. 12.7) – to assess vertebral involvement – and the severity of scoliosis, whereas lordosis or kyphosis is best assessed from the sagittal spinal view. Hemivertebra can be an isolated finding or can be associated with other structural anomalies and is a component of the VATER or VACTERL complex. Exclusion of hemivertebra is not an expectation of the routine 18–22 week anomaly scan.

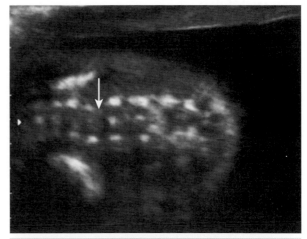

Fig 12.7 • A coronal view of the spine of a 22 week fetus demonstrating a scoliosis caused by a hemivertebra (arrow).

THE LIMBS

The limb buds start to appear in the embryo at around 26 days after conception – that is, at a gestational age of around 5⁺⁵ weeks. The upper limb buds appear first, with the lower limb buds appearing 1–2 days later. By the end of the sixth week the completed cartilaginous models of the various bones of the skeleton are present, including the digital rays of the rudimentary hands and feet. Two weeks later, by the end of the eighth week, the limbs are formed but not yet ossified. The process of ossification starts at around 8 weeks, in the clavicles, followed by the vertebral bodies and mandible at 9 weeks, in the frontal bones between 10 and 11 weeks and in the long bones at 11 weeks.

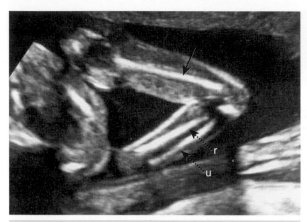

Fig 12.8 • A fetal arm at 20⁺ weeks showing the full length of the humerus (solid arrow). The radius (r) and ulna (u) can also be seen, but their proximal ends are poorly shown because of shadowing.

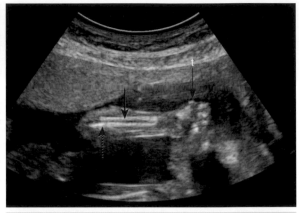

Fig 12.9 • The bones of the lower arm at 19⁺ weeks. The radius (solid arrow) is shorter than the ulna (dashed arrow), which extends further towards the elbow. The radius and thumb are on the same side of the forearm. Part of the proximal phalanx of the thumb (t) can be seen. Note the position of the hand relative to the lower arm in this normal fetus.

THE HUMERUS

The humerus is located and measured in the same way as the femur. Return to the section demonstrating the four-chamber view of the heart and slide the probe in a cranial direction until the clavicles are visualized. At this point a cross-section of the humerus is usually seen. By keeping this bright echo from the humerus in view, rotate the probe slowly until the full length of the humerus is obtained. You may need to make a *small* sliding movement after each rotational movement to bring the humerus back into view. To ensure that you have the full length of the humerus and that your section is not oblique, soft tissue should be visible beyond both ends of the humerus and the bone should not appear to merge with the skin of the upper arm at any point (Fig. 12.8).

THE RADIUS AND ULNA

The radius and ulna are visualized as follows. Keeping the lower end of the humerus (at the elbow) in view, rotate the probe slowly until some part of the two bones of the lower arm is seen. Continue to rotate the probe until both the radius and ulna can be seen in the same image (Fig. 12.9). You may need to accompany each rotational movement with a small sliding movement of the probe to keep the bones of the lower arm in view. The radius and ulna differ in appearance and this

should be noted. The ulna is longer, thinner and extends further towards the elbow or humerus than the radius. Remember that the radius and the thumb are on the same side of the lower arm. Ensure that the radius and ulna are straight and not bowed and are of similar echogenicity to the other long bones. As with the femur, ensure that you have obtained the maximum length of each bone before making your assessment or measurement. Should measurements be required, you should obtain images of the radius and ulna separately. As with other paired structures, attempting to measure both radius and ulna from the same image will rarely provide optimal sections of both bones.

THE HANDS

Patience is required to assess each hand properly, as the arms are often moving and the hands may either remain closed or may open and close very rapidly. Obtain a section of the lower arm in which part of the hand can be seen. The carrying angle of the hand relative to the lower arm can be assessed from this view (Fig. 12.9). Rotate or angle the probe, keeping this part of the hand in view until the full hand can be seen. You may need to add compensatory small sliding movements after you have rotated the probe to keep the image of the hand on the screen.

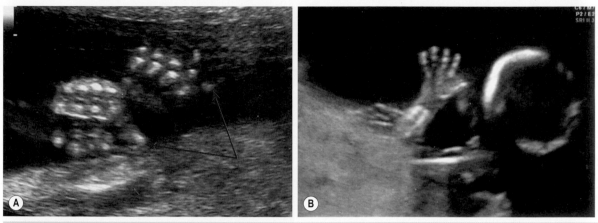

Fig 12.10 • A. The hands showing the fingers and thumbs of each hand in a 21 week fetus. Although the fingers are not fully extended, the thumbs (arrows) can be seen on both hands. B. A normal carrying angle of the hand with the wrist and forearm at 20 weeks.

Counting fingers is difficult, as the fetus often has a closed fist. Useful information can still be obtained when the fist is closed, however, as it is often possible to exclude overlapping of the fingers using this view (Fig. 12.10A). The outstretched hand view is necessary to confirm the normal appearance of the four fingers and thumb (Fig. 12.10B). Expecting to obtain this view with every fetus during the routine 18–22 week scan is unrealistic.

Abnormalities of the Hands

Abnormalities of the hand that can be identified with ultrasound relate to the position of the hand relative to the lower arm or its 'carrying angle' and the number and appearance of the fingers.

Fixed flexion of the hands

A hand that is held in a permanently inwardly flexed position is abnormal (Fig. 12.11). Identifying fixed flexion is usually obvious from observing both hands for a short time. This condition is usually bilateral and is associated with trisomy 18 and also with arthrogryposis.

Polydactyly

Polydactyly refers to the presence of more than five digits. In postaxial polydactyly, which is the more common form, there is an extra digit on the ulnar side of the hand. The extra digit will therefore be present beside the little (or fifth) finger. With

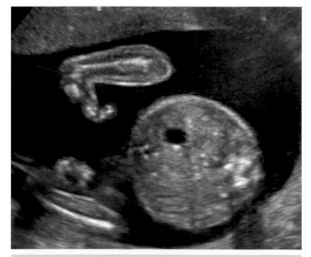

Fig 12.11 • Fixed flexion deformity of the hand (arrow) in a 20 week fetus with trisomy 18.

preaxial polydactyly the extra digit is located on the radial side and will therefore be present adjacent to the thumb (or first finger). Most commonly the extra digit is a simple skin tag, which is difficult to visualize on ultrasound. Postaxial polydactyly is an appearance seen in trisomy 13.

Syndactyly

Syndactyly refers to soft tissue or bony fusion of adjacent digits and is difficult to recognize on ultrasound unless the fetus opens its hands, allowing you to confirm, or otherwise, the normal separation of each finger from its neighbour. Syndactyly is an appearance seen in triploidy.

Clinodactyly

Clinodactyly refers to the permanent deviation of one or more fingers. Bilateral hypoplasia of the middle phalanx of the fifth finger produces clinodactyly of that finger, and this has been described in association with Down's syndrome. Clinodactyly can be seen on ultrasound if an image of the three phalanges of all four fingers can be obtained. It is, however, also a relatively common finding in chromosomally normal individuals, being described in up to 3% of normal Caucasians, so the implications of suspecting or identifying this appearance at 18–22 weeks need to interpreted with caution.

Overlapping fingers

In the normal closed hand the four fingers lie parallel to each other. *Overlapping fingers,* not surprisingly, describes the condition where one or more fingers permanently overlaps its, or their, neighbours. A fetus with overlapping fingers will not open its hands normally, so this is a condition that you are likely to suspect from imaging the fingers of the hand when closed. As with confirming fixed flexion of the hands, overlapping fingers is usually obvious from observing the fingers of both hands for a short time. This condition is usually bilateral and is associated with trisomy 18.

THE FEMUR

The techniques required to locate and measure the femur are described in Chapter 8. It is only normally necessary to measure one femur (see Fig. 8.16 and Fig. 12.12), but both should be visualized to confirm they are similar in length and appearance.

THE TIBIA AND FIBULA

The tibia and fibula are visualized as follows. Keeping the lower end of the femur (at the knee) in view, rotate the probe slowly until some part of the two bones of the lower leg is seen. Continue to rotate the probe until a view of the lower leg,

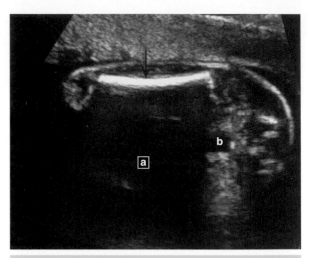

Fig 12.12 • Acoustic shadowing (a, dashed arrow) confirming normal ossification of the femur bone (arrow) in a 20 week fetus. b, bladder.

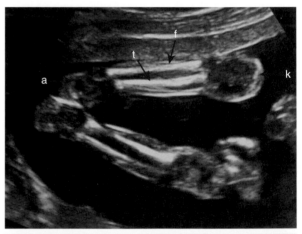

Fig 12.13 • A coronal view of the lower legs of a 21 week fetus demonstrating the normal appearances of the tibia (t) and fibula (f). The tibia is the broader and longer of the two bones and extends further towards the knee (k) than the fibula. The fibula extends further to the ankle (a).

demonstrating both the tibia and fibula, is obtained (Fig. 12.13). You may need to accompany each rotational movement with a small sliding movement of the probe to keep the bones of the lower leg in view. The differences in the appearances of tibia and fibula are more subtle than those of the radius and ulna. The tibia is longer and broader than the fibula and articulates with the femur. Thus the tibia extends further towards the knee than the fibula, which is thinner but extends further towards the ankle than the tibia. Ensure that the tibia and fibula are straight and not bowed and are of similar echogenicity to the other long bones. As with the femur, ensure that you have obtained the maximum length of each bone before making your assessment or measurement. Should measurements be required, you should obtain images of the tibia and fibula separately. As with other paired structures, attempting to measure both tibia and fibula from the same image will rarely provide optimal sections of both bones.

THE FEET

Less patience is required to assess the feet properly as, although the legs are often moving, the toes will present you with less of a challenge than the hands as the former are relatively motionless. Your aim is to assess the angle of the foot relative to the lower leg, and the plantar view of the foot. Two views of the lower leg are useful. As described earlier, the first, coronal section, in which the lower leg is viewed from the side, demonstrates both the tibia and fibula in longitudinal section. In this view only a cross-section of the talus of the foot (which articulates with the tibia and fibula to form the ankle joint) should be seen and *not* the whole foot. If the plantar or footprint view of the foot is obtained in this section, this is an abnormal finding.

The carrying angle of the foot can be assessed from the second, lateral view of the lower leg (Fig. 12.14). This section demonstrates only one (usually the tibia) bone well in longitudinal section. In this view the foot should be seen in sagittal section. A plantar view of the foot (sole of the foot) can be obtained by rotating the probe through 90° from this view (Fig. 12.15A). Although it can be difficult

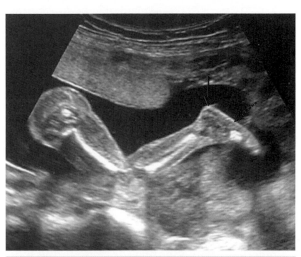

Fig 12.14 • Lateral view of the lower leg demonstrating the normal carrying angle of the foot in a 20 week fetus. Note the position of the foot, the shape of the normal heel (arrow) and of the normal sole (dashed arrow). The femur and parts of both the tibia and fibula also can be seen in this view.

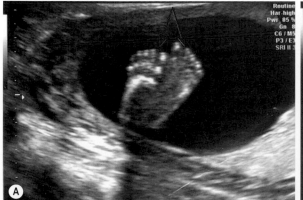
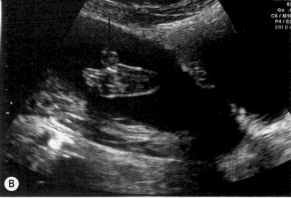

Fig 12.15 • A. Plantar view of the normal foot (left) in a 19 week fetus. Although this image was taken to demonstrate normal features of the foot to the left, it is clear that the appearance of the foot to the right is also normal, although not optimally seen here. Note the appearance of the toes, especially the normal spacing of the big toe and the second toe on both feet (arrow). B. The plantar view of one foot with an abnormal position and appearance of the big toe (arrow) in an 18 week fetus. The appearance of the fourth and fifth toes is also abnormal.

to count the toes on each foot, you should attempt to do so. It is usually fairly obvious if there are more than five toes, as the foot appears wider than usual. It is also important to look at the position of the big toe in relation to the second toe to exclude an abnormally wide space between the big toe and second toe called a sandal gap.

Measurement of the length of the foot can be made from the plantar view and is useful when a skeletal dysplasia involving the femurs is suspected. The length of the foot is obtained by placing the intersection of the cross of one calliper in the centre of the calcaneum (the heel) and the other at the distal end of the big toe, using the outer-to-outer technique.

In the normal second trimester fetus, the length of the femur and the length of the foot, as described earlier, are approximately equal. The ratio between femur length and foot length can be calculated with the resulting femur/foot ratio being approximately 1.0. Femur/foot ratio charts are available. The growth of the foot is not affected in skeletal dysplasias but, in some forms of severe skeletal dysplasias, that of the femur is. This will therefore be reflected in an abnormal decrease in the foot/femur ratio.

Abnormalities of the Foot

Abnormalities of the foot that can be identified with ultrasound relate to the position of the foot relative to the lower leg or its 'carrying angle', the shape of the foot and the appearance and number of the toes (Fig. 12.15B).

Talipes

Talipes is a congenital deformity of the ankle joint which results in medial deviation and inversion of the sole of the foot. The condition can be unilateral or bilateral. The relationship between the foot and the tibia and fibula in the normal fetus has been described earlier (Fig. 12.13 and Fig. 12.14). Talipes produces an abnormal carrying angle of the foot such that the plantar or semiplantar view of the foot is seen in the section which demonstrates the tibia and fibula in coronal section (Fig. 12.16). As it is fairly common for the feet to turn inwards into a position suggestive of talipes during both periods of fetal activity and inactivity, the false-positive diagnosis of talipes is

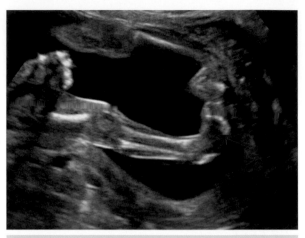

Fig 12.16 • Abnormal carrying angle of the foot at 20⁺ weeks, demonstrating talipes. Note that the coronal section tibia and fibula are imaged with the semiplantar view of the foot (arrow). Compare with the normal appearances shown in Fig. 12.13 and Fig. 12.14.

potentially high if the fetus is not observed for a sufficient period of time when it is active. Talipes is a relatively common finding in chromosomally normal fetuses, with a reported incidence of 1 in 1000. Persistent oligohydramnios increases the risk of positional talipes occurring during gestation. Talipes has a recognized association with trisomy 18, trisomy 13 and triploidy and may also be present in fetuses with spina bifida.

Rocker bottom foot

Rocker bottom foot describes the defect in which the foot has a prominent calcaneum or heel (Fig. 12.17) and an obviously convex sole. The carrying angle section in which the tibia is seen in longitudinal section and the foot is seen in sagittal section is required to exclude or confirm a rocker bottom foot. This condition is associated with trisomy 18.

Sandal gap

Separation of the big toe and second toe is described as a sandal gap (Fig. 12.18). The distance is assessed subjectively, from the plantar view of the foot, in which you will have observed that there is normally no gap or space between any of the toes, although some fetuses can be seen to flex their toes, producing an intermittent and short-lived sandal gap in one or both feet. Sandal gap has been described in cases of trisomy 21 and triploidy,

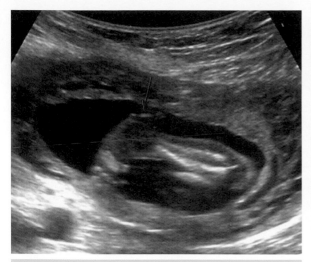

Fig 12.17 • Prominent heel (arrow) in a 17-week fetus. Note the presence of associated talipes.

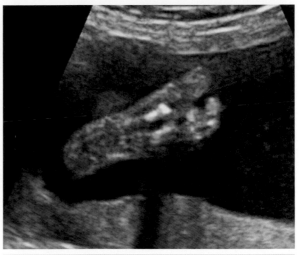

Fig 12.18 • Plantar view of a foot with a sandal gap, and abnormal toes. Note the wide space between the big toe and second toe (arrow). Compare with the normal image of Fig. 12.15A.

although the association is weak, especially in pregnancies at low risk of either condition. Interestingly sandal gap is described in up to 45% of children with Down's syndrome.

Polydactyly

See earlier. Although it is often difficult to count the toes, polydactyly of the feet is described in association with trisomy 13.

SKELETAL DYSPLASIA

Abnormal findings in the length or appearance of one or more of the long bones should raise the suspicion of a skeletal dysplasia. Skeletal dysplasia describes a generalized abnormality in bone formation. The conditions which include skeletal dysplasia are numerous and varied and may include abnormalities of not only the long bones but also the hands, feet, skull, face, chest and spine. Although the ultrasound appearances of some skeletal dysplasias are specific to that condition, there is often considerable overlap in the ultrasound appearances of other dysplasias, making an accurate prenatal diagnosis, and therefore postnatal prognosis, in such situations unfeasible. Making the correct diagnosis when abnormal skeletal findings are identified is therefore beyond the remit of the routine 18–22 week scan. The purpose of your routine 18–22 week examination of the fetal limbs is to identify and refer on those fetuses in which the skeletal findings are not normal.

A comprehensive description of the full range of the skeletal abnormalities is beyond the scope of this text, which gives a brief description of the ultrasound appearances and characteristic features of the more common skeletal dysplasias only.

For the purposes of ultrasound examination of the limbs, four criteria aid in the differential diagnosis of skeletal dysplasias:

- abnormal length of the bone
- bowing of the limb
- defective mineralization of the bone
- fractures of the bone.

ABNORMAL LENGTH

Complete or partial absence of a limb or limb segment is defined as follows:

- complete absence: *amelia*
- absence of a longitudinal segment of a limb: *hemimelia*

301

- absence of the three long bones with the relevant hand or foot attached to the body: *phocomelia.*

Shortening of one or more long bones is defined as follows:

- generalized shortening of the entire limb: *micromelia*
- shortening of the proximal long bone, i.e. the humerus and/or femur: *rhizomelia*
- shortening of the distal long bones, i.e. the radius and ulna and/or tibia and fibula: *mesomelia.*

As the femur length is affected in many of the severe skeletal dysplasias, a shortened femur provides the first clue that bone formation or growth is abnormal. The degree of shortening of the femur, and the time of the onset of poor limb growth, is specific for each skeletal dysplasia. Thus in achondrogenesis and osteogenesis imperfecta type II, severe shortening of all the limbs is apparent at 18–22 weeks, whereas in achondroplasia the shortening of the femur may not be obvious until after 22–24 weeks.

BOWING

In some skeletal dysplasias there is significant bowing of some or all of the long bones (Fig. 12.19). The normal femur is essentially a straight, hyperechoic complex, whereas a bowed femur may

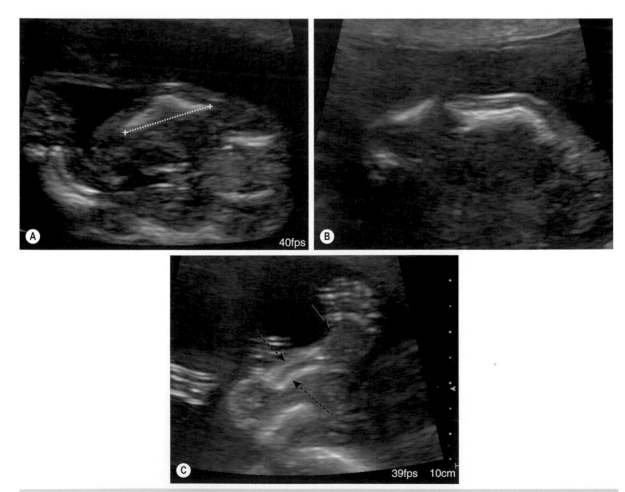

Fig 12.19 • A. A shortened and bowed femur at 17 weeks of gestation in a fetus with thanatophoric dysplasia. The callipers have been placed at either end of the obviously abnormal femur, which measured 15.5 mm. B. Bowing of the humerus in the same fetus. C. Bowing of the tibia and fibula bones (dashed arrows) in a different fetus, of a similar gestation. Note the abnormal position of the foot (arrow).

or may not demonstrate the same echogenicity but, by definition, is not straight. Bowing is a subjective assessment of a limb that will result in a length measurement that is reduced for the gestational age, the reduction depending on the degree of bowing present. Bowing can be associated with multiple fractures of the limbs which, when healed, produce bead-shaped irregularities of the bones. Pronounced bowing of the extremities is characteristic of campomelic dysplasia, thanatophoric dysplasia, osteogenesis imperfecta type II, achondrogenesis and hypophosphatasia.

DEFECTIVE MINERALIZATION

Acoustic shadowing is normally present from the edges of the cranium and the long bones (Fig. 12.12) when these bones are normally ossified. In skeletal dysplasias associated with hypomineralization this acoustic shadowing is absent. Reduced echogenicity suggestive of hypomineralization can affect the skull, limbs and vertebral bodies of the spine. Hypomineralization of the skull but not of the limbs is associated with osteogenesis imperfecta type II, whereas poor ossification of the spine but not of the skull is associated with achondrogenesis type II.

FRACTURES

Fractures of the long bones or ribs are identified by subtle but abnormal angulations of the bone together with bead-shaped irregularities along the bone, which represent healed fractures. Such fractures are characteristic of osteogenesis imperfecta type II (Fig. 12.20).

ADDITIONAL FEATURES

When a skeletal dysplasia is suspected, the hands and feet should be carefully examined, as abnormal appearances or extra digits such as preaxial (thumb side) or postaxial (fifth finger side) polydactyly are associated with some conditions but not others.

'Hitchhiker' thumbs, in which both thumbs are fixed in exaggerated abduction, is characteristic of diastrophic dysplasia, whereas postaxial polydactyly is characteristic of Ellis–Van Creveld syndrome (chondroectodermal dysplasia)

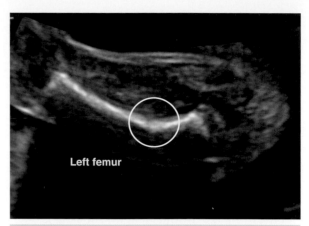

Fig 12.20 • Fracture of the left femur at 20 weeks in a fetus with osteogenesis imperfecta type II.

Abnormalities in appearance of the chest, skull and face together aid in reaching a specific rather than a differential diagnosis. Thanatophoric dysplasia is associated with a narrow chest but a trunk of normal length, whereas a small chest together with rhizomelic limb shortening is characteristic of asphyxiating thoracic dystrophy or Jeune syndrome.

Frontal Bossing

Frontal bossing describes the association of a prominent or bulging forehead with a depressed nasal bridge. This appearance is seen in some of the skeletal dysplasias including achondroplasia, thanatophic dysplasia and achondrogenesis and a number of craniosynostosis syndromes. These syndromes are characterised by premature closing of various of the skull sutures.

Nasal Bridge

The 'depth' of the bridge of the nose is assessed subjectively from the profile view. The bridge can be depressed, or lie deeper in the face than normal, in some skeletal dysplasias and craniosynostosis syndromes, although it is difficult to determine whether the nasal bridge appears depressed because of the frontal bossing or is in fact depressed in addition to the frontal bossing.

303

CHARACTERISTIC FEATURES

Characteristic features of the more common skeletal dysplasias are described next.

Thanatophoric Dysplasia

Thanatophoric dysplasia is the most common skeletal dysplasia, with a birth incidence of 1 in 30 000. It is lethal and is characterized by rhizomelic shortening, a small chest and frontal bossing. The femurs are extremely short and are shaped like old-fashioned telephone receivers. The thorax is narrow but the trunk is of normal length. The skull is often clover-leaf shaped and the fingers are short and sausage shaped.

Osteogenesis Imperfecta

Osteogenesis imperfecta can be divided into four types, with type II being the only type amenable to antenatal ultrasound detection. Type II is a lethal condition which is characterized by poor mineralization of the skull together with severe shortening of all the limbs, which are bowed as a result of multiple fractures. Fractures of the ribs are also common. Osteogenesis imperfecta (type II) is the second most common skeletal dysplasia with a birth incidence of 1 in 55 000.

Achondrogenesis

Achondrogenesis is a lethal condition characterized by severe shortening of all the limbs, a narrow chest, a large head and frontal bossing. There are two types of achondrogenesis. Type I is autosomal recessive and is associated with poor mineralization of both the skull and the vertebral bodies and with rib fractures. Type II demonstrates similar hypomineralization of the vertebra bodies only, the skull being normally mineralized, and there are no rib fractures.

Asphyxiating Thoracic Dystrophy

Asphyxiating thoracic dystrophy or Jeune syndrome is an autosomal recessive condition which is characterized by a narrow and bell-shaped thorax with short ribs. The long bones are normal or only minimally shortened and are not bowed. This condition is normally fatal as a result of respiratory failure.

Ellis–Van Creveld Syndrome

The long bones in Ellis–Van Creveld syndrome are similar to those of asphyxiating thoracic dystrophy. The severity of the chest constriction is less marked in Ellis–Van Creveld syndrome, which is also characterized by the presence of polydactyly.

Diastrophic Dysplasia

Diastrophic means twisted and describes the twisted shape of the body seen in diastrophic dysplasia. It is characterized by micromelia of the rhizomelic type, hitchhiker thumbs and severe talipes. The head and skull are normal but micrognathia is often present. Although this condition is nonlethal and intellect is not impaired, progressive kyphoscoliosis can lead to severe physical handicap.

Achondroplasia

Achondroplasia is an autosomal dominant condition in which the limbs, and particularly the femur, are shortened and bowed. The bones of the hands and feet are short and the fingers are divergent, producing what is called a 'trident' hand. Frontal bossing and a depressed nasal bridge are characteristic of this condition. Although the limbs are short, their decreased growth rate is rarely severe enough to be diagnostic of this condition at 18–22 weeks. Achondroplasia is therefore a condition which typically is only suspected in the late second or early third trimester.

MODES OF INHERITANCE

Skeletal dysplasias are rare and usually arise as new mutations. It is difficult to determine the mode of inheritance in those conditions which are lethal, but the nonlethal conditions are inherited either in an autosomal recessive or autosomal dominant rather than a sporadic pattern. The arbitors in making the final diagnosis are often the postmortem or a postnatal radiographic skeletal survey. Both these examinations are invaluable when attempting to counsel the parents on the recurrence risks for the condition in subsequent pregnancies.

The ultrasound features of the most common skeletal dysplasias are given in Table 12.1.

CONDITION	AMNIOTIC FLUID VOLUME	LONG BONES	FEMORAL BOWING	MINERALIZATION OF SPINE	THORAX	MINERALIZATION OF HEAD, SHAPE	HANDS/FEET	MODE OF INHERITANCE
Achondrogenesis type II	Polyhydramnios	Severe micromelia, fractures	No	Poor	Small	Normal, frontal bossing	Normal	AR
Osteogenesis imperfecta type II	Polyhydramnios	Micromelia, fractures	Yes	Normal	Short beaded ribs	Poor, brachycephaly	Normal	Thought to be AR
Thanatophoric dysplasia	Polyhydramnios	Severe micromelia	Yes, 'telephone receiver'-shaped	Flat vertebral bodies	Narrow but normal length	Large head, frontal bossing, clover leaf	Short, sausage-shaped fingers	Thought to be AR
Diastrophic dysplasia	Normal	Micromelia (rhizomelic), flexion deformities	No	Normal	Normal	Normal, micrognathia	Hitchhiker thumbs, severe talipes	AR
Achondroplasia	Normal	Rhizomelia, late presentation	Yes	Normal	Normal	Large head, frontal bossing, flattened nasal bridge	Trident hand	AD
Asphyxiating thoracic dystrophy/ Jeune's syndrome	Polyhydramnios	Mild rhizomelia or normal	No	Normal	Bell-shaped, narrow	Normal	Typically normal	AR
Ellis van Creveld syndrome	Polyhydramnios	Shortening of forearm and lower leg	No	Normal	Long and narrow	Normal	Postaxial polydactyly	AR

Table 12.1 Ultrasound features of common skeletal dysplasias

AD, autosomal dominant; AR, autosomal recessive

Assessing fetal growth, amniotic fluid, fetal and uterine artery Dopplers

13

CONTENTS

This chapter describes the assessment of fetal growth using fetal biometry, measurement of amniotic fluid and Doppler studies of the umbilical artery, fetal middle cerebral artery, fetal ductus venosus and uterine artery.

The aims of this chapter are to enable you to do the following:

- assess fetal growth
- assess amniotic fluid
- understand the causes of abnormal fetal growth
- identify with ultrasound the growth-restricted fetus and differentiate between the different types of fetal growth restriction (FGR)
- perform umbilical, fetal and uterine artery Doppler studies
- understand the role of umbilical, fetal and uterine artery Doppler studies in the assessment and monitoring of fetal well-being.

DEFINING GROWTH AND GROWTH VELOCITY

Growth is defined as an increase in size over time. Growth velocity is defined as the rate of that change over time. Growth can be described as normal if the size of the parameter being measured remains within the normal range for that parameter over the time frame under review.

The normal range is normally defined either by the 3rd and 97th centiles, the 5th and 95th centiles or the 10th and 90th centiles, the choice being determined by the author of the original data set. The growth velocity of that parameter is inferred as being normal if its size remains on the same centile over the time frame under review. Growth velocity is not normal if the centile on which the size of the parameter being measured lies changes. Units of size are, for example, centimetres or grams. Units of growth velocity are, for example, '3 cm/week' or '450 g/week'.

As you will be aware from considering the charts you are using in clinical obstetric ultrasound practice, 'fetal growth' is assessed by plotting measurement of size sequentially on a size chart and then evaluating whether the 'growth' or increase in size, which therefore implies the growth velocity, is 'normal'. A small number of growth velocity charts are available in the literature, usually published within texts which focus on statistical analysis. Velocity charts look very different from size charts and have the disadvantage, from a clinical perspective, of only providing information relating to change in growth over time. This can be inferred from a size chart, which, in addition, allows an estimation of size of that parameter relative to its normal range at a given gestation.

Because *fetal growth* is the term used in clinical practice to describe the combination of change in fetal size and growth velocity, this is the term adopted in this chapter.

ASSESSING FETAL GROWTH

Assessing fetal growth is clinically important because the perinatal mortality rate is higher in babies who weigh less than 2.5 kg at birth, weigh more than 4.0 kg at birth particularly if they are breech, those who are small for dates and those who are growth-restricted than in babies of normal weight and who have been growing normally.

Assessing growth relies on the accurate calculation of gestational age before 24 weeks. This is because the exact gestational age at the time of the later growth assessment must be known in order that the relative size, and therefore growth, of the fetus can be compared with the normal range for that gestational age.

Fetal growth is assessed primarily by comparison of the growth of the head circumference (HC) and abdominal circumference (AC). Assessment of amniotic fluid volume and inclusion of Doppler studies provide important additional information in the assessment of fetal well-being when the fetal growth is compromised.

Obtaining, plotting on the relevant charts and interpreting the measurements of the biparietal diameter (BPD), HC, AC and femur length (FL) are described in Chapter 8. The relative sizes of the HC and AC are of most importance in the assessment of fetal growth across a specific gestational age range. In the normal uterine environment, fetal growth will be normal and the size of the fetus will thus reflect the combination of its genetic potential and its environmental potential. Under abnormal uterine conditions, fetal nutrition, namely the availability of oxygenated blood from the placenta and the removal of carbon dioxide to the placenta, will be compromised. The fetus must adapt to these changes, and this is reflected in changes in its growth pattern.

Conditions which result in a decrease in available nutrition are more common than those that result in an excess. Uteroplacental insufficiency is the most common condition causing a decrease and poorly controlled maternal diabetes mellitus is the most common condition causing an increase in available nutrition. Against a background of reduced support and increasing fetal hypoxaemia, compensatory strategies occur to ensure that the most important organs of the fetus receive as normal a blood supply as possible and for as long as possible. Thus the blood supply to the most essential organs, namely the brain, heart and adrenals, increases, at the expense of that reaching the less essential splanchnic or visceral organs, which include the liver and the kidneys. The brain therefore continues to grow normally for as long as the environment will allow, but the growth of the abdomen slows because of the loss of subcutaneous fat, and kidney function decreases. In ultrasound terms, the resulting picture is of normal growth of the HC but a falling off of growth of the AC and, as urine output decreases, a reduction in amniotic fluid volume. It appears variable as to when, if at all, growth of the femur is affected in the environment of reduced support. Thus growth of the FL may mirror that of the HC or may exhibit some reduction in growth velocity, although it is rarely as marked as that of the AC.

Your task therefore is to measure, plot and interpret the HC and AC to assess fetal growth. In addition, you should include the FL and the BPD in order to calculate the estimated fetal weight (EFW),

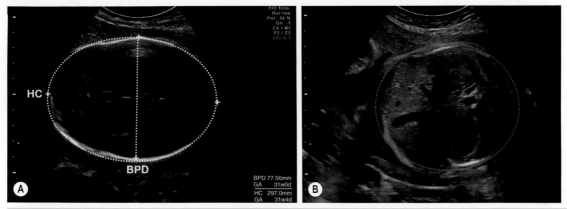

Fig 13.1 • A. Biparietal diameter (BPD) and head circumference (HC) measurement of a 31 week fetus. Note that the occipital region of the head is not easily visualized owing to the size and position of the head relative to the size of the probe's footprint. B. Abdominal circumference (AC) section of a 31 week fetus, with ellipse superimposed. The borders of the abdomen are readily identified, as the amniotic fluid volume in this pregnancy is normal. Note the difference between the outline of the fetal AC and the superimposed perfect ellipse. The match must be as close as possible but will rarely be exact.

as this is the parameter which often will determine whether or not a fetus should remain in utero or should be delivered.

Obtaining the correct sectional plane for measurement of the HC (Fig. 13.1A) and AC (Fig. 13.1B) tends to be more difficult in the later second or third trimester than at 18–22 weeks because of increasing fetal size within a more limited uterine space. Furthermore, in a cephalic presentation, the lower the fetal head lies within the pelvis, the more difficult it becomes either to image the entire head or to obtain the correct section from which to take measurements. Fibroids, scar tissue, obesity and the normal reduction in amniotic fluid towards term may all contribute detrimentally to the acoustic window available to you. It is better to abandon a measurement that is likely to be inaccurate because of difficulties in obtaining the correct section than to include an inaccurate measurement in your report. It is reasonable to assume that any information, including fetal biometry, included in an ultrasound report is accurate and therefore reliable. If the reported measurement is unreliable, it may encourage incorrect interpretation of your findings by a clinical colleague, which may, in turn, have serious consequences on the management of the pregnancy. You should therefore only ever include in your report measurements of images which will pass scrutiny by your peers.

DEFINING NORMAL GROWTH

We suggest that confirmation of 'normal' growth velocity should only be reported if the HC, AC and FL measurements sequential to those taken at the 18–22 week scan remain on their respective same centiles. In practice it is reasonable to use *normal growth* to describe the measurement subsequent to that taken at the 18–22 week scan that now plots between, we suggest, the 40th and 60th centiles. We suggest that growth velocity of a parameter is best described as *within normal limits* if the measurement subsequent to that taken at the 18–22 week scan now plots between either the 60th and 97th centiles or 40th and 3rd centiles using the relevant Chitty size chart (Fig. 13.2A and B). As with other fetal parameters, fetal growth should only be described as *abnormal* if the parameter being assessed lies outside the normal range.

Abnormalities of fetal growth are far more commonly encountered in clinical practice than fetal abnormalities, with poor fetal growth being more common than accelerated fetal growth. Fetal growth restriction, whatever the cause, is associated with a wide variety of adverse outcomes, from minor degrees of neonatal morbidity to intrauterine fetal death. As discussed earlier, the most common reason for fetal growth restriction is uteroplacental insufficiency. Chromosome abnormalities, some

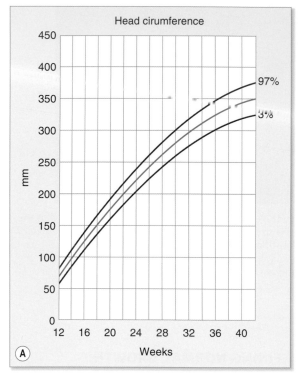

(A)

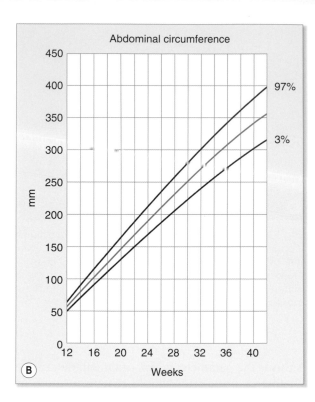

(B)

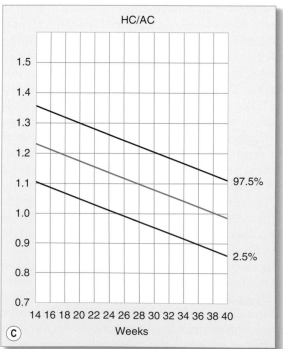

(C)

Fig 13.2 • A. Head circumference size chart.
(From Chitty L S, Altman D J, Henderson A, Campbell S. 1994 BJOG. Charts of fetal size: 2. Head measurements. 101 [1] 35–43.)
B. Abdominal circumference size chart.
(From Chitty L S, Altman D J, Henderson A, Campbell S. 1994 BJOG. Charts of fetal size: 3. Abdominal measurements. 101[2] 125–131.)
C. Head circumference/abdominal circumference (HC/AC) ratio chart.
(From Snijders R J M, Nicolaides 1994 Fetal biometry at 14–40 weeks gestation. Ultrasound Obstet Gynecol 4:34–48.)

fetal abnormalities and fetal infections can be associated with a reduction in growth velocity of varying severity. It is therefore important to be aware of the additional ultrasound features that aid in distinguishing among uteroplacental sufficiency, fetal abnormality and fetal infection as possible causes for fetal growth restriction. Distinguishing among these conditions effectively remains one of the most important ongoing challenges of fetal growth assessment. In addition, the relative frequency of fetal growth restriction and the anxiety it causes to both parents and medical carers necessitate a proper understanding of the diagnosis and management of this condition.

ESTIMATING FETAL WEIGHT

During the late second and third trimesters of an average, normal pregnancy, fetal weight gain is approximately 25 g per day or half a pound a week, decreasing slightly towards term. Genetic factors that influence birth weight include ethnicity, maternal weight and height, parity and gender. The baseline birthweight for a baby delivering at 40 weeks to an Anglo-European woman who is a nonsmoker, of average height (1.63 m) and booking weight (64 kg) and in her first pregnancy is 3480 g.

A large number of formulas from which to calculate the EFW have been published. The simplest algorithm estimates fetal weight using only the AC, whereas others include various combinations of BPD, HC, AC and FL. Weight estimations in this text have been calculated using one of the Hadlock formulas, which requires measurement of all four parameters described earlier. Whether or not you include measurement of the BPD when assessing fetal growth will depend on the formula you are using to derive the EFW.

The EFW is calculated numerically and, depending on the reporting system you are using, is also plotted electronically or manually on a birth weight chart (Fig. 13.3).

You may observe that an EFW which is 50th centile for gestational age as calculated from the Hadlock formula may not lie on the 50th centile when plotted on the EFW chart. This is most likely because the EFW chart on which the weight is plotted was not authored by Hadlock and the data sets therefore differ in their weight-equivalent centiles.

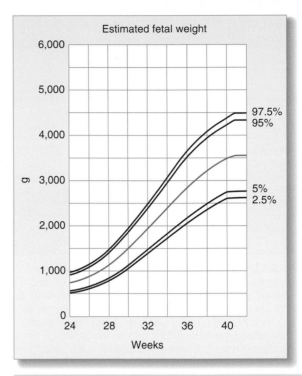

Fig 13.3 • Estimated fetal weight chart. *(From Yudkin P L, Aboualfa M, et al 1987 New birthweight and head circumference centiles for gestational ages 24 to 42 weeks. Early Hum Dev 15:45–52.)*

The proportions of a midtrimester fetus differ from those of a term fetus and thus departments may find that one birthweight formula provides greater accuracy in the EFW calculation of the 24–28 week fetus, whereas another is more accurate for the third trimester fetus. Should you wish to compare comparative EFWs from differing authors, you will discover that the same fetal measurements will produce a surprising range of birth weights, as demonstrated in Table 13.1.

The accuracy of fetal weight estimations carries a margin of error of 5–10% for those fetuses that are normal or small in size. The percentage inaccuracy increases significantly, however, in very large fetuses, such that any EFW calculated to be greater than 3.8 kg should be interpreted with great caution.

CUSTOMIZED GROWTH CHARTS

Because birth weight and gestational age at delivery show a degree of correlation with the previous

AUTHOR	EFW – CEPHALIC	EFW – BREECH
Hadlock BPD, HC, AC, FL	2609 g	2515 g
Hadlock AC, FL	2574 g	2574 g
Warsoff BPD, AC	2521 g	2132 g
Shepard BPD, AC	2610 g	No data presented
Difference All	89 g (3%–4%) 478 g	442 g (17%–20%)

TABLE 13.1 Fetal weight estimations as calculated by four data sets using a combination of BPD, HC, AC and FL, based on their average, 50th centile measurements at 36^{+0} weeks for a cephalic presentation (BPD 89.0 mm, HC 325.0 mm, AC 308.0 mm, FL 68.0 mm) and for a breech presentation where the BPD is on the 5th centile (as for the cephalic fetus but with a BPD of 81.0 mm). Note there is a 478 g difference between the largest (2610 g) and the smallest (2132 g) estimated fetal weight

NOTE: The Shepard data set does not enable an EFW to be calculated if the fetus is breech.
AC, abdominal circumference; BPD, biparietal diameter; EFW, estimated fetal weight; FL, femur length; HC, head circumference.

birth history, it would seem logical to use individualized growth charts to determine the expected growth velocity in the index pregnancy and therefore whether the growth of the current fetus is normal or not. Customized centile charts for symphysis fundal height measurement and estimated fetal weight were developed in the 1990s, based on the mother's height, weight, parity, ethnicity and the birth weights of her previous children. Such individualized or customized antenatal growth charts are increasingly being adopted into clinical practice, although they require internet access for the initial calculations and chart generation and are of less value in women who are in their first pregnancy than in multiparous women.

SGA AND IUGR

There is a close relationship between being small for gestational age (SGA) and being growth restricted, but being of small size does not automatically imply a reduced growth velocity. Thus these two terms are not interchangeable because not every fetus which is SGA is growth-restricted and not every growth-restricted fetus is SGA. Growth restriction is a major cause of neonatal morbidity and mortality, especially in SGA babies. Therefore, distinguishing between SGA fetuses and growth restricted fetuses is an important element of the examinations you perform to assess fetal growth.

Small for Gestational Age

Small for gestational age describes a fetus with an EFW which lies below a certain defined centile of weight or size for a specific gestational age. The 10th centile is commonly used to describe the lower end of the normal range for birth weight. Thus a fetus with an EFW on the 8th centile for gestational age would be described as SGA. By contrast, 8th centile HC and AC measurements used to calculate the EFW would be described as 'being within the normal range', or 'towards the lower end of the normal range' because the lower end of the normal ranges used for fetal biometry is commonly the 3rd or the 5th centiles. You should be aware of the potential problems that the differences in the normal ranges used with various ultrasound measurements, and therefore their clinical interpretation, could cause.

Intrauterine Growth Restriction

A fetus that demonstrates *intrauterine growth restriction* (IUGR) is one whose intrinsic growth rate potential is being modified by a particular pathological process, and therefore one whose growth velocity is less than normal. The growth velocity of a fetus with an EFW on the 95th centile which then falls to the 50th centile is certainly less than normal, as the EFW has crossed a significant number of centiles (namely 45) between the two examinations. This fetus therefore fulfils the criteria for IUGR. This is an important but a relatively uncommon pattern of IUGR. As average-sized fetuses are more common than large fetuses, the more common pattern of IUGR is demonstrated by a fetus with an AC on the 50th centile which then crosses the same number of centiles (i.e. 45) to the 5th centile. Deciding when to describe a slowing of growth as growth 'restriction' may also vary between individuals and/or departments. We recommend that the term *IUGR* is used when the AC alone, or the HC and AC fall below the normal range and that the term *reduction in growth velocity* is used when the parameter is still within the normal range.

Reduced fetal support and therefore growth restriction can be due to maternal factors or placental factors.

Maternal causes of growth restriction

Maternal causes of IUGR include the use of recreational drugs, alcohol and cigarettes, low maternal weight, hypoxia (such as caused by maternal heart disease or living at altitude) and severe undernutrition.

Placental causes of growth restriction

Placental causes of IUGR include reduced uteroplacental perfusion and reduced fetoplacental perfusion.

Reduced uteroplacental perfusion

Pre-eclampsia, autoimmune disease such as antiphospholipid syndrome and systemic lupus erythematosus (SLE), thrombophilias, renal impairment, diabetes, essential hypertension and multiple gestation all increase the risk of reduced uteroplacental perfusion. Since the introduction of combined screening in the first trimester, low levels of pregnancy associated plasma protein (PAPP-A) in the maternal serum have been found to be associated with an increased risk of IUGR.

Reduced fetoplacental perfusion

The presence of a single umbilical artery and twin-to-twin transfusion syndrome in a monochorionic-diamniotic twin pregnancy are conditions in which the risk of reduced fetoplacental perfusion is increased.

Identifying the High-Risk Population

There is a much higher prevalence of overall complications in women at increased or high risk for preeclampsia and IUGR than in the normal population. Such women are normally identified at booking and will constitute a group that requires additional ultrasound examinations to assess fetal growth during their pregnancies. Relevant risk factors include the following:

- previous SGA delivery
- low pre-pregnancy body mass index (BMI < 18)
- heavy smoker
- drug or alcohol abuser
- medical condition
- eating disorder
- low PAPP-A level at combined screening (the level varies, but <0.3 MoM is commonly used)
- multiple pregnancy
- abnormal uterine artery Doppler study at 22–23 weeks.

The Head/Abdomen Ratio

As discussed briefly in Chapter 9, the head/abdomen ratio (H/A) or head circumference/abdominal circumference (HC/AC) ratio, is obtained by dividing the HC by the AC to provide a single value. As can be observed in Fig. 13.2C, the HC is larger than the AC before 38 weeks of gestation. At 38 weeks the HC and AC are equal, and after 38 weeks the AC is larger than the HC. Thus the H/A ratio falls with gestation, being greater than 1.0 before 38 weeks, 1.0 at 38 weeks and less than 1.0 after 38 weeks.

When the HC and the AC values lie on the same centile, the H/A value will lie on the 50th centile. Thus the H/A ratio of a fetus with an HC and an AC on the 97th centile, with an HC and an AC on the 50th centile or with an HC and an AC on the 3rd centile will all have a 50th centile H/A ratio (Fig. 13.4 and Fig. 13.6). Applying simple arithmetic, you will realize that a fetus with an HC on the 97th centile and an AC on the 50th centile (Fig. 13.5) will have an H/A ratio above the 50th centile (Fig. 13.6), whereas a fetus with an HC on the 3rd centile and an AC on the 50th centile (Fig. 13.7) will have an H/A ratio below the 50th centile (Fig. 13.6). The H/A ratio chart is therefore useful in distinguishing between different types of abnormal fetal growth patterns.

Ultrasound Features of Intrauterine Growth Restriction

There are two main types of IUGR identified by ultrasound assessment – symmetrical and

313

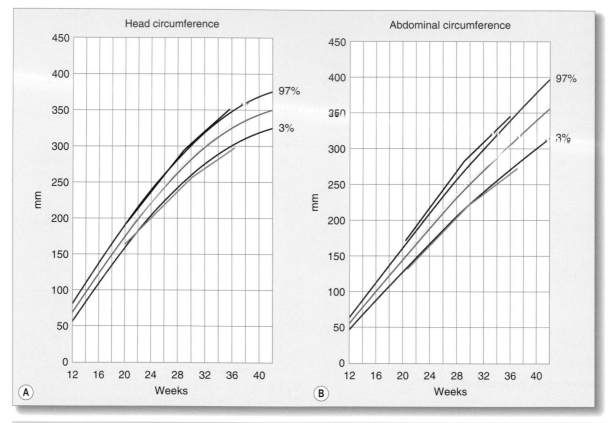

Fig 13.4 • Head circumference and abdominal circumference values are shown plotted along the 3rd centile, 50th centile and 97th centile. These are denoted by the orange, yellow and black lines, respectively. The head/abdomen (H/A) value will lie on the 50th centile for all three cases as shown in Fig. 13.6. *(From Chitty L S, Altman D J, Henderson A, Campbell S. 1994 BJOG. Charts of fetal size: 2. Head measurements. 101[1] 35–43; Chitty L S, Altman D J, Henderson A, Campbell S. 1994 BJOG. Charts of fetal size: 3. Abdominal measurements. 101[2] 125–131.)*

asymmetrical. They are both characterized by small AC measurements and distinguished by the size of the HC.

Symmetrical intrauterine growth restriction

Symmetrical IUGR is the description given to the equivalent reduction in growth velocity of both the head and abdomen and therefore the HC and AC. Thus although both the HC and AC cross centiles with gestation, the number of centiles they cross is the same (Fig. 13.8). The ratio between the HC and AC therefore remains unchanged and the H/A ratio falls normally (Fig. 13.6). In the majority of pregnancies this picture represents a constitutionally small fetus which is fulfilling its genetic potential. In a very small number of pregnancies, symmetrical IUGR occurs in pathological pregnancies.

The constitutionally small fetus

Constitutionally fetuses typically demonstrate decreasing growth velocity initially but then maintain a normal growth pattern along their 'chosen' centile. They are typically structurally normal with a normal amniotic fluid volume and uterine, umbilical and fetal Doppler values within the normal range.

The pathologically small fetus

Pathologically small fetuses have been exposed to an insult or injury in early pregnancy or are chromosomally abnormal. The majority of these pregnancies have severe early onset uteroplacental insufficiency or karyotypic abnormalities, typically triploidy. The growth velocity in these pregnancies continues to fall with increasing gestation,

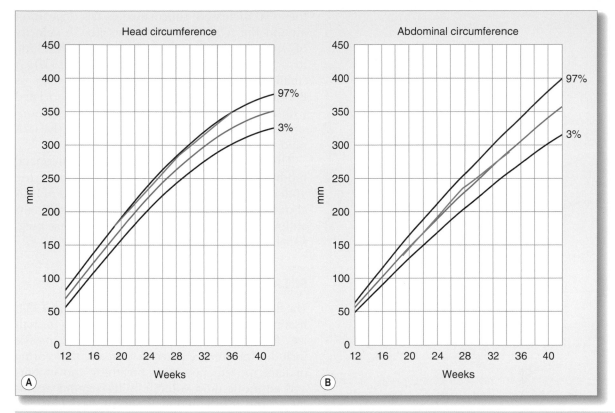

Fig 13.5 • The head circumference values are shown plotted along the 97th centile (left panel). The abdominal circumference values are shown plotted along the 50th centile (right panel). The corresponding head/abdomen (H/A) ratio will lie above the 50th centile (Fig. 13.6). *(From Chitty L S, Altman D J, Henderson A, Campbell S. 1994 BJOG. Charts of fetal size: 2. Head measurements. 101[1] 35–43; Chitty L S, Altman D J, Henderson A, Campbell S. 1994 BJOG. Charts of fetal size: 3. Abdominal measurements. 101[2] 125–131.)*

resulting in severe IUGR and very poor pregnancy outcome. Umbilical and fetal Doppler studies may be normal or abnormal depending on the underlying cause. In cases of fetal abnormality or infection, the uterine artery Dopplers and the amniotic fluid volume are normal unless the urinary tract is involved. In these situations, consideration should be given to prenatal diagnosis of chromosomal abnormality or congenital viral infection.

Asymmetrical growth restriction

Asymmetrical IUGR is the description given to a differential reduction in growth velocity of the fetal head and the abdomen. In the vast majority of cases, asymmetrical fetal growth restriction is a consequence of uteroplacental insufficiency. The H/A ratio increases (Fig. 13.6) as a result of arterial redistribution of blood flow preserving head growth, and therefore the normal size of the HC, and loss of subcutaneous fat around the trunk, reducing growth of the AC (Fig. 13.9). These physiological changes are reflected in changes in the umbilical artery and fetal Doppler studies.

LARGE FOR DATES

Large for dates (LGA) describes those fetuses with an EFW above the 90th centile for gestational age. They can also be described as macrosomic. The fetal biometry measurements lie at the upper limit of, or above, the normal range but do not cross centiles; thus the growth velocity in these pregnancies increases initially but then remains normal. Similar to the SGA group, the majority of fetuses

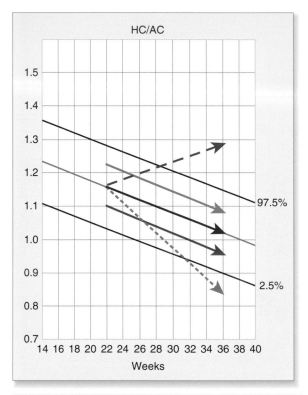

Fig 13.6 • Head circumference/abdominal circumference (HC/AC) ratio chart is shown with various growth patterns plotted.

- Red denotes normal growth where the HC and AC remain on the same centiles (growth patterns shown in Fig. 13.4 and symmetrical growth restriction (growth pattern shown in Fig. 13.8).
- Turquoise denotes large head circumference with normal abdominal circumference (growth pattern shown in Fig. 13.5).
- Dark blue denotes small HC with normal AC (growth pattern shown in Fig. 13.7).
- Purple (dashed) denotes asymmetrical growth restriction (growth pattern shown in Fig. 13.9).
- Green (dashed) denotes poor diabetic control (growth pattern shown in Fig. 13.10). *(From Snijders RJM, Nicolaides K H et al 1994 Fetal biometry at 14–40 weeks gestation. Ultrasound Obstet Gynecol 4:34–48.)*

in this group are constitutionally rather than pathologically large. A proportion are large for extrinsic reasons such as poor glycaemic control in maternal diabetes and gestational diabetes. Such cases demonstrate accelerated fetal abdominal growth, as

there is increased subcutaneous fat deposition around the fetal trunk. Thus the growth velocity of only the AC increases (Fig. 13.10), resulting in a reduction in the H/A ratio (Fig. 13.6). A small number of genetic conditions, such as Beckwith Wiedemann syndrome, are associated with increased fetal growth. As such cases demonstrate accelerated but generalized growth, the H/A ratio remains normal.

The risk of intrapartum maternal and neonatal morbidity increases when the EFW is above the 90th centile. Therefore, antenatal diagnosis of LGA allows clinicians to plan the delivery accordingly, although providing an accurate EFW in these pregnancies is challenging, as discussed earlier.

FETAL BIOPHYSICAL PROFILE

The first biophysical profile was published in 1984, its aim being the use of a scoring system to formalize fetal behavioural assessment. The profile includes four or five criteria. These are the scoring of fetal movements, tone, breathing movements and amniotic fluid volume by ultrasound assessment. The fifth criterion is the subjective assessment of the fetal heart rate pattern. Healthy fetuses would demonstrate good tone, general movement, breathing movements, amniotic fluid volume and a reactive heart rate pattern. Each criterion is allocated a maximum score of 2. The maximum biophysical profile score therefore is 10 if all five criteria are used and 8 if heart rate assessment is excluded.

A review of randomized trials has concluded that there is insufficient evidence to support the use of the biophysical profile as a test of fetal well-being in high-risk pregnancies.

It is included here because a modified type of biophysical profiling – the reporting of fetal movements and amniotic fluid volume, for example – is used in many departments in the assessment of fetal well-being. Reduced biophysical profile and/or modified profiling scores are found in growth-restricted pregnancies that already demonstrate abnormal umbilical and fetal Doppler findings.

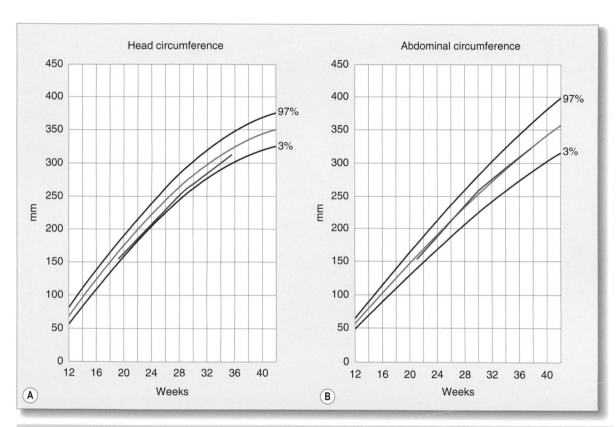

Fig 13.7 • The head circumference values are shown plotted along the 10th centile (left panel). The abdominal circumference values are shown plotted along the 50th centile (right panel). The corresponding head/abdomen ratio will lie below the 50th centile (Fig. 13.6). *(From Chitty L S, Altman D J, Henderson A, Campbell S. 1994 BJOG. Charts of fetal size: 2. Head measurements. 101[1] 35–43; Chitty L S, Altman D J, Henderson A, Campbell S. 1994 BJOG. Charts of fetal size: 3. Abdominal measurements. 101[2] 125–131.)*

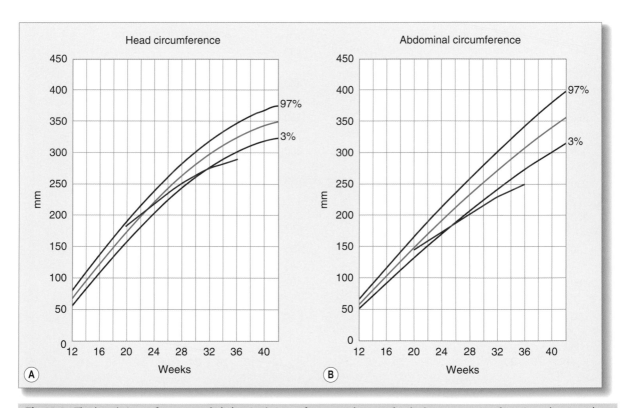

Fig 13.8 • The head circumference and abdominal circumference values are both shown crossing from just above and on the 50th centile at 20 weeks of gestation respectively to below the 3rd centile at 36 weeks of gestation. This growth pattern is typical of symmetrical growth restriction (Fig. 13.6). *(From Chitty L S, Altman D J, Henderson A, Campbell S. 1994 BJOG. Charts of fetal size: 2. Head measurements. 101[1] 35–43; Chitty L S, Altman D J, Henderson A, Campbell S. 1994 BJOG. Charts of fetal size: 3. Abdominal measurements. 101[2] 125–131.)*

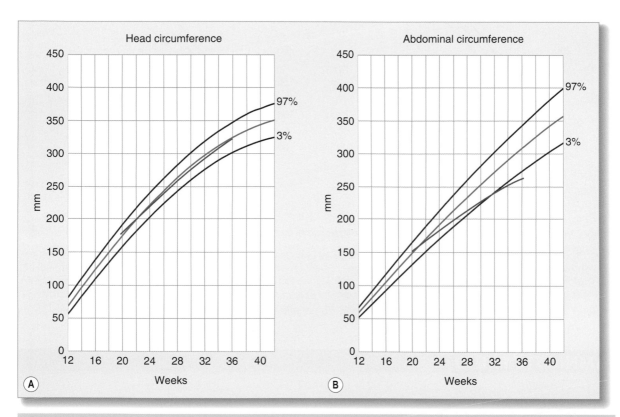

Fig 13.9 • The head circumference values are shown plotted along the 50th centile (left panel). The abdominal circumference values are shown crossing from the 50th centile at 20 weeks of gestation to below the 3rd centile at around 33 weeks of gestation. This growth pattern is typical of asymmetrical growth restriction (Fig. 13.6). *(From Chitty L S, Altman D J, Henderson A, Campbell S. 1994 BJOG. Charts of fetal size: 2. Head measurements. 101[1] 35–43; Chitty L S, Altman D J, Henderson A, Campbell S. 1994 BJOG. Charts of fetal size: 3. Abdominal measurements. 101[2] 125–131.)*

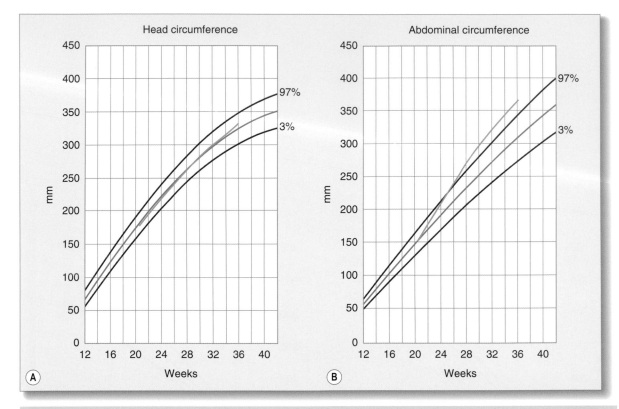

Fig 13.10 • The head circumference (HC) values are shown plotted along the 50th centile (left panel). The AC values are shown crossing from the 50th centile at 20 weeks of gestation to above the 97th centile at around 27 weeks of gestation. This growth pattern is typical of poor glycaemic control in maternal diabetes (Fig. 13.6). *(From Chitty L S, Altman D J, Henderson A, Campbell S. 1994 BJOG. Charts of fetal size: 2. Head measurements. 101[1] 35–43; Chitty L S, Altman D J, Henderson A, Campbell S. 1994 BJOG. Charts of fetal size: 3. Abdominal measurements. 101[2] 125–131.)*

AMNIOTIC FLUID

As discussed briefly in Chapter 8, from approximately 16 weeks of gestation the majority of amniotic fluid is fetal urine. The amniotic fluid volume increases from approximately 250 ml at 16 weeks to 1000 ml at 34 weeks, decreasing thereafter to approximately 800 ml at term. The amniotic fluid volume reflects the status of both the mother and the fetus and is altered in many physiological and pathological conditions. Ultrasound has a potential role in the management of such conditions by the assessment of amniotic fluid volume.

ASSESSMENT OF AMNIOTIC FLUID VOLUME

There are three methods for assessing amniotic fluid volume.

- subjective assessment
- single deepest pool
- amniotic fluid index.

Subjective Assessment

With experience, it is possible to classify amniotic fluid volume into the broad categories of absent, low, normal, increased and excessive. Although reliable in the hands of an experienced operator, this method has proved impossible to standardize in clinical and research terms.

Single Deepest Pool

The size of the deepest cord free pool of amniotic fluid is assessed with the ultrasound probe held

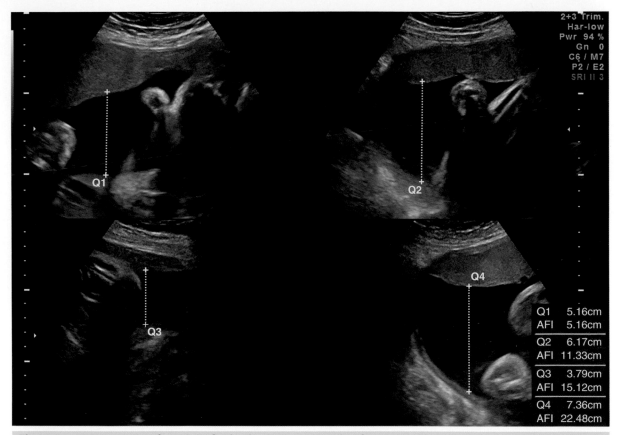

		2+3 Trim.
Q1	5.16cm	Har-low
AFI	5.16cm	Pwr 94 %
Q2	6.17cm	Gn 0
AFI	11.33cm	C6 / M7
Q3	3.79cm	P2 / E2
AFI	15.12cm	SRI II 3
Q4	7.36cm	
AFI	22.48cm	

Fig 13.11 • Measurement of amniotic fluid index (AFI) at 28 weeks of gestation. The AFI measured 22.48 cm, which is approaching the upper end of the normal range.

perpendicular to the anteroposterior (AP) axis of the uterus. It does not matter whether you are imaging the uterus in a longitudinal, transverse or oblique section. The vertical depth of the largest pool is measured. The pool may extend from the anterior uterine wall to the posterior uterine wall or may extend from the chorionic plate of an anterior or posterior placenta to part of the fetus. Using this method, *anhydramnios* describes the absence of any cord free pools. *Oligohydramnios* is defined as a single deepest pool of less than 2.0 cm and *polyhydramnios* as a single deepest pool greater than 8.0 cm. The normal range for amniotic fluid using the single deepest pool technique is therefore 2.0–8.0 cm.

Amniotic Fluid Index

The amniotic fluid index is a semi-quantitative technique for assessing amniotic fluid volume. The maternal abdomen is divided into four quadrants and the ultrasound probe placed on the maternal abdomen to obtain a longitudinal section of the uterus. The depth of the largest vertical pool, perpendicular to the AP axis of the uterus, is measured in each quadrant. The sum of these measurements represents the amniotic fluid index (AFI) (Fig. 13.11). If the fetus is very active, you will soon realize that the fluid depth in each quadrant can easily change before you have time to complete all four measurements.

The AFI is known to vary with gestational age and decreases towards term. Between 24 and 37 weeks the normal range for AFI is 10.0–24.0 cm, and after 37 weeks it is 7.0–24.0 cm. An AFI of less than 10.0 cm up to 37 weeks and less than 7.0 cm after 37 weeks is defined as *reduced* and less than 5.0 cm between 24 weeks and term as *oligohydramnios*. An AFI greater than 24.0 cm between

321

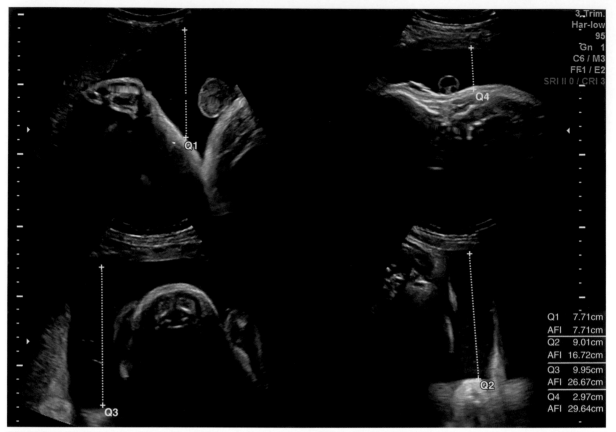

Q1	7.71cm
AFI	7.71cm
Q2	9.01cm
AFI	16.72cm
Q3	9.95cm
AFI	26.67cm
Q4	2.97cm
AFI	29.64cm

Fig 13.12 • Measurement of amniotic fluid index (AFI) at 32 weeks of gestation. This is a case of polyhydramnios, as the AFI measures 29.64 cm.

24 weeks and term is defined as *polyhydramnios* (Fig. 13.12).

Various authors have published AFI charts which vary quite considerably in their respective normal ranges and also how they correspond to charts of deepest pool. From a clinical perspective this is problematic, as an AFI of 8.0 cm at 34 weeks is within the normal range on chart A, borderline on chart B and below the 5th centile on chart C. Because action is usually required if a measurement falls outside the normal range, plotting AFI values on chart C is very likely to result in a percentage of pregnancies with a normal AFI being referred for further ultrasound assessment by clinical colleagues. Unless you are using an AFI chart in which the normal range equates to the values given here, we recommend that the numerical value of AFI is reported only and an AFI chart is not used.

Deepest Vertical Pool or AFI?

There is disagreement among authors as to whether measuring the deepest vertical pool or the AFI in singleton pregnancies is the more sensitive test to assess amniotic fluid volume. There is acceptance, however, that measuring the deepest vertical pocket is the recommended method in multiple pregnancies.

OLIGOHYDRAMNIOS/ANHYDRAMNIOS

There are three main pathological reasons for the finding of reduced or absent amniotic fluid:

- *abnormal renal function* – Unilateral renal problems in the fetus are usually associated with a normal amniotic fluid volume. Conversely, bilateral renal agenesis; polycystic kidney disease, which by definition is bilateral; bilateral multicystic dysplasia; and bladder outflow obstruction characteristically present with severe oligohydramnios or anhydramnios on ultrasound (see Fig. 11.23B)

- *amniotic membrane rupture* – The maternal history of persistent vaginal loss and dampness would suggest a diagnosis of prelabour or premature rupture of membranes (PROM). This is often associated with anhydramnios (Fig. 8.19) rather than oligohydramnios. The finding of normal amniotic fluid volume or oligohydramnios, however, does not exclude this diagnosis. In cases of PROM which have been confirmed by speculum examination, ultrasound is useful in confirming or otherwise the presence of a normal amniotic fluid volume
- *uteroplacental insufficiency* – The reduction in blood supply to the fetal kidneys results in decreased urine production and consequently oligo- or anhydramnios. Associated features are symmetrically or asymmetrically small fetal size and abnormal Doppler studies.

Prognosis

Anhydramnios or severe oligohydramnios, as a consequence of midtrimester PROM or renal pathological conditions, is often associated with a poor prognosis owing to the pulmonary hypoplasia that is a consequence of early and prolonged lack of amniotic fluid. Where the oligohydramnios is due to uteroplacental insufficiency, the management will depend on the severity of the growth restriction and the gestation of the pregnancy.

POLYHYDRAMNIOS

Polyhydramnios is defined as excess amniotic fluid volume for a given gestation of pregnancy. This is an idiopathic 'physiological' finding in approximately 1% of pregnancies in the third trimester and will be identified relatively frequently during third trimester growth scans.

Pathological Causes of Polyhydramnios

Polyhydramnios can occur as a result of increased fetal urine production, the most common causes for this being maternal diabetes mellitus and constitutional fetal macrosomia. This is most typically a third trimester finding in these pregnancies.

Polyhydramnios during the second trimester is uncommon and is most typically associated with a pathological fetal condition or fetal structural abnormality. Pathological conditions that predispose to a fetal hyperdynamic circulation, include fetal anemia resulting from rhesus disease or parvovirus infection.

Fetal abnormalities associated with second trimester polyhydramnios include the following:

- conditions in which the fetal chest is small, such as in asphyxiating thoracic dystrophy
- conditions in which swallowing and the normal absorption of amniotic fluid in the gastrointestinal tract are compromised. This usually is due to an atretic section of the tract, such as in oesophageal or duodenal atresia, and is more typically a feature of the third trimester rather than the second
- conditions in which a structural abnormality results in a hyperdynamic fetal circulation, such as sacrococcygeal teratoma (see Fig. 12.6)
- conditions in which the fetus appears structurally normal but is small or very small. Polyhydramnios in association with an apparently normal but small second trimester fetus, especially one which shows very few movements, is associated with chromosomal abnormalities or neurogenic disease
- conditions in which chorioangioma of the placenta at the cord insertion is present (see Chapter 14).

Prognosis

The prognosis for polyhydramnios is dependent on the cause of the condition. When the cause is idiopathic, the prognosis is usually very good, with the only complication being premature delivery as a result of uterine overdistension.

AFI IN THE TERM AND POST-TERM PREGNANCY

There is a well-recognized association among prolonged or post-term pregnancy, reduced amniotic fluid volume and poorer fetal and neonatal outcomes compared with outcomes from pregnancies with normal amniotic fluid which were delivered at term. As discussed previously, amniotic fluid volume decreases with advancing gestation, and this is reflected in the lowering of the normal range of AFI values towards term. Clinical management of women who decline induction towards or at term is likely to include assessment of AFI on a weekly or twice weekly basis in these post-term pregnancies. As the AFI measurement in such cases is extremely important, we recommend that you repeat the AFI measurements three times in every examination to ensure that your reported measurement is as accurate as possible.

RECOMMENDED SCANNING INTERVALS

The interval between ultrasound examinations is dependent on the variability, and therefore the 'accuracy', of the measurement being taken and the change in size of the parameter being measured over time. A time interval of 2 weeks is generally considered to be the minimum time interval between two ultrasound examinations where measurements of the HC, AC and FL are taken to assess fetal growth. This time interval should only be adopted in cases where the same operator, using the same equipment, performs the two scans. A 3 week time interval is preferable, and acceptable, for the majority of cases.

When oligohydramnios is present in the preterm pregnancy, serial assessment of the amniotic fluid volume can be performed on a weekly basis. Twice weekly assessment of amniotic fluid is recommended in the post-term pregnancy, as discussed earlier.

When polyhydramnios is present, serial assessment of amniotic fluid volume can be performed every 2 weeks.

Doppler studies are the only ultrasound examinations that may need to be carried out more frequently than weekly.

PERFORMING DOPPLER ULTRASOUND STUDIES

'Doppler' ultrasound includes, in the order in which they were developed for clinical use, continuous wave, pulsed wave or spectral, colour flow and power Doppler modalities. The principles of these techniques are described in Chapter 1.

Spectral and colour Doppler techniques are routinely used in current obstetric ultrasound practice, with 'Doppler' providing an important additional tool in the clinical management of the late second and third trimester compromised pregnancy.

Continuous wave Doppler imaging is used to perform M (for motion) mode fetal cardiac studies and is beyond the scope of this text.

Power Doppler imaging is used in obstetric imaging as an adjunct to colour Doppler.

The following text describes how to obtain, apply and interpret waveforms using colour and spectral Doppler techniques.

As you will be aware from Chapter 1, colour flow and power Doppler imaging both enable blood vessels to be imaged and information relating to blood flow within them to be assessed. Both permit blood vessels to be distinguished from other fluid collections. Colour flow imaging provides information about direction of flow, whilst power Doppler imaging displays information which is nondirectional but relates to the energy or power within the blood vessel. Power Doppler imaging processes the Doppler signal differently than colour flow imaging, and this results in the ability of power Doppler to image much smaller vessels and those with lower flow rates than colour Doppler. Power Doppler imaging therefore could be considered as the more sensitive of the two modalities but, as direction of flow is an important component of Doppler examinations, colour flow imaging remains the default modality of the two techniques. For this reason this text therefore refers primarily to colour flow Doppler imaging.

Once the required vessel has been identified using colour Doppler, spectral Doppler is applied. The resulting waveform is then assessed both qualitatively and quantitatively, with the clinical significance of either the shape of the waveform or the measurements taken depending on the specific vessel under interrogation.

In practice, therefore, colour Doppler and spectral Doppler complement each other. As colour and spectral Doppler images are produced in different ways, it is important to understand how to manipulate the ultrasound controls that affect the appearances of both the colour image and the spectral trace to maximize image quality and minimize measurement errors.

Your first task is to decide which vessel you wish to interrogate, followed by your second task, which is finding it. Let us assume that the grey scale image in front of you demonstrates the vessel you are seeking.

In brief, you now need to activate the colour flow control, often helpfully labelled 'C'. This superimposes a box of predetermined size on the screen, within which colour flow will appear. You then must activate the spectral trace or pulsed-wave control, often helpfully labelled 'PW'. This control superimposes a vertical sampling line on the screen. A 'gate', represented by two small horizontal lines, is present along this line. The spectral trace is then obtained by activating the 'go' or 'update' control. By adjusting the colour box, sampling line and gate correctly you will produce a, hopefully, perfect waveform from the vessel you wish to interrogate, which you can then assess and measure.

These steps are explained in more detail next.

COLOUR FLOW

Colour flow uses the shift in Doppler frequencies resulting from blood flow to produce a directional map of flow within the vessels being interrogated. This colour map is superimposed over the B mode grey scale image. The colours assigned show the direction of the blood flow. Typically, red is used to indicate flow towards the probe, and therefore the ultrasound beam, and blue for blood flowing away from the probe. The colours can be reversed if desired, by selecting the invert control so that blue now denotes the flow towards and red away from the probe. The shade of the red and blue is an indicator of the mean velocity of flow within the vessel. As velocity and angle are two

components of the Doppler equation, it should come as no surprise that the intensity of the colour displayed is dependent on the angle of the insonant ultrasound beam to the vessel. You can test the effect of this angle by dipping the probe – thus changing the angle of the blood vessel under investigation relative to the ultrasound beam – and observing the colour changes within the vessel.

Applying colour Doppler increases the total power to which the fetus is exposed. It is therefore important that you learn how the thermal index (TI) changes when you activate the colour control and also when you change the dimensions of the colour box.

The four points you must consider when using colour flow are as follows:

- the position and size of the colour box or region of interest (ROI)
- the angle of insonation
- the colour flow scale or pulse repetition frequency (PRF)
- the colour flow gain.

The Position and Size of the Colour Box

The colour box defines the area within which examination and/or sampling of the vessels of interest takes place. Having activated the colour flow control, you must now move the colour box over the vessels of interest using the tracker ball control. The position and depth of the box affect the sensitivity of the colour information displayed and also the power output of the examination.

The Doppler shift is influenced by the depth of the target vessel – or the distance of the colour box from the face of the probe – and therefore go/ return times. The time taken for the incident frequency signal to go from, and the shifted frequency signal to return to, the probe in turn influences the PRF. The PRF influences the velocity of blood flow that can be detected within a blood vessel. Thus the position and size of the colour box can be considered to be inversely proportional to the quality of the colour image – as the deeper the colour box, both in terms of its own vertical size and its vertical position relative to the probe, the lower the PRF available.

The width of the colour box also affects the potential quality of the colour image, as it determines the number of lines which need to be examined for evidence of Doppler shift within a certain time period and thus the frame rate.

You are unable to influence the position of the colour box relative to the probe, as this is obviously determined by the position within the uterus or maternal pelvis of the vessel being interrogated. You can, however, influence colour image quality by reducing the width and depth of the box as much as possible by using the horizontal and vertical colour box size adjustment controls.

Although the reducing the size of the colour box increases the colour Doppler resolution, the amount of power concentrated within the region of interest increases as the size of the box decreases. You must make sure, therefore, that the TI remains within safe limits – that is, less than 0.7 ideally and certainly less than 1.0 – irrespective of the size of the colour box. You may also observe that changing the depth of the colour box has a greater influence on the TI than changing its width.

Angle of Insonation

The optimum angle of insonation is 0°, or complete alignment of the beam with the direction of flow within the vessel. This is often difficult, so the angle should be made as small as possible, and certainly less than 60°, in order to obtain informative waveforms. The probe movement required to minimize the angle of insonation is dipping. Where the angle of insonation approaches 90° the Doppler shift is minimal, resulting in an ambiguous and/or unclear 'colour map' of the vessel within which little or no flow is demonstrated.

The reasons why the angle of insonation is important in terms of the Doppler equation are explained in Chapter 1.

Colour Flow Scale or Pulse Repetition Frequency

The principles behind colour flow scale or PRF in Doppler imaging and B mode imaging are broadly similar, the difference being that in the former it is the frequency shift that is being analyzed, whereas in the latter it is the difference in acoustic impedance across an interface. The PRF is the frequency of pulses generated by the probe. Note that this is not the same as the frequency of the probe. The PRF determines the maximum and minimum flow speeds within which the examination will be informative and therefore accurate.

The Doppler frequency shift cannot be estimated correctly unless the PRF is high enough for a sufficient number of samples along the beam to be analyzed. You will not be able to detect vessels with low velocity flow if you set the PRF too high. Conversely, setting the PRF too low will result in aliasing in those vessels with high velocity flow. Using colour to identify the umbilical artery, for example, requires a higher PRF setting than when locating the pulmonary veins entering the fetal heart.

Aliaising

Aliasing describes the effect of applying a PRF setting that is too low for the flow in the blood vessel being interrogated. It results in artefactual information being displayed in both the colour Doppler image and the spectral waveform. The maximum Doppler frequency that can be detected is one half of the PRF. This is known as the Nyquist criterion. Where higher frequency signals are present, then the sampled waveform cannot be reconstructed properly and the flow within the vessel is represented by incorrectly coloured pixels. The blood flow in the vessel is displayed as a mixture of colours including blue, red, yellow and green rather than the anticipated single colour. The information relating to flow and its direction in these situations is therefore inaccurate.

Aliaising is a useful tool, however, in identifying turbulent or high velocity flow within a vessel. This may be unexpected and therefore can be used as an indication of a potentially important clinical finding – regurgitant flow at an atretic valve, for example. Alternatively, it may be a normal feature of the vasculature at a specific anatomical point and is thus very helpful in the location of that area – identifying the ductus venosus, for example.

When colour flow is used to visualize the umbilical cord, for example, and the PRF is set correctly, both the lower flow in the vein and the higher velocities in the arteries will be clearly demonstrated. When the PRF is set too low, flow will be detected in the vein as previously, but aliasing will be present within the umbilical arteries. Setting the PRF too low will result in flow in the arteries being seen but no flow apparent in the vein.

Colour Flow Gain

Colour flow gain is used to adjust the overall sensitivity to the blood flow signals. Setting the gain too high results in extraneous colour flow signals or noise from surrounding tissue appearing as a random display of coloured dots or speckle across the whole colour box. This makes identification of the vessel and flow within it difficult. Setting the gain too low results in loss of potential flow information within vessels or being able to 'see' other vessels.

We recommend adjusting the PRF before adjusting the gain, as this sequence will maximize the sensitivity of your Doppler examination. In some circumstances the flow states may be such that the initial settings produce an image with far too much noise or, alternatively, insufficient information to visualize the vessel properly. Should this be the case, make a small adjustment of the gain first, then maximize the PRF for the required vessel and then optimize the image with the gain control.

SPECTRAL OR PULSED WAVE DOPPLER

The use of colour flow imaging alone provides directional information, but more detailed assessment of direction of flow and calculation of indices to inform clinical management require the use of spectral or pulsed wave (PW) Doppler. This produces the waveforms from which such assessment and calculations can be made.

Spectral Doppler increases the total power to which the fetus is exposed. Although the power outputs from colour and spectral Doppler imaging vary between manufacturers, the output from spectral Doppler is generally greater than from colour Doppler in the same machine. It is therefore important that you learn how the TI changes when you activate the spectral Doppler control.

You have now obtained a colour map of the vessel from which you wish to obtain a spectral trace. Your task now is to produce a waveform which will provide you with accurate and clinically helpful qualitative and quantitative information. To do this you must consider the following:

- the sampling line
- position and size of the sample gate
- activating the spectral trace
- the PW scale or PRF
- the PW gain

- the baseline
- wall motion filter
- sweep speed
- measuring the waveform.

The above are described in more detail in the following sections.

Sampling Line

Having placed the colour box over the required vessel, you need to produce the sampling line. This is done by activating the spectral trace or PW control. This control superimposes a vertical sampling line on the screen which should be positioned across the vessel, using the tracker ball. This line represents the direction of the insonant beam to the vessel and should, ideally, be down the barrel of the vessel, or as close to 0° as possible.

Position and Size of the Sample Gate

You will notice the sample 'gate', represented by two small horizontal lines positioned along the sampling line. The gate defines the size of the sample volume from which your waveform will be produced. The size of the sample volume can be adjusted by increasing or decreasing the vertical size of the gate. The range of velocities present within the waveform is dependent on how much of the vessel is sampled. The velocities in the centre of the vessel are higher than those towards the vessel walls. The angle of the sampling line to the vessel will also determine whether you have the option of opening the gate so that the sample volume extends to, or includes, the vessel wall on either side. This is a possibility if the angle between the vessel you are sampling and your sampling line is wide, approaching 60°, as the sampling gate is in approximate alignment with the barrel of the vessel. However, if the sampling line and vessel are in complete alignment, changing the gate size gives you no control over how much of the width of the vessel you are sampling, as the gate is at 90° to the barrel of the vessel.

It is advisable to start with a relatively wide sample gate to make sure that the maximum velocities throughout each cardiac cycle are recorded. As discussed later, the exact positioning of the gate along a vessel varies depending on the specific vessel being interrogated.

327

Activating the Spectral Trace

Having positioned the gate correctly, activate the spectral trace. Machines vary as to how the waveform and the colour flow image with sampling line and gate are displayed. The colour flow image is conventionally displayed in the upper half of the screen with the waveform displayed in the lower half of the screen. The relative sizes of both displays can be altered on some machines. It is also possible to toggle between the colour flow image filling the screen and the waveform filling the screen. Pressing the control of the display which is not required a second time will remove that display from the screen.

Showing both displays together in real time has a significant effect on frame rate. The machine is therefore usually set up so that the colour flow image is frozen while the spectral trace is running and vice versa. The colour flow image can be reactivated by using the 'update' control, which will then freeze the spectral trace display. Pressing either the update control or the PW control a second time, which will depend on the machine being used, will freeze the colour flow image and set the spectral trace to run again.

PW Scale or Pulse Repetition Frequency

As discussed earlier, the PW scale, or PRF, should be adjusted to suit the flow conditions within the vessel so that the waveform is clearly defined and easy to interpret. A low PRF setting will allow visualization and measurement of low velocity vessels but, as with colour flow imaging, will result in aliasing if used with vessels with high velocity flow. Altering the PRF adjusts the scale on the y axis of the spectral trace, resulting in a change in the height of the waveform displayed. The PRF should be set so that the waveform fills at least 75% of the screen. Setting the PRF too low may result in the loss of the systolic peaks of the waveform in the correct channel and their appearance in the opposite channel. This is due to aliasing. When the PRF is too high, the waveform displayed is too shallow for its shape to be interpreted or measured accurately.

PW Gain

The PW gain should be adjusted so that the waveform can be clearly visualized against a background display that is free from noise. The waveform should display shades of grey or gradations of a selected colour. Whether shades of grey or of a colour are shown will depend on the display format selected. The shades of colour reflect the range of frequencies that can be identified within the vessel and should be obvious within the waveform. When the gain is set correctly, the overall waveform should be neither too bright nor too dark. An overbright waveform removes the distinction between the differing frequencies, whereas a waveform that is too dark provides inadequate information for subsequent analysis.

Baseline

You will notice that the spectral trace which you have now produced has a horizontal line running through it. This is called the baseline and represents zero Doppler shift. The baseline indicates the watershed between forward flow, normally shown in the channel above the baseline, and reverse flow, normally shown in the channel below the baseline. The velocity scale displayed on the y axis, to the left and the right of the horizontal waveform, confirms which channel displays positive velocities and which displays negative velocities. Using normal settings, flow towards the probe, as represented by red in the colour map, will produce a waveform above the baseline, interpreted as forward flow. Flow away from the probe, as represented by blue in the colour map, will produce a waveform below the baseline, interpreted as reverse flow. The invert control for either colour flow or for PW will reverse the channel in which the waveform is displayed. This control is useful when sampling a tortuous vessel, the direction of which keeps changing.

The baseline also allows flow within a cardiac cycle to be categorized as forward or reverse. Flow during the majority of one cardiac cycle may be above the baseline, therefore indicating forward flow, but may drop below the baseline at one or more intervals during the cardiac cycle, indicating reverse flow. A waveform demonstrating forward and reverse flow is normal in some blood vessels, such as the maternal iliac arteries, but is abnormal in the umbilical artery or the fetal ductus venosus.

Where you position the baseline is dependent on the vessel you are interrogating. Where reverse flow is not a characteristic of the vessel – the uterine artery or middle cerebral artery are examples – then the baseline can be positioned at the bottom of the display. This allows you to use the complete display for the trace from the upper channel. Where you are actively looking for reverse flow – the umbilical artery or ductus venosus are examples – then the baseline should be positioned more towards the centre of the display to allow flow in both channels to be assessed.

Wall Motion Filter

The wall motion filter, or the 'low velocity reject' control, is used to eliminate noise produced by movement of the vessel walls. It is not a control that you will normally need to adjust, as it will usually have been set as low as possible (50–60 Hz) by the manufacturer in order to retain the flow information near to the baseline within the displayed waveform. When the motion filter is set too high, the diastolic component of the waveform may not be displayed because these velocities are so low they have been rejected by the machine's software. The resulting waveform, in which end-diastolic frequencies are absent, could be interpreted incorrectly, leading to inappropriate clinical management decisions being made. Adjusting the wall motion filter is usually only necessary where absent end diastolic flow is suspected, to determine whether the frequencies at the end of diastole are truly absent or are so low that they have been rejected because the wall motion filter setting is too high to record them within the waveform.

Sweep Speed

Sweep speed describes the speed at which the spectral trace moves across the screen and therefore the number of cardiac cycles which are represented on the screen at any one time. A slow sweep speed results in a large number of waveforms being shown. This makes assessment and measurement of individual waveforms unreliable. A very fast sweep speed will only show two or three waveforms on the screen at once. This is an insufficient number to ensure that the trace you have obtained is representative of true flow in that vessel over time. Thus the sweep speed should be fast enough to allow you to distinguish easily between the waveforms from successive cardiac cycles. The number of compete cardiac cycles that should be displayed on the moving or frozen image at any one time will depend

to some extent on the vessel being interrogated. Ideally the display should show at least three, but no more than 10, complete cardiac cycles.

Measuring the Waveform

You should now have a spectral trace of between three and 10 waveforms running across the ultrasound screen. Each blood vessel produces a characteristic waveform which has specific characteristics when normal and abnormal. Some of these features require visual interpretation, whereas others are assessed through measurements, as discussed later.

The spectral trace is assessed from the frozen image, which must display individual waveforms that are all consistent in shape. Thus before freezing the image, observe the running trace for a few seconds to ensure that the waveform remains consistent over time. The spectral trace from a fetus that is actively breathing, for example, produces successive waveforms of differing shapes and sizes. The measurements taken from such a trace therefore would be unreliable.

The outline of the waveform can be measured automatically or by hand. The automatic frequency follower can be adjusted to outline the whole trace displayed on the screen or a portion of the trace. It should be positioned so that the trace envelope it outlines contains only consistent waveforms, but with as many of them displayed sequentially on the screen as possible. This method is preferable to tracing the outline of one waveform by hand, although this may be necessary in situations where it is difficult to achieve a waveform that is consistent enough for the automatic frequency follower to trace accurately. A number of measurements will be automatically displayed on the screen when you press the 'enter' control after the outline has been traced. Alternatively, you can set up the frequency follower to run continuously with the moving trace. In this situation the same set of measurements, as calculated from the waveforms shown in the frozen trace, will be shown when you activate the freeze control.

The indices that have been used to measure the variations in flow during a cardiac cycle are the pulsatility index (PI), resistance index (RI) and A/B or S/D ratio. How these are calculated is discussed in Chapter 1. As the PI is the only one of these indices that remains informative when reverse flow is present, it is the measurement that is most commonly used in clinical practice and the one used in this text.

Angle correction

The value of the PI is not altered by the angle of the vessel to the ultrasound beam. Thus you do not need to take this into consideration when using PI measurements as they do not need to be 'angle corrected'. The angle correction control superimposes a thin line over the sample gate. The position of this line can be manipulated using the tracker ball control. Where angle correction is required, the bar should be positioned so that it lies within the lumen of the vessel being assessed, thereby measuring the angle of flow within that vessel to the insonant beam.

As velocity measurements are influenced by the angle of the vessel to the ultrasound beam, angle correction must be applied to obtain accurate measurements in such cases. Peak systolic velocity (PSV) measurements are taken of the middle cerebral artery in cases where fetal anaemia is present or suspected. These measurements are easy to perform, although it is unlikely that ultrasound management of anemic fetuses would be part of the routine workload.

UMBILICAL ARTERY DOPPLER

Doppler waveforms represent vascular impedance to flow downstream from the sampling site. Thus the umbilical artery waveform represents placental, not fetal, vascular resistance, as the direction of blood flow in this vessel is from the fetus to the placenta. Vascular impedence in the umbilical arteries falls with advancing gestation as a result of continuing development of the placental vascular system during pregnancy. Thus the PI falls with increasing gestation (Fig. 13.13). With uteroplacental insufficiency the umbilical artery impedance is increased only when a significant proportion of the placental vascular bed is obliterated. Characteristic umbilical artery waveforms have been found to correlate to various degrees of fetal hypoxaemia and acidaemia. Thus, as umbilical artery Doppler assessment is now a standard tool in the assessment of the growth restricted fetus, this is the vessel that you will interrogate most often when performing Doppler studies.

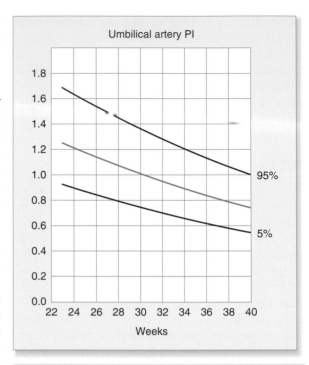

Fig 13.13 • Umbilical artery pulsatility index (PI) reference range. The 5th, 50th and 95th centiles are displayed. The PI values fall with increasing gestation.

Finding and Measuring the Umbilical Artery

There is a significant difference in PI values measured at the placental end, the fetal end or from a free loop of the cord, with impedance being highest at the fetal end. Absent or reversed EDF are therefore more likely to be seen first at this site. In practice, however, measurements are normally taken from a free loop of cord.

As the Doppler shift will be greatest when the ultrasound beam and blood flow are aligned, try to find a loop of cord in which one or both of the umbilical arteries lie vertically, rather than horizontally, on the screen. Despite the spiralling nature of the two umbilical arteries around the single vein, it is usually possible to obtain a small angle of insonation by dipping the probe to obtain a vertical position of the arteries. Alternatively, a different portion of umbilical cord in a more favourable position can be used where there is a smaller angle of insonation. Although both arteries may be well seen in your image, you only need to sample one of them.

Proceed through the steps described earlier to obtain a spectral trace displaying consistent waveforms. Once a satisfactory waveform of between four and six peaks of uniform size is displayed, freeze the image, select the part of the waveform to be measured, measure the PI and evaluate the waveform to determine whether or not EDF is present.

The umbilical artery PI should be calculated using the waveform envelope of four to six waveforms. As with all fetal measurements, umbilical artery PI measurements should be reproducible. We recommend, therefore, that you obtain PI values from three traces, each obtained separately, and that there should be no more than a 10% difference in PI values between the three. You should record the value from the most consistent trace, or the largest value if all the traces are of similar quality. The PI should be plotted on a data reference range and reported as being within, above or below the normal range for gestational age. Where previous PI measurements have been plotted, any obvious trend, especially if the PI is increasing, should be reported.

The Normal Umbilical Artery Waveform

The normal umbilical artery waveform is roughly triangular, with the apex representing peak systolic flow. Forward flow should be present throughout the cardiac cycle; thus the complete waveform of each cardiac cycle should be seen above the baseline (Fig. 13.14).

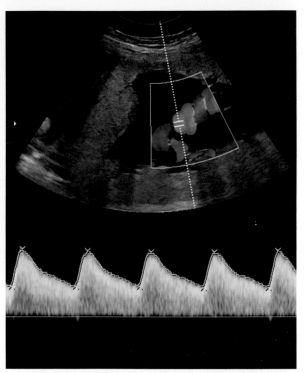

Fig 13.14 • A normal umbilical artery Doppler waveform at 30 weeks of gestation. The pulsatility index is 0.73. The colour flow mapping demonstrates flow in the umbilical arteries as red, confirming flow is towards the probe. Thus the spectral trace shows the waveform above the baseline. Note the triangular shape of the waveforms, with significant diastolic flow present at the end of each cardiac cycle.

The Abnormal Umbilical Artery Waveform

Abnormal findings of the umbilical artery waveform, in increasing severity, are a PI above the 95th centile, absent frequencies during or at the end of diastole and reversed flow during diastole. The latter are described as absent (Fig. 13.15) or reversed end-diastolic flow (EDF), respectively (Fig. 13.16).

Loss of end diastolic frequencies occurs only when more than 75% of the placental vascular bed has been obliterated. Loss of end diastolic frequencies before 36 weeks is associated with an 85% chance that the fetus will be hypoxaemic and a 50% chance that it will also be acidaemic. This is therefore a clinically significant finding and one which you must ensure is genuine and not artefactual. It is important to note that normal umbilical artery waveforms after 36 weeks of gestation do not exclude fetal hypoxaemia and acidaemia, although the significance of absent or reversed EDF towards term remains unchanged.

Thus when end diastolic frequencies appear absent, you must first exclude this finding being technique related. You should reduce the vessel wall filter to its lowest setting, or turn it off if possible. Dip the probe relative to the maternal abdomen to reduce the angle of insonation and increase the chance of the low frequencies in diastole being detected. If end diastolic frequencies are still absent, you should then attempt to obtain the signal from a different site, as this is likely to result in a different angle of insonation. Finally, fetal bradycardia is associated with decreased end diastolic frequencies, so ensure that the fetal heart rate is in the normal

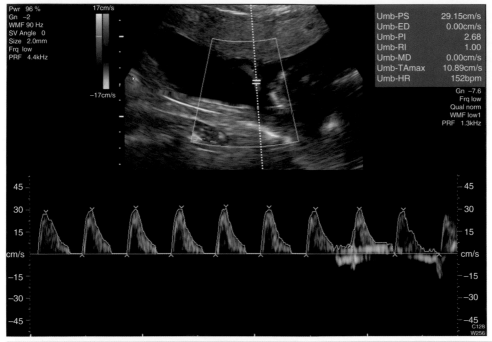

Fig 13.15 • Absent end diastolic flow in the umbilical artery at 24 weeks of gestation. The height of the systolic peak and the absence of flow through diastole are consistent across the first six cardiac cycles, after which the trace becomes unreliable. Note the raised pulsatility index (PI) value of 2.68. This measurement is likely to be unreliable, as the waveforms are not consistent in their appearance, especially the three at the right of the measured trace. This artery should be resampled to confirm the consistent finding of absent end diastolic flow.

range. A consistent finding of absent EDF after these techniques have been applied should be considered to be a genuine finding and reported as such.

The Umbilical Artery Waveform in Clinical Practice

A normal umbilical artery study, in which continuous forward flow and a normal PI are present, is a clinically reassuring finding in the growth restricted fetus before, but not after, 36 weeks of gestation.

A growth restricted fetus with normal umbilical artery waveforms before 36 weeks will not be acidaemic but has a 10% chance of being hypoxaemic. The pregnancy is very unlikely to develop loss of end diastolic frequencies within a 7–10 day period; therefore, Doppler monitoring can be performed weekly. It is important to note that normal umbilical artery waveforms after 36 weeks of gestation do not exclude fetal hypoxaemia and acidaemia.

Absent or reversed EDF in the umbilical artery is commonly associated with severe IUGR. The perinatal mortality rate in growth restricted fetuses with reversed EDF is 10 fold higher than in growth restricted fetuses with normal umbilical artery waveforms. Reversed EDF in such fetuses is considered to be a serious and preterminal condition. Few, if any, such fetuses will survive without delivery.

Although umbilical artery waveforms are invaluable in the management of fetal growth restriction, they are of little or no value as a screening test for the small for gestational age fetus. Additionally, umbilical artery Doppler studies do not appear to predict unexplained antepartum stillbirths or placental abruption.

Despite being commonly requested, umbilical artery Doppler studies are not of established value in the management of antepartum haemorrhage, preterm rupture of membranes, Rhesus isoimmunized, post term or multiple pregnancies, unless these coexist with fetal growth restriction.

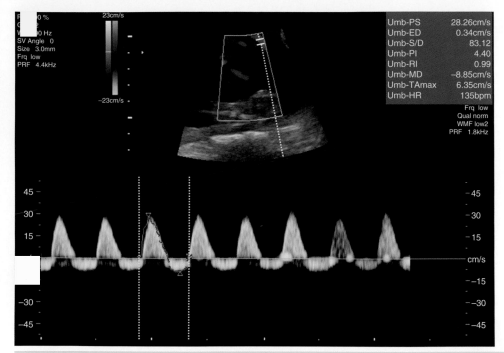

Fig 13.16 • Reversed end diastolic flow (EDF) in the umbilical artery at 23 weeks of gestation. The systolic and diastolic appearances are consistent across the trace. Note the raised pulsatility index (PI) value of 4.40, caused by the combination of the increased peak systolic values and the reversal of flow across the baseline, into the negative channel. This artery should be resampled to confirm the consistent finding of reversed EDF.

MIDDLE CEREBRAL ARTERY DOPPLER

The middle cerebral artery (MCA) carries more than 80% of the cerebral circulation. In normal circumstances the cerebral circulation is one of high impedance which increases up to 28 weeks of gestation, and then slowly decreases towards term, as reflected in the reference range for PI (Fig. 13.17A).

In cases of continued and progressive fetal hypoxia, blood flow to the fetal brain, heart, kidneys and adrenal glands is increased, with a reduction in flow to the peripheral circulation. This 'brain-sparing effect' results in dilation of the intracranial blood vessels and their decreasing impedance to flow. These adaptive strategies are reflected in changes in the normal MCA waveform.

In cases of Rhesus isoimmunization the maternal antibodies pass into the fetal circulation, causing destruction of the red cells, resulting in fetal anaemia. This leads to a hyperdynamic circulation within the fetus of increased cardiac output and increased velocity in the arterial circulation.

The degree of fetal anaemia correlates well with velocity measurements of the MCA, and a reference range for the peak systolic velocity (PSV) of the MCA is available for this purpose (Fig. 13.17B).

Finding and Measuring the Middle Cerebral Artery

The MCA forms part of the circle of Willis which lies slightly below, or caudal to, the HC plane. Obtain a transverse section of the fetal brain at the level of the HC and manipulate the image, by dipping the probe if necessary, so that the midline echo lies in the horizontal plane and therefore at 90° to the ultrasound beam. Slide the probe very slightly caudally to obtain the section in which the thalamus is seen in the centre of the brain, adjacent to the wing of the sphenoid bone which lies immediately anterior to it. Place the colour box over the centre of the brain. Blood flow will delineate the roughly circular circle of Willis, from which the

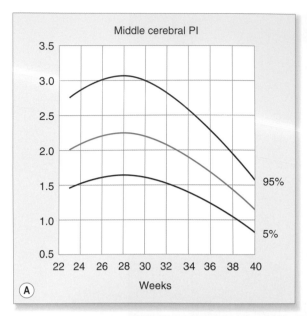

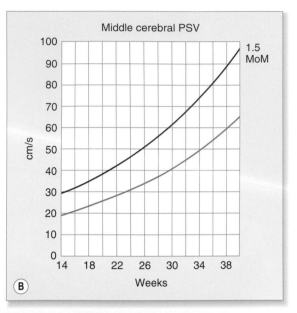

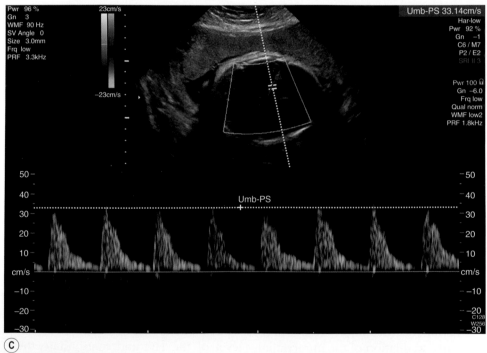

Fig 13.17 • A. Middle cerebral artery pulsatility index (PI) reference range. The 5th, 50th and 95th centiles are displayed. The PI values fall after 28 weeks of gestation. B. Middle cerebral artery (MCA) peak systolic velocity (PSV) reference range. C. Normal MCA Doppler waveform showing measurement of the PSV. Note the position of the angle correction bar (red line) parallel to the direction of the MCA, confirming that angle correction has been applied. The PSV value can therefore be taken as accurate. *(From Parra-Cordero M, Lees C, Missfelder-Lobos H, Seed P, Harris C 2007 Fetal arterial and venous Doppler pulsatility index and time averaged velocity ranges. Prenat Diag 27:1251–7.)*

posterior and middle cerebral arteries can be identified. The MCA is the more anterior of the two vessels and is on the same, frontal, side of the HC section as the cavum septum pellucidum (CSP). It leaves the circle of Willis at about 11 o'clock when the CSP is on the left of the screen (Fig. 13.18) or at about 1 o'clock when the CSP is on the right. As blood is flowing from the circle of Willis to the periphery of the brain, flow in the MCA will appear red. It is almost always possible to obtain a small angle of insonation on the MCA of less than 20° once the correct section of the head is obtained with the midline at 90° to the beam.

The MCA should be sampled within the proximal third of the vessel – that is, the portion nearest to its origin with the internal carotid artery of the circle of Willis – as velocities decrease with distance from this point. Optimize the waveform as described earlier, freeze the image and measure the PI. An angle correction is not necessary when measuring the PI of the MCA.

You must make sure that you apply as little pressure as possible to the probe, as increased probe pressure affects flow in the MCA, falsely increasing the PI. This is likely to become significant when the position of the fetal head makes it difficult to obtain an HC, which can only be achieved with acute angling of the probe or significant dipping to bring the midline into a position approaching the horizontal. The more pressure you need to apply to the probe to obtain the HC in these situations, the more likely it is that the PI from the MCA will be falsely increased and therefore falsely reassuring. As discussed previously, you should only report measurements that are accurate, and it may therefore be preferable not to include measurement of the MCA, with an explanation as to why, in such cases, than to take, record and report an unreliable measurement.

Velocity measurements of the MCA can be obtained by selecting the highest point of the waveform as the PSV. The auto trace option should be

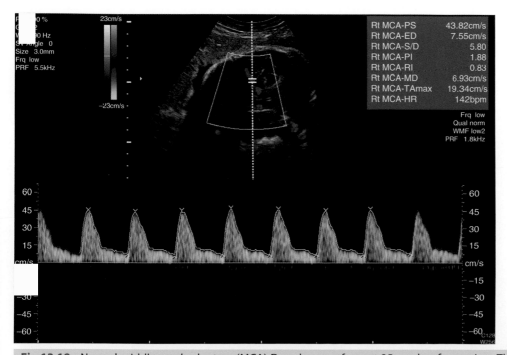

Fig 13.18 • Normal middle cerebral artery (MCA) Doppler waveform at 25 weeks of gestation. The MCA is visualized in red leaving the circle of Willis at about 11 o'clock. The pulsatility index (PI) measures 1.88. This is below the 50th centile but well within the normal range. This is explained by the presence of, rather than no, end diastolic frequencies.

used, rather than manual tracing, as the former more closely approximates to the published reference range used in clinical practice. Angle correction must be performed when velocity measurements are required, so do this before placing the horizontal bar of the PSV auto trace function at the highest, or most consistent, systolic peak of the waveform. The PSV is reported in centimetres per second (cm/s) (Fig. 13.17C). A PSV which is 1.5 times higher than the mean value for gestation is considered abnormal and therefore suggestive of anaemia.

The Normal Middle Cerebral Artery Waveform

The normal MCA waveform is monophasic with a sharp systolic peak and little or no end diastolic frequencies (Fig. 13.18). The degree of EDF varies with gestation, with little or no EDF being a normal finding before 28 weeks.

The Abnormal Middle Cerebral Artery Waveform

The MCA is the only vessel of the four commonly interrogated during pregnancy in which fetal compromise is associated with a decrease, rather than an increase, in PI (Fig. 13.19). This is because of the brain sparing effect, which reduces impedance in the MCA, and thus causes a decrease in the PI. *Fetal arterial redistribution* or 'redistribution' is the term used when the PI of the MCA falls below the normal range and is associated with fetal hypoxia.

Increased blood flow in the MCA can be identified by simply observing the appearance of the vessel before sampling. Because more blood is flowing through the MCA in a compromised fetus, the vessel is much more obvious when colour is applied than in the normal fetus. It has been described as 'lighting up like a Christmas tree'. The PI in such a vessel is highly likely to be abnormally low, indicating that the fetus is redistributing its blood supply.

With progressive and severe hypoxia, the brain sparing effect is lost and diastolic flow returns to the normal level; thus the PI will increase. The brain may then become oedematous, leading to reversal of diastolic flow as a result of raised intracranial tension. This suggests a grave and irreversible fetal

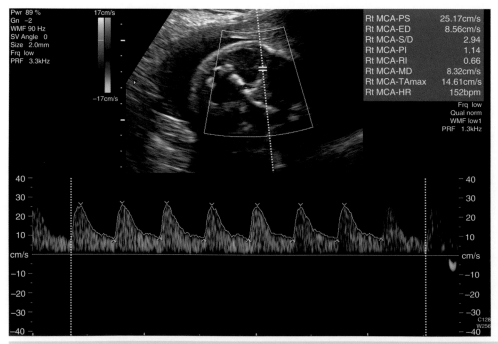

Fig 13.19 • Abnormal middle cerebral artery (MCA) Doppler waveform at 25+ weeks of gestation. The pulsatility index (PI) measures 1.14, which lies below the 5th centile.

neurological outcome. Such situations are very rare as the fetus would normally be delivered before reaching this state.

The Middle Cerebral Artery Waveform in Clinical Practice

The MCA should always be assessed in the growth restricted fetus to determine whether or not redistribution is present. A growth restricted fetus which is redistributing and has an abnormal umbilical artery waveform requires more intense surveillance than such a fetus with a normal MCA but an abnormal umbilical artery waveform or such a fetus with normal Doppler studies of both these vessels.

The angle corrected PSV should be measured in fetuses at risk of anaemia (Fig. 13.17C).

FETAL VENOUS DOPPLER

The two veins which are examined in the fetus, outside specialized examination of the fetal heart, are the ductus venous and the umbilical vein.

The Ductus Venosus

The ductus venosus is the main vessel through which highly oxygenated blood returning from the placenta is directed to the fetal heart, via the left portion of the inferior vena cava, just below the diaphragm, and the right atrium. It originates at the portal sinus where the umbilical vein and the extrahepatic portal vein meet, giving rise to the left portal vein, the right portal vein and the ductus venosus (Fig. 13.20). Blood flow through the ductus venosus is regulated by a muscular sphincter in the duct, close to its origin with the umbilical vein. Impedance to flow decreases with increasing gestation in the ductus venosus and is reported as the pulsatility index for veins (PIV). The PIV reference range is shown in Fig. 13.21.

As discussed earlier, worsening fetal hypoxaemia is associated with abnormal umbilical artery waveforms and fetal arterial redistribution, as reflected in the MCA. A further adaptation of the fetal circulation is an increase in flow of the highly oxygenated blood from the umbilical vein through the ductus venosus to the right atrium. This adaptive strategy is reflected in various changes in the

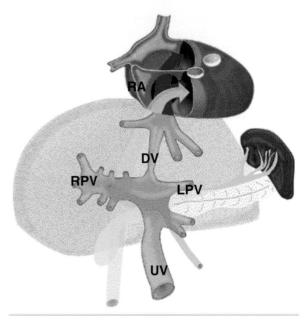

Fig 13.20 • The relationship between the umbilical vein (UV) and the ductus venosus (DV). LPV, left portal vein; RA, right atrium; RPV, right portal vein.

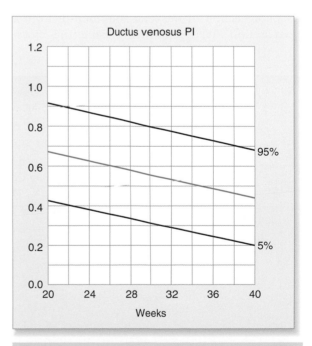

Fig 13.21 • Ductus venosus pulsatility index (PI) reference range. The 5th, 50th and 95th centiles are displayed. The PI values fall with increasing gestation. *(From Hecher K, Campbell S, Snijders R, Nicolaides K 1994 Reference ranges for fetal venous and atrioventricular blood flow parameters. Ultrasound Obstet Gynecol 4: 381–90.)*

normal ductus venosus waveform. Hence, interrogation of the ductus venosus may be used to monitor fetal compensatory responses to progressively deteriorating placental function.

Finding and Measuring the Ductus Venosus

In the normally grown fetus, flow through the ductus venosus is such that the vessel can be difficult to image, so manipulating the probe or the fetus to produce the most favourable position possible of the vessel in question is important if you are to be successful. The ductus venosus is most easily imaged, and therefore measured, when the fetal spine is posterior, the umbilical vein is therefore positioned almost vertically on the screen, providing alignment of the ductus venosus and the insonant beam, and access is unobstructed by one or more fetal limbs. In practice this is often impossible, but the vessel can usually be interrogated successfully when the fetal spine is between 3 o'clock and 5 o'clock, or 9 o'clock and 7 o'clock.

The ductus venosus can be sought either from a sagittal section of the fetal abdomen or from a cross-section. We recommend using the cross-sectional approach. Obtain a transverse section of the fetal abdomen at the level of the AC. Rotate the probe until you are imaging the entire length of the umbilical vein from the umbilicus to its anastomosis with the portal sinus. Dip the probe or slide the probe round the maternal abdomen so that the umbilical vein is as vertical as possible. Place the colour box over the intrahepatic portion of the umbilical vein. The ductus can be identified as it originates from the intrahepatic end of the umbilical vein by the aliasing resulting from the high velocities present in this narrow vessel. The sample gate should be placed over the area of aliasing (Fig. 13.22).

The ductus venosus waveforms are readily corrupted by signals from nearby vessels, so accurate positioning and the correct size of the sample gate are important. The gate needs to be as small as possible. Do not make it too small, however, as you will find that any slight fetal movements are likely to result in the gate moving out of the vessel, requiring you to start the whole imaging process again. Having placed the appropriately sized gate correctly over the vessel, run the spectral trace to obtain the waveform. As the sampling site is small,

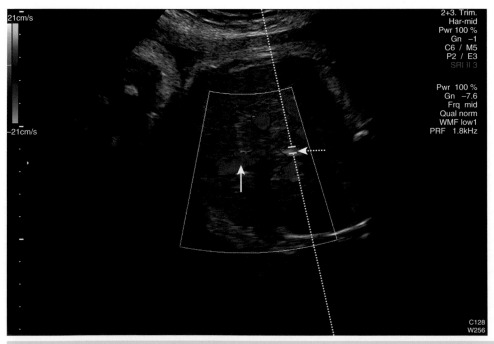

Fig 13.22 • Transverse section of the abdomen of a 32 week fetus. The umbilical vein (solid arrow) and ductus venosus (dashed arrow) are shown.

it is easily contaminated from adjacent vessels and previously quiescent fetuses have a habit of moving vigorously when you wish to interrogate the ductus, you will need to develop a relatively speedy technique with time if you wish to be successful.

The PIV should be calculated using the waveform envelope of three to six waveforms and should be reproducible. We suggest that you plot this on a data reference range. In addition to measuring the PIV, you should also assess the waveform to confirm forward flow throughout each cardiac cycle.

Do not measure the ductus venosus during fetal breathing movements. The changes in the intrathoracic pressure during breathing movements have a profound influence on flow velocity waveforms. The ductus venosus waveform should therefore only be measured during periods of fetal apnoea.

The Normal Ductus Venosus Waveform

The normal ductus venosus waveform has a characteristic M-shaped or biphasic waveform with positive end diastolic flow. With experience you will learn to recognize the distinctive sound of this vessel. The first peak of the waveform corresponds to ventricular systole, the second, smaller peak corresponds to early diastole and the lowest point in the waveform to the atrial contraction in late diastole. This is equivalent to the EDF used in the reporting of the umbilical artery and MCA. In the normal fetus continuous forward flow is present in the ductus venosus throughout each cardiac cycle (Fig. 13.23).

A normal ductus venosus waveform in a growth restricted fetus suggests that fetal compensation is currently adequate for the assumed underlying uteroplacental insufficiency.

The Abnormal Ductus Venosus Waveform

Abnormal findings in the ductus venosus are associated with severe growth restriction. An abnormal ductus waveform in the growth restricted fetus is associated with an increased neonatal mortality rate. As discussed earlier, arterial redistribution, as evidenced from the MCA, is associated with moderate acidaemia, whereas abnormal venous Dopplers are associated with severe fetal acidaemia.

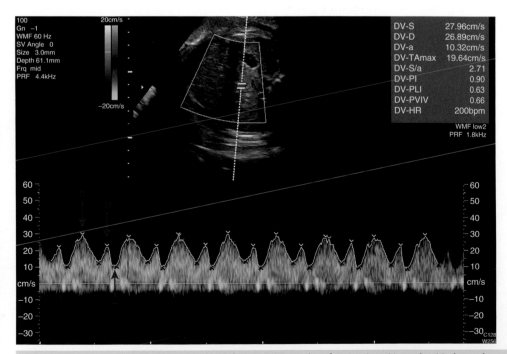

Fig 13.23 • Normal ductus venosus waveform at 28 weeks of gestation. Note the M-shaped waveform with positive end diastolic flow. *S, the highest peak, representing peak ventricular systole. D, the lower peak of early diastole; A, the lowest part of the waveform representing late diastole.*

Blood flow in the ductus venosus reflects the physiological status of the right ventricle. In the growth restricted fetus, when there is progressive hypoxia and worsening contractility of the ventricles and atria secondary to myocardial ischaemia, the ductus venosus shows a progressive decrease in forward flow. Absent or reversed flow in the ductus during atrial contraction occurs when fetal physiological responses fail to prevent the development of fetal hypoxia.

Compensatory changes in the ductus venosus are reflected as an increase in peak systolic forward flow, and therefore an increase in the PIV, and reduced, absent or reversed flow in the atrial contraction part (A) of the waveform. *Flow* in a ductus relates to forward flow during atrial contraction. Where the A wave extends to the baseline, forward flow is described as *absent* and where it is below the baseline it is described as *reversed* (Fig. 13.24).

The Ductus Venosus Waveform in Clinical Practice

Having identified the growth-restricted fetus during routine assessment of fetal growth, the ultrasound management of such a fetus is unlikely to remain within the routine setting, especially where compensatory arterial redistribution is evident through the MCA. This should not deter you from assessing flow in the ductus in a fetus in which the AC or EFW is at the lower limit of, or below, the normal range for gestation. Confirmation that the PIV is normal and forward flow is present in the ductus is helpful information in the clinical management of the small fetus.

The umbilical vein

The technique for interrogating the umbilical vein mirrors that for the umbilical artery.

The normal umbilical vein exhibits low velocity continuous flow with no pulsatility present. Its assessment is not normally included in Doppler studies of the fetus. When severe fetal compromise or heart failure are present, pulsatile blood flow may be seen in the umbilical vein. This is due to atrial pressure being transmitted through the ductus venosus to the umbilical vein and occurs just before the development of abnormal fetal heart rate patterns. The neonatal mortality rate is at least 60% in the growth restricted fetal population when umbilical vein pulsations are present.

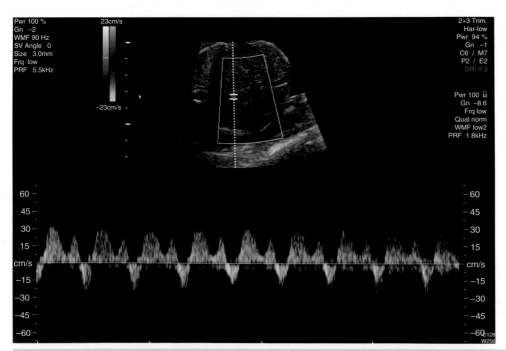

Fig 13.24 • Abnormal ductus venosus waveform at 28 weeks of gestation. Note the reversed end diastolic flow.

This can be compared with a 20% rate in the growth restricted fetal population when umbilical vein pulsations are absent.

Active fetal breathing is the most common cause for pulsations being identified in the umbilical vein waveform. You will observe this often during interrogation of the umbilical artery and so will soon recognize the typical, episodic waveform pattern produced by the actively breathing fetus. Interrogation of the umbilical vein for nonbreathing pulsatile activity is indicated in the severely compromised fetus in which abnormal flow in the ductus is already present.

UTEROPLACENTAL DOPPLER

The blood supply to the uterus derives from the right and left uterine arteries which arise from the internal iliac arteries. The uterine arteries branch extensively into arcuate and radial vessels, which eventually terminate as spiral arteries. The uterine artery is unique among the maternal vessels in that it has a remarkable ability to increase its capacity during pregnancy.

Resistance to blood flow in the uterine arteries falls with advancing gestation because of trophoblastic invasion of the spiral arteries, as reflected in the reference range for uterine artery PI (Fig. 13.25).

Failure or poor trophoblastic invasion is characteristic of pre-eclamptic and growth restricted pregnancies. Thus assessment of uterine artery blood flow is an established screening test for pregnancies at higher risk of developing either or both of these conditions. This is normally performed between 22 and 24 weeks of gestation. Uterine artery Doppler examination is of limited value in the normally grown fetus in later gestations.

The timing of this screening test is important, as high resistance uterine artery waveforms with post-systolic notching, which are features of an abnormal uterine artery Doppler study, are three times more likely to be present at 20 weeks of gestation than at 24 weeks, when they occur in about 5% of pregnancies.

Finding and Measuring the Uterine Artery

The uterine artery is most easily found by first locating the external iliac artery. To find the left uterine artery, place the probe in the midline to

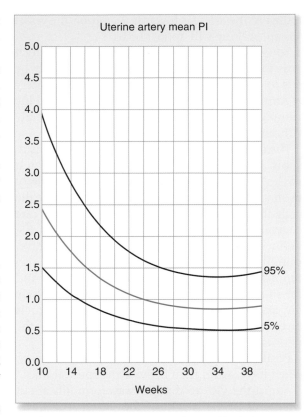

Fig 13.25 • Uterine artery pulsatility index (PI) reference range. The 5th, 50th and 95th centiles are displayed. The PI falls with increasing gestation. (From Gomez O, Figueras F, Fernandez S et al 2008 Reference ranges for uterine artery mean pulsatility index at 11–41 weeks of gestation. Ultrasound Obstet Gynecol 32: 128–132.)

obtain a sagittal section of the maternal pelvis. Slide the probe towards the maternal left side until the left side of the uterus is no longer in view. Rotate the probe clockwise, through approximately 30°. You should now see the tubular structures of the external iliac artery and vein crossing the screen from roughly 2 o'clock to 7 o'clock. Your aim is to sample the uterine artery just anterior to, or downstream from, where the uterine artery crosses the external iliac artery. Unfortunately this position varies considerably between left and right uterine arteries in the same woman and between women. Activate the colour box and use the colour map to identify what you anticipate to be the uterine artery. A reasonably large colour box is helpful to allow you to search across about half the visible length of the iliac artery at one time. As flow in the uterine artery is towards the probe, the vessel you are seeking will appear red.

You may find that there are several vessels which cross the external iliac artery and you will only be able to determine which vessel is the uterine artery by running a spectral trace. Adjust the PRF and the colour gain to display the flow in the vessels clearly without any aliasing.

The direction of the uterine artery varies considerably, but it is commonly almost vertical when it crosses the iliac artery, producing a small angle of insonation at the sampling site. You can reduce the angle if necessary by dipping the probe. Take care to avoid sampling the iliac artery instead of the uterine artery, both of which have distinctive-sounding and very different waveforms. It is also important that you sample the uterine artery and not an arcuate branch, as this may lead to a falsely low assessment of impedance. The resistance is lower in vessels that are further away from the uterine artery.

Position the sample gate across the uterine artery, adjust its size and then activate the spectral trace.

Adjust the PRF so that the waveform fills about two thirds of the height of the screen. The waveform itself will contain a range of frequencies, represented by a range of differing colours within it. If the waveform obtained appears very bright, contains few colours and the background is noisy, reduce the spectral gain until the optimal balance is obtained.

The PI should be calculated using the waveform envelope of three to six waveforms and should be reproducible. We suggest that you plot this on a data reference range. In addition to measuring the PI, you should also assess the waveform to confirm forward flow throughout each maternal cardiac cycle. Subjective assessment of the waveform should also be performed to assess the presence or absence of a notch at the end of systole.

Having successfully measured the left uterine artery, repeat the process for the right uterine artery.

It is not uncommon for the PI values from the left and right uterine arteries to differ quite considerably; this is thought to relate to placental position with resistance to flow and therefore the PI being lower in the uterine artery which is closer to the placenta.

The findings of the uterine arteries should be reported separately.

The Normal Uterine Artery Waveform

The normal uterine artery waveform is monophasic with positive end-diastolic flow. There is a smooth transition from the end of systole to diastole with forward flow present throughout each maternal cardiac cycle (Fig. 13.26). With experience you will learn to recognize the distinctive sound of this vessel and be able to distinguish between a normal and an abnormal waveform.

The Abnormal Uterine Artery Waveform

An increase in the peak systolic frequencies, causing an increase in the PI, a notch at the end of systole and reduced end diastolic frequencies describe the abnormal findings of the uterine artery waveform (Fig. 13.27). Loss of end diastolic frequencies in the uterine artery is extremely rare.

There are no criteria that define a uterine artery notch, and this remains a subjective diagnosis. Significant notches are very easy to confirm with certainty, but smaller notches present more of a challenge. In a situation where you are suspicious that a notch is present, repeat your sampling twice more, as advised previously. Where the appearance is consistently present from three separate samplings, you should report this finding as 'a possible notch present on the left/right/both side(s)'.

The Uterine Artery Waveform in Clinical Practice

Uterine artery Doppler studies are normally only performed in women at increased risk of pre-eclampsia or who have previously delivered a growth restricted fetus. Such studies are performed between 22 and 24 weeks of gestation.

The subsequent management of such pregnancies in which the uterine artery Doppler study is normal will vary between different departments. Some will arrange no further ultrasound follow-up, whereas others will arrange a growth scan at around 34 weeks.

The subsequent management of such pregnancies in which the uterine artery Doppler study is abnormal will normally involve serial growth scans, the frequency of which depends on the severity of the uterine artery findings. Growth scans at 30 and 34 weeks, for example, may be arranged

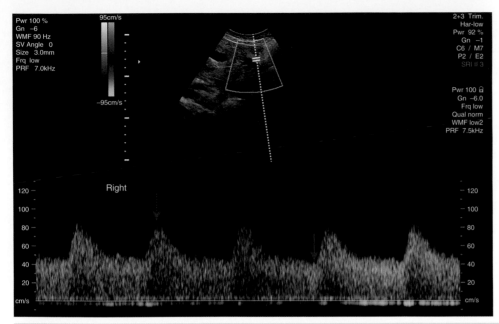

Fig 13.26 • Normal uterine artery (right) Doppler waveform at 24 weeks of gestation. Note the amount of end diastolic flow (solid arrow) and compare with that of Fig. 13.27. Peak systole is shown by the dashed arrow

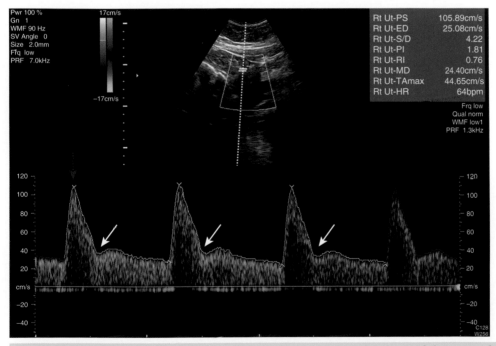

Fig 13.27 • Abnormal uterine artery Doppler waveform. Compare the shape of these waveforms, with high peak systolic peaks (dashed arrow) and reduced end diastolic flow, producing a pulsatility index (PI) value of 1.81. This value lies above the 95th centile. Note also the presence of the consistent uterine artery notch (arrowed).

where the findings at 22–24 weeks are of bilateral borderline raised PI values with no notches. The findings at 22–24 weeks of bilateral notches with raised PI values would typically involve three or four weekly growth scans.

Further reading

Bhide A, Acharya G, Bilardo CM, et al 2013 ISUOG practice guidelines: use of Doppler ultrasonography in obstetrics. Ultrasound Obstet Gynecol 41:233–239

Loughna P, Chitty L, Evans T, Chudleigh T 2009 Fetal size and dating: charts recommended for clinical obstetric practice. Ultrasound 17:161–167

Royal College of Obstetricians and Gynecologists 2013 Small for gestational age fetus: investigation and management. Green-top Guideline No. 31. RCOG Press, London

Placental and cervical imaging

14

CONTENTS

This chapter addresses the ultrasound examination of the placenta, with particular reference to the second and third trimesters of pregnancy, and ultrasound assessment of the cervix in pregnancy.

The aims of this chapter are to enable you to do the following:

- recognize the ultrasound appearances of the normal placenta
- identify and report the position of the placenta within the uterus
- measure accurately the distance between the leading edge of the placenta and the internal os
- distinguish between normal and abnormal appearances of the placenta
- image and assess the cervix using the transvaginal route
- measure accurately the cervical length.

DEVELOPMENT OF THE PLACENTA

The endometrium of the uterus undergoes a decidual reaction in response to pregnancy, resulting in an increase in the size and number of stromal cells, blood vessels and glands within it. Three regions of the decidua are recognized, according to their position relative to the site of implantation of the chorionic sac. The decidua underlying the site of implantation, and the area which will form the maternal component of the placenta, is called the decidua basalis. The superficial decidua, which lies between the sac and the uterine cavity, is called the decidua capsularis. The remaining decidua is called the decidua parietalis.

Up to about the 10th week of gestational age, or the 8th week after fertilization, the whole surface of the chorionic sac of the developing embryo is covered with villi. As the chorionic sac grows, only the villi associated with the decidua basalis persist. They form the villous chorion or the fetal component of the future placenta. With the increasing size of the chorionic sac during the first trimester, the villi associated with the decidua capsularis become compressed, their blood supply therefore decreases and they start to degenerate. The resulting chorion lacks villi and is therefore termed *smooth chorion*.

As discussed in Chapter 5, the amniotic sac develops within the chorion sac, with the former growing more rapidly than the latter. The two membranes fuse during the early part of the second trimester to form the amniochorionic membrane. This membrane fuses with the decidua capsularis and then with the decidua parietalis, obliterating the uterine cavity. By about 24 weeks of gestation the reduced blood supply to the decidua capsularis results in it degenerating and then disappearing (Fig. 14.1).

NORMAL PLACENTAL APPEARANCES

As will be obvious from the discussion earlier, the ultrasound appearances of the chorionic sac and its surrounding decidua (capsularis, parietalis and basalis together) early in the first trimester of pregnancy will be very different from the appearances towards the end of the first trimester when the villous chorion and the decidua basalis have developed sufficiently to produce a definitive placenta. This can be appreciated by comparison of the rather symmetrical appearance of the decidua surrounding the chorionic sac shown in the 6⁺ week pregnancy with the more definitive placental site seen on the lateral wall of the 8 week pregnancy and at the fundus of the 20 week pregnancy as shown in Fig. 14.2.

In addition to the appearance of the placenta evolving during the first trimester, the uterus itself grows during early pregnancy, and its position relative to the cervix and its orientation within the pelvis can both change. These factors can result in the position of the placenta appearing to change in location within the uterus, and relative to the internal os, during the first and early second trimesters, and therefore between the dating scan and the routine anomaly scan.

However, with the exception of women undergoing chorion villus sampling, accurate assessment of placental position in the first trimester uterus is not necessary. We therefore do not recommend reporting placental position in normal circumstances until the routine 18–22 week scan. Localizing and reporting placental position in the second trimester is described in Chapter 8. We recommend that you avoid using the term *placenta praevia* to describe a placenta that appears to extend to and/or cover the internal os until after the lower uterine segment has formed for the reasons discussed in Chapter 8.

LOCALIZING THE PLACENTA AT 18–22 WEEKS

As discussed in Chapter 8, the placenta should be localized and the relationship between its lower edge and the internal os determined. Approximately 95% of women will have a placenta which clearly lies in the upper portion of the uterus at 18–22 weeks and therefore are not at risk of placenta praevia in later pregnancy (Figs. 14.2C and 14.3).

The remaining 5% will have a placenta which appears to extend to, and/or cover, the assumed internal os at 18–22 weeks, as assessed with transabdominal imaging (Fig. 14.4). One in five of these women will have a true placenta praevia at, or towards, term (Fig. 14.5). The critical factor in determining whether or not the placenta will encroach

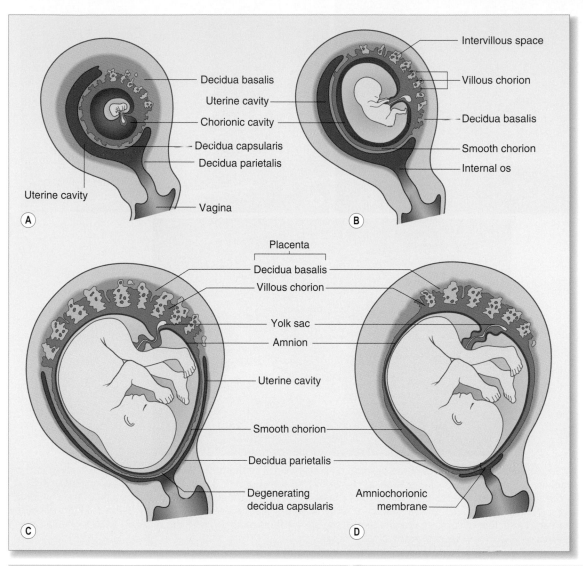

Fig 14.1 • Sagittal sections of the pregnant uterus at 6 weeks (Fig. A), 10 weeks (Fig. B), 20 weeks (Fig. C) and 24 weeks (Fig. D) weeks of gestation demonstrating the developing placenta and the changing relationship between the amnion, chorion and the three regions of the decidua. In D the amnion and chorion have fused with each other and the decidua parietalis, thus obliterating the uterine cavity. Note that the villi only persist where the chorion is associated with the decidua basilis, thus forming the fetal component of the placenta.

on or cover the internal os at delivery is the lower segment. This develops between the internal os and the body of the uterus and plays a vital role in natural labour and delivery. The lower segment starts to develop from around 26 weeks and is fully formed by approximately 36 weeks. Its significance, in terms of ultrasound imaging, lies in its effect on the distance between the lower edge of the placenta and the internal os because, as the lower uterine segment develops, this distance has the potential to increase. The placenta therefore appears to 'move' away from the internal os, although any specific part of the placental tissue obviously remains implanted into the same part of the uterine wall throughout the pregnancy. Placental tissue that implants below the area of formation of the lower segment will not be influenced by its development and will therefore remain adjacent to or covering the internal os.

347

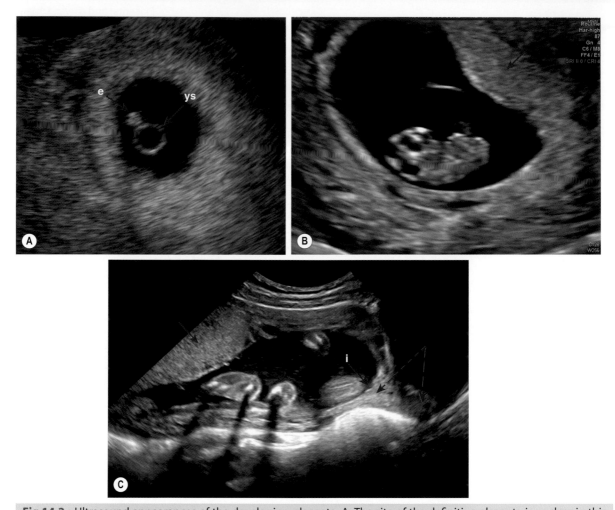

Fig 14.2 • Ultrasound appearances of the developing placenta. A. The site of the definitive placenta is unclear in this transvaginal image at 6 weeks of gestation, as the outline of the chorionic sac is still relatively symmetrical. B. By 8 weeks the site of the developing placenta (arrow) can be identified by the asymmetry in the outline of the chorionic sac and surrounding decidua (transvaginal scan). C. By 20 weeks the placental site is clearly defined. In this transabdominal sagittal section the placenta can be seen at the uterine fundus (arrow) with the cervical canal (dashed arrows) and internal os (i) also well seen. e, embryo; ys, yolk sac.

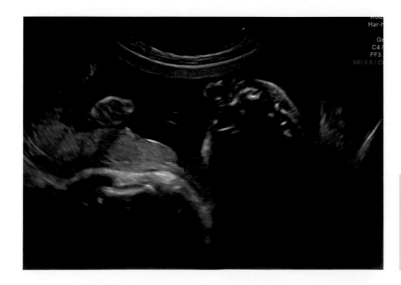

Fig 14.3 • Transabdominal scan demonstrating the placenta on the posterior wall of the uterus in this 20 week pregnancy. It is clearly in the upper part of the uterus, with its leading edge (arrow) above the fetal head, which is in a direct OP position. OP, occipito-posterior.

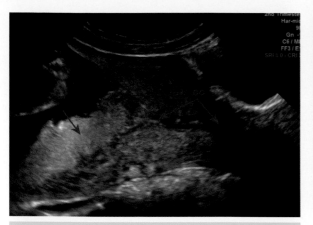

Fig 14.4 • Transabdominal scan showing the posterior placenta (arrow) clearly extending to and covering the internal os (dashed arrow) at 19⁺ weeks of gestation. cc, cervical canal.

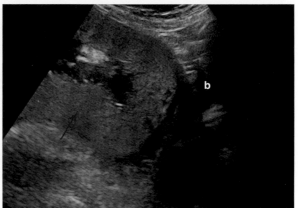

Fig 14.5 • Transabdominal sagittal scan at 35 weeks of gestation. Although the maternal bladder (b) is empty and the internal os (dashed arrow) and cervical canal cannot be clearly identified, the position of the posterior placenta (arrow) is obvious, extending from the posterior uterine wall, across the internal os and onto the anterior wall. These findings suggest a major placenta praevia, which should then be confirmed with a transvaginal scan in order to image the position of the internal os and its relationship to the placenta accurately.

PLACENTA PRAEVIA

CLASSIFICATION

Placenta praevia describes a placenta which implants wholly or partially into the lower segment of the uterus.

Major praevia describes a placenta which lies over the cervical or internal os. *Minor praevia* describes a placenta with which the leading edge is in the lower segment but does not cover the internal or cervical os. This classification is unrelated to whether or not the woman is in early labour and is therefore applicable in the third trimester.

THE CLINICAL PROBLEM

It is obvious that if the placenta overlies the internal os, vaginal delivery can only occur through the placenta. With a major degree of placenta praevia,

life-threatening bleeding can occur when the uterus contracts and the placenta separates from it. In some cases this will not occur until the woman goes into labour; alternatively it may occur any time during the pregnancy either spontaneously or in response to premature contractions. Women known to have a major placenta praevia may be kept in hospital and are delivered by elective Caesarean section at about 39 weeks, or earlier if they have had a large vaginal bleed, which is assumed to be related to the position of the placenta.

THE RELATIONSHIP BETWEEN THE PLACENTAL EDGE AND THE INTERNAL OS

The lower uterine segment is an anatomical entity, but its ultrasound appearance is indistinguishable from that of the body of the uterus. As it is covered

349

anteriorly by the bladder, the position of the anterior lower segment can be assumed by using the transabdominal approach and a reasonably full maternal bladder. The posterior aspect of the lower segment can then be determined by projecting the upper edge of the bladder onto the posterior wall of the uterus. However, being able to determine the extent of the lower segment with ultrasound imaging is of less clinical value than assessing the relationship between the leading edge of the placenta and the internal os, as this is key to distinguishing between a major praevia, a minor praevia and a placenta which is not low-lying.

The transvaginal route is the preferred method for assessing this relationship and should always be performed if there is any doubt as to placental position using the transabdominal route. The main disadvantage of using the transabdominal approach with a moderately full maternal bladder is the common difficulty of reliably imaging the position of the internal os. When the internal os and the leading edge of the placenta can be clearly seen transabdominally, such that the distance between the two can be measured accurately, then it is reasonable to perform a transabdominal scan only before 36 weeks (Fig. 14.6). This is not the case at 36 weeks, however, as important clinical decisions

relating to delivery will be dependent on the scan findings from what is likely to be the final scan before delivery. Thus unless all the placental tissue is quite clearly in the upper half of the uterus at 36 weeks and there is no evidence of either a succenturiate lobe or a vasa praevia on colour flow mapping, a transvaginal scan should always be performed to image accurately the internal os and the leading edge of placenta relative to it. This is because of the potentially catastrophic consequences of failing to identify a low-lying placenta in the third trimester.

Irrespective of whether you are performing a transvaginal or a transabdominal scan, the internal os must be identified (see Assessment and Measurement of Cervical Length later) so that the linear callipers can be placed correctly to measure the distance between the leading edge of the placenta and the internal os.

WHEN TO SCAN IN THE THIRD TRIMESTER

In pregnancies where the placenta is centrally placed over the internal os, or extends to and covers the internal os, at 18–22 weeks, a major degree of placenta praevia towards term is likely. Such pregnancies should be rescanned at 32 weeks to assess the placental position. When the placenta is obviously still covering the internal os as assessed transabdominally, there is little additional clinical value to be obtained by confirming this with a transvaginal scan. If you are unable to identify the leading edge of the placenta transabdominally at 32 weeks, it is imperative that you proceed to a transvaginal scan in order to determine whether or not a further scan is required at 36 weeks.

When the placenta is still low-lying at 32 weeks, a further scan should be arranged at 36 weeks to exclude either a major or minor placenta praevia. Because the definition of 'low' may vary between clinicians, it is preferable for you as the sonographer to report the position of the leading edge of the placenta in terms of its distance from the internal os, and not to use a subjective or qualitative description. A placenta that is covering the internal os at 32 weeks should obviously be rescanned at 36 weeks, whereas a placenta with a leading edge which is at least 3.0 cm from the internal os does not need to be reviewed at 36 weeks, as there is no

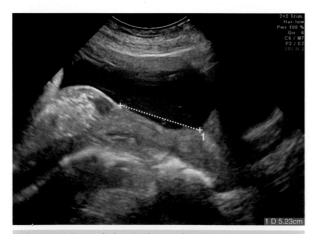

Fig 14.6 • Transabdominal scan demonstrating the relationship between the leading edge of the posterior placenta and the internal os at 32 weeks of gestation. The distance, of 52.3 mm, can be accurately measured, as no fetal part obscures the required view. A transvaginal scan is not required in this case. As this placenta is no longer low-lying, rescanning at 36 weeks to exclude a minor praevia is not necessary.

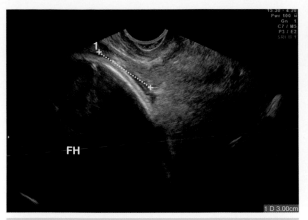

Fig 14.7 • A transvaginal scan at 32 weeks of gestation. The position of the leading edge of the anterior placenta was unclear on the transabdominal scan. No placental tissue is seen covering the internal os nor within 3.0 cm from the internal os, as shown by placement of the two callipers. As this anterior placenta is not low-lying at 32 weeks it does not need to be rescanned at 36 weeks to exclude a minor praevia. FH, fetal head.

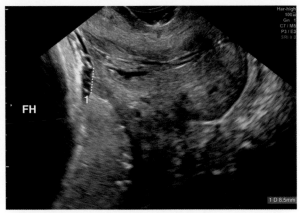

Fig 14.8 • A transvaginal scan at 31⁺ weeks of gestation. The position of the leading edge of the posterior placenta is 8.5 mm from the internal os, as shown by the two callipers. As this placenta is low-lying at 32 weeks it needs to be rescanned at 36 weeks to exclude a minor praevia. FH, fetal head.

risk of such a placenta being praevia at term (Fig. 14.6 and Fig. 14.7).

A decision needs to be made regarding the ultrasound management of those placentas which are neither extending to or covering the internal os nor very clearly no longer low-lying – namely the group in which the leading placental edge is between 3.0 cm and 0.0 cm from the internal os.

It is a matter for local discussion and agreement as to what the minimum distance should be between the placental leading edge and the internal os at 32 weeks for you to report that placenta as 'no longer low-lying' or 'not low'. It is therefore also a local decision as to the maximum distance between the leading placental edge and the internal os that should generate rebooking that woman for a 36 week scan. Clinicians may use 2.0 cm, or err on the side of caution and use 2.5 cm, at 36 weeks of gestation as the leading placental edge to internal os measurement, above which they would consider natural labour and delivery to be an acceptable aim and below which delivery by elective Caesarean section would be a likely consideration. Thus it would seem reasonable to adopt the same, more cautious watershed of 2.5 cm to identify those 32 week placentas which should be reviewed again at 36 weeks. A woman therefore with a placenta which is 2.4 cm from the internal os at 32 weeks should be rebooked for a 36 week

scan, but this will not be required if the distance is 2.6 cm. Those women in whom the placenta remains less than 2.5 cm from the internal os at the 36 week scan should be referred to the clinical team as soon as possible so that a decision regarding delivery can be agreed and a management plan put in place in case of a preterm delivery (Fig. 14.8).

In those women in whom the placenta is extending to but not overlying the internal os at 18–22 weeks, the resulting placenta praevia, if present, is likely to be minor rather than major. Such women should be rescanned at 36 weeks to assess whether or not a minor placenta praevia is present (Fig. 14.9).

In the event of a woman experiencing vaginal bleeding, the timing of any scans should be arranged according to the individual clinical need.

REPORTING PLACENTAL SITE AT 32 AND 36 WEEKS

At 32 Weeks

We suggest that a placenta which is centrally placed over the internal os, or extends to and covers the internal os, at 32 weeks be reported as follows: *'The anterior/posterior placenta is centrally positioned over the internal os extending onto the posterior/anterior wall as assessed by transvaginal/transabdominal imaging. A further scan has been arranged at 36 weeks to exclude a major placenta praevia.'*

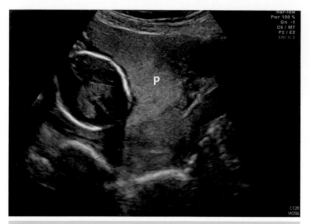

Fig 14.9 • Transabdominal scan at 19⁺ weeks of gestation demonstrating an anterior placenta (p), the leading edge (arrow) extends almost to, but does not cover, the internal os (dashed arrow). The site of this placenta should be reviewed at 36 weeks to exclude a minor placenta praevia.

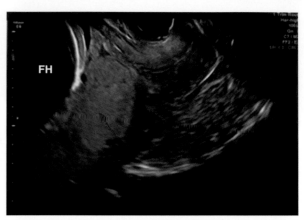

Fig 14.10 • A transvaginal scan at 36 weeks of gestation. The leading edge of the posterior placenta (arrow) can be seen extending across the internal os (dashed arrow). This appearance is therefore indicative of a major placenta praevia. FH, fetal head.

Where the placenta remains low-lying but does not extend to or cover the internal os, we suggest reporting its position as follows: *'The anterior/posterior placenta remains low-lying, with its leading edge 1.9 cm from the internal os as assessed by transvaginal/transabdominal imaging. A further scan has been arranged at 36 weeks to exclude a minor placenta praevia.'*

Where the placenta is no longer low-lying and therefore does not extend to or cover the internal os, we suggest reporting its position as follows: *'The anterior/posterior placenta is no longer low-lying. The distance between its leading edge and the internal os is greater than 3.0 cm, as assessed transabdominally.'*

At 36 Weeks

We suggest that a placenta which remains centrally placed over the internal os, or extends to and covers the internal os, at 36 weeks (Fig. 14.10) be reported as follows: *'The anterior/posterior placenta remains centrally positioned over the internal os extending onto the posterior/anterior wall as assessed by transvaginal imaging. These appearances are consistent with a major placenta praevia. Ms X has been referred to the day assessment unit for discussion with the consultant on call regarding her further management. No further scan appointment has been made.'*

The placenta that remains low-lying but does not extend to or cover the internal os requires very similar ultrasound management. We suggest reporting its position as follows: *'The anterior/posterior placenta remains low-lying, with its leading edge 2.2 cm from the internal os as assessed by transvaginal imaging. Ms X has been referred to the day assessment unit for discussion with the consultant on call regarding her further management. No further scan appointment has been made.'*

VARIATIONS IN PLACENTAL MORPHOLOGY

The majority of placentas exhibit a very similar range of appearances through gestation. Although arguably the most important feature of the placenta is its position relative to the internal os, you also need to be aware of the less common morphological features of the placenta, as described next.

PLACENTAL LAKES

Placental lakes are one of the most readily identified of the less common placental appearances. They describe hypoechoic areas that lie immediately under the chorionic plate, when they are best described as subchorionic lakes, or lie within the bulk of the placenta. They are often multiple and of varying and changeable size. They are filled with slowly moving blood which can be observed either on grey scale image or with very low velocity colour flow mapping. They are thought to represent inter-villous spaces in areas lacking chorionic villi. His-torically, there was thought to be a relationship between the presence of placental lakes, raised serum AFP, uteroplacental insufficiency and poor fetal growth. It was conjected that growth restric-tion was attributed to the reduced surface area available for interchange within the intervillous space because of the reduced number of villi present in the fetal component of the placenta. This relationship, however, was not supported in the literature. Placental lakes therefore can be assumed to be of limited clinical significance and their presence does not require any change in ultra-sound management of the pregnancy.

SUCCENTURIATE LOBE

The *succenturiate lobe* is an, or more than one, accessory lobe of the placenta that is attached to the bulk of the placenta by blood vessels. Making the diagnosis is important, as it is possible to have a fundal placenta together with a succenturi-ate lobe that is centrally placed over the internal os. These women have the same problems as those with placenta praevia. Alternatively, neither the main body of the placenta nor the succenturi-ate lobe is low-lying, but the course of the vessels connecting the two is across the internal os. This condition is described as a vasa praevia, type II. A succenturiate lobe may be retained after delivery and may be the source of postpartum haemor-rhage or infection.

Having identified the site of the main placental mass, a thorough survey of the rest of the uterus, paying particular attention to the appearance of the rest of the uterine wall, should ensure that you have not overlooked an additional area of placen-tal tissue that would raise your suspicions of a succenturiate lobe.

Should you identify a succenturiate lobe, you should first assess its position relative to the internal os, as you have already done with the main body of the placenta. Next you should attempt to trace the vascular connection between the accessory lobe and the main body of the pla-centa using colour flow mapping to determine whether or not the vessels run close to the internal os. Your assessment of both of these should be included in your ultrasound report.

AMNIOTIC BAND

Amniotic band is one of the most common of the less common appearances associated with the pla-centa. As the name suggests, an amniotic band is a band of amnion that floats within the amniotic fluid. It most typically presents as a thin, rather hyperechoic band across a corner of the uterus (Fig. 14.11). It is thought to be due to the partial rupture of the amniotic sac in early pregnancy. Only the amniotic membrane is involved in the rupture; the chorionic membrane remains intact. The band may encircle or trap part of the fetus. As the preg-nancy progresses, the fetus will grow but the band does not. Constriction of, and reduction in blood supply to, the affected fetal part may result in an anomaly or a 'natural amputation'. Such condi-tions are described as examples of amniotic band syndrome.

Amniotic band syndrome can range from minor indentations in the skin of a digit to severe facial anomalies resulting from a band becoming attached to the face during early development.

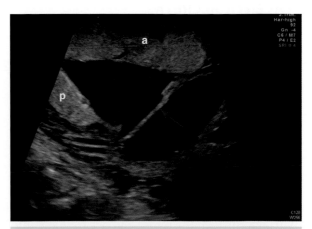

Fig 14.11 • Transabdominal scan of 19⁺ week uterus in transverse section. An amniotic band (arrow) can be seen extending from the edge of the anterior (a) com-ponent to the edge of the posterior (p) component of this right lateral placenta. Note there are no fetal parts visible near the band.

ULTRASOUND FEATURE	VISIBLE ON GREY SCALE	VISIBLE WITH COLOUR
Abnormal direction of blood vessels in retroplacental zone		y
Abnormal number of placental lakes	y	
Area(s) of hypervascularity between placenta and maternal bladder		y
Area(s) of increased vascularity in retroplacental zone		y
Focal mass invading into maternal bladder	y	
Irregularity of hypoechoic retroplacental zone	y	
Loss of hypoechoic retroplacental zone	y	
Thinning of tissue between placenta and maternal bladder	y	
Turbulent flow within placental lakes		y

Table 14.1 Ultrasound appearances associated with the diagnosis of placenta accreta using grey scale imaging and colour flow mapping

An amniotic band is of no clinical significance providing you are able to confirm that the fetus appears structurally normal and that its head, body and all its limbs, including both hands and both feet, are moving freely and are not constricted in any way by the amniotic band.

MORBIDLY ADHERENT PLACENTA/ PLACENTA ACCRETA

A *morbidly adherent placenta* describes the invasion of placental tissue through the decidua basalis into the myometrium. There are three types of morbidly adherent placenta, namely placenta accreta, placenta increta and placenta percreta, with their classification being dependent on the degree of invasion.

Placenta accreta describes a placenta that is adherent to the myometrium but does not invade into it. In *placenta increta* the chorionic villi invade into the myometrium only, whereas in *placenta percreta* the placental villi invade through the myometrium, through the serosa and occasionally into adjacent organs such as the bladder. The term *placenta accreta* is often used to describe all three types of adherent placenta.

Women with a history of a previous Caesarean section and a current placenta praevia or in whom there is an anterior placenta overlying the site of the previous Caesarean section scar are at risk of placenta accreta. When a low-lying anterior placenta is identified at the 18–22 week scan in a woman who has had a previous Caesarean section, it is important that the pregnancy is reviewed at around 24 weeks to exclude the ultrasound features of placenta accreta. The ultrasound criteria used for the diagnosis of placenta accreta are shown in Table 14.1.

The diagnosis of placenta accreta is beyond the scope of a routine screening examination and should be made by a specialist. Despite the well-recognized ultrasound features associated with placenta accreta, it is acknowledged that this condition is often difficult to diagnose and the ultrasound examination therefore is inconclusive. The use of magnetic resonance imaging in diagnosing placenta accreta is becoming more widespread and is now commonly recommended for women in whom the ultrasound findings are inconclusive.

CHORIOANGIOMA

Chorioangioma is a very rare vascular tumour of the placenta. Such tumours vary both in appearance and in size and occasionally appear to be

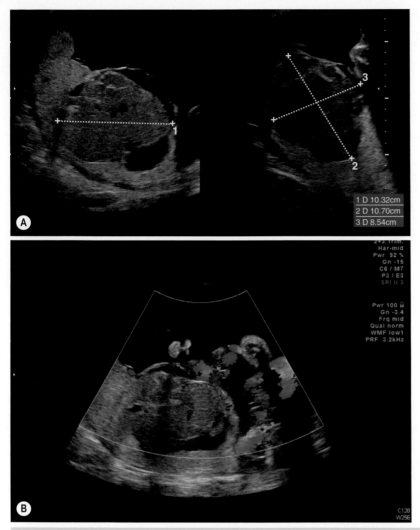

1 D 10.32cm
2 D 10.70cm
3 D 8.54cm

2+3.Trim.
Har-mid
Pwr 92 %
Gn -15
C6 / M7
P3 / E3
SRI II 3

Pwr 100 Ø
Gn -3.4
Frq mid
Qual norm
WMF low1
PRF 3.2kHz

C128
W256

Fig 14.12 • Transabdominal scan of a 31 week pregnancy demonstrating (A) a large chorioangioma measuring 10.7 × 10.3 × 8.7 cm at the site of the cord insertion. B. Colour flow mapping aids in the identification of the cord insertion at the apex of the mass, which has a complex and mixed echo pattern.

separate from the placenta. They are usually benign and, if less than 5.0 cm in diameter, are rarely of clinical significance. They are also infrequently detected with ultrasound. Larger tumours are very vascular, and may act as a fetal arteriovenous anastomosis (Fig. 14.12). In this situation, a fetal hyperdynamic circulation can result in high-output cardiac failure with subsequent polyhydramnios and hydrops fetalis. Such cases obviously require close monitoring with a low threshold for delivery.

PLACENTAL GRADING

Placental grading is a classification of the normal changes that occur in the placenta during the course of a pregnancy; it is often known as Grannum grading after its author (Fig. 14.13). Originally it was suggested that a Grannum grade III placenta was associated with mature fetal lungs and placental dysfunction. This concept has been largely rejected, and placental Grannum grading is therefore of no value in assessing fetal lung

355

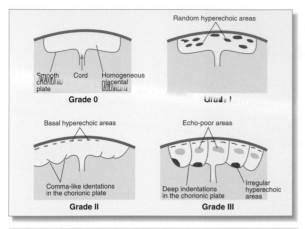

Fig 14.13 • Diagram of the ultrasound appearances of placental grading. (Adapted from Grannum et al 1982.)

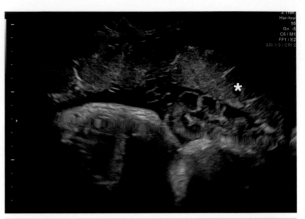

Fig 14.14 • Transabdominal scan of a Grannum grade III placenta at 35 weeks of gestation. Basal hyperechoic areas can be seen (arrows) together with the outlining of the individual cotyledons (dashed arrows). Echo poor areas are also present (*).

maturity. It does illustrate the varying appearances of the normal placenta as it matures and still finds favour in some circles as a method of describing placental aging (Fig. 14.14).

PLACENTAL ABRUPTION

About 3% of the pregnant population will bleed after 28 weeks of gestation. Approximately one third of these women will have suffered a placental abruption, in which all or some of the placenta separates from the underlying myometrium before the fetus has been delivered. A major abruption is usually clinically apparent because of abdominal pain and a peculiar 'woody hardness' to the uterus. Ultrasound has no place in the diagnosis of major abruption, although it may be needed to determine whether the fetus is still alive.

Minor abruption may produce few or no clinical symptoms. The woman presents with slight abdominal pain and/or an antepartum haemorrhage. The diagnosis is difficult to make clinically and has no features that can be reliably identified with ultrasound. The main role of ultrasound in these cases is in excluding placenta praevia, although it is hoped that the placental site has already been reported accurately at the 18–22 week scan.

It must be stressed, therefore, that ultrasound is unreliable in refuting or confirming the diagnosis of either major or minor abruption and should not be part of the routine management of either of these clinical diagnoses.

Recurrent antepartum haemorrhage and abruption can be associated with uteroplacental insufficiency. Ultrasound assessment for fetal growth is therefore indicated in pregnancies with this clinical history.

CORD INSERTION INTO THE PLACENTA

The umbilical cord normally inserts into the centre of the placental mass, and it is good practice, although not normally an expectation of routine screening, to confirm this at the 18–22 week scan.

Scan across the surface of the placenta, using sliding probe movements in either longitudinal or transverse sections of the uterus, and note where the smooth edge of the chorionic plate is disrupted by the vessels of the umbilical cord inserting into the placenta. The cord insertion can then be confirmed with colour flow mapping by applying the colour box over the site. The cord typically branches as it inserts into the chorionic plate of the placenta (Fig. 14.15A).

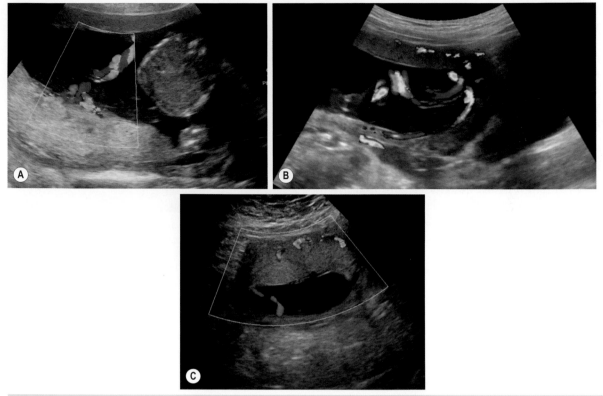

Fig 14.15 • A. Insertion of the umbilical cord centrally into a posterior placenta at 19 weeks of gestation. Colour flow mapping demonstrates the branching of the vessels as they insert into the placenta. B. Velamentous insertion of the cord into the amniochorionic membrane, away from the body of the placenta at 24 weeks of gestation. C. Marginal insertion of the cord into an anterior placenta. Colour flow mapping identifies the site at the right margin of the anterior placenta at 23 weeks of gestation.

Ensure that the cord inserts into the centre of the placental mass, rather than at its margin or into the membranes. Make sure that you are not mistaking a free loop of cord for the cord insertion by ensuring that the vessels you are imaging insert into the placental mass. If you are unable to identify the cord insertion using a transabdominal approach, you should consider the possibility of a velamentous cord insertion.

VELAMENTOUS CORD INSERTION

Velamentous cord insertion describes a cord that inserts into the chorioamniotic membranes outside the placental margin, travelling to the placental mass between the amnion and the chorion (Fig. 14.15B). Although the fetal membranes afford the cord some protection, it is effectively unprotected because of the absence of Wharton's jelly within

the membranes and is therefore at increased risk of damage, especially during labour and delivery.

The incidence of velamentous cord insertion is approximately 1% in singleton pregnancies and around 9% in twin pregnancies overall, the incidence being on the order of 15% in monochorionic twins.

Velamentous cord insertion is one of the causes of vasa praevia.

Exclusion of velamentous cord insertion is not normally part of a routine screening examination. However, if you are unable to identify a normal cord insertion centrally within the placental mass and are therefore suspicious of a potential velamentous insertion, we recommend that you use colour flow mapping to exclude fetal vessels coursing across the internal os. Place the colour box over the lower uterus and internal os and activate the colour map. If there are no vessels seen crossing

357

the area of the internal os, the examination can be considered normal. Should you identify vessels crossing the area of the internal os, you must first make sure you are not imaging a piece of normal umbilical cord in the amniotic fluid. Having excluded this possibility, you should consider a type I vasa praevia and the woman should be managed accordingly.

MARGINAL CORD INSERTION

Marginal cord insertion describes a cord that inserts close to the margin of the placenta rather that at its centre (Fig. 14.15C). Some authors use an insertion distance of less than 2.0 cm from the margin of the placenta to define a marginal cord insertion, whereas others use a distance of less than 1.0 cm.

A marginal cord insertion may evolve into a velamentous cord insertion as the pregnancy progresses.

VASA PRAEVIA

Vasa praevia describes the condition in which fetal vessels within the chorioamniotic membranes course over the internal os below the fetal presenting part (Fig. 14.16). These vessels are unprotected by either Wharton's jelly or placental tissue and are at risk of tearing, with the potentially devastating consequence of fetal exsanguination when the cervix dilates or the membranes rupture during labour.

Vasa praevia is thought to occur in approximately 1 in 2500 births, although this rises to 1 in

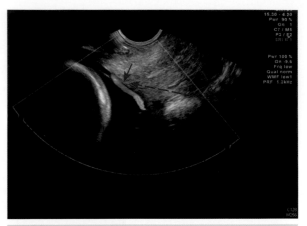

Fig 14.16 • A transvaginal scan using colour flow mapping to demonstrate the vessels from a type 1 velamentous cord insertion crossing the internal os (arrow) of the cervical canal (dashed arrows) in a case of vasa praevia at 21 weeks of gestation.

300 in in vitro fertilization pregnancies. Unlike placenta praevia, vasa praevia carries no risk to the mother but poses a significant risk to the fetus. The fetal mortality rate in cases which are not detected antenatally is reported to be between 60% and 95%. Antenatal detection is associated with a survival rate of up to 97%. Risk factors for vasa praevia include placenta praevia, succenturiate lobe, assisted conception pregnancies and multiple pregnancy.

To summarise, there are two types of vasa praevia: *Type 1* is secondary to a velamentous cord insertion. *Type 2* is associated with fetal vessels which run between a placenta and a succenturiate lobe.

THE CERVIX

Premature birth is the main cause of perinatal death and disability. As a short cervix is associated with an increased risk of preterm labour, measurement of cervical length has been used to assess the risk of preterm labour and birth in women considered to be at higher risk of this condition. Women at increased risk of preterm labour include those who have had a previous preterm birth; those who have undergone previous cervical surgery, including, for example, cone biopsy; and

those who are currently pregnant with a multiple pregnancy.

ASSESSMENT AND MEASUREMENT OF CERVICAL LENGTH

The cervical length as measured with ultrasound describes the distance between the internal os and the external os. Although the cervix and cervical canal can be visualized transabdominally, accurate visualization of the positions of either the internal os and/or external os is usually difficult, making measurement of the intervening cervical length inaccurate. Assessment of the cervix and measurement of the cervical length should always be performed using the transvaginal route.

The preparation and technique required for a transvaginal examination have been described in detail in Chapter 4. The text assumes that you, the operator, are sitting to the left of, or at the foot of, the scanning couch, holding the probe in your right hand; that the woman is lying to your right side or directly in front of you; and that you are facing each other. The image is orientated so that the apex of the image is displayed at the top of the ultrasound monitor.

It is important that the maternal bladder is emptied immediately before the examination. Even a slightly full bladder can contribute to an inaccurate cervical length measurement. A longitudinal section of the cervical canal (i.e. the full length of the cervix from the internal to external os) should be demonstrated in one plane. The cervix is often slightly deviated to the right or left of the midline and also dextrorotated. Having obtained a sagittal section of the lower uterus and cervix, small panning or rotational movements of the probe are therefore required to best achieve this view. Undue pressure should not be applied by the probe, as this can cause an alteration to the cervical length. The cervical canal is usually visualized as a thin hyperechoic line, with the surrounding endocervical glands apparent as a hypoechoic halo. The image should be magnified sufficiently so that the cervix occupies 50–75% of the screen (Fig. 14.17).

Provided the previously described orientation is adopted, the internal os will be visualized to the left of the image. Using the surrounding amniotic fluid as an acoustic window, the internal os can be identified as a subtle notch at the uterine end of the cervical canal, where the anterior and posterior lips of the cervix meet. The internal os may be less easy to identify if the fetal presenting part is in close proximity to the cervix. In such situations, raise the foot of the scanning couch in an attempt to move the fetal presenting part away from the lower uterus. The external os is identified as a triangular area at the vaginal end of the cervical canal, where the anterior and posterior lips of the cervix

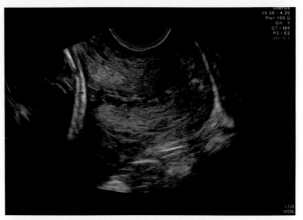

Fig 14.17 • Transvaginal scan of the cervix at 24 weeks of gestation. The opposing walls of the cervix produce a thin hyperechoic line centrally within the canal (arrow). The internal os (dashed arrow) appears as a dimple at the uterine end of the canal. The external os appears as a triangular-shaped area at the vaginal end of the canal (dotted arrow). The cervix is closed with no evidence of funnelling at its uterine end.

meet together (Fig. 14.17). The intersection of the cross of the on-screen linear callipers should be placed on the internal os and external os, respectively, as shown in Fig. 14.18A. As the cervix is a dynamic structure, at least three measurements should be made, ideally over a 5 minute period, and the best, shortest measurement recorded.

Applying pressure to the cervix with the tip of the vaginal probe is easily done and will falsely reduce its length. Make sure, therefore, that you apply as little pressure as possible to the cervix with the probe. You will be able to assess the effect of the pressure you are applying by withdrawing the probe slightly once you are imaging the cervix. Your aim should be to ensure that the width of the cervical tissue above the cervical canal is the same as that below the canal in the image you are assessing, before you attempt to measure the cervical length (Figs. 14.17, 14.18B and 14.19). A discrepancy between the thickness of the two cervical walls, with the upper wall being thinner than the lower, is due to excess pressure from the probe tip.

When the cervical length measures more than 25.0 mm, the cervix will be curved in more than half of cases. The linear measurement will thus be an underestimate of the true cervical length. An

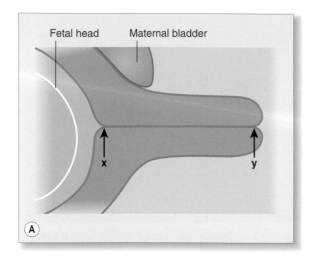

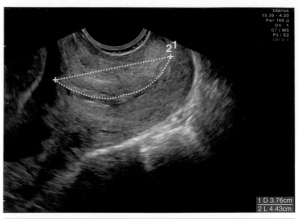

Fig 14.19 • Transvaginal scan demonstrating the two methods of measuring a cervical length when the cervix is curved. (1) The linear measurement of 3.76 cm has been obtained by placing the intersection of the cross of each linear calliper at the internal os and external os, respectively. (2) The measurement of 4.43 cm has been obtained by tracing the actual length of the cervical canal between the internal os and the external os. Most authors recommend using method 1.

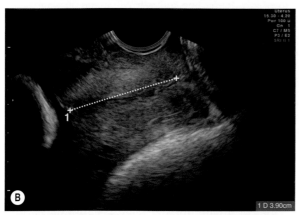

Fig 14.18 • A. Schematic diagram of measurement of the cervical length from internal os (x) to external os (y). B. Transvaginal scan demonstrating measurement of the cervical length from the internal os to the external os (3.9 cm) in a 20 week pregnancy. The cervix is normal in appearance, being long with no evidence of funnelling. Note the width of the cervix above and below the canal is equivalent, indicating that undue pressure has not been applied to the tip of the vaginal probe while obtaining this image.

published. To et al. reported a mean cervical length of 36.0 mm between 22 and 24 weeks. This can be compared with that reported by Salomon, of 41.0 mm at 22 weeks and 40.0 mm at 24 weeks. As important as the mean length for gestational age is the association between a shortened cervical length and the risk of preterm delivery. A review by Honest of five studies using cervical length measurements between 20 and 24 weeks, and cut-offs of between 20.0 mm and 30.0 mm, to predict preterm labour before 34 weeks, reported positive likelihood ratios from 2.3 for 30.0 mm to 7.6 for 20.0 mm.

The definition of, and subsequent clinical management of a woman with, a short cervix will be locally agreed. In the absence of definitive local guidance, we suggest that a woman with a singleton pregnancy and a cervical length which has been properly measured and is less than 2.0 cm at any gestation between 16 and 24 weeks should be referred for consultant review as soon as possible.

Although a normal cervical length is reassuring at the time of the examination, you are unable to predict whether or not these findings will remain such over time. For this reason, the clinical management of women at increased risk of preterm

option is to attempt to follow the curve of the cervix, provided that the measurement software within your machine allows you to do so (Fig. 14.19). However, when the cervix is shortened it will always be straight and the linear measurement will be an accurate one. For these reasons the problem of how to measure a curved cervix is not thought to be clinically significant.

Various reference ranges describing cervical length from 16 weeks to 36 weeks have been

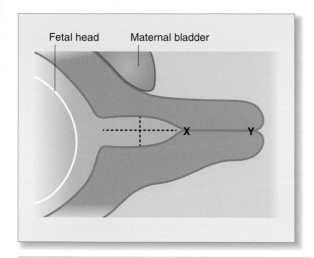

Fetal head   Maternal bladder

X   Y

Fig 14.20 • Schematic diagram demonstrating funnelling measured by two linear measurements, internal os (x) and external os (y).

delivery, and for whom cervical length screening is appropriate, may require regular cervical length assessment every 2 weeks up to 24 weeks of gestation. This is because clinical management up to 24 weeks may include rescue cerclage. As this is not normally the treatment of choice for a shortened cervix after 24 weeks of gestation, cervical length assessment is not normally undertaken after this time.

CERVICAL FUNNELLING

Funnelling of the cervix describes the dilation of the internal part of the cervical canal, reduction in cervical length and prolapse of the fetal membranes into the cervical canal. The appearance of the normal, closed cervical canal and dimple of the internal os at its internal end is lost and is replaced by a V- or U-shaped appearance at the internal end of the cervical canal (Fig. 14.20). Although funnelling is thought by some to be an additional risk factor for preterm labour, studies have suggested that funnelling without a shortened cervix should not be considered as a risk factor. Cervical mucus can accumulate within the cervical canal and is a normal finding; care must be taken not to mistake this for funnelling. It can be difficult to distinguish between the features of the normal lower uterine body/lower segment, and a funnelling cervix as the demarcation between the cervical and uterine tissue is usually too subtle to be appreciated on transvaginal imaging in the routine setting.

Further reading

Daly-Jones E, Jones A, Leahy A, McKenna C, Sepulveda W 2008 Vasa praevia: a preventable tragedy. Ultrasound 16(1):8–14

Honest H, Bachmann LM, Coomarasamy A, Gupta JK, Kleijnen J, Kahn K 2003 Accuracy of cervical transvaginal sonographer in predicting preterm birth, a systematic review. Ultrasound Obstet Gynecol 22:305–322

Kagan K O, Sonek J 2015 How to measure cervical length. Ultrasound Obstet Gynecol 45:358–362

Royal College of Obstetricians and Gynaecologists 2011 Placenta praevia, placenta praevia accreta and vasa praevia: diagnosis and management. Green-Top Guideline No. 27. RCOG Press, London

Salomon L J et al 2009 Reference range for cervical length throughout pregnancy: non-parametric LMS-based model applied to a large sample. Ultrasound Obstet Gynecol 33:459–464

To MS, Skentou C, Liao AW, Cacho A, Nicolaides KH 2001 Cervical length and funneling at 23 weeks of gestation in the prediction of spontaneous early preterm delivery. Ultrasound Obstet Gynecol 18:200–203

Multiple pregnancy

CONTENTS

This chapter addresses the ultrasound diagnosis, examination and reporting of twin pregnancies.

The aims of this chapter are to enable you to do the following:

- understand the differences between zygosity and chorionicity
- determine chorionicity
- understand the issues that are specific to twin pregnancies when screening for Down's, Edwards' and Patau's syndromes
- understand the issues that are specific to twin pregnancies when assessing fetal anatomy and fetal growth in twin pregnancies.

This chapter primarily discusses twin pregnancies, as they are the most commonly encountered type of multiple pregnancy.

The clinical management of a twin pregnancy does not depend on whether or not the twins are 'identical' or 'nonidentical' – that is, its *zygosity*. What is important is the number of placentas present – that is, its *chorionicity* – and, where only one placenta is present, the number of amniotic sacs present – that is, its *amnionicity*. Thus zygosity is often of great importance to the parents but normally of only passing interest to the clinician, for whom correct assessment of the chorionicity by you, the sonographer, is critical. The issue of zygosity is of great importance to the clinician, however, when genetic testing is sought or indicated.

PLACENTATION OF THE SINGLETON PREGNANCY

In order to understand chorionicity and amnionicity in twin pregnancies, it may be helpful to revisit the comparative processes in a singleton pregnancy.

At ovulation the egg is released from the ovary and enters the Fallopian tube, where it is fertilized. The zygote starts to divide as it travels down the Fallopian tube towards the endometrial cavity of the uterus. This journey takes 3–4 days, during which time cleavage (division of the zygote into a cluster of cells that has the same size as the original zygote) takes place, resulting in a solid ball of cells called the morula. At approximately 4 days after fertilization, a cavity starts to develop within the morula separating a small number of cells, the inner cell mass, from the rest. This hollow ball of cells is called the blastocyst; the cavity within it is the precursor of the chorionic cavity and the inner cell mass is the precursor of the embryo. The cells surrounding the chorionic cavity, the trophoblast cells, will give rise to the chorionic membrane or chorion and the fetal component of the placenta.

It is a blastocyst that enters the endometrial cavity 4–5 days after fertilization and starts to embed into the endometrium. The placenta develops at the site of implantation, from the invasion of the cells of the blastocyst called the trophoblast into the endometrium and the subsequent maternal response of the endometrial cells adjacent to this invasion.

The blastocyst starts to implant into the endometrium 5–6 days after fertilization and is fully embedded below the surface of the endometrium approximately 10 days after fertilization. Approximately 7 days after fertilization, a second cavity, the amniotic cavity, develops between the inner cell mass and the invading trophoblast (Fig. 15.1). The cells surrounding this cavity will give rise to the amniotic membrane or amnion. The amnion is attached to the margins of the embryonic 'disc', as it is now termed. Due to the folding of the future embryo, the amnion surrounds the embryo and sheaths the umbilical cord, thus separating the early embryo from its yolk sac. The embryo therefore lies in the amniotic cavity and its yolk sac lies in the chorionic cavity.

Initially the amniotic cavity is obviously much smaller than the chorionic cavity, but it grows more rapidly, such that by 14 weeks the two cavities are the same size. The filling of the chorionic cavity by the amniotic cavity allows the outer chorion to fuse with the inner amnion, thus forming the double-layered 'membranes', the rupture of which has significant sequelae in later pregnancy.

All singleton embryos could therefore be described as *monochorionic* and *monoamniotic*, as they are surrounded by an outer single chorion and an inner single amnion, although these terms are not used in clinical practice.

ZYGOSITY

As discussed in Chapter 5, a zygote is a cell which results from the union of a sperm and an egg or ovum. *Zygosity* therefore refers to the number of fertilized eggs that produce the multiple pregnancy. A twin pregnancy arises in one of two ways. Either it results from the fertilization of two eggs or from one egg which then divides. A pregnancy that results from the fertilization of two eggs is termed *dizygotic (DZ)*. Ovulation of the two eggs can occur simultaneously from either the same or each ovary.

A pregnancy that results from the fertilization of one egg that subsequently divides to form two or more genetically identical conceptuses is termed *monozygotic (MZ)*.

DIZYGOTIC TWINS

As dizygotic twins result from the fertilization of two eggs, they are as genetically similar as two siblings who happen to be developing in the uterus at the same time. Approximately half of DZ twin pairs will be the same sex and approximately half will be of different sexes.

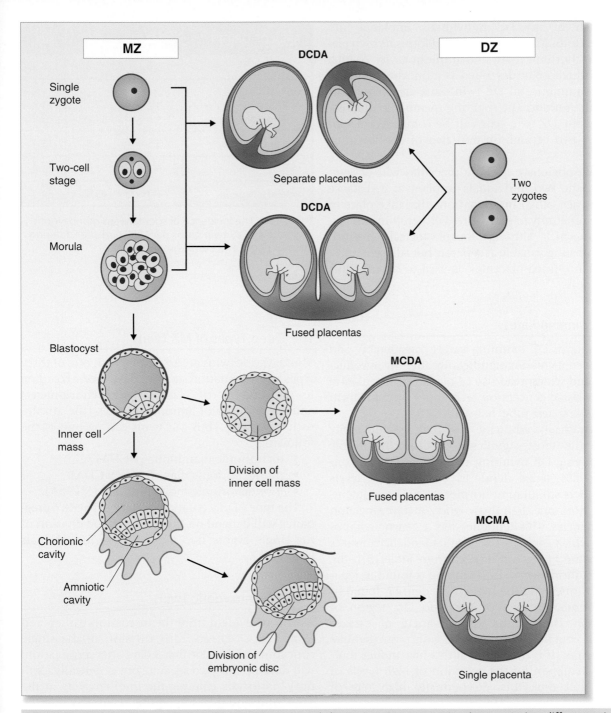

Fig 15.1 • Embryological pathways for monozygotic and dizygotic twin pregnancies demonstrating differences in chorionicity and amnionicity in dichorionic and the three types of monochorionic twinning. DCDA, dichorionic diamniotic; DZ, dizygotic; MCDA, monochorionic diamniotic; MCMA, monochorionic monoamniotic; MZ, monozygotic.

Each of the DZ individuals implants into the endometrium separately and forms its own placenta, chorionic cavity and amniotic cavity. As each individual can be described as monochorionic and monoamniotic, all DZ twin pairs are dichorionic and diamniotic. The resulting membrane that separates the DZ twin pair will be composed of four layers, two of amnion and two of chorion (Fig. 15.1).

Two obviously separate placentas will develop when the two individuals implant at a distance from each other. Implantations that take place in close proximity to each other will result in two placentas which, although morphologically distinct, are indistinguishable as separate but adjacent units. The term 'fused placentas' is used to describe this situation.

AREA OF ORIGIN	MZ	DZ	ALL
Japan	3.0	1.3	4.3
United States White Afro-Caribbean	4.2 4.7	7.1 11.1	11.3 15.8
England & Wales	3.5	8.8	12.3
India	3.3	8.1	11.4
Western Nigeria	5.0	49.0	54.0

Table 15.1 The incidence of spontaneous monozygotic, dizygotic and all twin births per 1000 births for differing areas of origin and ethnic groups
Adapted from MacGillivray 1986.
DZ, dizygotic; *MZ*, monozygotic.

DZ Twinning Rates

The rate of DZ twinning varies considerably and has been increasing significantly after the introduction and widespread use of ovulation stimulation and assisted conception techniques since the birth of the first 'test tube' baby in 1978.

Historically, ethnicity, maternal age and parity were the most significant predisposing factors underlying DZ twinning rates. Women who conceive DZ twins tend to have higher levels of follicle stimulating hormone (FSH) and luteinizing hormone than those who conceive singleton pregnancies. This tendency has a genetic component which explains the familial tendency towards DZ twinning. As can be seen from Table 15.1, the lowest incidence of DZ twinning is found in Japanese women and the highest incidence is found in the Yoruba women of the Igbo Ora region of Nigeria. The Yoruba eat a variety of cassava which contains a component with oestrogen-like properties. It is thought that this may induce multiple ovulation by the secretion of high levels of FSH and thus this exceptionally high rate of twinning.

MONOZYGOTIC TWINS

As MZ twins arise from the division of a single fertilized egg, both conceptuses are almost always, as discussed later, genetically identical and therefore will be the same sex.

The Three Types of MZ Twins

Monozygotic twins are associated with one of three types of placentation and are described according to the number of placentas (the chorionicity) and the number of amniotic cavities (the amnionicity) present. Thus MZ twins can be one of the following:

- dichorionic diamniotic (DCDA)
- monochorionic diamniotic (MCDA)
- monochorionic monoamniotic (MCMA).

The type of placentation present in the MZ pregnancy will depend on the timing of the division of the single zygote into two or more individviduals (Fig. 15.1).

DCDA Monozygotic Twins

As will be evident from the discussion earlier, and from Fig. 15.1, very early division of the single conceptus, within the first 3 days after fertilization, will develop into two separate but genetically identical blastocysts entering the uterine cavity at the same time and then implanting separately into the endometrium. The placentation of such MZ twins will therefore be the same as that of all DZ twin pairs. These monozygotic individuals will each have their own placenta, chorionic cavity and amniotic cavity, resulting in a DCDA twin pair.

As the two genetically identical conceptuses enter the endometrial cavity from the same

Fallopian tube, they are likely to implant into the endometrium in close proximity to each other and therefore have what appears to be a single placenta rather than two distinct placentas.

Approximately 25–30% of MZ twins will be DCDA, with placentation that is the same as all DZ twin pairs. The only way that the zygosity of DCDA twin pairs can be established with ultrasound is by establishing the presence of a male fetus and a female fetus. Such a pregnancy is DZ. It is not possible to assign zygosity in a twin pair of the same sex, as 50% of DZ twin pairs will be of the same sex and 50% will be of different sexes.

MCDA Monozygotic Twins

The most common type of MZ twins are formed by the splitting of the single conceptus 4–8 days after fertilization, after the formation of the chorionic cavity but before the formation of the amniotic cavity.

A single blastocyst therefore implants into the endometrium, initiating the development of a single placenta and a single chorionic cavity with its surrounding chorionic membrane. The inner cell mass within the blastocyst divides. The two genetically identical individuals will share the same placenta and chorionic cavity and therefore will be monochorionic. They will then each develop their own amniotic cavity, surrounded by its own amniotic membrane, and will therefore be diamniotic. The membrane dividing the MCDA monozygotic twin pair will be composed of two layers of amnion only (Fig. 15.1).

Monochorionic diamniotic twin pairs are the most common type of MZ twins and constitute approximately 70–75% of MZ pregnancies.

The twins share the same placenta, and this sharing may not always be equal. Unequal sharing of the placenta predisposes MCDA twins to the condition of twin to twin transfusion syndrome (TTTS).

These twin pregnancies are also at risk of another severe condition, twin reversed arterial perfusion syndrome (TRAP).

MCMA Monozygotic Twins

The least common type of MZ twins is formed by the splitting of the single conceptus between approximately 9 and 13 days after fertilization. As with the MCDA twins, a single blastocyst implants into the endometrium, initiating the development of a single placenta and a single chorionic cavity with its surrounding chorionic membrane. The amniotic cavity forms together with its surrounding amniotic membrane. The embryonic disc, which now lies within its amniotic cavity, then divides. The two genetically identical individuals will share the same placenta and chorionic cavity and will therefore be monochorionic. They will also share the same amniotic cavity surrounded by its amniotic membrane and will therefore also be monoamniotic. Because both individuals lie within the same amniotic cavity, there will be no membrane dividing this type of MZ twin pair (Fig. 15.1).

Monochorionic monoamniotic twin pairs comprise approximately 1–2% of MZ pregnancies and approximately 5% of MC twins.

The loss rate of MCMA twins varies between authors, with 10–40% being reported in one series and 50–75% in another. The high loss rate is due to a combination of fetal malformations, polyhydramnios and preterm delivery together with complications of acute TTTS. These are thought to arise because of the proximity of the two umbilical cords within the shared amniotic sac.

Conjoined twins

Incomplete division of the embryonic disc results in conjoined or 'Siamese' twins. This type of MCMA twinning is very rare and occurs in between 1 in 30 000 and 1 in 100 000 live births. Seventy percent of conjoined twins are females. Conjoined twins are classified according to the site of fusion, with the thoraco-omphalopagus type, where the two bodies are fused from the upper chest to the lower chest, being the most common, constituting approximately 25–30% of cases of conjoined twins.

The prognosis for conjoined twins depends on the site and extent of organ sharing. Approximately 50% of conjoined twin pregnancies are stillborn. Of those born alive, approximately 30% will have severe defects for which no surgery is possible.

Incomplete and asymmetrical division of the embryonic disc results in a parastic twin, where one twin is much smaller or less formed than the other and dependent on its larger co-twin.

MZ Twinning Rates

The rate of MZ twinning is fairly constant across the world (Table 15.1) and is reported to be around 3.5/1000 deliveries. Monozygotic twinning is unaffected by ethnicity, maternal age or parity. Recent evidence suggests that the assisted conception technique of intracytoplasmic sperm injection (ICSI) confers a two to three fold increase in the rate of MZ twinning. This is thought to be due to damage to the zona pellucida during the in vitro fertilization (IVF) process which then stimulates splitting of the single conceptus.

THE IMPLICATIONS OF TWINNING

The early identification of an ongoing twin pregnancy is important because of the following:

- monozygotic twin pregnancies have a higher risk of structural abnormalities than dizygotic or singleton pregnancies
- monochorionic twin pregnancies have the unique risk of TTTS and TRAP sequence
- the risk of chromosomal abnormalities is higher in twin pregnancies that in singleton pregnancies
- the risk of fetal growth restriction (FGR) is 10 times higher in twin pregnancies than in a singleton pregnancy
- the birth weight of at least one of the twin pair being below the 5th centile for gestational age is likely to occur in 30–35% of MC twin pairs and in 20–25% of DC twin pairs
- the perinatal mortality rate in twin pregnancies is six times the singleton rate, mainly because of prematurity-related complications.

Thus because all twin pregnancies are at increased risk of both growth-related problems and premature delivery, all twin pregnancies should be monitored more closely than singleton pregnancies, and by staff experienced in the clinical management of twin pregnancies.

RISKS OF CHROMOSOMAL DEFECTS

The prevalence of a chromosomal abnormality being present in one or both of a twin pair overall is expected to be approximately 1.6 times that in a singleton pregnancy. This is based on the proportion of spontaneous DZ to MZ twins in the United Kingdom being approximately 2 : 1.

DZ Twins

Each fetus of a DZ twin pair has the same risk of a chromosomal abnormality as a singleton. The chance of at least one of the twin pair having a chromosomal abnormality is twice that of the individual risk in a singleton pregnancy. The chance that both of the twin pair will be affected is derived by squaring the singleton risk.

As the rate of DZ twinning increases with maternal age, the proportion of twin pregnancies in which a chromosomal abnormality is present is higher than in singleton pregnancies.

MZ Twins

The risk of an MZ twin pair having a chromosomal abnormality is the same as that of a singleton pregnancy. As the two fetuses are genetically identical, both fetuses will be affected in the vast majority of cases.

Discordance does occur in chromosomally abnormal MZ twin pairs, with the most common discordance being 45X0 (Turner's syndrome) and 46XX/XY. A mosaic, rather than a complete, abnormal karyotypic pattern is the more common in these cases.

DC Twins

As confirming zygosity is only reliable in a small percentage of twin pregnancies, using chorionicity as a guide to the likelihood of one or both of the twin pair having a chromosomal abnormality is more practical.

Let us assume that the maternal age-related risk for trisomy 21 in a DC twin pregnancy is 1 : 100. This mother would therefore be about 40 years of age at the time of her (term) delivery. The risk of one twin of a DC pair being affected with Down's syndrome would be $1:50$ ($1:100 + 1:100$), whereas the risk of both of the DC pair being affected would be $1:10,000$ ($1:100 \times 1:100$). This, however, does not take into account the percentage of DC twin pairs that are MZ and is therefore an oversimplification, but a useful one.

ESTABLISHING CHORIONICITY AND AMNIONICITY

As soon as it is possible to identify a pregnancy within the uterus it should be possible to determine whether one or two gestation sacs are present. Similarly, it should be possible to confirm the presence of heart pulsations in two embryos as early in gestation as in a single embryo.

DIAGNOSING THE EARLY TWIN PREGNANCY

It is possible to identify the presence of two separate gestation sacs from around 5 weeks of gestation transvaginally and about a week later transabdominally. Two separate sacs indicate the presence of a dichorionic twin pregnancy – which may be DZ or MZ (Fig. 15.2). As with a single gestation sac, both gestation sacs should be measured in three orthogonal planes and assessed internally to determine whether a yolk sac or embryo can be identified.

Between 6 and approximately 9 weeks of gestation the tissue mass separating the two sacs in a DC twin pregnancy is thick, giving the appearance of two obviously separate gestation sacs (Fig. 15.2A). This area becomes progressively thinner as the intertwin membrane develops. It remains at the placental interface, to form the triangular 'lambda' or 'delta' sign that provides the characteristic appearance of a DCDA pregnancy (Fig. 15.2B), as discussed in more detail later.

A single gestation sac in very early pregnancy in which you can visualize two yolk sacs suggests a MCDA twin pregnancy rather than a singleton pregnancy (Fig. 15.3).

Once the presence of two embryos within a single gestation sac can be confirmed, the diagnosis of an MC, and therefore MZ, twin pregnancy can be made. However, the complete assessment of an MC pregnancy includes assessment of its amnionicity. This is difficult to establish accurately before 7–8 weeks, as the amniotic membrane is very difficult to identify within the gestation sac before this time (Fig. 15.4). As the amniotic cavity surrounding each twin increases in size, the two-layered intertwin amniotic membrane becomes distinguishable

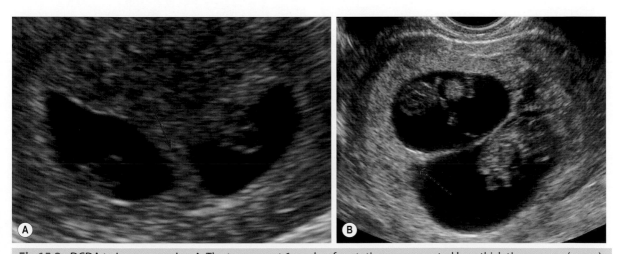

Fig 15.2 • DCDA twin pregnancies. A. The two sacs at 6 weeks of gestation are separated by a thick tissue mass (arrow). B. By 9 weeks of gestation the two sacs are now separated by a membrane. This is composed of 4 layers, two of amnion, separated by two of chorion. The membranes/placental interface of the DCDA twin pregnancy produces the typical lambda sign (dashed arrow). DCDA, dichorionic diamniotic.

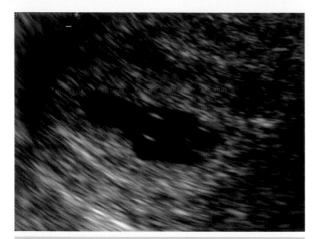

Fig 15.3 • A MC twin pregnancy at 5 weeks of gestation. Two yolk sacs can be seen but it is too early to identify the two embryos. Subsequent scans confirmed a MCDA twin pregnancy. MC, monochorionic; MCDA, monochorionic diamniotic.

Gestational age (weeks)	DCDA	MCDA	MCMA
5	○ ○	○	○
6			
7			

○ = gestation sac   ⬭ = amniotic sac   ▮ = embryo

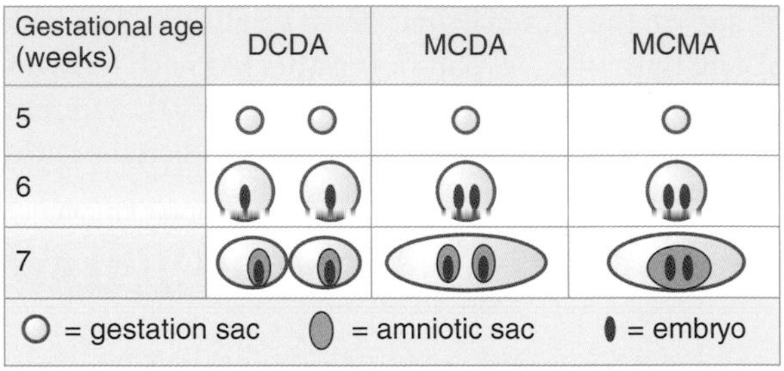

Fig 15.5 • Schematic diagram showing gestational ages at which chorionicity and amnionicity in early twin pregnancies can be recognised. DCDA, dichorionic diamniotic; MCDA, monochorionic diamniotic; MCMA, monochorionic monoamniotic.

within the chorionic cavity, enabling the amnionicity of the twin pregnancy to be established (Fig. 15.5).

The inability to identify an intertwin membrane, together with the presence of only one yolk sac, raises the possibility of an MCMA twin pregnancy (Fig. 15.6). As the intertwin membrane can be very thin, and therefore difficult to identify in early pregnancy, we recommend that the diagnosis of a MCMA twin pregnancy is not made until after these early appearances have been reviewed, and confirmed, at 12 weeks at the earliest.

As with every early pregnancy, whether singleton or multiple, you should be guarded in your prognosis until you are able to confirm heart activity in the embryo or both embryos is present. As discussed in Chapter 5, apparently empty sacs in a multiple pregnancy may regress spontaneously before the embryo develops. This "vanishing twin"

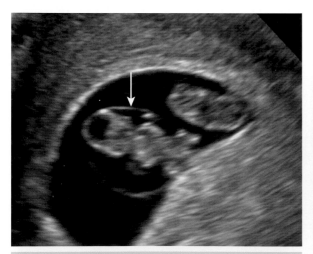

Fig 15.4 • MCDA twin pregnancy at 8⁺³ weeks of gestation. The two embryos can be seen within the same gestation sac (chorionic cavity). The amnion (arrow) can be clearly seen surrounding one of the embryos, indicating that each embryo lies within a separate amniotic cavity and therefore confirming that this is an MCDA twin pregnancy. MCDA, monochorionic diamniotic.

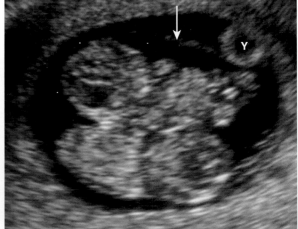

Fig 15.6 • MCMA twin pregnancy at 9 weeks of gestation. Both embryos are seen to lie within one amniotic cavity. The amnion (arrow) surrounds both embryos. The single yolk sac (y) is seen to lie outside the amniotic cavity, within the chorionic cavity. MCMA, monochorionic monoamniotic.

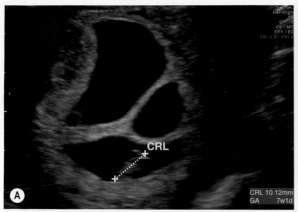 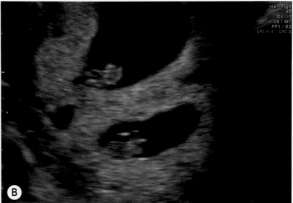

Fig 15.7 • A. Three gestation sacs identified in a pregnancy five weeks after three day 3 blastocysts were transferred. B. A live embryo was present in only two of the three gestation sacs, indicating an ongoing DC twin pregnancy. CRL, crown rump length; DC, dichorionic.

phenomenon has been reported to affect up to 20% of multiple pregnancies. Although this figure may be an overestimate, this further supports delaying the diagnosis of multiple pregnancy until a live embryo can be identified in both sacs.

Having diagnosed a twin pregnancy, always make sure you have not missed an elusive triplet (Fig. 15.7). The woman's confidence tends to falter if another fetus is discovered at every ultrasound examination. She will rarely return for a fourth appointment.

Problems

Not all cystic areas within the uterus are gestation sacs, and it is important to distinguish between the following:

- a genuine multiple gestation (Figs. 15.2, 15.3, 15.4 and 15.6)
- an implantation bleed or subchorionic haematoma accompanying a singleton pregnancy. The gestation sac is usually anechoic, whereas blood usually has low-level echoes (Fig. 15.8)
- a kidney shaped gestation sac will produce the appearance of twin sacs when viewed in certain sections. If this is a single sac, then the two 'sacs' must join at together at some point, to form the true single sac. Careful scanning of the sac(s) in several planes perpendicular to each other will determine whether this is truly a multiple gestation.

Fig 15.8 • Singleton pregnancy at 5 weeks of gestation demonstrating the gestation sac and yolk sac (arrow) with an implantation bleed adjacent to it (dashed arrow) mimicking the second gestation sac of a dichorionic twin pregnancy.

DETERMINING CHORIONICITY

You will now understand why it is so important to establish the chorionicity of a twin pregnancy as early in gestation as possible.

The optimal time to distinguish between DC, MCDA and MCMA twin pairs using ultrasound is between 10 and 14 weeks of gestation.

The presence of two gestation sacs in which each has a separate placenta indicates the presence of a DCDA twin pregnancy (Fig. 15.9).

The presence of an apparently single placenta can indicate either a DC pregnancy with adjacent implantation of the two placentas or an MC pregnancy with a single placenta. In such a situation the chorionicity should be established. Locate the insertion of the chorional membranes into the placenta. As noted earlier, a dichorional placenta will demonstrate the 'lambda' or 'delta sign' (Fig. 15.10). This appearance arises from the tongue of placental tissue, which projects between the amniotic and chorionic membranes of one twin and the two membranes of the other. This causes a slight separation between the two sets of membranes at their insertion site into the placenta. This small area of separation has the appearance of the Greek letters delta (Δ) or lambda (λ). This type of twinning is therefore DCDA.

A monochorional placenta will demonstrate a 'T sign' at the placental insertion of the amniotic membranes (Fig. 15.11). The T is composed of two layers of amnion which constitute the intertwin membrane inserting into the shared placenta of an MCDA twin pregnancy. This type of twinning is therefore MCDA. Care should be taken to distinguish between placental insertion of the amniotic membrane and its appearance at the uterine wall, as the latter often have an appearance that is very similar to a T sign (see Fig. 15.10).

If no dividing membrane can be identified between the two fetuses, then MCMA twins should

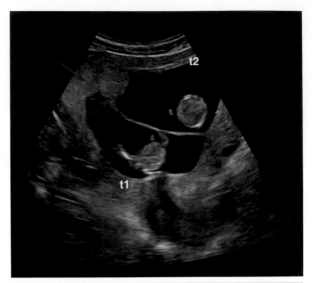

Fig 15.10 • A twin pregnancy at 12 weeks of gestation in which a single fundal placenta can be seen (arrow). The interface between the placenta and the intertwin membrane forms a lambda or delta shape (dashed arrow) because of a tongue of placental tissue separating the two layers of chorion between the two sacs. This is therefore a DCDA twin pregnancy. Note the appearance of the intertwin membrane at the uterine wall, opposite the placenta, mimicking the T sign of a MCDA twin pregnancy. DCDA, dichorionic diamniotic; MCDA, monochorionic diamniotic; t1, twin 1; t2, twin 2.

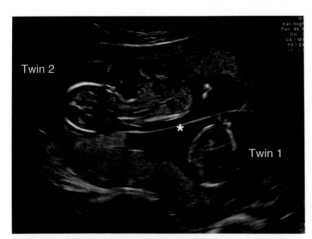

Fig 15.9 • A twin pregnancy at 13+ weeks of gestation in which a separate placenta in each of the two sacs can be clearly identified. Twin 1 has a posterior placenta (arrow) and twin 2 has an anterior placenta (dashed arrow). This is therefore a DCDA twin pregnancy. The intertwin membrane (*) is relatively thick, as it is composed of four layers. It is most likely to be dizygotic, although 12% of DCDA twin pregnancies will arise from the early division of a single zygote. DCDA, dichorionic diamniotic.

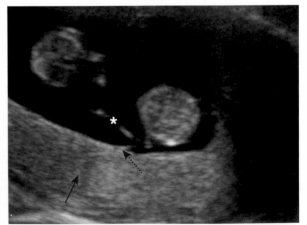

Fig 15.11 • A twin pregnancy at 13 weeks of gestation in which a single posterior placenta can be seen (arrow). The interface between the placenta and the intertwin membrane forms a T shape (dashed arrow). The site of insertion is often difficult to locate owing to the thinness of the membrane (*), which is composed of only two layers of amnion. This is therefore a MCDA twin pregnancy and must also be monozygotic. MCDA, monochorionic diamniotic.

ZYGOSITY	DCDA ALL	DCDA PLACENTAS SEPARATE	DCDA PLACENTAS FUSED	MCDA	MCMA	TOTAL
MZ	10	6	4	19	1	30
DZ	70	42	28	0	0	70
All	80	48	32	19	1	100

Table 15.2 The relationship between zygosity and types of placentation in 100 spontaneously conceived twin pairs
DCDA, dichorionic diamniotic; *DZ*, dizygotic; *MCDA*, monochorionic diamniotic; *MCMA*, monochorionic monoamniotic; *MZ*, monozygotic.

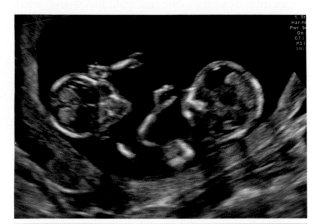

Fig 15.12 • A MCMA twin pregnancy at 15+ weeks. No interwin membrane was identified at the combined screening scan performed 3 weeks earlier. No membrane could be identified at the second scan, thus confirming the diagnosis. MCMA, monochorionic monoamniotic.

be suspected. As the dividing membrane between MCDA twins is very thin and mobile, it may be difficult to visualize in the first trimester twin pregnancy. Conversely, reverberation artefacts may lead to the incorrect diagnosis of a dividing amniotic membrane in a true MCMA twin pregnancy. Confirmation of an MCMA pregnancy should therefore always be made in the second trimester in order that the correct advice can be given to the parents (see Fig. 15.12). Note that the apparent absence of an intertwin dividing membrane in the second trimester or later may be a sign of TTTS because of the ultrasound features of the stuck twin.

The relationship between zygosity and chorionicity can be summarized by considering the chorionicity and amnionicity of 100 spontaneously conceived twin pairs in which we assume the MZ rate is 30%. Of the 100 twin pairs, 70 pairs will therefore be DZ. Of these 70 DCDA twin pairs, their placentas will be separate in 42 cases and fused, thus demonstrating a lambda sign, in the remaining 28 cases. Of the 30 MZ twin pairs, 10 pairs will be DC. Their placentas will be separate in six cases and in four cases will be fused, thus demonstrating a lambda sign. Of the remaining 20 MZ twin pairs, all will be MC, 19 pairs will be MCDA, thus demonstrating a T sign, and one pair will be MCMA in which no intertwin membrane will be present, as shown in Table 15.2.

TRIPLOIDY SCREENING IN A TWIN PREGNANCY

Triploidy screening in a twin pregnancy is performed either by combined or quadruple screening using maternal serum or ultrasound imaging.

COMBINED SCREENING

Combined screening can be performed in a twin pregnancy as with a singleton pregnancy. A risk therefore can be calculated for Down's syndrome alone, only for Edwards' and Patau's syndromes together or for Down's syndrome and Edwards' and Patau's syndromes together as for a singleton pregnancy. A single risk for each condition being screened for will be reported for a MC twin pregnancy, whereas a risk for each fetus will be reported for each condition being screened for in a DC twin pregnancy.

Measuring NT in a Twin Pregnancy

Measuring the nuchal translucency (NT) of the fetuses in a twin pregnancy requires the same techniques as for a singleton pregnancy. The pregnancy being dated from the larger crown rump length (CRL), unless this is an IVF pregnancy (see Chapter 5). What differs in a twin pregnancy is the calculation of the risk of chromosomal abnormality. The risk of a chromosomal abnormality in a twin pregnancy relates to the zygosity of the pregnancy. Because all MC twin pregnancies are MZ, the chromosomal risk in these cases is calculated and reported for the pregnancy, not for each individual fetus.

As the assumption is that both twins of a MC pair are genetically identical and that the size of the NT is a reflection of the karyotypic status of the fetus, it would be reasonable to expect not only the CRL of both fetuses to be essentially the same, but also the NT. It should be remembered that increased NT in both fetuses will increase the risk of a chromosomal abnormality but is also a marker for cardiac abnormalities, genetic syndromes and early TTTS. When only one of the MC twin pair demonstrates an increased NT, greater than 3.5 mm, remember that MC twins are more likely to be discordant than concordant for nonkaryotypic abnormalities. Thus discrepant NTs in a MCDA pregnancy increase not only the risk for congenital heart disease in the fetus with the increased NT but also for TTTS in the remainder of the pregnancy.

In a DC twin pair, the assumption is that both fetuses are genetically dissimilar and therefore a risk will be calculated for both individuals separately. As approximately 12% of DC twin pairs are MZ and are therefore genetically identical, but cannot be identified before combined screening, the sensitivity of NT in screening for chromosomal abnormalities in a DC twin pregnancy is less than for a singleton pregnancy. An increased NT measurement in one of a DCDA twin pair is associated with an increased risk of a chromosomal, genetic or cardiac abnormality as with singleton or MC twin pregnancies. When one twin demonstrates an increased NT, it is important to report the placental sites and relative positions of the two gestations within the uterus, as this aids in further distinguishing between the two fetuses later in the pregnancy. Remember that increased NT is essentially a feature of the late first trimester fetus and, although nuchal oedema may be present in the same fetus after 14 weeks, this is not always the case and therefore cannot be relied upon as the only means of identifying the potentially abnormal twin.

The Twin Pregnancy With One Live Fetus and One Empty Sac

Combined screening can be performed in a twin pregnancy in which one sac contains a live fetus and the other is completely empty – that is, in which *no* evidence of an embryo, fetus or yolk sac can be seen.

The Twin Pregnancy With One Live Fetus and One Dead Fetus

Where ultrasound shows a twin pregnancy in which one sac contains a live fetus and the other contains tissue remnants, a yolk sac or a recognizable dead embryo or fetus is present, combined screening should *not* be performed. This is because there may still be a contribution to the hormone levels being measured from the dead twin, and this will affect the accuracy of the biochemical component of the risk result. In such cases, the chromosomal risk should be calculated from the NT and maternal age only.

QUADRUPLE TEST SCREENING

The risks for chromosomal abnormality based on NT cannot be calculated when the CRL of one or both fetuses is greater than 84.0 mm. Quadruple test screening can be offered in such cases but can only be used to screen for Down's syndrome in a twin pregnancy. A single risk is reported for the pregnancy, irrespective of the chorionicity of the pregnancy.

The second trimester screening test for Edwards' syndrome and Patau's syndrome is ultrasound examination and not, currently, the quadruple test.

Quadruple Testing in an MC Twin Pair

As both fetuses in an MC twin pregnancy are assumed to be genetically identical, the sensitivity of the quadruple test for an MC twin pregnancy is comparable to that of a singleton pregnancy, namely a detection rate of 80% for a standardized screen-positive rate of 3%.

Quadruple Testing in a DC Twin Pair

The sensitivity of the quadruple test for Down's syndrome in a DC twin pregnancy is affected by the uncertainty of the zygosity of the pregnancy. Quadruple test screening for Down's syndrome in a DC twin pregnancy has a detection rate of 40–50% for a standardized screen-positive rate of 3%.

ULTRASOUND LABELLING OF TWINS

To ensure consistency of assessment of a twin pregnancy throughout gestation it is important that each twin can be correctly identified. The position of the two gestation sacs relative to the cervix remains unchanged with gestation, and for this reason we recommend the following method of labelling: The twin in the sac closer to the cervix should be identified as Twin 1 or Twin A and the twin in the sac further from the cervix as Twin 2 or Twin B. This notation should be *strictly* applied from the very beginning of pregnancy.

It was common practice to label twins as Twin 1 and Twin 2, the connotation being that Twin 1 (closer to the cervix) would be delivered first. A potential discrepancy exists between the pre- and postnatal labelling of twins. The postnatal labelling of the twins relates to the time of their deliveries; the first baby delivered is referred to as Twin 1 and the second as Twin 2. To overcome this, labelling the twins in the antenatal period using A and B has been widely adopted. It can be difficult to determine which twin lies closer to the cervix in the first trimester. In such situations it is preferable to identify the fetuses as 'left' and 'right' or 'upper' and 'lower' and leave labelling them as A or B until this can be done with accuracy a little later in the pregnancy. Remember that it is the relative positions of the sacs to the cervix which determines which pregnancy is A and which B and not the position of the embryo or fetus within the sac. It is therefore possible, although unusual, for the presenting part of the twin in sac B to be lie closer to the cervix at the time of your scan than that of the twin in sac A. Do not be tempted to reassign the labelling in such a situation, but you may wish to comment on this finding in your report.

Identifying each fetus by the position of its placenta (e.g. anterior, posterior, fundal) is of value in a DC pregnancy where the implantation sites of the two placentas can be identified separately but of no value in MC gestations where the placenta is shared. The relative position of the twins (e.g. left, right or upper, lower) is useful in the majority of cases, and we recommend this is recorded as confirmation that the correct labelling has been applied.

It should be noted that none of these parameters can be applied to MA twin pairs which are the same gender, share a single placenta and develop within the same sac. Monoamniotic twins can only be distinguished if they demonstrate differential growth rates or are discordant for a structural abnormality.

THE IMPLICATIONS OF MONOCHORIONIC TWINNING

As stated earlier, one or both of the pair of MC twins are not only more likely to be smaller at birth than DC twins but both have a prenatal mortality rate that is three to four times higher than DC twins. This is due primarily to TTTS.

Monochorionic twinning is considered by some authors to be an abnormality in its own right. This should not detract from the fact that MZ twin pregnancies (and therefore a small proportion of the DC pregnancies you will scan) have a rate of structural abnormalities – in particular anencephaly and congenital heart disease – that is, between two and four times higher than DZ twin pregnancies or singleton pregnancies.

Both twins being concordant for the same abnormality is uncommon in all types of twins but occurs in 20% of MC twins compared with 10% of DC twins. The observant reader will have noticed that some authors refer to *zygosity*, whereas others refer to *chorionicity*, and this is an issue that you should be aware of when considering literature relating to twin pregnancies in future.

The complications unique to monoamniotic MC twins have been discussed earlier.

As stated earlier, MC twin pairs are uniquely at risk of TTTS and TRAP, with both these conditions being far less common in MCMA twin pairs than MCDA twin pairs.

TWIN TO TWIN TRANSFUSION SYNDROME

Within the shared placenta of an MCDA twin pregnancy, anastomoses, or natural communications, occur between either arteries of the two fetoplacental circulations (arterioarterial [AA]), between veins (venovenous) or between an artery from one fetoplacental circulation and a vein in the other (arteriovenous [AV]). In 10–15% of MC twin pregnancies, an imbalance of net blood flow across the

AV communications from one fetus, the donor, to the other, the recipient, and this results in TTTS.

Why only some MCDA twin pairs develop TTTS is poorly understood. One theory is that the development of the part of the placenta which supports the donor twin is abnormal and may cause an increased resistance in the placental circulation of this twin, promoting the shunting of blood from the donor to the recipient. As the donor twin is supporting the circulation of the recipient twin, the donor suffers from hypovolaemia and anaemia together with hypoxia as a result of placental insufficiency. The recipient becomes hypervolaemic and may develop high-output cardiac failure as a result. Increased urine output in the recipient results in an abnormally large bladder and polyhydramios with the subsequent increased risk of preterm labour. The reduced blood flow in the donor results in a decrease in urine output, which in turn results in a very small or absent bladder and oligo- or anhydramnios (Fig. 15.13).

THE INTERTWIN MEMBRANE

Observation of the intertwin membrane is an important component of your assessment for TTTS. In the presence of a normal amniotic fluid volume in both sacs, you will see the intertwin membrane floating freely between the two fetuses. In severe

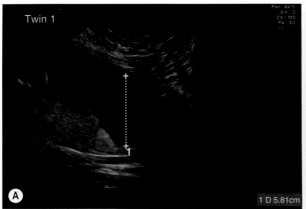
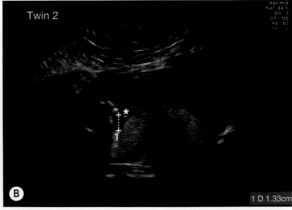

Fig 15.13 • A. Increased fluid in the sac of twin 1 of a pair of monochorionic diamniotic (MCDA) twins with a posterior placenta (arrow) at 17+ weeks of gestation. The deepest pool of amniotic fluid measures 5.81 cm. This is in marked contrast to the reduced fluid noted in the sac of twin 2. This discrepancy is suggestive of early twin-to-twin transfusion syndrome. Twin 1 is the recipient and twin 2 the donor. B. Decreased fluid in the sac of twin 2 of the same pair of MCDA twins. The deepest pool of amniotic fluid measures 1.33 cm. The intertwin membrane (*) is in close proximity to twin 2.

TTTS, the oligohydramnios or anhydramnios present in the donor sac results in the intertwin membrane adhering so closely to the affected twin that the fetus appears 'shrink-wrapped', and, as it is effectively immobolized against the uterine wall or the placenta, it is commonly described as 'stuck'.

An early indicator of a discrepancy in amniotic fluid volume between the two amniotic sacs is the folding of the intertwin membrane onto itself. Thus instead of the intertwin membrane appearing as freely floating 'thread' between the two fetuses, the folded part of the membrane has an appearance similar to an arrowhead, with the point of the arrowhead directed towards the increased amniotic fluid volume in the recipient's sac and away from the decreased amniotic fluid volume in the donor's sac (Fig. 15.14).

The ultrasound features associated with TTTS are shown in Table 15.3.

Signs of TTTS can develop at any stage of pregnancy although they are most likely to occur between 16 and 24 weeks of gestation. There is no 'automatic' progression of TTTS once present. In some cases, mild TTTS may be identified in the second trimester and may remain unchanged through gestation. In other, rarer cases, progression can occur extremely rapidly, often with severe and catastrophic consequences. Severe TTTS, apparent between 16 and 24 weeks, causes the death of both fetuses in approximately 90% of cases.

Twin-to-twin transfusion syndrome can be classified as mild, moderate or severe depending on the ultrasound appearances. A more subjective

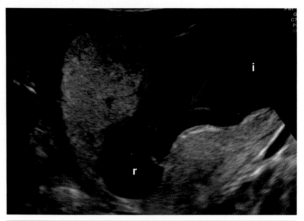

Fig 15.14 • Appearance of possible early intertwin membrane folding at 15 weeks of gestation in a monochorionic diamniotic twin pregnancy with a single anterior placenta and T sign (dashed arrow). The folding is artefactual, as the point of the 'arrowhead' (arrow) is directed towards the sac with reduced amniotic fluid (r) rather than towards the sac with increased amniotic fluid (i), as should be the case in twin-to-twin transfusion syndrome.

GESTATIONAL AGE	DONOR TWIN	RECIPIENT TWIN
11–14 weeks	NT within normal range Very small or absent bladder	NT above 95th centile Enlarged bladder
15–17 weeks	Folding of intertwin membrane, pointing away from sac	Folding of intertwin membrane, pointing towards sac
2nd trimester onwards	Absent bladder	Large bladder
	Oligohydramnios	Polyhydramnios
	Growth restriction	Ascites/hydrops
		Cardiomegaly
	Echogenic bowel	
	Absent EDF in umbilical artery	
	Absent/reversed flow in ductus venosus	

Table 15.3 Ultrasound and Doppler appearances associated with twin-to-twin transfusion syndrome and the gestational ages at which these features may be identified
EDF, end-diastolic flow; *NT*, nuchal translucency.

QUINTERO STAGE	ULTRASOUND FEATURES	DOPPLER STUDIES
1	Bladder of donor visible	Normal
2	Bladder of donor not visible during full length of examination	Not critically abnormal
3	As above	Critically abnormal in one or both twins: Umbilical artery – absent or reverse EDF Ductus venosus – reverse flow Umbilical vein – pulsatile flow
4	Recipient – ascites, pericardial or pleural effusion, scalp oedema or hydrops	As above
5	One or both dead	

Table 15.4 The staging of twin-to-twin transfusion syndrome as described by Quintero

Adapted from Quintero R, Morales W, Allen M, Bornick P, Johnson P, Krueger M 1999 Staging of twin-twin transfusion syndrome. Journal of Perinatology 19:550–555.
EDF, end-diastolic flow.

method of classifying TTTS, into five stages, was developed by Quintero in 1999. This classification uses a combination of ultrasound appearances and Doppler studies of the umbilical artery, umbilical vein and ductus venosus of both twins, as shown in Table 15.4.

These classifications are included for completeness, as the ultrasound management of MCDA twin pregnancies with TTTS, once identified, is beyond the scope of this text.

Once the structural normality of both twins has been established, the role of ultrasound management of MCDA twin pregnancies is to assess fetal growth and to exclude features of TTTS. Such scans should take place at 2 weekly intervals from 16 weeks to 24 weeks. Many departments will scan MCDA twin pregnancies every 2 weeks from 16 weeks until delivery, at around 36 weeks, whereas others may reduce the scanning frequency somewhat, and will, for example, only scan at 26 weeks and 30 weeks if clinically indicated.

TWIN REVERSED ARTERIAL PERFUSION

The most extreme form of TTTS is twin reversed arterial perfusion or acardiac twinning, which occurs in approximately 1% of MC pregnancies. It is thought to result from AA anastomoses between the two fetoplacental circulations. The perfused twin, the recipient, has no direct vascular connections with the placenta but receives its blood supply through a single umbilical artery, with the blood exiting via the umbilical vein – hence the reversed arterial perfusion of the condition. The lower body of the recipient receives a better oxygenated blood supply than the upper body and head and thus the abnormalities present are most severe in the upper body of the recipient in TRAP. The perfused recipients are commonly acardiac, hence their being described as 'acardiac monsters', and all die as a result of the associated multiple malformations. Approximately 50% of the donors die as a result of congestive heart failure or severe preterm delivery caused by polyhydramnios.

Your Role in the Scanning of MCDA Twin Pregnancies

Although it is unlikely that you will be responsible for the ultrasound management of a twin pregnancy with TTTS, it is highly likely that you may be the sonographer identifying the MCDA twin pregnancy for the first time or performing the scan in which the features of TTTS are present for the first time. You must, therefore, be aware of the early and later ultrasound signs of TTTS across gestation (see Table 15.3), understand how important it is to assess every MCDA pregnancy you scan for one or more of its features associated with the condition and realize that you must refer the woman for more specialized ultrasound management immediately when you suspect TTTS is present.

Normal Ultrasound Findings in MCDA Twin Pregnancies

The ultrasound features that indicate normal appearances in an MCDA twin pregnancy from 16 weeks onwards are as follows:

- normal growth velocity of both fetuses
- the bladder of both fetuses is seen and both are of equivalent and normal size

- normal amniotic fluid volume is present in both amniotic sacs
- the intertwin membrane is seen to be moving freely.

We recommend that your reporting of each ultrasound examination performed after 16 weeks of an MCDA twin pregnancy that is normal should include the previous comments.

DIAGNOSIS AND ASSESSMENT OF CHORIONICITY OF TWINS AFTER 14 WEEKS

As the majority of women will have had at least one scan in the first trimester, it is unlikely that a twin pregnancy will be diagnosed at the time of the 18–22 week anomaly scan, unless the woman is a late booker. The same methodology should be applied when assessing chorionicity as is used in the first trimester.

It is more difficult to distinguish between a delta and T sign later in gestation. It is also more difficult to differentiate between a single and two separate placentas. Thus, if chorionicity cannot be established with certainty – whether this is in the first trimester or subsequently – the pregnancy should be assumed to be MC, and managed as such, until proven otherwise.

THE 18–22 WEEK SCAN IN A TWIN PREGNANCY

Assessing the fetal anatomy in a twin pregnancy is likely to take approximately twice as long as the time required to assess the anatomy in a singleton pregnancy. Thus it is important that the appropriate appointment time interval is arranged for the 18–22 week examination of all twin pregnancies. As a 30-minute time interval is recommended for the routine 18–22 week anatomical assessment of a single fetus, we recommend allocating 1 hour for this assessment of a twin pregnancy.

The main difficulty of examining both fetuses in a twin pregnancy is making sure the anatomy you are assessing and the various measurements you are taking relate to the same fetus. This can be problematic for the novice when both fetuses are very active or they are both lying so close together that it is difficult to distinguish between them. A disciplined scanning technique is required. Sliding your probe up and down the (same) fetus to move from one section you are seeking to the next is likely to be more successful than taking your probe

off the maternal abdomen and hoping you will be examining the same fetus when you replace it on her abdomen. Remember that the head, body and femur of one fetus are all attached to each other in sequence, so you should always be able to get from one end of the same fetus to the other by sliding slowly through the fetus in cross-sections.

Structural Abnormalities in a Twin Pregnancy

As has been stated earlier, the risk of structural abnormalities in a DZ twin pregnancy is no greater than in a singleton pregnancy. However, you will also now be aware that the risk of structural abnormalities is higher in MC twin pregnancies, because these pregnancies are MZ, and there are a small group of abnormalities that are unique to MC twinning.

Congenital anomalies in twin pregnancies therefore fall into two groups:

- abnormalities that are not unique to twin pregnancies but occur more commonly in MZ twins, such as cardiac anomalies and anencephaly
- abnormalities unique to MC twinning, namely conjoined twins and TRAP.

Although every anomaly scan should be performed to a rigorous standard, you need to be aware of the increased potential for structural abnormalities in every twin pregnancy. This is because you are unlikely to know at the start of your examination of a DC twin pregnancy whether or not it is DZ or MZ. You should therefore assume that it is MZ, and thus at the same risk of structural abnormalities as an MC twin pregnancy, until proven otherwise.

ASSESSMENT OF FETAL GROWTH IN A TWIN PREGNANCY

The majority of twin individuals are smaller than their singleton counterparts at birth. However, most are constitutionally small rather than growth-restricted. As abdominal palpation is of little value in multiple pregnancy, it is appropriate for serial ultrasound scans to be performed in twin pregnancies for assessment of fetal growth.

As discussed earlier, MC twin pregnancies should be assessed for growth and signs of TTTS every 2 weeks from 16 weeks onwards. As DCDA twin pregnancies are not at risk of TTTS, they do not require such intense surveillance. Many departments assess growth in DCDA twin pregnancies on a monthly basis, namely at 24, 28, 32 and 36 weeks when the growth velocity of both fetuses is normal and more frequently (2–3 weekly) if one or both demonstrates growth restriction.

MEASURING AMNIOTIC FLUID IN A TWIN PREGNANCY

Amniotic fluid volume in each sac of a twin pregnancy is assessed by measurement of the deepest vertical pool in each sac rather than by amniotic fluid index. Normal fluid volume is expressed by a deepest vertical pool in each sac of a twin pregnancy of between 2.0 cm and 8.0 cm after 24 weeks of gestation.

Intertwin Growth Discrepancy

A difference in growth rate between the two twins is considered significant when the intertwin discrepancy is 20% or greater. This is most easily calculated by comparison of the two estimated fetal weights. As twins act as 'internal controls', such a discrepancy suggests a pathological cause, with uteroplacental insufficiency or TTTS being the most likely. Such pregnancies should be referred for more detailed examinations that are likely to include further anatomical assessment together with umbilical and fetal Doppler studies.

Pitfalls

In some situations a fetus that had been growing poorly over several examinations demonstrates what appears to be a sudden catch-up in growth. Conversely a fetus that had been growing normally demonstrates what appears to be an unexpected fall-off in growth. Although both scenarios are possible, both can arise because of poor technique or human error. Make sure the sections you have selected for measurement are correct, you have measured them correctly and they have been entered into the reporting package correctly. Make sure that you have labelled the twins correctly. You should not assume that the previous measurements or labelling will always be correct, so the information, including the measured images, provided from previous scans should also be rechecked. Only when you are satisfied that your interpretation of your findings and those of the previous scans are correct should you decide on the significance of your scan findings.

Further reading

National Institute for Health & Clinical Excellence 2011 Multiple pregnancy. The management of twin and triplet pregnancies in the antenatal period. Nice Clinical Guideline 129. www.nice.org.uk/guidance/cg129

Public Health England 2015 NHS Down's, Edwards' and Pataus' syndromes screening programme. Handbook for Laboratories, version 1.0. NHS Fetal Anomaly Screening Programme (Public Health England). www.screening.nhs.uk

Scanning the non pregnant pelvis

CONTENTS

This chapter explains the normal ultrasound appearances of the pelvic organs assessed during a gynaecological scan.

The aims of this chapter are to enable you to do the following:

- describe the ultrasound appearances of the pelvic organs
- understand the normal findings in order to appreciate the equivocal and abnormal findings
- report the findings of a gynaecological scan.

The primary focus of a gynaecological ultrasound examination is to answer the clinical question posed. Requests for ultrasound examinations will be predominantly from three main sources – the general practitioner (GP), the gynaecologist or the subfertility team. The GP will often seek basic information to establish the cause of the most common gynaecological complaints, namely dysfunctional uterine bleeding or pelvic pain. The gynaecologist will generally require more detailed information relating to possible pathological conditions, whereas the subfertility team will be seeking specific information relating to subfertility.

The basic scan undertaken should be the same, irrespective of who makes the request. However, the difference between the examinations will tend to be in the level of detail required and the manner in which the scan findings are interpreted and reported back to the original referrer. The operator's role in answering the clinical question is to identify the key clinical features and link them with the corresponding ultrasound appearances, to understand the range of normal, 'not normal' and abnormal findings and their overlap and ultimately to translate the findings into a clinically useful report.

The ultrasound appearances of the uterus and ovaries will vary depending on the woman's menstrual status, type of contraception and any exogenous hormone treatment. You need to be aware of these factors and understand the implications they have on the ultrasound appearances of the structures you are examining. Your role is to understand the range of normal, 'not normal' and abnormal findings in these varying situations and to interpret the ultrasound findings in their correct context.

This chapter describes the typical ultrasound appearances and measurement of the normal uterus, cervix and ovaries in the premenopausal and postmenopausal woman.

We recommend that all ultrasound examinations be only performed after the receipt of a written request. The minimum information which you as the operator require, and therefore which should be included, is the woman's age, the date of her last menstrual period (or years since the menopause), details of any contraception or exogenous hormones, the relevant clinical information and the clinical questions posed. Unfortunately, request forms are often poorly completed and therefore you may need to question the woman further to obtain all the information you need.

Once you have established the clinical question being asked and are confident you have the necessary relevant information, the examination can be started. Irrespective of the questions asked, you should adopt a systematic approach to every examination you undertake. This ensures that the pelvic organs will be assessed thoroughly and in a standardized, and therefore reproducible, manner.

As described in Chapter 4, we recommend assessment of the pelvic organs in the following order:

- uterus and cervix, longitudinal sections followed by transverse sections
- ovaries and adnexae
- Pouch of Douglas.

In the majority of cases, imaging a structure properly is only part of the ultrasound examination. Your assessment of a structure will involve a subconscious assessment of its size, and this information is important in your evaluation of its normality or otherwise. You must be able to measure that structure accurately and in a reproducible fashion. There are many situations where serial measurements contribute to the clinical relevance of your examination and the report it generates.

This text assumes that you, the operator, are sitting to the left of, or at the foot of, the scanning couch, holding the transvaginal probe in your right hand, that the woman is lying to your right side and that you are facing each other.

THE UTERUS AND CERVIX

ANATOMY

The uterus is a retroperitoneal organ and is therefore covered with peritoneum for most of its length. It is a hollow, pear-shaped muscular organ, which consists of four anatomical parts – the fundus, corpus or body, isthmus and cervix. The fundus is the superior, dome-shaped portion of the uterus, above the ostia. The ostia are the openings of the Fallopian tubes into the uterus. The corpus or body constitutes the main part of the uterus and is delineated inferiorly by the internal os. The isthmus is the junction between the body and cervix. It is the site of the development of the lower uterine segment in pregnancy but is not visualized with ultrasound in the nonpregnant woman. The cervix extends from the isthmus into the vagina. It is delineated superiorly by the internal os and inferiorly by the external os.

The parametrium is the outer layer of the uterus and represents an incomplete covering of peritoneum. The anterior portion of the cervix is bare of peritoneum to allow movement of the bladder. The reflection of the peritoneum from the posterior surface of the uterus posteriorly to the rectum forms the rectouterine space, commonly called the Pouch of Douglas.

The myometrium is the muscular middle layer of the uterus.

The endometrium is the innermost layer of the uterus.

Ultrasound Appearances

The normal premenopausal uterus has a characteristic ultrasound appearance, which enables delineation between the parametrium, myometrium, endometrium and cervix. The normal postmenopausal uterus is essentially similar in ultrasound appearance, the main differences being in its size and the appearance of the endometrium.

The sagittal section of the uterus will demonstrate the following features:

The parametrium is easily recognizable because the peritoneal layer provides an identifiable hyperechoic border.

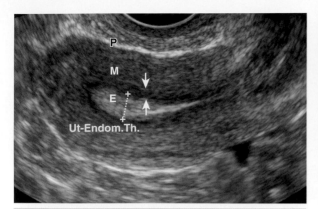

Fig 16.1 • Sagittal view of the uterus demonstrating the parametrium (P), myometrium (M), junctional zone (arrowed) and endometrium (E), measured with on-screen callipers. Ut-Endom. Th., uterine endometrial thickness.

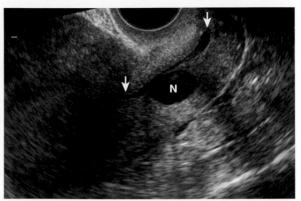

Fig 16.2 • Sagittal view of the uterine cervix. Mucus within the cervix highlights the cervical canal (arrowed). A Nabothian cyst (N) is located within the posterior cervical wall.

The myometrium typically demonstrates homogeneous midrange echoes. Small cystic spaces may be identified towards its outer borders. These are the arcuate blood vessels and will demonstrate low-velocity flow if colour/power Doppler is applied.

The endometrium varies in appearance depending on the stage of the menstrual cycle and in response to cyclical hormone influences. The endometrium is normally hyperechoic and should be regular in its outline. The thin, regular, brighter *'cavity line'* is produced by the apposition of the anterior and posterior endometrial layers. The premenopausal and postmenopausal endometrial appearances are described in detail in Chapter 17.

The junctional zone is an important area to identify, although it is not always apparent. The junctional zone represents the inner muscle layer of the myometrium (i.e. the zone between the endometrium and the outer myometrial muscle layer). The ultrasound appearances are of a hypoechoic halo, which surrounds the hyperechoic basal layer of the endometrium (Fig. 16.1). A common error is to overmeasure the endometrium by including the junctional zone.

The cervix should be homogeneous in its echotexture, and similar to that of the myometrium. This makes it difficult to use echogenicity alone in distinguishing between the lower uterine body and the upper cervix.

The most obvious feature of the cervix is the thin, regular hyperechoic 'cavity line' produced by the opposing layers of the anterior and posterior cervical walls. This effectively should be continuous with the cavity line of the endometrium, as the uterine cavity and the cervical canal are only separated by the internal os. A slight discontinuity of 'endometrial/cervical cavity line' may be present, indicating the assumed position of the internal os. If the cervical glands produce mucus, the cervical canal will be more readily identified as an anechoic canal. Nabothian cysts are mucus-filled cysts that can form within the cervical wall (Fig. 16.2). Cysts will be seen as spherical anechoic structures within the cervical wall. Nabothian cysts are not thought to be of any clinical significance.

Caesarean Section Scar

The increasing prevalence of Caesarean section births means an increasing likelihood that a previous Caesarean section scar will be visualized during an ultrasound examination. The ultrasound appearances of a Caesarean section scar are typically of a wedge-shaped anechoic area or hyperechoic distortion in the lower anterior uterine wall. The scar will be located midway between the utero-vesical fold (visualized as a hyperechoic line positioned at the posterior bladder wall) and the internal os (Fig. 16.3).

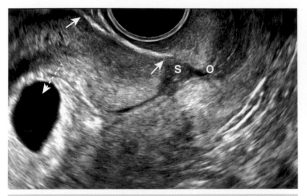

Fig 16.3 • Sagittal view of the lower uterus and cervix in an early pregnancy demonstrating a previous Caesarean section scar (S). The scar lies between the edge of the uterovesical fold, seen as a hyperechoic line (arrowed) and the internal os (O). A gestation sac can be seen normally positioned in the uterus (dashed arrow).

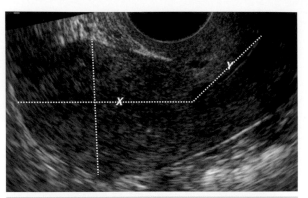

Fig 16.4 • Sagittal view of the uterus demonstrating the longitudinal and anteroposterior diameter of the uterus. The longitudinal measurement includes the fundus, body and cervix by summation of the two lengths x and y (method A) using the 'outer to outer' technique.

MEASURING THE UTERUS

Practices differ as to the value of measuring the dimensions of a normal uterus. The gynaecologist is rarely interested in the size of a normal uterus, but rather the presence or otherwise of abnormal findings. However, you as the operator must be able to measure a uterus consistently so that you know where to place your calliper when you suspect the size to be abnormal.

Practices also differ as to how these measurements should be taken, the principal point of contention being the uterine length, as discussed later. It is obviously important that all operators in a centre employ the same method of measuring, which ideally should be according to a referenced technique.

The longitudinal, anteroposterior (AP) and transverse diameters of the uterus are measured in three planes, orthogonal to each other. The callipers should be positioned to obtain an 'outer-to-outer' measurement for each diameter.

Longitudinal Diameter

Obtain a sagittal section of the uterus in which the endometrium is clearly visualized. The longitudinal diameter should be measured from the midpoint at the fundus to either the external os or the internal os, following the line of the endometrium. The former measurement includes the fundus,

body (isthmus) and cervix (method A), whereas the latter will, in effect, be a measurement of the fundus and body only (method B).

In reality, defining the absolute position of both the internal os and external os can be challenging. In the pregnant uterus the 'dimple' of the internal os is delineated by the amniotic fluid above it. In the nonpregnant uterus discriminating between the cervical canal and the endometrium is difficult, thus reducing the accuracy with which the internal os can be identified. Similarly, defining the absolute position of the external os is often as difficult. In addition, the angle between the uterine body and the cervix may be as great as 30°. This makes it impossible to obtain an accurate measurement using method A if one linear measurement is used. To overcome the change in angle, and to avoid obtaining an undermeasurement, two measurements may be required. The first measures the distance from the uterine fundus to the internal os and the second measures the distance from the internal os to the external os (Fig. 16.4). We therefore recommend method B (Fig. 16.5), which can be obtained with reasonable accuracy, using the standard technique of applying linear callipers.

A third method, method C, measures the distance from the uterine fundus to the lower posterior uterine wall. This measurement is, in effect, an overestimated length of the uterine body while not including the cervix. We do not, therefore, recommend using method C.

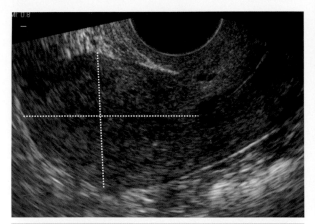

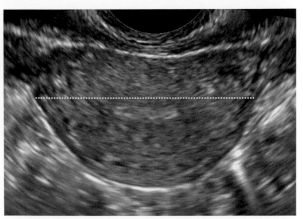

Fig 16.5 • Sagittal view of the uterus demonstrating the longitudinal and anteroposterior diameters of the uterus. The longitudinal measurement includes the fundus and body only (method B) using the 'outer to outer' technique.

Fig 16.6 • Transverse section of the uterus. The transverse diameter is measured across the widest part of the uterine body using the 'outer to outer' technique.

DIAMETER	NULLIPAROUS (mm)	MULTIPAROUS (mm)	POSTMENOPAUSAL (mm)
Longitudinal (fundus – internal os) (method B)	<45	<55	<30
AP	<35	<45	<25
Transverse	<40	<50	<30

Table 16.1 Average measurements of the uterus taken in three planes, using the transvaginal route and using the 'outer to outer' technique, relating to menstrual status and parity

AP, anteroposterior; <, less than.

AP Diameter

Using the same section as earlier, the AP diameter should be measured across the widest point of the uterine body, perpendicular to the longitudinal axis of the uterus and endometrium and therefore the longitudinal diameter (Figs. 16.4 and 16.5).

The AP diameter measurement should *not* be taken in the transverse plane, as this will result in an overestimation of the measurement. As discussed in Chapter 4, this is due to the oblique view of the uterus obtained in the transverse plane when scanning transvaginally.

Transverse Diameter

Obtain a transverse section of the uterus and endometrium by rotating the probe through 90°

from the longitudinal section described earlier. The transverse diameter should be measured across the widest part of the uterine body, from the left lateral border to the right lateral border (Fig. 16.6).

The size of the uterus varies with menstrual status and parity. Typical values are given in Table 16.1.

ASSESSMENT OF THE ENDOMETRIUM

Examination of the endometrium is performed in the sagittal and transverse planes. The variation in endometrial thickness between the pre- and postmenopausal status is 1.0–15.0 mm. A transvaginal ultrasound examination, where not contraindicated, is therefore the examination of choice because of the superior resolution it affords. Every attempt should be made to manipulate the probe to display the endometrium in a horizontal

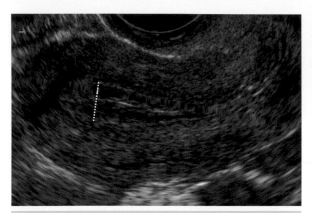

Fig 16.7 • Sagittal view of the uterus and endometrium. Callipers demonstrate the anteroposterior measurement of the endometrium using the 'outer to outer' technique.

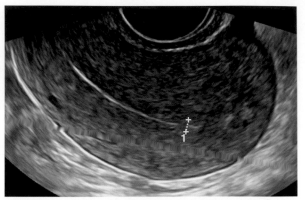

Fig 16.8 • Sagittal view of a retroverted uterus demonstrating the endometrium in a postmenopausal woman. The cavity line is readily identified. The endometrium is isoechoic. Placement of the callipers is difficult, as the endometrial myometrial interface is not clearly delineated (measured using the outer to outer technique).

position. This is because optimal ultrasound information is obtained from structures lying at 90° to the ultrasound beam.

The image can be further optimized by using as high a frequency as is possible, narrowing the sector width, applying multiple focal zones and manipulating the harmonics settings. Applying additional image-processing techniques – which tend to be manufacturer-specific – may improve the image further.

Measuring Endometrial Thickness

A sagittal section of the uterus should be obtained with the long axis of the endometrium imaged in as horizontal a plane as possible. The thickest part of the endometrium, which is usually located just below the fundus, should be measured. The callipers should be placed across the hyperechoic endometrium only, to obtain an 'outer-to-outer' measurement. Care should be taken to ensure that the measurement is made at 90° to the long axis of the endometrium (Fig. 16.7).

As discussed in Chapter 4, measurement of the endometrial thickness should always be taken from a sagittal image and should never be measured from a 'transverse' section of the pelvis. Measurements taken in this plane are likely to be an overestimation and therefore inaccurate. The ease with which the interface between the endometrium and myometrium is identified is dependent on the contrast in echogenicity between the two. The

endometrium may be isoechoic relative to the myometrium so that the interface can be difficult to delineate, and consequently it may be difficult to decide where to place the callipers (Fig. 16.8).

The endometrium is generally hyperechoic compared with the surrounding myometrium, and, if visualized, the junctional zone lying between the endometrium and the outer myometrium is hypoechoic.

The endometrial thickness represents the thickness of the anterior layer and the thickness of the posterior layer of the endometrium added together. Where the endometrial cavity is empty, the apposition of the two endometrial layers creates a hyperechoic line described as the 'cavity line'. Fluid and/or clot within the endometrial cavity will distend the cavity, separating the two endometrial layers. The contents within the endometrial cavity can be measured, using the same method as described for the endometrial thickness. In such instances the measurement of the endometrial contents should be subtracted from the total measurement to obtain the true thickness of the endometrium (Fig. 16.9).

Subjective Assessment of the Endometrium

It is not sufficient to simply obtain an endometrial thickness measurement and write on the report, *'The endometrium measures x cm'*, without assessing the appearance of the endometrium.

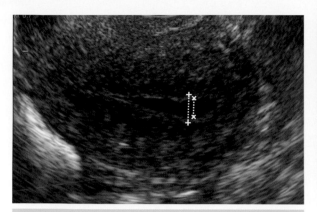

Fig 16.9 • Sagittal view of a retroverted uterus. There is intracavity fluid present. The fluid depth (x – x) should be subtracted from the total measurement (+ – +) in order to measure the endometrium only.

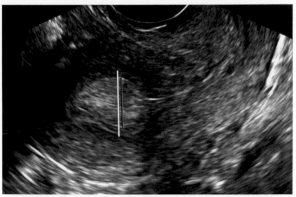

Fig 16.10 • Sagittal view of endometrium. No cavity line can be seen towards the fundus. This is due to the presence of an intracavity lesion – an endometrial polyp. The endometrium has been measured using the 'outer to outer' technique (yellow line). The AP diameter of the polyp has been measured (red line).

We suggest that, in addition to the measurement, a subjective appraisal is made of the endometrium. An assessment of the following specific features will help you establish normality or otherwise of the endometrium:

- is the hyperechoic intracavity line clearly visible, in which case it can be reported as *'defined'* (Figs. 16.7 and 16.8)? Separation of the two layers will occur if there are intracavity contents – for example, fluid (Fig. 16.9), blood or an endometrial polyp (Fig. 16.10). In these cases, you will be unable to define the intracavity line because the endometrial cavity is distended
- is the endometrium *hyperechoic* (Figs. 16.1 and 16.9), *isoechoic* (Fig. 16.8) or *hypoechoic* compared with the surrounding myometrium? An isoechoic endometrium often occurs in the menopause. The similar echotexture of the endometrium and myometrium can make it difficult to decide where to place the callipers for measurement of the endometrium
- is there a three-layer pattern to the endometrium? This is a typical appearance in the premenopausal woman (Fig. 16.7) and in women taking hormone replacement therapy. The three-layer pattern is described more fully in Chapter 17
- is the endometrial/myometrial interface distinct and undistorted (Figs. 16.1 and

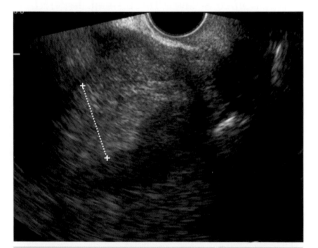

Fig 16.11 • Sagittal view of the endometrium. The endometrium is markedly thickened (32.2 mm) and heterogeneous in appearance. There is no intracavity line present. The contour of the endometrium is irregular, with an ill-defined endometrial myometrial interface. Histological testing confirmed endometrial cancer.

16.7), or is there is any irregularity or distortion present (Fig. 16.11)?

Chapter 18 discusses in further detail some of the commonly encountered endometrial pathological conditions.

THE POSTMENOPAUSAL UTERUS

The size of the postmenopausal uterus is smaller than that of the premenopausal uterus.

Furthermore, the uterus atrophies throughout the menopause so that the uterine size in a woman who has been menopausal for 20–30 years will be much smaller compared with a woman who is 2–3 years postmenopausal. It can be difficult to visualize a small postmenopausal uterus either transvaginally or transabdominally. Withdrawal of the transvaginal probe a few centimetres, ensuring that the cervix is not compressed and increasing the depth control, will improve the likelihood of successful visualization.

The postmenopausal cervix is proportionally large compared with the uterine body, thus the corpus/cervical length ratio is decreased.

The postmenopausal myometrium has a typical ultrasound appearance of homogeneous midrange echoes. A not infrequent finding in the postmenopausal uterus is foci of calcification within the outer myometrial layer. These small, hyperechoic areas are due to atherosclerosis, which causes the arcuate arteries to calcify (Fig. 16.12).

The postmenopausal endometrium in established menopause is atrophic because of the cessation of cyclical hormonal stimulation. The low levels of oestrogen after the menopause cause thinning of the endometrium. The ultrasound appearance reflects this change, the typical findings being of a hyperechoic, thin endometrium with a thickness of less than 3.0 mm. It is often difficult to differentiate between the bright echo of the cavity line and the atrophic endometrium itself (Fig. 16.12).

THE PERIMENOPAUSAL UTERUS

The physiological changes expressed through the gradual transition from menstruation to the postmenopausal period are reflected in the ultrasound appearances of the perimenopausal endometrium. There is therefore no typical appearance of the perimenopausal endometrium, but rather a gradation between those described earlier.

CONGENITAL UTERINE ANOMALIES

The uterus forms from the fusion of paired Müllerian ducts during embryogenesis. Congenital uterine anomalies may occur as a result of abnormal development of the ducts, in that there is a failure of the ducts to fuse or canalize, or a failure of septal resorption at some point in their development. The most commonly encountered anomalies are bicornuate, septate and arcuate uterus.

A transverse sweep of the uterus which demonstrates an apparent dividing of the endometrial cavity echo into two separate endometrial echoes towards the fundal aspect of the uterus is an abnormal finding (Fig. 16.13). Such an appearance suggests that a uterine anomaly may be present.

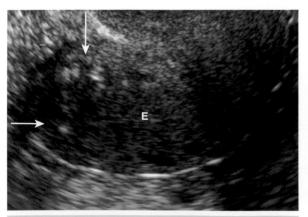

Fig 16.12 • Sagittal view of a postmenopausal uterus, foci of calcification arrowed in the anterior and fundal uterine wall represent calcified arcuate arteries. The endometrium (E) is thin.

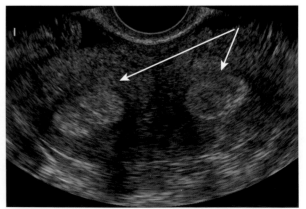

Fig 16.13 • Transverse view of the uterus showing two endometrial cavities (arrowed). A 3D scan subsequently demonstrated a septate uterus.

Although it may be tempting to suggest the type of uterine anomaly from your two-dimensional (2D) scan, this should not be attempted. A three-dimensional (3D) scan is required to confirm and classify the anomaly. If a 3D scan is not available, then your report should suggest that there is a uterine anomaly and that confirmation, if needed, requires a 3D scan and interpretation of the acquired 3D volume.

Interpretation of a 3D Volume

A '3D' scan acquires a volume of 2D ultrasound in a data set. This stored volume can then be manipulated and displayed in a multiplanar format. The multiplanar format demonstrates the three cross-sectional planes of the uterus that are orthogonal to one another. Two of them can be acquired on standard 2D scanning (i.e. the sagittal and transverse sections). The third plane is the coronal section, which is not achievable on 2D scanning because of the restriction of probe movement within the vagina.

A coronal plane of the uterus demonstrates the outline of the fundus, the shape of the endometrium and the continuity of the cervix. It is the coronal image which is required to determine whether or not a uterine anomaly is present and its type.

It is likely that, before the introduction of 3D ultrasound, an assumption was made of the finding of two split endometrial cavities on a transverse scan being due to a bicornuate uterus. This resulted in an over reporting of bicornuate uteri and an under reporting of septate uteri,

Three-dimensional ultrasound is a technique that should be learned once you have gained a moderate degree of skill and experience in 2D gynaecological ultrasound. An accurate and appropriately performed 2D ultrasound is in many respects more important than the 3D scan, as it is the information acquired from the 2D scan which determines whether a 3D scan is needed.

It is beyond the scope of this text to explain the technique of 3D ultrasound. However, it is perhaps useful to describe the coronal plane appearances

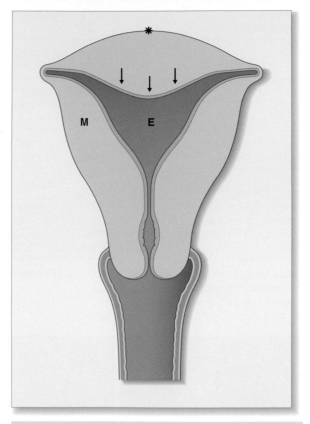

Fig 16.14 • Schematic diagram of a coronal view of the uterus. The fundal contour of the endometrium (arrows), external contour of the fundus (*), endometrium (E) and myometrium (M) are shown.

of the more common anomalies so that you aware of the role that 3D plays in the interpretation.

In 1988, the American Fertility Society produced an extensive classification of Müllerian duct (uterine) anomalies, which has been widely adopted by clinicians. Salim et al. have developed criteria for ultrasound features to be assessed on the coronal view of the uterus as acquired on 3D ultrasound.

There are two areas of the uterus that are specifically considered: first, the fundal contour of the endometrium and, second, the external contour of the uterus (Fig. 16.14). The features that are present with the various uterine congenital anomalies are shown in Table 16.2 and Fig. 16.15.

UTERINE MORPHOLOGY	FUNDAL CONTOUR OF THE ENDOMETRIUM	EXTERNAL CONTOUR OF THE FUNDUS
Normal (Fig. 16.15A)	Straight or convex	Uniformly convex or with indentation <10 mm
Arcuate (Fig. 16.15B)	Concave fundal indentation with central point of indentation at an obtuse angle (>90°)	Uniformly convex or with indentation <10 mm
Subseptate (Fig. 16.15C)	Presence of septum, which does not extend to the cervix, with central point of septum at an acute angle (<90°)	Uniformly convex or with indentation <10 mm
Septate (Fig. 16.15D)	Presence of uterine septum that completely divides the cavity from fundus to cervix	Uniformly convex or with an indentation <10 mm
Bicornuate (Fig. 16.15E)	Two well-formed uterine cornua	Fundal indentation >10 mm dividing the two cornua
Unicornuate with or without a rudimentary horn	Single well-formed uterine cavity with a single interstitial portion of Fallopian tube and concave fundal contour	Fundal indentation >10 mm dividing the two cornua if rudimentary horn present

Table 16.2 Ultrasound features obtained from 3D imaging of the uterus used for the classification of uterine congenital anomalies

Adapted from Salim et al 2003.

3D, three dimensional; <, less than; >, more than.

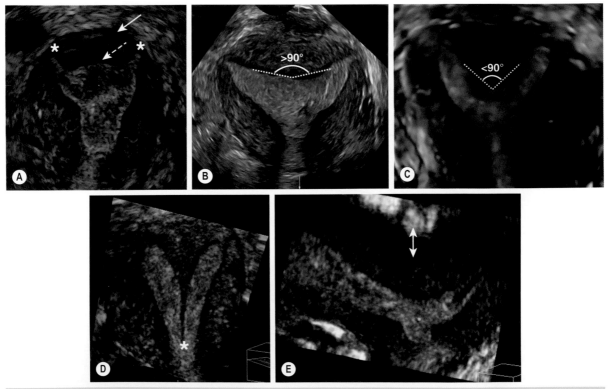

Fig 16.15 • A. A 3D coronal view demonstrating a normal uterine shape. The external contour (solid arrow) is convex and the fundal contour (dashed arrow) is convex. The interstitial portion of each Fallopian tube is denoted (*). B. 3D coronal view demonstrating an arcuate uterus. There is an obtuse angle (>90°) at the fundal contour of the endometrium. C. Coronal view of subseptate uterus. The septum does not extend to the cervix, and the central point of the septum is at an acute angle (<90°). D. 3D coronal view demonstrating a septate uterus. The cavity is divided at the cervix by the uterine septum (*). E. 3D coronal view demonstrating a bicornuate uterus. The fundal indentation (arrowed) is greater than 10 mm. It is also difficult to demonstrate both cornua in one image as they can be moderately divergent in this anomaly.

THE ADNEXAE

The adnexae refers to any structures that are adjacent or near to the uterus within the pelvis. Adnexae is the plural of adnexa the *right* and *left adnexa* describe the respective areas to the right and left of the uterus. This area includes the ovaries, Fallopian tubes, blood vessels and broad and round uterine ligaments. The only structures that are usually visualized with ultrasound in the adnexae are the ovaries and blood vessels. A pelvic ultrasound examination should always include assessment of both adnexae even if the woman gives a history of oophorectomy. On occasion an ovary is present, as previous surgery may have been of a cyst removal (cystectomy) rather than an oophorectomy. Furthermore, there is a risk of recurrence of malignancy if an ovary was removed because of malignancy.

THE OVARIES

The ovary is an almond-shaped organ which lies within the posterior layer of the broad ligament, lateral to the uterus, below the Fallopian tube and medial and anterior to the internal iliac vessels. Unfortunately, for the beginner, the positions of the ovaries can vary both within and between individuals.

The ovary consists of follicles embedded within a vascular stroma which is surrounded by a thin capsule. The capsule allows the outline of the ovary to be identified and therefore allows measurements of ovarian size to be taken relatively easily.

Ultrasound Appearances

The ultrasound appearance of the premenopausal ovary is characterized by a heterogeneous echo pattern caused by the varying size of the developing follicles, the differing appearances of the corpus luteum (if present) within the stroma and the stroma itself.

The premenopausal ovarian appearances vary throughout the menstrual cycle and are explained in detail in Chapter 17. The follicles are spherical in shape and anechoic. The smallest follicles that can be resolved with ultrasound are 1.0–2.0 mm in mean diameter, with the largest typically reaching a maximum of 25.0 mm before ovulation. Peripheral vascularity, as identified with colour or power Doppler, is not a feature of the developing follicle.

The ultrasound appearance of the supporting stroma is typically of a homogeneous midrange echo pattern.

The corpus luteum (plural, corpora lutea) demonstrates a range of appearances. Most typically it is spherical and anechoic, similar, therefore, in size and appearance to a developing follicle. Peripheral vascularity, sometimes referred to as a 'ring of fire', and as identified with colour or power Doppler, is characteristic of the corpus luteum, thus enabling it to be distinguished from a developing follicle. Alternatively, the corpus luteum may appear collapsed or haemorrhagic.

Measuring Ovarian Size and Volume

The ability to measure the ovaries accurately is important, as disparity in size or volume relative to the normal reference range or a disparity in size or volume between the two ovaries can be of value in aiding the gynaecologist to reach a diagnosis.

The longitudinal, AP and transverse diameters of both ovaries are measured in three planes, orthogonal to each other. The callipers should be positioned to obtain an 'outer-to-outer' measurement for each diameter. Ovarian size may be reported as linear measurements or as a volume. The volume may be calculated by software in the machine or in the computer database and software package if used.

Alternatively, the volume can be calculated using the following formula, which is derived from the formula for calculating the volume of a sphere:

$$\text{Ovarian volume (ml)} = d1 \times d2 \times d3 \times 0.5233$$

d1 = longitudinal diameter (mm)
d2 = AP diameter (mm)
d3 = transverse diameter (mm).

Longitudinal Diameter

Obtain a sagittal section of the ovary which demonstrates the maximum length of the ovary. Remember that additional small panning, angling

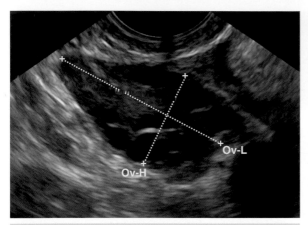

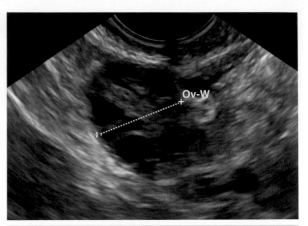

Fig 16.16 • Sagittal view of the right ovary demonstrating measurement of the longitudinal (Ov-L [33.2 mm]) and anteroposterior (Ov-H [18.5 mm]) diameters.

Fig 16.17 • Transverse view of the right ovary demonstrating measurement of the transverse (Ov-W [16.5 mm]) diameter.

MEASUREMENT	PREMENOPAUSAL	POSTMENOPAUSAL
Longitudinal	25–40 mm	20.0 mm
AP	15–30 mm	15.0 mm
Transverse	15–30 mm	10.0 mm
Volume	6–12 ml	<4.0 ml

Table 16.3 Average measurements of the ovary taken in three planes, using the transvaginal route and the 'outer-to-outer' technique, relating to menstrual status.

AP, anteroposterior.

and rotational movements of the probe will confirm that you have indeed obtained the optimal sagittal section of the ovary for measurement. The longitudinal diameter should be measured by placing the callipers at each end of the long axis of the ovary using the 'outer-to-outer' technique (Fig. 16.16).

AP Diameter

Using the same section as earlier, the AP diameter should be measured across the widest part of the ovary, perpendicular to the longitudinal axis, using the 'outer-to-outer' technique. We recommend that the AP diameter is taken from the longitudinal rather than the transverse section of the ovary. This is because the AP diameter measured from a

transverse section of the ovary is less likely to be orthogonal to both the longitudinal and transverse planes than if it is measured from a longitudinal section of the ovary (Fig. 16.16).

Transverse Diameter

Obtain a transverse section of the ovary by rotating the probe through 90° from the longitudinal section described earlier. The transverse diameter should be measured across the largest diameter of the ovary, from the left lateral border to the right lateral border, using the 'outer-to-outer' technique (Fig. 16.17).

The size of the ovary varies with menstrual status and the size of any developing follicles or the corpus luteum, as shown in Table 16.3.

The size of the ovary varies with menstrual status and the size of any developing follicles or the corpus luteum. If there is any ovarian pathological condition present, such as one or more cysts, the size of the ovary will be increased.

Where an ovarian cyst is identified, it should be measured in three orthogonal planes, using the method as described earlier for measurement of the ovary. The 'inner to inner' technique should be used. The most commonly occurring cysts – for example, simple cysts or haemorrhagic cysts – tend to be relatively round. Thus there will be little difference in the three diameters of such masses. A cyst volume can be calculated using the same formula used for ovarian volume.

A significant proportion of gynaecological ultrasound examinations referred from GPs will be normal. Thus, only a small proportion of ultrasound examinations will demonstrate the presence of an adnexal mass. An adnexal mass must be measured and described and, where possible, a differential diagnosis should be given. It can be daunting to the novice operator as to how best to interpret abnormal findings. The more commonly encountered ovarian abnormalities are discussed in Chapter 18. As with the endometrium, there are terms and definitions used to describe the ultrasound features of adnexal pathological conditions. These are discussed in Chapter 19.

Paraovarian cysts

A not uncommon incidental finding is of a paraovarian cyst. These originate from either the embryonic Müllerian or Wolffian ducts. A paraovarian cyst is separate from the ovary and Fallopian tube. It will appear either exophytic to the ipsilateral ovary or more obviously separate. The cyst is thin-walled with no surrounding ovarian tissue and the internal content is hypoechoic. Paraovarian cysts are usually small, measuring between 10.0 mm and 40.0 mm in diameter. A positive sliding sign will confirm that the cyst is paraovarian. Paraovarian cysts are usually asymptomatic and are of no clinical significance.

THE FALLOPIAN TUBES

Each Fallopian tube lies within the broad ligament and extends from the cornua of the uterus to its

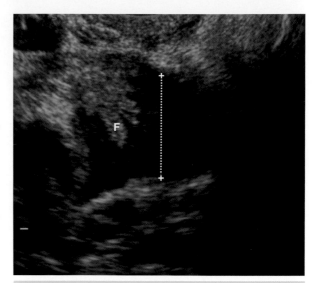

Fig 16.18 • Peritoneal fluid (depth 15.9 mm) surrounded the infundibulum portion of the left Fallopian tube. The fimbriae (F) can easily be seen at the outermost part of the tube.

fimbrial ends, which are usually located superior to the ovary. The Fallopian tube is made up of four parts: the interstitial portion, the isthmus, the ampulla and the infundibulum. The interstitial portion is located within the body of the uterus and may be seen as a hyperechoic line extending from the lateral uterine angle to the origin of the broad ligament. It may be visualized on the coronal view of a 3D scan (Fig. 16.15A). Visualization of the whole tube is possible after distension either with contrast media or because of fluid, blood or pus present within the tube in cases of hydro-, haemo- or pyosalpinx, respectively. The infundibulum may also be seen if free fluid surrounding the tube is present in the pelvis (Fig. 16.18).

THE POUCH OF DOUGLAS

The Pouch of Douglas is a blind-ended potential space. It is only apparent on ultrasound when there is an accumulation of fluid within it of a minimum vertical depth of 5–10 mm. Fluid is released from the dominant follicle at ovulation. This fluid can typically be identified as an anechoic triangular area within the Pouch of Douglas. A larger collection of fluid in the Pouch of Douglas may be indicative of a pathological condition (Fig. 16.19). The maximum vertical depth of free fluid present should always be measured, the quantity subjectively assessed and both included in the report. Our suggested method for subjective assessment is given in Chapter 6.

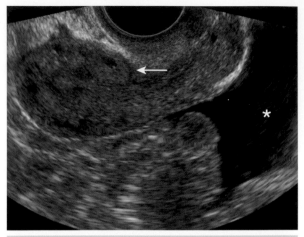

Fig 16.19 • Sagittal view of the uterus. Free fluid containing blood demonstrable by low-level echoes (*) in the Pouch of Douglas consistent with recent cyst rupture. Note previous Caesarean section scar (arrowed).

WRITING THE REPORT

A template facilitates a consistent and structured approach to the report and ensures that all relevant features and measurements are included and then summarized in a conclusion. The writing of the report for abnormal findings is discussed in Chapters 18 and 19.

We suggest the following template of information that should be included for a gynaecological scan report:

- the reason for the examination
- the menstrual status, the date of the last menstrual period and the use of any oral contraception or exogenous hormones
- the approach used, whether transvaginally, transabdominally or both
- recording of a latex allergy and documentation of appropriate management
- measurement of the uterus
- documentation of the uterine orientation (i.e. anteverted, retroverted or axial; see Chapter 4)
- documentation of the uterine appearances
- measurement of the endometrium
- documentation of the endometrial appearances
- interpretation of whether or not the endometrial appearances are consistent with

the menopausal status and hormonal use of the woman (see Chapter 17)

- measurement of the ovaries
- documentation of the ovarian appearances
- a conclusion of the scan findings
- documentation of any other relevant management after the scan
- recommendations for the purpose and timing of a further scan
- the name and professional role of the operator/supervisor
- the name and status of a trainee if performing any aspect of the examination.

Further reading

Leone F P G, Timmerman D, Bourne T et al 2010 Terms, definitions and measurements to describe the sonographic features of the endometrium and intrauterine lesions: a consensus opinion from the International Endometrial Tumor Analysis (IETA) group. Ultrasound Obstet Gynecol 35:103–112

Salim R, Woelfer B, Backos M, Regan L, Jurkovic D 2003 Reproducibility of three-dimensional ultrasound diagnosis of congenital uterine anomalies. Ultrasound Obstet Gynecol 21:578–582

The American Fertility Society 1988 The American Fertility Society classification of adnexal adhesions, distal tubal occlusion, tubal occlusion secondary to tubal ligation, tubal pregnancies, Müllerian anomalies and intrauterine adhesions. Fertil Steril 49:944–955

The menstrual cycle, the menopause and the effects of exogenous hormones

CONTENTS

The aims of this chapter are to enable you to do the following:
- describe the ultrasound appearances during the menstrual cycle
- describe the ultrasound findings during the menopause

- understand the different ultrasound findings encountered with the following:
  - hormonal contraception use
  - ovulation induction and oocyte donation
  - hormone replacement therapy use
  - tamoxifen use.

THE MENSTRUAL CYCLE

From the menarche until the menopause the female reproductive tract is subject to cyclical physiological changes in response to hormonal signals and influences. The role of the menstrual cycle is threefold: to initiate the maturation and release of a mature ovum or egg, to prepare the uterine endometrium for implantation of the blastocyst after fertilization of the ovum and to support the development of the early embryo.

This chapter considers in detail the pelvic ultrasound findings of the premenopausal and postmenopausal woman and the effects of the exogenous hormones which the woman may be taking.

Knowledge of the woman's menstrual status together with her current clinical history are key to the correct interpretation of the ultrasound findings. For example, the endometrium at the start of the menstrual cycle has a characteristic appearance that is dramatically different from that at midcycle. However, these 'normal' midcycle appearances will be different in a woman who is taking an oral contraceptive and may differ again in a woman with a contraceptive implant. Conversely, the endometrial appearances of a woman undergoing infertility treatment tend to be treatment-specific and may therefore differ from the appearances of a 'normally menstruating' woman. Furthermore, women who are peri- or postmenopausal may be using exogenous hormones – that is, hormone replacement therapy (HRT). It is important that you are aware of the effect these hormones can have on the endometrial appearances in order to confidently differentiate between normal findings and pathological conditions.

The effects of exogenous hormones on the endometrium and ovaries are perhaps easier to appreciate once the ultrasound findings during the menstrual cycle are fully understood. The menstrual cycle is, on average, 28 days long. The time leading up to ovulation is called the *proliferative phase* when referring to the endometrium and, confusingly, the *follicular phase* when describing changes in the ovary. Ovulation, in a 28 day cycle, typically occurs on day 14. The time after ovulation is called the *secretory* or *luteal phase*, depending again on whether reference is being made to the endometrium or the ovary.

In a 28 day cycle, therefore, the proliferative/follicular and secretory/luteal phases are both of equal length, namely 14 days. However, not every cycle is 28 days in length. It is the secretory or luteal phase that tends to remain constant at 14 days, with the subsequent variation taking place in the proliferative or follicular phase. Thus ovulation will typically take place on day 7 in a 21 day cycle and on day 21 in a 35 day cycle.

The physiological changes that occur within the endometrium and ovaries during the menstrual cycle take place in response to variations in circulating hormone levels. The operator needs to appreciate this synchrony in order to put the ultrasound appearances in perspective and thus to interpret them correctly. We feel it is easier to appreciate the rather complicated interactions between the hormones, endometrium and ovaries if they are considered as a whole, as this reflects the real life situation you, as the operator, will encounter. For this reason, they are described together and in a day by day format.

THE ENDOMETRIUM

The endometrium is composed of two layers, the deep basal layer or zona basilis and the superficial functional layer or zona functionalis (Fig. 17.1). The zona functionalis is divided into the deeper and thicker stratum spongiosum and the more

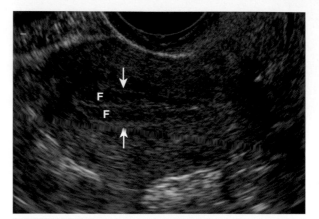

Fig 17.1 • Sagittal section of the endometrium demonstrating the zona basilis (arrowed) and the thicker zona functionalis (F).

superficial and thinner stratum compactum. The basal layer contributes approximately 25% of the thickness of the endometrium and varies little in depth and appearance during the menstrual cycle. The functional layer contributes the remaining 75% of the maximum thickness, and it is this layer that undergoes physiological change during the menstrual cycle.

Oestrogen and progesterone are produced by the ovaries in a cyclical manner. It is the specific levels of these circulating hormones that influence the physiological changes of the endometrium during the menstrual cycle.

DAYS 1–5

Day 1 of the menstrual cycle describes the first day of vaginal bleeding. Menstruation is initiated by a reduction below a specific threshold in the circulating levels of oestrogen and progesterone. Once this threshold is reached, the spiral arteries of the stratum spongiosum undergo vasoconstriction, which in turn initiates necrosis and desquamation of the functional layer.

Menstruation typically lasts 5 days and the endometrial appearances on day 1 will differ from those on day 5. At the start of menstruation the ultrasound appearances of the endometrium are effectively the same as those of day 28, as the thick functional layer is yet to be shed. By the cessation of menstruation, the thick functional layer will have been shed in its entirety, resulting in a thin endometrium composed of the basal layer only.

The Endometrium

On day 1 the endometrium is 'thick', with an irregular outline but with a homogeneous and hyperechoic echopattern. The 'cavity line', which represents the interface between the opposing layers of the endometrium, is often poorly visualized at this stage. This makes it difficult to distinguish between the anterior and posterior elements of the endometrium. The maximum thickness of the endometrium at this stage is 10.0–15.0 mm. By the end of bleeding and the sloughing off of the functional layer by day 5, the endometrium is 'thin', as it is composed of the basal layer only. It now has a regular outline while retaining its hyperechoic echopattern. Its maximum thickness is 3.0–4.0 mm.

Modern transvaginal ultrasound probes afford high resolution imaging which enables visualization of wavelike contractions of the endometrium. These wavelike contractions are in fact caused by the contractility of the myometrium. Before menstruation, high frequency endometrial contractions may be observed travelling from the uterine fundus to the cervix. This process facilitates the shedding of the endometrium at menstruation.

It is clear, therefore, that the appearances of the endometrium will change substantially between days 1 and 5. In addition, the endometrial cavity, which separates the two thicknesses of endometrium, may be distended with blood that will appear echo-poor. Blood clot within the cavity may also be present and can be differentiated from frank blood by its low-level echoes (Fig. 17.2). Retrograde bleeding, through the Fallopian tubes, may occur during menstruation, resulting in blood collecting in the Pouch of Douglas, posterior to the uterus.

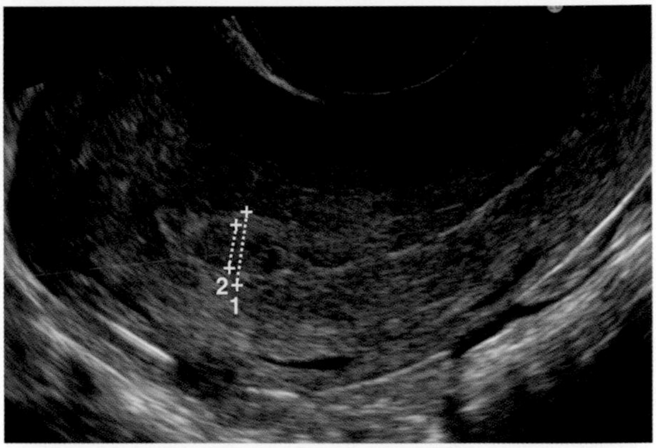

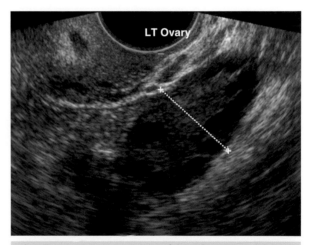

Fig 17.2 • Sagittal section of the endometrium on day 2 of the menstrual cycle. The 'endometrial thickness' (5.5 mm) has been measured (calipers 1) together with the depth of menstrual blood (4.2 mm) (calipers 2). The actual endometrial thickness therefore is 1.3 mm.

Fig 17.3 • Transverse section of the left ovary in the early follicular phase, demonstrating multiple small follicles (day 5 of the menstrual cycle).

The Ovary

Follicular growth in the ovary is initiated by secretion of follicle stimulating hormone (FSH) by the anterior pituitary in response to falling levels of oestrogen, from the ovarian thecal cells, and progesterone, from the failing corpus luteum, in the latter part of the preceding luteal phase. Immature, quiescent follicles can always be seen randomly distributed throughout the cortex of the ovary. Under stimulation from FSH, a cohort of 5–10 follicles is recruited towards the end of the preceding cycle. On day 1 of the cycle the mean diameter of the small follicles in this cohort is in the region of 1.0–2.0 mm. They are seen as distinct spherical, unilocular and anechoic structures within the more hyperechoic ovarian cortex. These follicles can vary in size but will all grow by approximately 0.5–1.0 mm per day. They will all continue to grow so that, by day 5, the same 5–10 follicles will be readily visualized, their mean diameter varying between 3.0 and 6.0 mm (Fig. 17.3).

Unfortunately, the cyclical changes that occur in the ovary do not always follow the rules. Thus those structures that should have disappeared during the previous cycle may not necessarily have done so by the start of the next. This can cause some confusion to the ultrasound interpretation in that a persistent corpus luteum or an unruptured follicle from an earlier cycle may be present within the ovary in this new cycle.

DAYS 6–12

The cessation of menstruation marks the start of the proliferative or follicular phase. The cohort of follicles secretes oestrogen which, in turn, initiates and supports the growth of a new functional layer of endometrium.

The Endometrium

The appearance of the endometrium continues to change, reflecting the development of the functional layer as mentioned earlier. Differentiation of the layers of the endometrium now becomes possible. The thin, hyperechoic basal layer can be distinguished from the functional layer, which now appears hypoechoic. The latter increases in thickness because of the enlargement of the glands and dilation of the blood vessels within it. On day 6 the endometrium measures 3.0–4.0 mm (Fig.

17.4) and by day 12 has reached a thickness of 8.0–12.0 mm (Fig. 17.5).

The endometrium is described as having a 'triple line' appearance from the early proliferative phase until midcycle (Fig. 17.6). The apposition of the hypoechoic anterior and posterior functionalis layers accentuate the hyperechoic appearance of the resulting 'cavity line' - this is the middle line of the three. The two outer lines are formed by the hyperechoic anterior and posterior basilis layers.

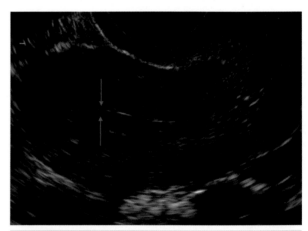

Fig 17.5 • Sagittal section of the endometrium, in the late proliferative phase (day 12 of the menstrual cycle). Note the thickening zona functionalis layers (arrows) when compared to that shown in Fig. 17.4.

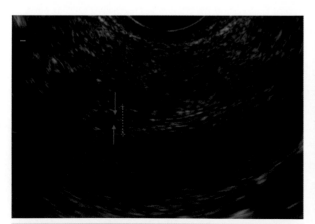

Fig 17.4 • Sagittal section of the endometrium, in the early proliferative phase (day 6 of the menstrual cycle). Note the thin zona functionalis layers (arrows). The callipers demonstrate the measurement of the endometrium (3.8 mm).

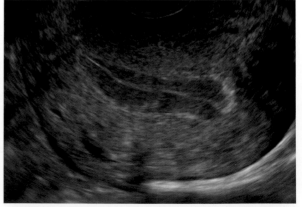

Fig 17.6 • Sagittal section of the endometrium in a retroverted uterus demonstrating the typical appearances at periovulation.

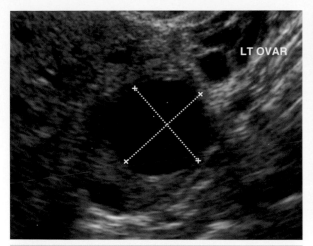

Fig 17.7 • Sagittal section of the left ovary, in the late follicular phase (day 11 of the menstrual cycle), with a dominant follicle measuring 16.3 × 15.7 mm.

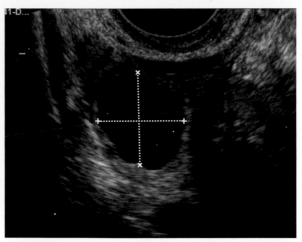

Fig 17.8 • Transverse section of the right ovary, in the periovulation phase, immediately prior to ovulation. The dominant follicle measures 19.2 × 22.3 mm.

The Ovary

The principal aim of ovarian function is to release a mature egg at ovulation. Normally only one follicle will ovulate, the ovulation of more than one follicle leading potentially to a multiple, dizygotic pregnancy. For ovulation to be achieved, one follicle, the 'dominant follicle', must be selected from the cohort of those that start to grow at the beginning of the cycle. The follicle selected is the largest and therefore presumably the most developed (Fig. 17.7). The size discrepancy between the dominant follicle and the others becomes increasingly obvious, enabling the dominant follicle to be identified from around day 8, when its mean diameter is approximately 10.0 mm. Its rate of growth thereafter is approximately 2.0 mm per day. By day 12 its mean diameter is therefore around 18.0 mm. During this period oestrogen levels are rising, causing a negative feedback on the secretion of FSH. The reducing FSH levels are thus concentrated on developing this one dominant follicle, with subsequent growth of the remaining follicles in the cohort ceasing.

DAYS 13–14

The dominant follicle secretes increasing amounts of oestrogen, the level of which peaks in the late follicular/periovulation phase. It is the oestrogen level reaching a threshold peak which exerts a positive feedback on luteinizing hormone (LH) levels. The resulting and dramatic surge in LH occurs approximately 12 hours before ovulation. The FSH level rises to a peak in synchrony with the LH surge.

The Endometrium

At periovulation the endometrium has a very pronounced triple line appearance. The functionalis layers are very glandular rich, enhancing their hypoechoic appearance, which contrasts with the hyperechoic basilis layers (Fig. 17.6).

In a fashion similar to that observed during menstruation, high frequency contractions occur within the endometrium during the periovulatory phase. The periovulatory contractions are observed to start from the cervix and move up the uterine body to the fundus. This phenomenon is thought to facilitate sperm transport to the Fallopian tubes.

At periovulation, the cervical glands secrete mucus. The mucus can be recognized as an anechoic stripe within the cervical canal.

The Ovary

Immediately before ovulation the mean diameter of the dominant follicle is between 20.0 and 25.0 mm in diameter (Fig. 17.8). Occasionally the

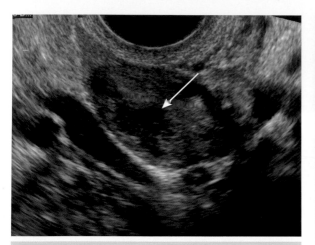

Fig 17.9 • Sagittal section of the right ovary, postovulation. This is evident because the dominant follicle is no longer present. The corpus luteum is collapsed with a crenulated wall (arrow).

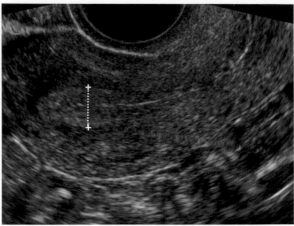

Fig 17.10 • Sagittal section of the endometrium, in the early secretory phase (day 18 of the menstrual cycle). The endometrium measures 8.9 mm. Note the loss of the triple line effect and the less distinct cavity line.

cumulus oophorus can be visualized 12–24 hours before ovulation. The cumulus oophorus is the mass of cells which surrounds the oocyte within the dominant follicle. It is identified within the dominant follicle as a small, irregular hyperechoic focus at the follicular wall.

It is the LH surge which initiates ovulation, although it is thought that the midcycle surge in FSH contributes to the freeing of the oocyte from the wall of the follicle. The dominant or Graafian follicle swells and ruptures at ovulation, releasing the oocyte into the peritoneal cavity. Ultrasound imaging performed before and after ovulation should demonstrate the presence and then absence of the dominant follicle. The postovulatory collapsed follicle often demonstrates a thickened crenulated wall (Fig. 17.9). Ovulation is thought to occur in a random fashion from either ovary and not necessarily from alternate ovaries during consecutive menstrual cycles.

After ovulation, a normal physiological finding is a small amount of free fluid within the dependent area of the pelvis, namely the Pouch of Douglas. In the case of a retroverted uterus, this will correspond to the area around the uterine fundus.

DAYS 15–22

Following ovulation the corpus luteum starts to secrete large amounts of progesterone.

The Endometrium

During the secretory phase, the endometrium is maturing – that is, secretory changes are occurring within the endometrial glands and the blood supply to the endometrium is increasing. These changes are in preparation, in the event of fertilization, for reception of the fertilized egg or blastocyst, which will start to implant into the endometrium between days 20 and 23. If fertilization does not occur, the progesterone level falls, leading ultimately to menstruation.

Within the first 7 days after ovulation the thickness of the endometrium normally remains unchanged, measuring 8.0–12.0 mm. The ultrasound appearance of the secretory phase endometrium is quite distinct from that of the proliferative and periovulatory phases. The triple line appearance of the periovulatory endometrium changes, gradually, to one characterized, at the end of the secretory phase, by a homogeneous, hyperechoic appearance with the cavity line becoming less distinct (Fig. 17.10).

The Ovary

The *luteal phase* refers to the luteinization of the remaining components of the ruptured follicle, now termed the corpus luteum. The cells surrounding the ruptured follicle proliferate and undergo luteinization. This is the accumulation of lutein, a yellow pigment, hence the name *corpus luteum* or 'yellow body'. Secretion of progesterone by the corpus luteum causes negative feedback on the levels of LH and FSH, which subsequently fall. In the event of nonfertilization of the oocyte, the corpus luteum ceases to function at around day 22, resulting in a decline in its production of oestrogen and progesterone. Over the following days the corpus luteum regresses, normally having disappeared by the end of the luteal phase.

The appearances of the corpus luteum are many and varied (see Fig. 1.33 and Fig. 5.10A and B). Its internal contents may vary from anechoic through to haemorrhagic, the latter being more readily identified immediately after ovulation. Its size may vary from 5.0 to 40.0 mm in mean diameter and its overall appearance may vary from 'small and collapsed' (see Fig. 5.10B) to 'large and cystic' (see Fig. 1.33). Nevertheless it is important to remember that this confusing range of appearances all describe a normally functioning corpus luteum.

The corpus luteum is not always readily identified by ultrasound, even when being sought by an experienced operator. Improvements in the resolution of equipment have undoubtedly increased the likelihood of visualizing the corpus luteum. It is likely that an unidentified corpus luteum is haemorrhagic in nature, with subtle appearances, which are difficult to differentiate from the surrounding ovarian tissue.

Vascularization of the corpus luteum ensures that it has a rich blood supply in order to function. The area of angiogenesis is well demonstrated with colour or power Doppler and typically is seen as a circumferential ring of flow, the 'ring of fire', around the corpus luteum (see Figs. 1.33 and 5.10A). Vascularization peaks at around day 22, coinciding with the time of implantation, assuming fertilization had occurred. Colour or power Doppler can assist in the visualization of the more subtle appearances of haemorrhagic corpus luteum (see Fig. 5.10A).

DAYS 23–28

In the absence of implantation, the activity of the corpus luteum ceases. Subsequently the circulating

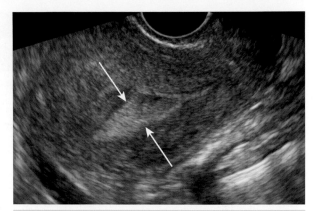

Fig 17.11 • Sagittal section of the endometrium (arrows), in the late secretory phase (day 25 of the menstrual cycle). Note that there is no cavity line present towards the fundus.

levels of oestrogen and progesterone fall, removing the negative feedback on FSH. Levels of FSH start to rise and follicular growth is initiated in preparation for the next cycle.

Falling levels of progesterone and oestrogen initiate the involution of the endometrium and ultimately menstruation. Around days 25–26 the spiral arteries start to vasoconstrict, resulting in the ischaemia which may cause early uterine cramps before the impending menstruation.

The Endometrium

The appearance and thickness of the endometrium in the last few days of the cycle remain essentially unchanged to that described at day 22, namely homogeneous and hyperechoic, with little distinction between the functional and basal layers. This lack of distinction is due to the endometrial glands become increasingly tortuous and dilated, with the subsequent increase in echogenicity of the functional layer so that it approaches that of the basal layer in ultrasound appearance. In addition, the cavity line will not be identified (Fig. 17.11).

The Ovary

The corpus luteum regresses in size and becomes atretic, evolving into the corpus albicans or white body. The corpus albicans is not readily identified on ultrasound, making it difficult to identify the

DAY	HORMONE LEVEL	ENDOMETRIAL APPEARANCE (THICKNESS)	FOLLICULAR SIZE, MEAN DIAMETER	CORPUS LUTEUM
1	FSH ⇧ Oestrogen = Progesterone =	Hyperechoic basal & functional layers (ET 10–15 mm)	Follicle(s) 1–2 mm	May be present from previous cycle (inactive)
5	FSH = Oestrogen ⇧ Progesterone =	Hyperechoic basal layer (ET 2–3 mm)	Follicle(s) 3–6 mm	As above
6	FSH ⇧ Oestrogen ⇧ Progesterone =	Predominantly hyperechoic basal layer & hypoechoic functional layer (ET 3–4 mm)	Follicle(s) 4–7 mm	
12	FSH ⇩ Oestrogen ⇧ Progesterone =	Hyperechoic basal layer & hypoechoic functional layer (ET 8–12 mm)	Dominant ~18.0 mm follicle	
13	LH surge FSH ⇧ Oestrogen ⇧ Progesterone =	Triple line echo sign representing the hyperechoic basal layer, hypoechoic functional layer & hyperechoic interface	Dominant follicle ~22.0 mm	
14	LH ⇩ FSH ⇩ Oestrogen = Progesterone ⇧	Appearances essentially unchanged from day 13	Dominant follicle absent	
15–22	LH ⇩ FSH ⇩ Oestrogen ⇧ Progesterone ⇧	Little difference in hyperechoic appearances of functional & basal layers (ET 8–12 mm)	Follicle(s) 1–2 mm	Corpus luteum can be anechoic, haemorrhagic, collapsed. Vascularization peaks at day 22
23–28	LH = FSH = Oestrogen ⇩ Progesterone ⇩	As days 15–22, endometrium possibly thicker	Follicle(s) 1–2 mm	Corpus luteum appearances as above, although less likely to be haemorrhagic

Table 17.1 The principal hormonal changes that occur during days 1–28 of the normal menstrual cycle, together with associated ultrasound appearances

ET, endometrial thickness; *FSH*, follicle stimulating hormone; *LH*, luteinizing hormone; ⇧, hormone level rising; ⇩, hormone level falling; =, hormone level unchanged.

site of the corpus luteum towards the end of the luteal phase. In some cycles, however, the corpus luteum may persist in an inactive state into the follicular phase of the next cycle.

The principal hormonal changes that occur during the menstrual cycle, together with the associated ultrasound appearances, are tabulated in Table 17.1.

HORMONAL CONTRACEPTION

The effect on the ultrasound appearances of the endometrium and ovaries is dependent on the type of hormonal contraception used. Most hormonal

contraception prevents pregnancy by inhibiting ovulation, thinning the endometrium and thickening mucus in the cervical canal. However, not all

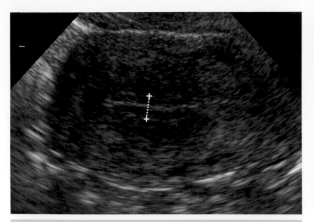

Fig 17.12 • Sagittal section of the endometrium, measuring 3.8 mm, as shown by the callipers, on day 8 in a woman using the combined pill. Note the isoechoic appearances of the endometrium and myometrium.

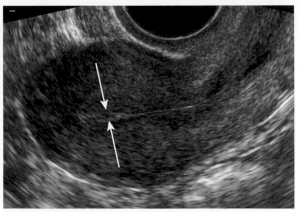

Fig 17.13 • Sagittal section of the endometrium (arrows) in a woman with a contraceptive implant. Note the thinness of the endometrium.

inhibit ovulation, so it is useful to be aware of which do and which do not.

THE COMBINED PILL

The most common oral contraceptive pill currently in use is the combined pill containing oestrogen and progesterone. These are usually taken for the first 21 days of the cycle, followed by a pill-free interval of 7 days to allow shedding of the endometrium. The endometrial appearances are uniform throughout the cycle.

After prolonged use of the combined pill, the endometrium typically is thin. It becomes more difficult to differentiate it from the myometrium as their echogenicity is typically similar i.e. isoechoic (Fig. 17.12). Ovulation is inhibited, so the ovaries will contain multiple small antral follicles with no evidence of follicular growth or corpora luteal cysts.

THE PROGESTERONE ONLY PILL

The progesterone only pill provides contraception primarily by thickening the cervical mucus and thinning the endometrium. Inhibition of ovulation occurs in about 50% of users of lower dose progesterone pills. Approximately 97% of users of higher dose progesterone pills, however, have anovulatory cycles. The progesterone only pill is taken continuously, without a pill free interval. The

woman's periods may stop, her periods may be irregular or she may experience spotting. Typically the endometrium will be thin, the ultrasound findings therefore being similar in appearance to those seen in women using the combined pill. If ovulation does occur, follicular growth will be apparent and a corpus luteum may be visualised.

THE CONTRACEPTIVE IMPLANT

The contraceptive implant is a progesterone only, single rod contraceptive device which is inserted, subdermally, into the inner side of the upper arm. The progesterone is released slowly and continuously, at the same rate over the device's lifespan, which is a period of up to 3 years.

For the implant to be effective from the first day of use, it must be inserted within the first 5 days of the cycle. Contraception is achieved by blocking the LH surge and therefore inhibiting ovulation. Thus the endometrium will usually be thin, measuring no more than 2.0–3.0 mm (Fig. 17.13). The implant can cause periods to stop. Alternatively, women may experience irregular bleeding, spotting or heavier periods.

The ovaries may contain follicles, measuring up to a maximum of 13.0–15.0 mm in diameter. Occasionally an escape ovulation can occur, particularly towards the end of the contraceptive implant's life cycle. This would be evidenced by visualization of a corpus luteum when present.

DEPO-PROVERA

Depo-Provera (depot-medroxyprogesterone acetate) contains a synthetic progesterone and is given in the form of an intramuscular injection, usually every 3 months. Depo-Provera works by inhibiting ovulation. The endometrium will therefore be very thin and hyperechoic, and similar in appearance to that shown in Fig. 17.13. Most women using this method of contraception either will not menstruate at all or have light periods.

IUCDs

As its name suggests, the intrauterine contraceptive device (IUCD) is a device that is inserted into the uterine cavity. Its function is to prevent implantation of the blastocyst into the endometrium. Modern devices secrete progesterone while the older types did not. The most commonly used hormone secreting device at present is the levonorgestrel-releasing intauterine system (IUS) or Mirena®. This has a polyethylene frame consisting of a vertical stem and a horizontal portion consisting of two arms. The stem has a reservoir which contains progesterone that is slowly released. In some women the level of circuiting progesterone inhibits ovulation, but the majority of women will continue to ovulate. Pregnancy is prevented by thinning of the endometrium and thickening of cervical mucus. It is common for women to experience irregular bleeding or spotting, particularly in the first 6 months of usage. This irregular bleeding may continue, although the majority of women find that their periods stop altogether.

In addition to its contraceptive effect, the Mirena® is often used as treatment for women with menorrhagia.

Correct placement of the Mirena® requires the cranial end of the device to be positioned in the fundal region of the endometrium. This results in the caudal end lying in the lower uterine body towards the internal os. Earlier versions of the Mirena® were difficult to visualize on ultrasound compared with the older non hormone-releasing IUCDS. These older devices were of three main types: the copper 7, the copper T or the Lippes' loop. Each had very characteristic ultrasound appearances. The copper 7 had a single arm, as its name suggests, and the copper T had two arms, whereas the Lippes' loop was spiral shaped. You are

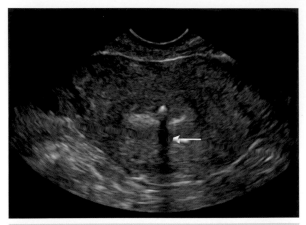

Fig 17.14 • Transverse view of uterus with a Mirena® intrauterine system in situ. Note the posterior acoustic shadowing (arrow).

very unlikely to examine a woman still fitted with one of these older devices, but you may come across images of them in historical ultrasound textbooks.

A common indication for an ultrasound scan of a woman fitted with a Mirena® is to confirm the correct placement of it. You should be aware that identifying a Mirena® might be an incidental finding in an ultrasound scan performed for entirely different reasons.

The strings of the older first generation Mirenas® were readily identified within the cervix on ultrasound, as they appeared hyperechoic, but the shaft was difficult to locate confidently. Newer versions of the Mirena®, however, have a more easily identifiable shaft. Providing the ultrasound beam is perpendicular to the axis of the shaft, the shaft produces a strong acoustic shadow. A sagittal section of the uterus and endometrium will demonstrate the full length of the Mirena's® shaft. The shaft produces a marked acoustic shadow which is rectangular in shape. Transverse sections of the uterus and endometrium will demonstrate the Mirena® in transverse section as a hyperechoic focus, producing an acoustic shadow posteriorly (Fig. 17.14). A transverse section towards the fundus should demonstrate the two arms of the device, giving the appearance of a thin horizontal, hyperechoic stripe situated within the fundal aspect of the endometrium and producing an acoustic shadow.

It may not be possible to assess or measure the endometrium satisfactorily if there is an IUCD in situ. A comment should be made to this effect in the report.

THE ROLE OF ULTRASOUND IN SUBFERTILITY

Subfertility investigations form a specialized area of gynaecology and usually fall within the remit of assisted conception units. Increasingly, however, ultrasound departments are being requested to scan women who are undergoing ovulation induction or oocyte donation. The medications used for these procedures have specific desired effects upon the endometrium and ovaries. As the primary focus of this chapter is the appreciation of the varying appearances of the endometrium and ovaries, it is appropriate to consider those effects at this point. The features that need to be assessed and included in the ultrasound report are discussed later.

For a more in depth understanding of the role of ultrasound in the investigation and treatment of subfertility and infertility, we suggest that specialist texts should be consulted.

OVULATION INDUCTION

Failure to ovulate is a common cause of sub-fertiilty. In such cases, the woman is given medication to stimulate follicular development and ovulation. The medication is usually clomiphene citrate to stimulate follicular development, followed by human chorionic gonadotropin (hCG) to induce ovulation. Ultrasound is used to monitor the size of the follicles and the endometrial thickness.

Clomiphene treatment is normally started between 3 and 5 days after the first day of the last menstrual period (LMP) and is continued for 5 days. An ultrasound scan is normally performed around day 8 post LMP. At this stage it should be easy to identify and measure the dominant follicle. It is good practice to measure all follicles of diameter greater than 8.0 mm.

Ideally, the longitudinal, anteroposterior (AP) and transverse diameters of the follicle should be measured in three planes, orthogonal to each other. In practice however, it is more common only to measure the diameter of each follicle in two planes, from a transverse section of the ovary. The follicles should be measured using the 'inner to inner' technique, and the mean follicular diameter calculated.

Scanning is repeated until the leading follicle is between 16.0 and 18.0 mm in mean diameter. At this stage, a single injection of hCG is given. The hCG induces maturation of the oocyte and ovulation approximately 36 hours after the injection. Giving the hCG at this follicular size enables the couple to time intercourse or an insemination procedure with either the male partner's or donor's semen.

It is not uncommon for a woman to produce multiple follicles. In this situation caution should be exercised. This is because of the risk of a multiple pregnancy if the treatment continues in the presence of two or three follicles of 16.0 mm mean diameter or greater.

Occasionally the follicles fail to grow and do not attain the required size to induce induction. The treatment then has to be abandoned. Increasing the clomiphene dose may have the required effect, so the woman may return for another cycle to once again assess the response of the ovaries to stimulation.

Clomiphene is an antioestrogenic agent. Thus although the endometrium thickens, it will not attain the same thickness as that of an untreated cycle at the comparative times in the cycle.

OOCYTE DONATION

The use of donor oocytes has extended the boundaries of fertility treatment so that age is no longer a limiting factor for a woman wishing to achieve a pregnancy. Essentially the process involves the collection of oocytes from a known or anonymous donor who undergoes a cycle of in vitro fertilization (IVF) treatment.

The endometrium of the recipient must be prepared and be ready to receive the embryos at the correct phase of the donor's cycle. Currently some recipients travel abroad to undergo embryo transfer in the country in which the donor has undergone a standard IVF cycle. Ultrasound monitoring of the recipient's endometrium is required to ensure that its priming is in tandem with the anticipated collection of the donor's eggs. This is of particular importance if the donor and recipient are separated geographically.

The recipient initially undergoes a period of downregulation, essentially a 'temporary menopause'. This takes about 2 weeks and improves the control of follicular development once superovulation of the donor begins. An ultrasound examination is performed to ensure that downregulation has occurred.

The appearances of downregulation are a thin endometrium less than 4.0 mm and quiescent ovaries containing only small follicles.

As the donor undergoes superovulation, the recipient starts to take oral oestrogen medication to thicken the endometrium. The recipient is scanned at intervals to ensure adequate endometrial growth. At day 8 the recipient's endometrium should measure 6.0 mm, so ideally, by the time the donor is ready for oocyte collection, the recipient's endometrium will measure 7.0–8.0 mm thick with a triple layer appearance.

THE MENOPAUSE

The menopause is defined as the permanent cessation of menstruation and ovarian follicular activity. The menopause can be said to have occurred once 12 months have elapsed since the final menstrual period. The perimenopause is the period before the menopause.

POSTMENOPAUSAL ENDOMETRIUM

The normal postmenopausal endometrium consists of the two basalis layers with no functionalis layer. The levels of oestrogen and progesterone fall in the postmenopausal woman; consequently the endometrium is thin, typically measuring 1.0–3.0 mm (Fig. 17.15).

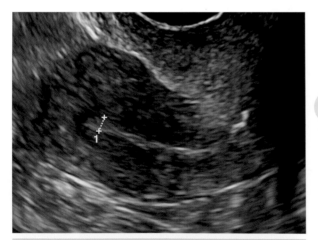

Fig 17.15 • Sagittal section of a postmenopausal uterus. The endometrium measures 2.4 mm. Note the relatively small size of the uterus compared to the premenopausal uterus in Fig. 17.5.

A not infrequent finding in postmenopausal women is the presence of intracavity fluid. The depth of fluid, which is usually only 2.0–3.0 mm, should be subtracted from the anteroposterior measurement of the endometrium, so that the resulting measurement represents endometrial tissue thickness only (see Fig. 16.9).

Fluid in the cavity is a benign finding and is of no clinical significance. The fluid can prove to be an advantage, as it can provide an acoustic window which aids visualization of the endometrium. This acoustic window mimics the view obtained with saline contrast hysterosonography. The purpose of this procedure is to examine the endometrial cavity, typically to exclude a uterine polyp or other similar pathological conditions of the cavity. Saline is infused into the uterine cavity through the cervix, using a fine flexible catheter under direct ultrasound control, to distend the cavity and allow better visualization of its borders.

POSTMENOPAUSAL OVARIES

The ovaries will atrophy throughout the menopause and are described as quiescent when no discernible follicles are present, as demonstrated by the ovary shown in Fig. 4.9. This lack of follicular activity makes identification of the ovaries in the menopause difficult for the novice operator. Knowing where to expect to find the postmenopausal ovaries will be gained from examining premenopausal ovaries, the more the better. Knowing where their locations are most likely to be should increase your confidence in finding postmenopausal ovaries.

HORMONE REPLACEMENT THERAPY

Hormone replacement therapy (HRT) describes the use of cyclical oestrogen and progesterone. Various combinations of HRT are commonly prescribed for women who are peri- and postmenopausal. The appearances of the endometrium are dependent on whether the woman is taking cyclical or sequential oestrogen and progesterone or continuous combined oestrogen with progesterone.

Cyclical HRT

Women who are perimenopausal or who are going through the menopause and are having irregular periods often use cyclical HRT.

Cyclical HRT causes changes in the endometrial appearance which may be evident on ultrasound depending on when in a cycle the woman is examined. Assessment of the endometrium in a women taking cyclical HRT ultrasound should be performed 7 days after the last progesterone pill. At this time the criteria for assessment of the endometrium are similar to all other premenopausal women.

Continuous HRT

Women who are definitively menopausal tend to use the continuous combined therapy. With continuous combined therapy, the endometrium should be uniformly thin – that is, less than 4.0 mm – and similar in appearance to that of a postmenopausal woman who is not taking HRT.

ENDOMETRIAL HYPERPLASIA

Endometrial hyperplasia results from the prolonged action of oestrogens that are unopposed by progesterone. The uterus of a postmenopausal woman taking HRT, or tamoxifen for breast cancer, will demonstrate thickening of the endometrium as a result of the stimulatory effect of the oestrogen. Thickening of the endometrium is also associated with endometrial cancer.

A postmenopausal woman who is experiencing vaginal bleeding is described as symptomatic. The current cut-off for normal endometrial thickness varies between 4.0 and 5.0 mm, depending on the individual centre. Evidence suggests that applying a cut-off of 4.0–5.0 mm has a high negative predictive value for the presence of cancer.

Accurate measurement and assessment of the endometrium is essential for the reasons stated earlier. Where it is not possible to image the endometrium clearly, and therefore to obtain an accurate measurement of the combined anterior and posterior layers of the endometrium, this must be documented in the report. It is not acceptable to assume an unmeasurable endometrium is normal.

TAMOXIFEN

Tamoxifen is used as an antioestrogen in the treatment and prevention of breast cancer. Its oestrogenic properties cause proliferation of the endometrium. There is an increased risk of endometrial cancer with the use of tamoxifen.

The endometrium in a woman taking tamoxifen typically will appear thickened and hyperechoic. Multiple small cystic structures are often present within it and its outline may be irregular.

Tamoxifen therapy in postmenopausal women with breast cancer is associated with a high incidence of endometrial polyps. The polyps tend to be large and fill the entire endometrial cavity. This makes it difficult to distinguish the polyp from the endometrium unless intracavity fluid is present. As described earlier, hysterosonography may be a useful additional examination in such cases.

Several investigators have concluded that there is an increased risk of endometrial pathological conditions, including endometrial cancer, in women undergoing tamoxifen therapy and when a thickened endometrium of 8.0 mm or greater is present.

Futher Reading

Endometrial Hyperplasia Management of (green-top Guideline no 67). RCOG 2016

Menopause: diagnosis and management (NG23). NICE 2015

Uterine and ovarian anomalies

18

CONTENTS

The more common abnormalities of the uterus, adnexae and ovaries are described in this chapter.

The aims of this chapter are to enable you to do the following:

- appreciate the ultrasound appearances of the more common abnormalities of the uterus, ovaries and adnexae
- report the findings of the scan
- appreciate the importance of a clinically relevant report.

This text assumes that you, the operator, are sitting to the left of, or at the foot of, the scanning couch, holding the transvaginal probe in your right hand, that the woman is lying to your right side and that you are facing each other. It also assumes that you are able to find and examine the normal uterus, ovaries and adnexae and are therefore able to recognize the range of normal ultrasound appearances within the pelvis.

You are now therefore able to recognize appearances in the female pelvis which are not normal. The following text will hopefully equip you with the skills you require to reach as accurate and as clinically useful an interpretation of your examination as possible.

UTERINE FIBROIDS

Uterine fibroids, or leiomyomas, account for a significant proportion of the uterine pathological conditions that you will encounter when scanning women referred for gynaecological ultrasound assessment. Fibroids are the most common gynae-cological tumour and have such a low malignancy potential that they are considered benign.

INCIDENCE

The reported incidence of uterine fibroids is vari able, as it is dependent on the imaging modality used and the population being studied. We quote the findings of one typical study, which demon-strates an increasing incidence with increasing age, as shown:

- in women aged between 20 and 30 years, the incidence is approximately 4%
- in women aged between 30 and 40 years, the incidence is 11–18%
- in women aged between 40 and 50 years, the incidence is approximately 33%.

Fibroids are more common in black, Afro-Caribbean women than Caucasian or Asian women. They are more common in nulliparous and obese women than in parous or women of normal weight.

Fibroids tend to increase in size during preg-nancy and regress in size during the menopause.

SYMPTOMS

Fibroids are often a coincidental finding on ultra-sound examination and are thus present in both asymptomatic and symptomatic women. Symp-toms typically associated with fibroids are menor-rhagia, pain, subfertility and pressure symptoms.

Despite its frequent presentation, the fibroid uterus can prove technically difficult to scan. Thus translating the findings into a clinically relevant report can be challenging, even for the most expe-rienced operator.

ULTRASOUND APPEARANCES

Fibroids are benign tumours of the smooth muscle of the uterus. They are composed of smooth muscle fibres and fibrous connective tissue which are arranged in concentric rings. The dense arrange-ment of the muscle fibres produces the character-istic ultrasound 'whorled' appearance of the mass of the fibroid. The fibroid is surrounded by a pseu-docapsule which produces a clear border to the mass. The ultrasound appearance of a fibroid

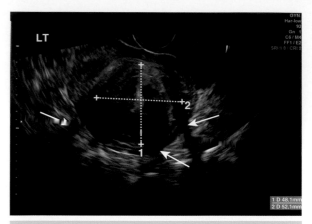

Fig 18.1 • Left lateral intramural fibroid. The fibroid is isoechoic with the endometrium, and is, surrounded by a hyperechoic border. The maximum diameters of the fibroid have been measured in its sagittal section. Note the acoustic shadowing (arrows).

therefore is typically of a rounded, homogeneous mass which is either hypoechoic or isoechoic com-pared with the surrounding myometrium, sur-rounded by a relatively hyperechoic border (Fig. 18.1). The dense nature of the abnormal smooth muscle of the fibroid often results in acoustic shad-owing posteriorly.

A common feature of the fibroid is calcification, particularly in the postmenopausal woman. This can either appear as small foci scattered through-out the fibroid or as a rim or partial rim of calcification surrounding the fibroid (Fig. 18.2). The calcified material causes posterior acoustic shadowing, and this can make measurements of such fibroids inaccurate, as the entire outline of the fibroid is difficult to define.

When applying colour Doppler to a fibroid, blood flow typically is seen circumferentially around the fibroid. There is usually little or no blood flow detected in the centre of the fibroid.

LOCATION

The vast majority of fibroids are situated within the uterine body. They may be seen less commonly in the cervix and broad ligament. Discussing such fibroids is beyond the scope of this text.

Uterine fibroids should be described in terms of their relationship to the uterine layers (i.e. the endometrium, myometrium and serosa). There are three possible locations of fibroids: submucosal,

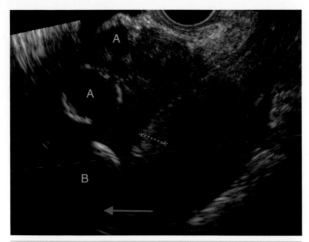

Fig 18.2 • Sagittal section of the uterus containing several intramural fibroids in the anterior uterine wall. Note the calcified fibroids (A) with circumferential calcified rim and (B) with crescent-shaped anterior calcified rim and posterior acoustic shadowing (arrow). The endometrium is demarcated by the two calipers.

subserosal and intramural, in addition to pedunculated fibroids, as shown in Fig. 18.3.

Submucosal

Submucosal fibroids project from the inner surface of the myometrium and distort the uterine cavity. They are often associated with menorrhagia and dysmenorrhoea. Submucosal fibroids can contribute to subfertility, as the distortion of the endometrium which they may cause results in an unfavourable environment for implantation of the fertilized ovum. Submucosal fibroids have been reported to contribute to an increase in the miscarriage rate and, when in close proximity to the placenta, are often associated with early pregnancy bleeding.

Submucosal fibroids are classified into a further three types:

- type 0: pedunculated and lying entirely within the cavity (Fig. 18.4)
- type 1: sessile, with less than 50% of the fibroid lying within the myometrium (Fig. 18.5)
- type 2: sessile, with more than 50% of the fibroid lying within the myometrium.

The term *sessile* describes a structure that has a broad base.

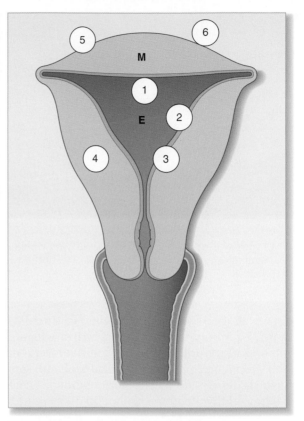

Fig 18.3 • Coronal pictorial image of the uterus demonstrating the most common locations of fibroids. *1*, Type 0 submucosal; *2*, type 1 submucosal; *3*, type 2 submucosal; *4*, intramural; *5*, subserosal; *6*, pedunculated. E, endometrium; M, myometrium.

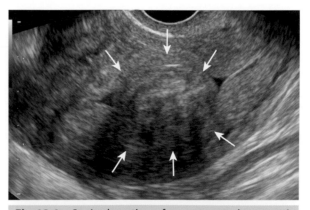

Fig 18.4 • Sagittal section of an anteverted uterus. A submucosal type 0 fibroid (arrows) lies entirely within the uterine cavity. A trace of fluid is present within the cavity, which helps delineate the fibroid.

411

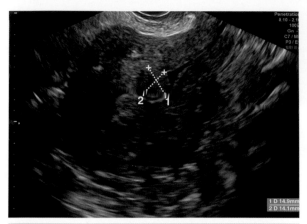

Fig 18.5 • A submucosal fibroid type 1, measuring 14.9 × 14.1 mm with less than 50% of the fibroid lying within the myometrium. The fibroid arises from the anterior uterine wall.

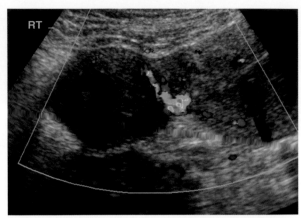

Fig 18.7 • A right sided pedunculated subserosal fibroid. The colour Doppler demonstrates the vascular stalk which connects the fibroid to the uterine body.

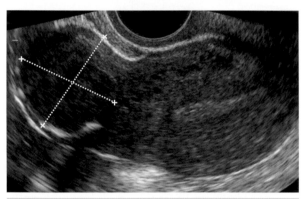

Fig 18.6 • Transverse view of the uterus. A subserosal (calcified) fibroid measuring 32 × 33 mm is present within the right lateral uterine wall.

Subserosal

A *subserosal* fibroid is so named because it lies under the serosal surface of the uterus and therefore projects out from the outer surface of the uterus (Fig. 18.6). The degree of projection is subjective and will vary. There seems to be no agreed definition of 'serosal' as opposed to 'subserosal' and, confusingly, these terms are used interchangeably. We have adopted the term 'subserosal' throughout this text.

Intramural

An *intramural* fibroid (see Fig. 18.1) lies within the myometrium and does not distort the uterine cavity. If the degree of distortion of the uterine surface is less than 50%, this is classified as an intramural rather than subserosal fibroid.

Pedunculated

A fibroid can be attached to the myometrium by a relatively thin stalk and is then termed *pedunculated*. A pedunculated submucosal fibroid therefore will be positioned within the uterine cavity, whereas a pedunculated subserosal fibroid (Fig. 18.7) will be exophytic to, or outside, the uterus. Confirming continuity of the fibroid with the myometrium via its stalk is important in both situations.

As the stalk is relatively narrow, a pedunculated fibroid can undergo torsion. The resulting compromise to its vascular blood supply may result in acute pain. A pedunculated subserosal fibroid may be confused with an adnexal mass. To avoid such confusion it is important to identify both ovaries separately from the mass.

Pathophysiological processes can result in atypical ultrasound appearances of uterine fibroids, as detailed next.

DEGENERATION

Degeneration is the breaking down of all or part of the tissue of the fibroid mass and takes place when the fibroid increases in size such that it outgrows

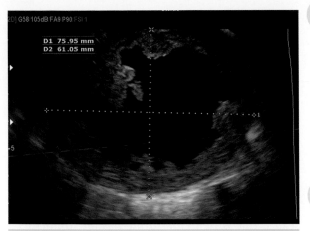

Fig 18.8 • An example of red degeneration within a fibroid, associated with a 16 week pregnancy. The mass is large, measuring 76.0 × 61.0 mm, with an irregularly shaped anechoic centre.

its blood supply. There are three types of degeneration: red, hyaline and myxoid.

Red degeneration is so called because the gross pathological appearance of the degenerating fibroid resembles red meat. This can be caused by the high levels of circulating oestrogen found during pregnancy. A haemorrhagic infarction occurs as a result of obstruction of the draining veins. The necrosis results in altered ultrasound appearances, namely a central disorganized, anechoic area, which is irregular in outline, within the fibroid mass (Fig. 18.8).

Red degeneration may cause symptoms of pain, tenderness and fever. Red degeneration is rare but it is important to differentiate such a finding from an ovarian pathology.

Hyaline degeneration is the most common type of degeneration in the nonpregnant woman and describes the replacement of the fibrous and muscle tissues by hyaline tissue. As with red degeneration, the echo texture of the fibroid with hyaline degeneration appears disorganized and part liquefied.

Hyaline degeneration does not usually give rise to symptoms.

Myxoid degeneration is the least common type and describes the breakdown of the fibrous and muscle tissues into a mass which is gelatinous in content.

Myxoid degeneration does not usually give rise to symptoms.

LIPOLEIOMYOMA

Lipoleiomyoma describes a fibroid or leiomyoma within which fatty changes have taken place. A lipoleiomyoma is a rare finding and most likely to occur in the postmenopausal woman. Its ultrasound appearance is of a well-defined mass which is hyperechoic compared with the surrounding myometrium. If the lipoleiomyoma is subserosal, it can be mistaken for a dermoid ovarian cyst.

LEIOMYOSARCOMA

Leiomyosarcoma is a rare uterine tumour which we include here because of the similarity in ultrasound appearances of this malignant tumour and a fibroid.

As fibroids do not normally increase in size during the menopause, a rapid increase in uterine size in a postmenopausal woman should always be investigated in order to exclude malignancy. Some authors report irregular peripheral and central vascularity when interrogating leiomyosarcoma with colour Doppler. Flow is typically high velocity with low impedance. Unfortunately fibroids also exhibit similar peripheral vascularity, so the use of Doppler to discriminate between the malignant and benign masses is not considered specific enough to be of clinical value in such cases.

ULTRASOUND EXAMINATION

Fibroids may be known, suspected or a coincidental finding. They can be single, multiple or conglomerate. *Conglomerate* refers to fibroids that are clustered together and are therefore difficult to identify confidently as being separate from each other.

Each fibroid identified should be described according to its location, as discussed and depicted in Fig. 18.3. Furthermore, the uterine position should be described – for example, whether the fibroid is anterior or posterior to the endometrium; whether it is to the right or the left of the endometrium; and whether it lies at the fundus, within the main body of the uterus or towards the lower uterine segment.

You must be able to identify the uterine cavity in its entirety to assess correctly the relationship of each fibroid to the cavity. The maximum diameter of each fibroid should be measured in three planes

413

orthogonal to each other, using the 'outer-to-outer' technique. Make sure you have obtained the sagittal and transverse sections of the uterus in which the maximum diameters of the fibroid are demonstrated. Fibroids are usually round, so the three diameters should all be of a similar size.

Describing the location, position and size of the fibroid is termed *mapping*. The relevance of fibroid mapping is discussed later in this chapter.

As discussed previously, ultrasound assessment of the uterine cavity and pelvic organs is usually best achieved using the transvaginal approach because of its superior resolution compared with the transabdominal route. We therefore recommend that every gynaecological examination starts with the transvaginal approach, unless contraindicated or where a previous ultrasound examination has reported the presence of fibroids causing uterine enlargement to such a degree that the uterine fundus reaches the umbilicus. In such cases we recommend starting the examination using the transabdominal approach.

Let us assume the examination is being performed transvaginally. Examination of the uterus and ovaries is undertaken as has been described in Chapter 4, and if any fibroids are present, they should be mapped. You must satisfy yourself as to whether your transvaginal examination has provided you with all the information you require or whether a transabdominal examination is also required. The need for transabdominal imaging will depend on the number, size, location and position of the fibroids and whether the ovaries and adnexae have been adequately imaged.

We suggest that you consider the following points in order to make that decision.

- has the uterine cavity been adequately imaged?

    The uterine cavity may be distorted by one or more fibroids to such a degree that it may not be possible to assess the cavity in its entirety
- have both ovaries been adequately imaged?

    Fibroids may cause the ovaries to be displaced laterally and therefore beyond the field of view of the transvaginal probe
- has the entire serosal surface of the uterus been adequately imaged?

    If the uterus is enlarged by the presence of multiple fibroids, it may not be possible to image the whole uterus within the field of view of the transvaginal probe
- have the fibroids all been adequately imaged?

    Fibroids attenuate sound, and especially if they are calcified; therefore the ability to image the fibroid or tissue posterior to it may be compromised by the relatively high frequency of the transvaginal probe.

If the answer to any of these questions is negative, then a transabdominal examination should be performed as an adjunct. It is not necessary to ask the woman to fill her bladder for a transabdominal scan if this is being performed as an adjunct to a transvaginal scan, as the fibroid uterus will be sufficiently enlarged that it lies above the symphysis pubis.

As the transabdominal probe operates at lower frequencies than the transvaginal probe, the sound beam has a greater penetration with which to examine the entire depth of uterus. The associated disadvantage of this approach is that the resolution of the resulting images will be poorer than with the higher frequency transvaginal probe.

Let us now assume that the decision has been taken to perform the initial examination transabdominally. Examination of the uterus and ovaries is undertaken as has been described in Chapter 5, and if any fibroids are present, they should be mapped. You must satisfy yourself as to whether your transabdominal examination has provided you with all the information you require or whether a transvaginal scan is also required as an adjunct examination. The need for the transvaginal scan will again be dependent on the number, size and location of the fibroids and whether you are satisfied that you have been able to assess the ovaries and adnexae adequately from the transabdominal approach.

We suggest that the following points are considered in order to make that decision:

- have both ovaries been adequately imaged?

    One or either of the ovaries may be located inferiorly and close to the lateral border of the uterus. The ovary may therefore not be amenable to visualization with the transabdominal probe but may be within the field of view of the transvaginal probe

- has the cervix been adequately visualized?

  If it is suspected that this is because there are fibroids located within the cervix, it is likely that these will be better visualized using the transvaginal approach

- has the uterine cavity been adequately visualized?

  If it is suspected that this is because one or more fibroids are obscuring the cavity, it will be better visualised using the transvaginal approach.

If the answer to any of these questions is negative, then a transvaginal examination should be performed as an adjunct.

Mapping and Reporting of Fibroids

We suggest using the template for a gynaecological ultrasound report described in Chapter 16. In addition, the fibroid should be reported according to its location, position and size. Comment needs to be included as to whether or not the uterine cavity is distorted by the fibroid. If there is a submucosal fibroid present, there will be distortion of the uterine cavity. The International Federation of Obstetricians and Gynaecologists (FIGO) recommends adopting a standardized system of reporting or mapping fibroids as described later.

It is not acceptable to use phrases such as 'bulky fibroid uterus' in your report. It is highly likely that the referring clinician has reached that conclusion from his or her physical examination of the woman before requesting the scan. He or she would be hoping to gain additional, clinically useful, information from your ultrasound examination.

'Early fibroid change' is also a phrase which should be avoided. If discrete fibroids are not identified but there is a loss of the homogeneous low-level echotexture of the myometrium, you need to consider whether the myometrial appearances are more in keeping with adenomyosis than fibroids.

We recommend the following as example reports that include the correct, clinically useful information relating to one or more uterine fibroids.

Example report A

Subserosal fibroid noted right/fundal aspect of the uterus, measuring 57 × 62 × 63 mm.

The uterine cavity is not distorted by the fibroid.

Example report B

Several fibroids are noted as described:

1 *intramural right/anterior, measuring 23 × 25 × 26 mm*
2 *intramural left/anterior/fundal, measuring 40 × 41 × 44 mm*
3 *subserosal left lateral, measuring 47 × 47 × 52 mm*
4 *submucosal, as <50% lies within the myometrium, mid/posterior, measuring 25 × 26 × 24 mm.*

The information that you provide for the clinician is important for three reasons:

- serial scans, performed to assess whether fibroids have grown, multiplied or regressed, can be directly compared
- the clinician can assess whether the fibroids are, or are not, likely to be the cause of the woman's presenting complaint or symptoms
- the mapping of fibroids aids in the management of the woman's fibroids where indicated.

Mapping and Reporting Difficulties

On occasion you will encounter a fibroid uterus where it is not possible to identify and map individual fibroids. Either it is not possible to identify the fibroids separately, as there is minimal myometrium which appears to be unaffected by fibroids, or there are too many fibroids to map.

When faced with the former scenario your report needs to include the uterine size, whether or not the uterine cavity has been visualized and, if it has, whether or not it is distorted. You should also document that the uterus contains multiple fibroids which are not possible to define individually and that there is little or no myometrium unaffected by fibroids.

In cases where multiple fibroids are present, the following approach should be employed:

- map the relevant fibroids (i.e. those likely to cause symptoms and those that are likely to be factored into a management decision). These would include all pedunculated subserosal fibroids, large subserosal fibroids, cervical fibroids and all submucosal fibroids
- make an approximate assessment of how many other fibroids remain to be mapped.

415

If there are too many to measure, select a cut-off measurement – for example, 15.0 mm in diameter. Map any fibroids greater than 15.0 mm in diameter

- the remaining fibroids should not be individually mapped. Instead attempt to give an approximate estimate of the size and number of the remaining fibroids. For example, *'The remaining fibroids, of which there are more than 10, are all intramural, are located within the anterior and posterior myometrium and all measure less than 15.0 mm in diameter'.*

Due to the composition of a fibroid, the incident ultrasound beam may be reflected at its anterior border, reducing the amount of sound available to image the fibroid tissue posteriorly. In addition, the fibroid tissue attenuates the sound beam more strongly than normal myometrium. Thus in cases of multiple large fibroids it may not be possible to produce a satisfactory image through the whole depth of the uterus to its posterior wall, despite using the lowest frequency setting available within the gynaecology presets. This difficulty is likely to be further compounded if the woman is obese. On these occasions selecting a preset that is not normally used for gynaecological ultrasound examinations may prove a useful alternative. Most machines will have a 'penetration' abdominal preset. This preset includes ultrasound parameter combinations normally used for the abdominal ultrasound examination of an obese male. These may facilitate visualization of the large fibroid uterus.

The uterine cavity may be obscured by fibroids, making it very difficult or impossible to visualize it in its entirety. Thus it will not be possible to accurately assess whether the fibroids are submucosal or intramural and where they lie relative to the cavity. A comment should be made in the report to this effect. It is important that you still map as many fibroids as possible using the approach described earlier.

Clinical Management

Management options for symptomatic fibroids include resection, embolization, myomectomy or hysterectomy. Discussion of these techniques is beyond the scope of this text.

Hysteroscopic resection of fibroids would be considered in cases of type 0 and type 1 submucosal fibroids but not in type 2 submucosal fibroids, where myomectomy would be considered the appropriate choice.

Large subserosal fibroids are not successfully reduced in size if embolization of fibroids is being considered as an option.

Myomectomy and hysterectomy are surgical options for management of fibroids. The ultrasound examination and accurate mapping of fibroids are contributory factors in that clinical decision.

ADENOMYOSIS AND ADENOMYOMA

Adenomyosis is a relatively common condition that is considered to be a variant of endometriosis. It occurs as a result of ectopic endometrial glands which have migrated from the basal layer of the endometrium into the myometrium. Endometriosis is discussed in more detail towards the end of this chapter.

Adenomyosis affects women of reproductive age, typically who are in the latter part of their reproductive years and are multiparous. It is found to coexist with endometriosis in up to 20% of women. The classical presenting symptoms are dysmenorrhoea and menorrhagia.

On physical examination an adenomyotic uterus is often enlarged and examination usually elicits pain.

Historically, adenomyosis has been a difficult condition to diagnose with ultrasound, only being made with confidence at hysterectomy. The advent of high resolution transvaginal ultrasound imaging has improved the ability to identify the subtle ultrasound characteristics associated with adenomyosis.

Adenomyoma is a focal area of adenomyosis.

ULTRASOUND APPEARANCES

Adenomyosis

The uterus is often enlarged and is described as 'globular' – that is, rounded. One uterine wall may be disproportionately large compared with the other, with the posterior wall being more commonly affected (Fig. 18.9).

The endometrial/myometrial interface may be so ill defined that it is difficult to decide where to place the callipers to measure the endometrial thickness. The ultrasound appearance of the myometrium is also altered.

In adenomyosis, the myometrium is typically heterogeneous, with hypoechoic striations often seen coursing from the endometrium into the myometrium, producing a 'sunburst' effect. Small anechoic areas of 1.0–5.0 mm in size may be present within the myometrium. These represent myometrial cysts and contain the remnants of menstrual flow from the ectopic endometrium (Fig. 18.10).

Recent studies have suggested that assessing the thickness and appearance of the junctional zone with 3D ultrasound may prove to be effective in the diagnosis of adenomyosis.

Adenomyoma

An *adenomyoma* is often mistaken for a fibroid. It can be distinguished from a fibroid because it does not possess the pseudocapsule of the fibroid nor does it exhibit peripheral blood flow when colour Doppler is applied (Fig. 18.11).

Confusingly, fibroids are a coexisting pathological condition with adenomyosis.

It is likely that fibroids are overdiagnosed, and consequently adenomyosis underdiagnosed, because of the difficulty in their differentiation.

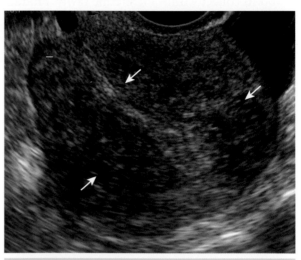

Fig 18.10 • A sagittal retroverted globular uterus. The myometrium is heterogeneous, multiple myometrial cysts (arrows) are present and the endometrial/myometrial interface is ill defined – appearances consistent with adenomyosis.

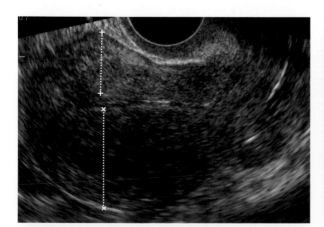

Fig 18.9 • Sagittal section of the uterus. The ultrasound findings are consistent with adenomyosis – the posterior uterine wall is disproportionately large (depth 33 mm) compared with the anterior uterine wall (depth 19 mm). The endometrial/myometrial interface is ill defined.

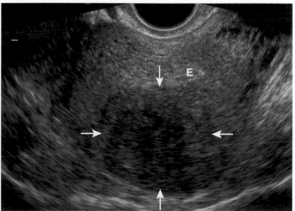

Fig 18.11 • Transverse section of the uterus. The endometrium (E) is ill defined. There is a localized area of adenomyosis in the posterior uterine wall (arrows) and subtle striations are seen – appearances are of an adenomyoma rather than a fibroid.

HAEMATOMETRA, HAEMATOCOLPOS AND HAEMATOSALPINX

Haematometra is the distension of the uterine cavity with blood. It can be caused by stenosis of the cervix or cervical surgery, these often being the causes of haematometra in the older woman (Fig. 18.12).

By contrast, an imperforate hymen can cause blood to collect within the uterine cavity, producing a haematometra. This presentation is typically seen in young girls with delayed menarche who have primary amenorrhoea and cyclical abdominal pain. Because of the young age at presentation, ultrasound examination in these cases is usually performed transabdominally.

Haematocolpos is the distension of the vagina with blood and may be an additional consequence of an imperforate hymen (Fig. 18.13).

Haematosalpinx is caused by the retrograde flow of blood into the Fallopian tubes, causing one or both of them to dilate, and is discussed in more detail later in this chapter.

ULTRASOUND APPEARANCES

The ultrasound appearances will depend on how much of the reproductive tract is distended with blood. The accumulated blood appears as a hypoechoic area within the vagina, uterine cavity or Fallopian tube and will be seen to contain low level echoes rather than being completely anechoic.

The uterus is typically hourglass in shape when a haematometra is present. The uterine cavity will appear distended with blood. It may be difficult to differentiate between the endometrium and myometrium, but every effort should be made to do so.

Only the vagina will be distended when a haematocolpos is present. The appearance of the accumulated blood will be as with a haematometra.

The haematometra is usually smaller than the haematocolpos.

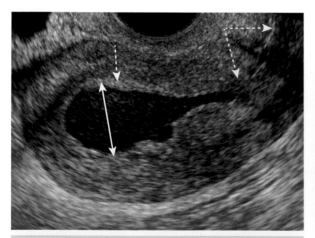

Fig 18.12 • A sagittal section of the uterus demonstrating a haematometra. The uterine cavity is distended with blood (arrows). The endometrium is thin (dashed arrow) and the cervix (yellow dashed lines) is closed.

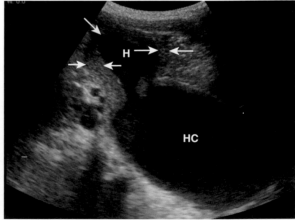

Fig 18.13 • Transabdominal scan. Sagittal view of the uterus and vagina. The haematometra (H) is smaller than the haematocolpos (HC). The posterior myometrium is more readily identified (left arrows) than the anterior myometrium (smaller right arrows). The uterine fundus is marked with the yellow arrow.

ENDOMETRIAL POLYP

The endometrial polyp arises from the basal layer of the endometrium and is usually vascularized by a single vessel that passes through its stalk. Unlike the endometrium from which it arises, the endometrial polyp tends to be unresponsive to steroid hormones. Its appearance therefore remains similar throughout the menstrual cycle.

Endometrial polyps are most commonly found in women who present with intermenstrual bleeding and in women with dysmenorrhoea or infertility. It is postulated that the polyp prevents implantation of the blastocyst into the endometrium. Polyps are a common finding in women between 35 and 50 years of age who present with abnormal vaginal bleeding and are identified in up to 10% of such cases. They may also be an incidental finding in asymptomatic women.

Endometrial polyps are often found as an isolated pathology. Alternatively, they may be present within areas of endometrial hyperplasia or in association with endometrial carcinoma. The incidence of endometrial carcinoma arising within a polyp is less than 1%.

ULTRASOUND APPEARANCES

Polyps tend to arise initially at the fundal aspect of the endometrium and therefore the first suggestion of their presence may be an area of focally thickened endometrium.

The typical ultrasound appearance of an endometrial polyp is of a distinct hyperechoic area within the endometrial cavity. This area may appear homogeneous or may have small cystic spaces throughout it (Fig. 18.14) and can vary in size from a few millimetres in mean diameter to a few centimetres. The polyp should be imaged in both the sagittal and transverse views and its longitudinal, anteroposterior and transverse diameters measured in planes orthogonal to one another, using the 'outer-to-outer' technique. The dimensions of the polyp should be included in the report.

As the endometrial polyp is an intracavity lesion, it separates the anterior and posterior endometrial layers. Where this separation is complete along the full length of the cavity, the intracavity line will not be visualized.

The endometrial thickness should be measured at its maximum diameter in the sagittal view (see Fig. 16.10). This measurement should be included in the report.

Colour or power Doppler applied to the endometrium may demonstrate vascularity of the single vessel within the stalk of the polyp. As the flow within the vessel is of low velocity, the colour Doppler controls need to be optimized to improve sensitivity. Before turning on the colour Doppler, obtain a high resolution image of the endometrium (see Chapter 16). Superimpose a small colour box, reduce the pulse repetition frequency and lastly increase the colour or power Doppler gain incrementally until flow is detected (Fig. 18.15).

Assessment of the endometrium for endometrial polyps is best performed between days 3 and 8 of the menstrual cycle, when the endometrium is at its thinnest. In addition, the hyperechoic polyp is optimally visualized in the proliferative phase of the menstrual cycle when it produces the greatest contrast relative to the hypoechoic functional layer of the endometrium.

It follows that it is difficult to diagnose an endometrial polyp in the secretory phase of the

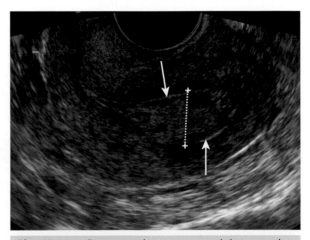

Fig 18.14 • Retroverted uterus containing a polyp within the cavity. The measurement of 10.4 mm includes the diameter of the polyp and the very thin layer of endometrium (arrows) on either side of it. Note the cystic areas within the polyp.

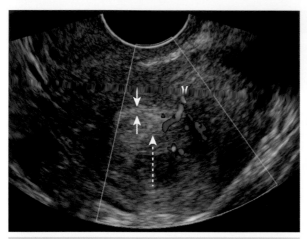

Fig 18.15 • Transverse view of the uterus showing the vascular stalk (V) of an endometrial polyp (dashed arrow), as detected with colour Doppler. The anterior layer of the endometrium is thin (arrows) and is slightly more hyperechoic than the polyp.

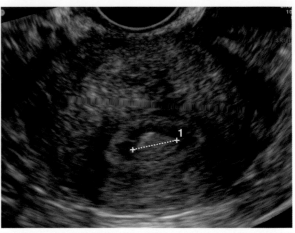

Fig 18.16 • Transverse view of the uterus showing a polyp within the uterine cavity. The polyp measures 10.4 mm in the transverse plane and is clearly delineated because of the presence of intracavity fluid. The echogenicity of the endometrium and the polyp are similar.

cycle, as the echogenicity of the polyp and the endometrium are similar. Fluid present within the cavity will aid in the delineation of the polyp from the endometrium (Fig. 18.16). Thus instillation of a small amount of fluid into the endometrial cavity under aseptic technique, a procedure known as saline instillation sonography, can aid in the identification of the polyp. Unfortunately, this technique is not usually readily accessible for practitioners performing gynaecological ultrasound examinations in the routine setting.

In practice, therefore, if an ultrasound scan is performed in the secretory phase of the cycle and an endometrial polyp is suspected but cannot be excluded, the examination should be repeated in the proliferative phase of a subsequent cycle. Ideally the follow up examination should take

place between 3 and 7 days after the first day of menstruation. In such a case your report should record that it was not possible to exclude an endometrial polyp, as the woman was in the secretory phase of her menstrual cycle.

The sensitivity of ultrasound in the detection of endometrial polyps is therefore dependent on the size and location of the polyp, the menstrual status, the phase of the menstrual cycle, the thickness of the endometrium and, of course, the sensitivity of the ultrasound machine and the experience of the operator. Thus not all endometrial polyps will be detected by ultrasound. However, an abnormally thickened endometrium should always be detectable, which, in a postmenopausal woman with vaginal bleeding, should warrant further investigation.

ENDOMETRIAL HYPERPLASIA

Endometrial hyperplasia is the excessive proliferation of glands and stroma within the endometrium because of the prolonged action of oestrogens that are unopposed by progesterone, and which results in abnormal thickening of the endometrium.

Endometrial hyperplasia is most commonly found in association with high circulating levels of oestrogen. Endometrial hyperplasia is therefore

most commonly found in women with polycystic ovarian syndrome as a result of anovulatory cycles, obesity or oestrogen-producing tumours such as a granulosa cell tumour of the ovary. Endometrial hyperplasia is also found in women who are perimenopausal and may be experiencing anovulatory cycles, women who are taking exogenous oestrogens as in hormone replacement therapy and women who are undergoing tamoxifen therapy (see Chapter 17).

The significance of endometrial hyperplasia lies not only in its symptomology but also because it may be a precursor of endometrial carcinoma.

ULTRASOUND APPEARANCES

The ultrasound appearance of endometrial hyperplasia is characteristic. The endometrium is hyperechoic with occasional small cystic, or hypoechoic, areas within it. Small hyperechoic areas representing endometrial polyps may also be present. The intracavity line is often not defined. The endometrium will be thickened. In the premenopausal woman the endometrium can attain thicknesses of 10.0–15.0 mm in the secretory phase during a normal menstrual cycle. In the postmenopausal woman an endometrial thickness greater than 5.0 mm, or 4.0 mm depending on the centre as discussed in Chapter 17, should raise the suspicion of endometrial hyperplasia. In the perimenopausal woman it is not always possible to differentiate between normal secretory endometrium and endometrial hyperplasia (Fig. 18.17).

The ultrasound features of endometrial hyperplasia are twofold, namely the heterogeneous appearance of the endometrium together with an increase in endometrial thickness to greater than 5.0 mm (or 4.0 mm).

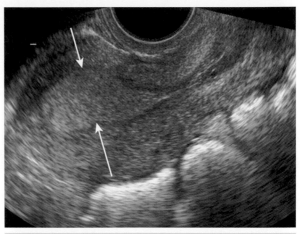

Fig 18.17 • Sagittal view of the uterus showing thickened endometrium (arrows) which measured 15.8 mm. Where the endometrium is homogeneous in appearance and the woman is perimenopausal, it may be incorrect to assume that this is a case of endometrial hyperplasia.

Endometrial hyperplasia is classified into four types: simple, complex, simple atypical and complex atypical. They are indistinguishable on ultrasound.

The final diagnosis of endometrial hyperplasia is only made histologically. Therefore in the presence of a history that is suggestive of endometrial carcinoma together with suspicious ultrasound findings, endometrial sampling is indicated. Complex atypical hyperplasia indicates a high risk of coexistent, or progression to, endometrial carcinoma.

ENDOMETRIAL CANCER OR CARCINOMA

Endometrial cancer is the most common gynaecological cancer in the developed world. It is rare in women who are younger than 45 years of age, with approximately 75% of cases occuring in women older than 55 years of age.

Risk factors include obesity and unopposed oestrogen stimulation of the endometrium. Postmenopausal women presenting with vaginal bleeding have an increased risk of endometrial cancer. The literature indicates that using an endometrial thickness cut off of less than 5.0 mm will exclude significant endometrial pathological conditions, and in particular endometrial cancer, in postmenopausal women. Postmenopausal women in whom the endometrial thickness measures 5.0 mm or more

will therefore require endometrial sampling. These facts underline the importance of being able to image the endometrium and measure it correctly.

ULTRASOUND APPEARANCES

The typical appearances of endometrial carcinoma are of hyperechoic and thickened endometrium – that is, equal to or greater than 5.0 mm.

A regular border between the endometrium and the myometrium suggests that tumour growth is confined to the endometrium. Invasive endometrial cancer may breach the endometrial/myometrial interface. The interface therefore may appear ill-defined. Increased vascularity as demonstrated with colour Doppler correlates with the more advanced stages of endometrial cancer which are typified by the process of angiogenesis.

In cases of endometrial cancer the endometrium is often heterogeneous (see Fig. 16.11). Conversely, in cases of endometrial hyperplasia, the endometrium is often homogeneous. Because there is considerable overlap in the ultrasound appearances of the endometrium in the two conditions, these appearances are not sufficiently reliable to allow accurate discrimination between them.

THE FALLOPIAN TUBE

The normal Fallopian tube is not visualized on ultrasound unless there is free fluid surrounding it (see Fig. 16.18) or it is distended by fluid, pus or blood, as described next.

HYDROSALPINX AND PYOSALPINX

Hydrosalpinx describes the distension of a Fallopian tube by serous fluid and is a sign of chronic tubal inflammatory disease. In the acute phase of tubal inflammatory disease the tube may dilate with pus rather than serous fluid. This is termed a *pyosalpinx*.

The diagnosis of the acute phase of pelvic inflammatory disease is normally made on clinical assessment and often without an ultrasound scan. A transvaginal scan would normally elicit pain, particularly when scanning on the ipsilateral side as the pyosalpinx.

Ultrasound Appearances

A hydrosalpinx usually appears as an anechoic and ovoidal or tubular structure, depending on whether it is imaged in longitudinal or cross-section. In the chronic phase of the tubal inflammatory disease the tubal walls and septae are thin. What appear to be incomplete septae are often seen within the tube. These represent the kinks in the distended tube as it folds over on itself (Fig. 18.18).

The endosalpingeal folds which form the internal wall of the Fallopian tube are flattened and fibrosed. If the tube is imaged in transverse section, the hyperechoic nodes are described as 'beads on a string'.

The distended Fallopian tube may be confused with an ovarian cyst owing to the incomplete septations within the tube, which mimic the loculations of a multilocular cyst. You should follow the tortuous course of the Fallopian tube, using rotational and sliding movements of the probe, in order to satisfy yourself that this is a tubular structure and not part of the ovary – which you must be able to identify as separate from the suspected hydrosalpinx.

The use of colour Doppler will ensure that you do not mistake a hydrosalpinx for a blood vessel.

A pyosalpinx contains pus rather than serous fluid and is an indicator of the acute phase of tubal inflammatory disease. In this condition the tubular structure will demonstrate the low level echoes that produce the course granular appearance typical of pus. The tubal walls are thickened and oedematous and the endosalpingeal folds produce a 'cogwheel' appearance when the tube is imaged in transverse section. This appearance is similar, but more dramatic, to that of hydrosalpinx described earlier.

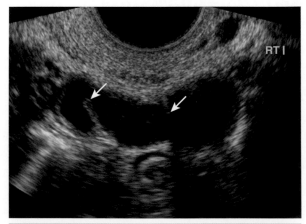

Fig 18.18 • Longitudinal section of a right hydrosalpinx. Note the typical appearances of the incomplete septae (arrows).

Haematosalpinx describes a Fallopian tube distended with blood and is found in cases of ectopic gestation rupture or in conjunction with haematometra.

The differences in the ultrasound appearances of blood and pus can be subtle and it is therefore difficult to differentiate between a pyosalpinx and a haematosalpinx. Both should be considered in the context of the presenting symptoms and other ultrasound findings.

TUBO-OVARIAN ABSCESS

Pelvic inflammatory disease is commonly caused by an infection, which ascends from the lower to the upper genital tract, potentially causing a hydrosalpinx or a pyosalpinx. If the infection breaches the ovary and the inflammatory process progresses to a more advanced and serious state, a tubo-ovarian abscess can form. Symptoms include abdominal pain with rebounding or guarding, fever, vaginal discharge or vaginal bleeding.

Ultrasound Appearances

A tubo-ovarian abscess typically appears as a multilocular, heterogeneous mass with thick and incomplete septations. It is often difficult to differentiate the ovary from the tube. The abscess presents as a mass of mixed echogenicity and is usually well vascularized. Tubo-ovarian abscess demonstrates a wide variety of ultrasound appearances and may therefore be a diagnosis of exclusion rather than certainty.

ABNORMAL APPEARANCES OF THE OVARY

FUNCTIONAL OR PHYSIOLOGICAL CYST

The majority of functional ovarian cysts are detected incidentally in asymptomatic women. They may result from an anovulatory cycle where the dominant follicle fails to collapse and ovulation therefore does not take place. Such cycles are seen most commonly at the extremes of reproductive life. A functional cyst can also result from a non dominant follicle that persists and does not regress.

Functional cysts are rarely symptomatic, although a large functional cyst can cause pelvic pain, and, infrequently, result in ovarian torsion.

Ultrasound examination of women with a history of irregular vaginal bleeding may reveal the presence of functional cysts.

Ultrasound Appearances

A functional cyst is similar in appearance to a follicle with thin, regular walls. It differs from a follicle in its size, being larger – that is, greater than 30.0 mm in mean diameter and occasionally reaching more than 100.0 mm in mean diameter (Fig. 18.19). The diameter of the cyst should be measured in three planes orthogonal to each other, using the 'inner to inner' technique, and the mean diameter calculated. A functional cyst is usually poorly vascularized. This aids in differentiating it from a luteal cyst, which has thicker and more irregular walls and typically is well vascularized circumferentially.

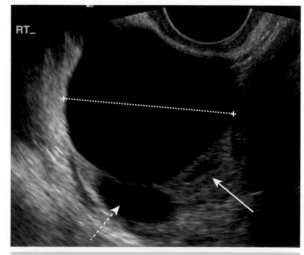

Fig 18.19 • A right ovarian functional cyst measuring 47.0 mm. A rim of normal ovarian tissue (arrow) together with a small follicle (dashed arrow) are also present in transverse diameter.

The ultrasound management of a functional cyst should be expectant, as the cyst will usually regress spontaneously. A repeat ultrasound examination after 6 weeks should be performed – that is, after the next menstruation and in a different part of the subsequent menstrual cycle – to confirm resolution.

HAEMORRHAGIC CYST

A haemorrhagic cyst result from bleeding or haemorrhage into a functional cyst or corpus luteum. The vessels within the wall of a newly vascularized corpus luteum are very fragile. If they rupture, a haemorrhagic corpus luteum ensues.

A haemorrhagic cyst can cause acute pain of sudden onset or otherwise can be an incidental finding.

Ultrasound Appearances

The sequence of events which take place within a haemorrhagic cyst are, first, acute haemorrhage, followed by clot formation and finally clot retraction. The ultrasound appearances of the cyst will therefore reflect this process.

In the acute stage of initial bleeding into the cyst, the cyst is typically more hyperechoic than the surrounding ovarian parenchyma. Over the course of the subsequent few days the haemorrhage becomes more hypoechoic as the constituent blood products break down. The internal architecture of a haemorrhagic cyst can give a fine reticular appearance or lacelike pattern (Fig. 18. 20). Gentle compression of the woman's abdomen will cause a 'jellylike wobble' of the fine strands.

As haemolysis occurs and clot formation takes place, the internal contents of the cyst may divide into two layers, with a sharp demarcation line present between the fluid above and the debris below. Eventually the blood clot retracts and separates from the anechoic serum. The blood clot can appear triangular or curvilinear. The internal contents of haemorrhagic cysts are avascular.

Resolution of the cyst occurs without any need for intervention and confirms the provisional diagnosis of a haemorrhagic cyst. A repeat scan performed after two or three menstrual cycles should confirm resolution.

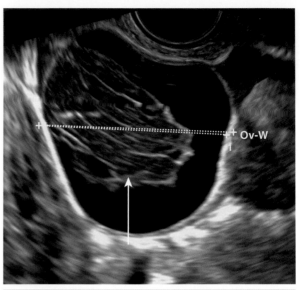

Fig 18.20 • A transverse section of a haemorrhagic cyst. The internal contents display a fine reticular appearance or lacelike pattern. Gentle compression of the woman's abdomen will cause a 'jellylike wobble' of the fine strands. There has been retraction of the clot (arrow). The transverse diameter of the ovary (Ov-W) together with the transverse diameter of the cyst (caliper 1) are shown.

POLYCYSTIC OVARIES

Polycystic Ovarian Syndrome (PCOS) was first described by Stein and Leventhal in 1905 and describes a triad of features, namely (1) clinical symptoms, (2) abnormal hormone profile and (3) a polycystic appearance of the ovaries on ultrasound.

Universal agreement on the definition of PCOS is problematic because of the broad spectrum of its clinical presentation. A group of international experts defined and agreed on the criteria for PCOS in 2003. The Rotterdam Consensus on Diagnostic Criteria for PCOS reflects this agreement.

The diagnosis of PCOS requires two of the following three criteria to be present:
- oligo- or anovulation
- clinical and/or biochemical signs of hyperandrogenism
- the ultrasound appearances of polycystic ovaries (PCO).

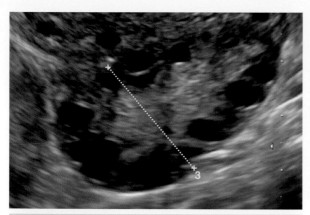

Fig 18.21 • Longitudinal section of a polycystic ovary with the AP diameter measured. There are more than 12 follicles, all of which measure 2.0–9.0 mm. The ovarian volume measures 14.0 mls. AP, antero-posterior.

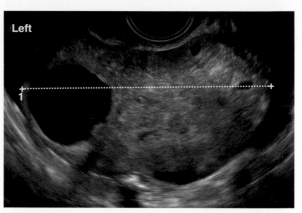

Fig 18.22 • Torsion of the left ovary. The ovary appears enlarged, with a transverse diameter of 53.6 mm (caliper 1), oedematous and 'featureless'. One follicle is seen at the periphery.

Ultrasound Appearances

The current ultrasound definition of PCO, based on the 2003 consensus, is an ovary that contains 12 or more follicles, each of which measures between 2.0 mm and 9.0 mm in mean diameter and/or has an increased ovarian volume, that is greater than 10.0 ml (Fig. 18.21).

The definition of PCO can still be applied where only one ovary fulfils the ultrasound criteria of PCO. Where there is a dominant follicle greater than 10.0 mm in mean diameter or a corpus luteum present, the ovarian volume will be falsely increased. The ultrasound examination should be repeated during the next cycle before making the diagnosis of PCO.

Previously, subjective assessment of the peripheral distribution of the follicles and an increase in the central stromal echogenicity were used as being indicative of PCO. This subjective assessment should no longer be used to define PCO.

OVARIAN TORSION

This is an acute event often diagnosed clinically without the need for an ultrasound examination. This is because surgery to detort the ovary should be performed as a matter of urgency to ensure that the ovary does not become necrotic.

Torsion of the ovary occurs when there is complete or partial rotation of the ovary on its ligamentous support. The arterial and venous supply to the ovary is compromised. The right ovary is affected more commonly than the left. The torsion may also include the ipsilateral Fallopian tube.

Ovarian torsion may occur if the ovary is previously enlarged because of the presence of an ovarian cyst such as a dermoid cyst.

Ultrasound Appearances

The torted ovary is increased in size and appears oedematous and generally 'hazy', with a loss of the normal architecture (Fig. 18.22). Follicles are displaced peripherally. Comparison of both size and appearance with the contralateral ovary is helpful in confirming the diagnosis of torsion. There is often accompanying free fluid in the pelvis.

A torted ovary will not demonstrate vascularity within its tissue whereas a normal ovary will. However, as the torsion can be intermittent, the presence of blood flow within the ovarian tissue may be falsely reassuring.

DERMOID CYST OR MATURE CYSTIC TERATOMA

A dermoid cyst contains tissue from two or three of the three germ cell layers, namely ectoderm, endoderm and mesoderm. The embryological cell lines differentiate into more mature tissue types within the cyst, producing, for example, clumps of long hair, pockets of sebum, blood, fat, bone, nails, teeth, eyes, cartilage and thyroid tissue. Dermoid cysts are most commonly found in women younger than 35 years of age.

Dermoid cysts are usually unilateral, being bilateral in only 10–15% of cases. Most are asymptomatic, but they are the most common tumour to cause torsion of the ovary. The majority are benign, with approximately 1–2% of dermoid cysts having a malignant component.

Ultrasound Appearances

As the contents of a dermoid cyst are very variable its ultrasound appearances are diverse. It is therefore not unexpected that a dermoid cyst is often misinterpreted as another ovarian pathological condition, with its ultrasound appearance being largely dependent on its content. Some features, however, are characteristic and include the following:

- the *Rokitansky nodule* or dermoid plug is a focal protuberance projecting from the wall of the cyst. It contains sebum and solid elements such as bone and teeth. Its ultrasound appearance will be dependent on the content of the nodule. Posterior acoustic shadowing, because of the bone and/or teeth, is a feature of a Rokitanksy nodule (Fig. 18.23)
- the *'dots and dashes'* sign is produced by the floating strands of hair within the cyst
- a *moderately hyperechoic appearance*, of mainly homogeneous echotexture, is caused by the sebum content of the mass. Strands of hair may also be present, which will produce 'dots and dashes' within the mass. Good transmission of sound is present, with no posterior acoustic shadowing. This is due to the sebum content (Fig. 18.24)
- the *'tip of the iceberg'* sign is produced by an area of acoustically highly reflective tissue, such as bone or teeth, situated anteriorly within the cyst. Acting in the same way as the calcified rim of a fibroid, the acoustic shadowing which this hyperechoic area produces may obscure most of the ultrasound features of the dermoid cyst posterior to it. The hyperechoic mass may

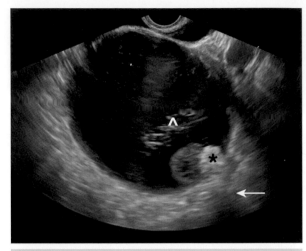

Fig 18.23 • Transverse section of a cyst. The cyst is unilocular, containing a Rokitansky nodule (*) with acoustic shadowing (arrowed). The 'dots and dashes' sign due to the presence of hair strands, can also be seen (^).

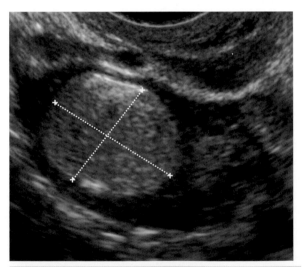

Fig 18.24 • A sagital section of the right ovary in which a dermoid cyst is present. The cyst measures 19 × 15 mm and appears solid and hyperechoic. However, the absence of acoustic shadowing posteriorly indicates that the cyst contains only sebum.

be mistaken for bowel and the dermoid cyst may be therefore missed. This mistake can be avoided if the mass is observed for signs of peristaltic movements typified by bowel but which are absent in a dermoid cyst.

ENDOMETRIOMA

Endometriosis arises as a result of the ectopic migration of endometrial tissue from the uterus. Symptoms of endometriosis can include any of the following: dysmenorrhoea, dyspareunia, dysuria, dyschezia (painful defecation), chronic pelvic pain and infertility. The extent of the disease assessed by staging poorly correlates with the severity of a woman's symptoms. Endometrial tissue can be located within the ovary or on any peritoneal surface within the pelvis.

An *endometrioma* is endometriotic tissue within a cyst positioned centrally within the ovary and will therefore be surrounded by normal ovarian tissue. An endometrioma is usually readily identified on ultrasound; however, endometriotic tissue separate from the ovary and in other locations is not. The mapping of endometriotic tissue is beyond the scope of this text.

Ultrasound Appearances

An endometrioma (plural, endometriomata) is usually easily recognizable by its characteristic ultrasound appearance. It is typically unilocular with regular internal walls and has a homogeneous internal echotexture resulting from the thick, old blood of which the cyst is composed. When examined histologically, this blood is dark in colour and explains why endometriotic cysts are commonly called chocolate cysts.

The blood within the cyst produces a characteristic ultrasound appearance of a moderately hyperechoic fluid, likened to ground glass (Fig. 18.25). Punctuate calcific foci may be present towards the periphery of an endometrioma.

There is no blood flow detectable from the internal contents of an endometrioma.

Endometriomata may be single or multiple and are often bilateral.

Endometriosis causes adhesions which may affect the relative positions of the uterus and ovaries. Both ovaries may be identified in the Pouch of Douglas and may adhere to each other, producing the distinctive 'kissing ovaries' sign. Alternatively, the ovary may be stuck to the uterus or pelvic sidewall as a result of the adherent endometriotic deposits.

Slight pressure towards the ovary with the ultrasound probe, which results in a negative sliding

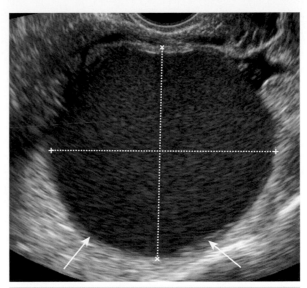

Fig 18.25 • A transverse section of the right ovary in which an endometrioma is present. The cyst measures 47 × 52 mm. Note the 'ground glass' appearance of its contents. There is a surrounding thin rim of normal ovarian tissue (arrows).

sign, is indicative of reduced mobility of the ovary or a fixed uterus. This can be used to aid in the assessment of the extent and the severity of the disease, particularly if surgery is considered.

Further reading

Jain K A 2002 Sonographic spectrum of haemorrhagic ovarian cysts. JUM 21:879–886

Luries S, Piper I, Woliovitch I, Glezerman M 2005 Age related prevalence of sonographically confirmed myomas. J Obstet Gynecol 25:42–44

Maizlin Z, Vos P, Cooperberg P 2007 Is it a fibroid? Are you sure? Sonography with MRI assistance. Ultrasound Quarterly 23(1):55–62

Munro M, Critchley H, Broder M, Fraser I 2011 The FIGO classification system (PALM-COEIN) for causes of abnormal uterine bleeding in non gravid women of reproductive age. International Journal of Gynaecology & Obstetrics 113:3–13

Rotterdam ESHRE/ASRM-Sponsored PCOS Consensus Workshop Group 2004 Revised 2003 consensus on diagnostic criteria and long-term health risks related to polycystic ovary syndrome. Fertil Steril 81:19–25

Salim S, Won H, Nesbitt-Hawes E, Campbell N, Abbot J 2011 Diagnosis and management of endometrial polyps: A critical review of the literature. Journal of Minimally Invasive Gynaecology 18(5):569–581

Timor-Tritsch I, Lerner J, Montteagudo A, Murphy K, Heller D 1998 Transvaginal sonographic markers of tubal inflammatory disease. Ultrasound Obstet Gynecol 12:56–66

Characterization of adnexal cysts, differential diagnoses of the pelvis and report writing

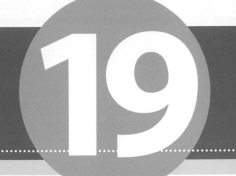

CONTENTS

There is considerable overlap between the ultrasound findings of the various benign and possibly malignant pathological conditions you will encounter while performing routine gynaecological ultrasound examinations. This chapter addresses the assessment of adnexal masses which you may not recognize as being typical of a specific pathological condition and, consequently, are unsure how to describe their ultrasound appearances and report your findings.

The aims of this chapter are to enable you to do the following:
- describe the ultrasound features of an adnexal mass using a standardized approach
- assess those features in order to characterize the mass
- construct a clinically useful report.

THE ADNEXAE

The adnexae describes the area of the true pelvis surrounding the uterus and that is posterior to the broad ligaments. The adnexae can be divided into the left adnexa and the right adnexa. From an ultrasound viewpoint, the adnexal structures that are of relevance are the ovaries, the Fallopian tubes, their supporting ligaments and the peritoneum.

DEFINING AN ADNEXAL CYST

A cyst can originate from within an ovary, the area around the ovary or the paraovarian area, the Fallopian tube or the peritoneum and all would be correctly described as adnexal cysts.

The term *cyst* is used interchangeably with mass, tumour or lesion. For the purposes of this chapter, and for the ease of learning for the beginner, we have used *cyst* in the ultrasound context to describe the ultrasound appearances of a primarily fluid-filled lesion and *mass* in the ultrasound context to describe the ultrasound appearances of a more solid lesion. You must remember that these descriptors should not necessarily be applied when classifying and characterizing adnexal masses according to accepted consensus criteria before writing your report.

THE PURPOSE OF YOUR ULTRASOUND EXAMINATION

Your first task is to recognize that a pelvic mass is present and then decide, if possible, whether it is uterine or adnexal in origin.

There are many different types of adnexal cyst, which vary in their location, characteristic appearances and malignancy potential. This text does not attempt to provide you with an exhaustive list of adnexal cysts, but rather to help you in differentiating as far as possible between the more common and/or significant pelvic masses. These therefore include both masses that are uterine in origin and adnexal cysts – as listed in Table 19.1 and described

TYPE OF ADNEXAL CYST	LOCATION	ULTRASOUND CHARACTERISTIC(S)
Dermoid cyst	Ovary	Varied appearance depending on content (see Chapter 18)
Endometrioma	Ovary, peritoneum	Unilocular with regular internal walls, homogeneous low level echoes, 'ground glass' appearance
Fibroma	Ovary	Unilocular, homogeneous low level echoes, 'stripey' reverberation Mild/moderate circumferential vascularity Large
Functional cyst	Ovary	Unilocular, thin, regular walls Large, poorly vascularized
Granulosa cell tumour	Ovary	Solid or multilocular, solid cyst Heterogeneous echopattern, similar to necrosis Moderate to high internal vascularity
Haemorrhagic cyst	Ovary	Unilocular, varying appearance dependent on time interval since internal bleed occurred
Hydrosalpinx	Fallopian tube	Tubular, anechoic, incomplete septae
Ovarian carcinoma	Ovary	Varied – solid or multilocular solid, irregular border, highly vascular
Mucinous cystadenoma	Ovary	Multiloculated; locules may have differing echogenicity
Paraovarian cyst	Adjacent to one ovary	Unilocular, anechoic
Pedunculated fibroid	Extrauterine, broad ligament	Unilocular, rounded, homogeneous, moderately hyperechoic Circumferential blood flow
Peritoneal pseudocyst	Variable within peritoneal cavity	Adopts shape of potential space Unilocular or multilocular
Pyosalpinx	Fallopian tube	Tubular, low-level echoes Incomplete septae
Serous cystadenoma	Ovary	Multilocular, anechoic locules and/or papillary projections
Tubo-ovarian abscess	Fallopian tube/ Fallopian tube and ovary	Multilocular, heterogeneous, thick and incomplete septations, usually well vascularized

Table 19.1 Types of adnexal cyst categorized by their location in the pelvis and their typical ultrasound appearances

in this chapter. Uterine, Fallopian and ovarian pathological conditions are also discussed in Chapter 18.

Cysts can be unilateral, bilateral, single or multiple. They may have the same pathology or different pathologies. Each cyst should be measured, described and characterized individually. Having identified one or more adnexal cysts, you should first attempt to determine their origins, then measure, classify and characterize them as discussed next.

HOW TO ESTABLISH THE ORIGIN OF AN ADNEXAL CYST

The adnexal cyst can be ovarian, paraovarian, tubal or peritoneal in origin. It can arise from either the left or the right of a pair of structures. The origin of some adnexal cysts will be very easy to determine, whereas others may be more challenging.

We suggest the following series of steps.

Are you able to identify both right and left ovaries, are they both normal in appearance and are they both clearly separate from the adnexal cyst? If the answer is yes to all three questions, consider the pathologies of paraovarian cyst, hydrosalpinx or pedunculated fibroid.

Paraovarian Cyst

A paraovarian cyst is an anechoic unilocular cyst adjacent to one ovary (Fig. 19.1). The sliding sign should be positive, as the paraovarian cyst is seen to move separately to the ipsilateral ovary when gentle pressure is applied with the transvaginal probe.

Hydrosalpinx

Hydrosalpinx is typically tubular when viewed in longitudinal section and circular in cross-section. The dilated tube folding on itself produces the appearance of incomplete septae. A positive sliding sign will confirm that the structure you are examining is separate to the ovary. However, in the case of pelvic inflammatory disease caused by the presence of adhesions, the hydrosalpinx may be adherent to the ovary (Fig. 19.2). If this is the case, there may be a negative sliding sign. It is possible to mistake the adherent hydrosalpinx for a multiloculated

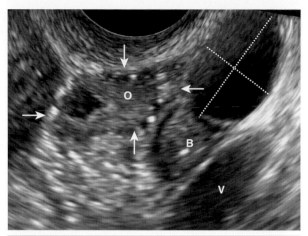

Fig 19.1 • A paraovarian cyst (marked with calipers) is seen separate from the left ovary (O) in a postmenopausal woman. The ovarian margins are identified (arrows) together with a loop of bowel (B) and the left iliac vein (V).

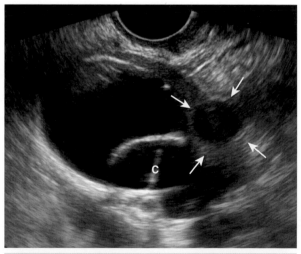

Fig 19.2 • Hydrosalpinx adherent to the left ovary. On this image the appearances could be mistaken for a multilocular ovarian cyst with an apparent complete septation (C). Careful scanning demonstrates that it is an incomplete septation. The ovary is arrowed.

ovarian cyst. A tortuous hydrosalpinx can lie in the midline in the Pouch of Douglas between the ovaries, so it is sometimes not possible to determine whether it is a right or left hydrosalpinx. In these cases you should describe the hydrosalpinx in the report and add that it is not certain whether it is arising from the right or left Fallopian tube.

431

Pedunculated Fibroid

Does the adnexal cyst look like a fibroid? If the answer is yes, it may well be because it is. Provided both ovaries are seen separately, then a mass, which may appear extrauterine, could be a pedunculated fibroid or a fibroid within the broad ligament. Colour Doppler can help identify the vascular supply and also demonstrate the typical circumferential flow around the fibroid.

Are you only able to identify the contralateral ovary as separate from the adnexal cyst? If the answer is yes, this suggests that the adnexal cyst arises from the ipsilateral ovary. If the cyst has a surrounding rim of ovarian tissue or exhibits the ovarian crescent sign, this is conclusive that the cyst is ovarian in origin. Adnexal cysts which are ovarian in origin include pathologies of fibroma, granulosa cell tumour and tubo-ovarian abscess.

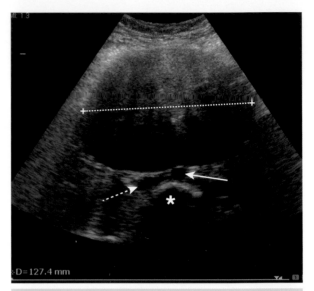

Fig 19.3 • A transabdominal scan of a large fibroma, with a transverse diameter of 127 mm. Note the moderately hyperechoic echotexture of the mass with 'stripey' acoustic shadowing. The woman's spine (*) is visualized posterior to the fibroma; the aorta (arrow) and inferior vena cava (dashed arrow) are seen in transverse section between the fibroma and the spine.

Fibroma

Does the mass look like a fibroid and the ipsilateral ovary is not identified? In this case a possible differential diagnosis is of a fibroma. Fibromas of the ovary are formed from the ovarian stromal tissue and are benign tumours. They can exhibit a variety of appearances, most commonly being round, oval or lobulated solid masses, of primarily homogeneous and moderately hyperechoic internal echotexture with acoustic shadowing best described as 'stripey' (Fig. 19.3). Fibromas typically demonstrate mild to moderate circumferential vascularity. They are often large, measuring up to 10.0–15.0 cm in diameter. They are usually an incidental finding, as they are seldom symptomatic.

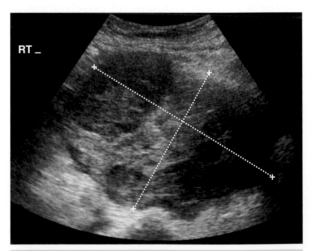

Fig 19.4 • A transabdominal scan of a right sided granulosa cell tumour, an example of a solid mass. The mass measures 146 × 94 mm.

Granulosa Cell Tumour

There may be no discernible ovarian tissue surrounding the mass, making it difficult to be certain that the mass is ovarian. The ultrasound appearance is typically of a mixed, moderately hyperechoic echopattern (Fig. 19.4).

In the absence of the ipsilateral ovary, it is not unreasonable to report the findings as 'probably arising from the right [or left] ovary, as a normal right [or left] ovary was not identified separately'.

Tubo-Ovarian Abscess

Normal ovarian tissue is often difficult to identify in cases of tubo-ovarian mass, as described in Chapter 18. Women with a tubo-ovarian abscess will be pyrexial and tender on clinical examination and also on scanning. The clinical presentation will normally indicate a high suspicion of tubo-ovarian abscess.

You should consider that if an adnexal cyst or mass is large it may be obscuring the ipsilateral ovary, making it difficult to visualize the ovary separately. In the postmenopausal woman the ipsilateral ovary is likely to be small, compounding the difficulties in determining whether or not the mass is separate from the ovary.

Does the cyst have clearly demarcated walls?

The cysts described earlier can be identified as discrete masses with boundaries that can be reasonably easily defined. If the answer to this question is no, you should consider the a peritoneal pseudocyst as a differential diagnosis.

Peritoneal Pseudocyst

A *peritoneal pseudocyst* is often mistaken for a multilocular ovarian cyst or a hydrosalpinx. This type of cyst occurs as a result of the formation of adhesions caused by pelvic surgery, endometriosis or pelvic inflammatory disease. Fluid is entrapped between the ovary, or ovaries, and the adhesions in the pelvic cavity, producing what is called a pseudocyst (Fig. 19.5A). The contour of the pseudocyst follows the outline of the pelvic organs and adhesions, with the trapped fluid effectively moulding itself to the pelvic wall (Fig. 19.5B). Peritoneal pseudocysts are almost always multilocular, with a chaotic internal arrangement. The locules are either anechoic or contain low-level echoes. The septae are thin and can often be seen to oscillate if pushed by the transvaginal probe, producing the 'flapping sails' sign. A normal ovary is usually seen separate from the pseudocyst but may be seen entrapped within the fluid collection of the pseudocyst.

MEASUREMENT OF AN ADNEXAL CYST

If the cyst is ovarian in origin, there will often be definable ovarian tissue surrounding the cyst. The ovarian size and volume should be calculated as described in Chapter 16.

Not all adnexal cysts are spherical, the peritoneal pseudocyst and the essentially tubular hydrosalpinx described earlier being good examples. The peritoneal pseudocyst, as discussed earlier, adapts a variable shape as fluid occupies the potential space

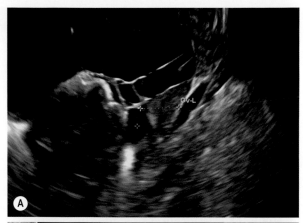

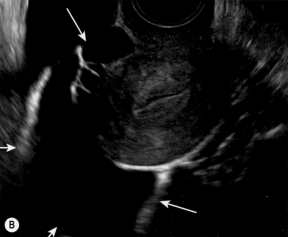

Fig 19.5 • A. A transverse section of the left ovary with its margins delineated (Ov-L). The ovary is surrounded by multiple locules of fluid trapped between the adhesions and the pelvic side wall indicating a pseudocyst. B. A peritoneal pseudocyst. The cyst moulds itself around the uterus (arrows). The appearances could be mistaken for ascites.

within the peritoneal cavity. Measurement of the dilated Fallopian tube can be further complicated if it is tortuous, as it often will be.

Measurement of such irregular adnexal cysts has to be made on the basis of the best estimate. Measurements from the three orthogonal planes should be taken from sagittal and transverse sections that demonstrate the maximum diameters of the cyst. Although this method is likely to lack the accuracy of measuring the size of a spherical cyst, it is important to document the measurements so that the clinician has an indication of the size of the cyst and, if serial examinations are requested, it will be possible to assess whether the cyst has increased, decreased or remains unchanged in size.

IOTA CLASSIFICATION

A wide spectrum of definitions and terminologies has been utilized to describe the ultrasound features of an adnexal cyst, with an overall lack of standardization in their description.

The International Ovarian Tumour Analysis (IOTA) group has proposed terms, definitions and measurements to describe the sonographic features of adnexal cysts in a structured and consistent way. We suggest adopting this terminology as described.

The IOTA classification uses four broad criteria, which are type, internal content, contour and vascularity.

TYPE

The cyst is classified according to one of five types according to the degree of solid material present and the number of locules present within the cyst. The five types are as follows:

- unilocular
- unilocular solid
- multilocular
- multilocular solid
- solid.

Solid material includes papillary projections, septae and loculations and is hyperechoic.

Cystic material is anechoic or hypoechoic and includes serous fluid, blood, mucin and pus.

A *papillary projection* is solid material which projects into the cyst from its internal wall. It is measured in two perpendicular planes, namely its height and base. The height of the projection must be 3.0 mm or more for it to be classified as a papillary projection.

A *septa* is a thin strand of tissue which crosses a cyst from one internal wall to another. A complete septa is one that can be seen to meet both internal walls in all scanning planes, whereas an incomplete septa does not.

A *locule* is defined as a cavity or compartment within a structure which, in the context of adnexal cysts, is separated by complete or incomplete septae.

Unilocular Cyst

A *unilocular cyst* is composed of one locule, without a complete septation, although an incomplete septation can be present. There should be no solid elements or papillary projections present within the cyst (Fig. 19.6).

The *pyosalpinx* is an example of a unilocular cyst. Thickening of the wall and septae are not classed as solid tissue. The internal content is cystic, comprising low-level echoes, which is consistent with the ultrasound appearances of pus. The septae within the pyosalpinx are incomplete in this plane (Fig. 19.7).

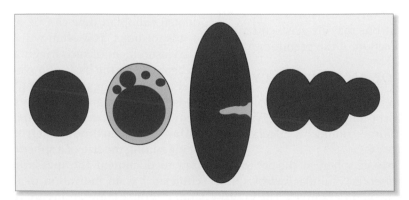

Fig 19.6 • The IOTA classification of unilocular cysts, from left to right: a single cyst, five cysts, a cyst with an incomplete septa, an irregularly shaped single cyst.

Unilocular Solid Cyst

A unilocular solid cyst is composed of one locule, within which there are solid elements which are large enough to be measured, and/or one or more papillary projections, the height of which is 3.0 mm or greater (Fig. 19.8).

The *borderline ovarian tumour* in Fig. 19.9 is an example of a unilocular solid cyst. The cyst is composed of one locule, with no septations present. Although the cyst is predominantly anechoic, papillary projections are present. In this example the smaller papillary projections have a smooth contour, whereas the larger papillary projection has an irregular contour. This is described as 'cauliflower-like'.

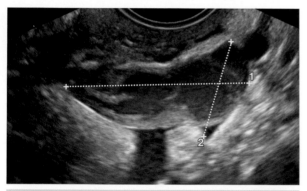

Fig 19.7 • A pyosalpinx (callipers 1 and 2) is an example of a unilocular cyst. The septations are incomplete. The internal echoes are low level, consistent with pus.

Multilocular Cyst

A multilocular cyst has at least one complete septation, therefore creating at least two locules. There should be no solid elements or papillary projections within the cyst (Fig. 19.10).

The *mucinous cystadenoma* in Fig. 19.11 is an example of a multilocular cyst. Multiple locules are present with no evidence of solid tissue within them. The cyst contains a mucin like substance which produces anechoic or low level echoes within differing locules. The locules therefore often demonstrate differing degrees of echogenicity. The low-level echoes can be subtle; thus their appreciation will depend on the sensitivity of the equipment. For this reason such mucin containing cysts may appear anechoic on transabdominal imaging, emphasizing the need to examine these cysts with the superior resolution of the transvaginal probe.

Multilocular Solid Cyst

A multilocular solid cyst is a cyst which has at least one complete septation, together with measurable solid elements and/or a papillary projection(s) which measures 3.0 mm or greater in height (Fig. 19.12).

The *serous cystadenoma* is an example of a multilocular cyst within which multiple anechoic locules and a papillary projection can be seen (Fig. 19.13).

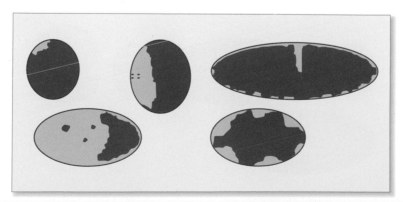

Fig 19.8 • The IOTA classification of unilocular solid cysts. The darker brown areas represent the cystic components and the lighter areas the solid components of the cyst.

Solid Cyst

A solid cyst is a cyst in which solid material occupies at least 80% of the cyst when assessed in two dimensions (Fig. 19.14).

The *granulosa cell tumour* is an example of a solid cyst in which the majority of the tissue is solid, with no evidence of cystic tissue (Fig. 19.4).

The ultrasound appearances of granulosa cell tumours are described as a solid cyst with a heterogeneous echopattern, similar to necrosis. Granulosa cell tumours can also be multilocular solid with a large number of small locules. They are moderately to highly vascular when assessed with colour Doppler.

The granulosa cell tumour is a sex cord stromal tumour with a low malignant potential. The majority of such tumours occur in postmenopausal women. As it is a hormone producing tumour, women can exhibit signs of hyperestrogenism in the form of abnormal vaginal bleeding patterns.

INTERNAL CONTENT

The internal contents of the cyst are next assessed. The dominant feature of cystic, as opposed to the solid, contents is described according to its ultrasound appearances. In solid cysts, any apparently cystic content should be described. The cystic content appearances together with examples are detailed in Table 19.2.

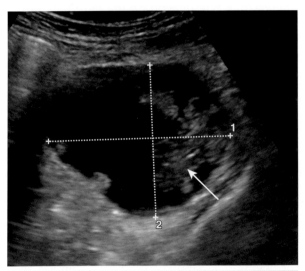

Fig 19.9 • A borderline ovarian tumour with papillary projections is an example of a unilocular solid cyst. The cyst measures 78 × 63 mm. The irregular contour of the larger papillary projection (arrow) is described as 'cauliflower-like'.

IOTA CYSTIC CONTENT	EXAMPLE
Anechoic (black)	Functional cyst
Low-level echoes	Pyosalpinx
Ground glass	Endometrioma
Haemorrhagic – reticular/lacy pattern	Haemorrhagic cyst
Mixed	Dermoid cyst

Table 19.2 Descriptors of the ultrasound appearances of the internal cystic contents of the adnexal cyst as recommended by IOTA, with an example of each
IOTA, the International Ovarian Tumour Analysis group.

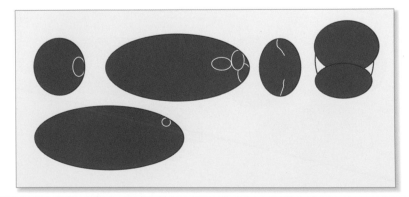

Fig 19.10 • The IOTA classification of multilocular cysts. The white lines indicate locules and the dark brown areas show that the cysts are entirely cystic, with no solid components.

CONTOUR

The contour of the internal or external wall of the cyst is next assessed. It is described as smooth or irregular (Fig. 19.15).

A papillary projection will distort the internal wall and, in such cases, the internal contour is therefore described as irregular. Where the cyst is solid, the internal wall is not discernible. In such cases the external wall contour is assessed and described as being either smooth or irregular.

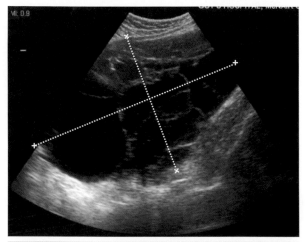

Fig 19.11 • Transabdominal scan of a mucinous cystadenoma, an example of a multilocular cyst. Note the locules containing low-level echoes in the near field. The cyst measures 221 × 144 × 158 mm.

VASCULARITY

The vascularity of the cyst is then assessed using colour Doppler to interrogate the wall of the cyst, the septae and any solid components with the cyst. The rationale for this assessment is that neoangiogenesis occurs in malignant tumours but not in benign tumours.

The early literature used spectral Doppler and reported low impedance blood flow in malignant tumours, with a resistance index (RI) of less than 0.4 being suggestive of malignancy. Later studies indicated that the RI was an insensitive discriminator between malignant and benign tumours, as there is considerable overlap in their RI values.

The current recommendation is that a subjective and qualitative rather than a quantitative assessment of the vascularity within the septa and cyst wall and in any solid component is made using colour Doppler. The gain and pulse repetition frequency need to be set in order to detect low flow rates. The subjective assessment of blood flow is made and a score from 1 to 4 assigned on that basis, as shown in Table 19.3.

FREE FLUID

Your examination should always include as assessment of the pelvis for the presence, or absence, of free fluid. Where frec fluid is present, you should attempt to assess the nature of the free fluid as both these factors are of clinical significance.

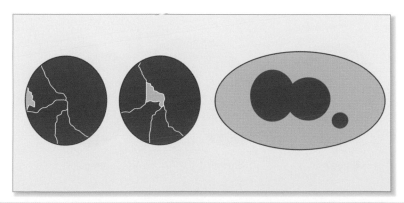

Fig 19.12 • The IOTA classification of multilocular solid cysts. The lighter areas represent solid components or septae within the cyst. The darker brown areas represent cystic components within the cyst.

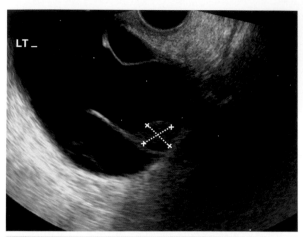

IOTA VASCULARITY SCORE	BLOOD FLOW
1	None
2	Minimal flow
3	Moderate flow
4	Highly vascular

Table 19.3 The IOTA score assigned to the vascularity of an adnexal cyst, based on the subjective assessment of the blood flow within its wall, septae and any solid components, using colour Doppler

IOTA, the International Ovarian Tumour Analysis group.

Fig 19.13 • Left sided serous cystadenoma, an example of a multilocular solid cyst. There are several locules; a papillary projection measures 14 × 14 mm.

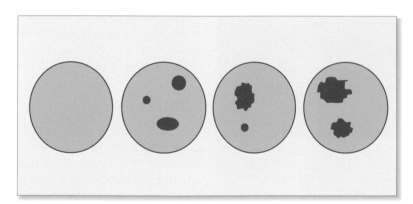

Fig 19.14 • The IOTA classification of solid cysts. The darker brown areas represent cystic components within the cyst.

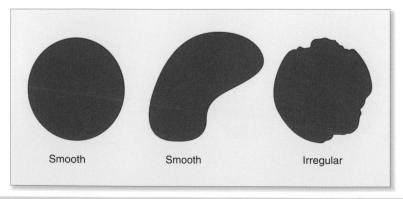

Smooth   Smooth   Irregular

Fig 19.15 • The IOTA classification of the contour of cysts. Note that the dark brown colour in this figure does not relate to the type or contents of the cysts.

For example, anechoic fluid localized within the Pouch of Douglas is most likely to be physiological and therefore of no clinical significance. A greater amount of free fluid which extends to the uterine fundus is very likely to be clinically significant and may represent ascites, which, in the presence of an adnexal cyst, is suspicious of malignancy.

CHARACTERIZATION FOR MALIGNANCY RISK

Characterization of an adnexal cyst includes an assessment of the likelihood of its being benign, malignant or borderline. The characterization of an adnexal cyst is important with regard to the management of a woman.

If the cyst is thought most likely to be benign, then it may be monitored expectantly, particularly if the woman is asymptomatic. This reduces morbidity and anxiety for the woman and the cost of her care. If the decision is to perform surgery to remove a benign adnexal cyst, this can be performed by a general gynaecologist. A borderline tumour of the ovary grows slowly and is usually diagnosed at an early stage when the abnormal cells are still encapsulated within the ovary. It has a low malignancy potential. In cases of advanced endometriosis with infiltration and adhesion, surgery is usually performed by a gynaecologist with a special interest in endometriosis often operating with a colorectal surgeon. Cysts that are suspicious of being malignant require referral to the gynaecology-oncology multidisciplinary team. This management pathway is known to optimize the woman's care and survival. Surgery performed by the gynaecology-oncology team can be conservative or radical according to the clinical indication for the individual woman. All cysts surgically removed undergo histopathological examination. It is the histopathological analysis which gives the final diagnosis.

The training and experience of any operator will affect their ability to identify abnormal findings confidently, construct a report and suggest the differential diagnoses. Given the wide range of features that can be encountered with some pathological conditions, it is unlikely that you will be able to identify the specific pathological condition on many occasions. Furthermore, even in the hands of experts other modality imaging is often required to make a provisional diagnosis. Unless you are working in a specialized gynaecological referral unit, it is likely that the majority of gynaecological scans you perform will either be normal or will identify benign ovarian tumours, as most adnexal cysts are not malignant. It is important, however, that you are aware of the various methods employed to assess the malignancy risk if only to reassure you that the adnexal cyst you have identified has a very low risk of malignancy.

ASSESSING THE MALIGNANCY RISK

Three methods of assessing malignancy are described next.

Ovarian Crescent Sign

Ovarian crescent sign describes the presence of normal ovarian tissue which lies adjacent to the adnexal cyst and which is contained within the ovarian capsule. The ovarian tissue adopts the shape of a crescent; hence the name. A negative sliding sign is present if gentle pressure of the transvaginal probe is applied – that is, no separation of the adnexal cyst from the ovarian tissue is demonstrated.

Observation of the ovarian crescent sign provides reassurance that the adnexal cyst arises from within the ovary. The ovarian crescent sign has been demonstrated to be a useful indicator that the adnexal cyst is likely to be benign.

Diagnostic Algorithms

Various diagnostic algorithms incorporating ultrasound features have been used to assess the likelihood of malignancy. The adnexal cyst is assessed for evidence of certain ultrasound features. The algorithm is then applied to determine the risk of malignancy. The risk of malignancy index (RMI) and the simple rules algorithm are described next.

Risk of Malignancy Index

The RMI is not part of the IOTA classification but has been included here as an adjunct in the discussion of malignancy risk. The RMI analysis combines the presence or absence of certain ultrasound features (U), menstrual status (M) and the ovarian tumour marker CA125 (CA).

The ultrasound features of the adnexal cyst that are scored as present or absent are as follows:

- the cyst is multilocular
- the cyst contains solid areas
- there is evidence of metastatic spread
- ascites is present
- the adnexal cysts are bilateral.

Metastatic spread describes the presence of malignant cells from a cancer in sites distant from the primary location. Metastatic spread from an ovarian cancer occurs along the greater omentum, the fatty peritoneal sheet which extends from the stomach onto the lower abdomen. Any evidence of solid tissue or discrete nodules between the peritoneum and bowel is indicative of metastatic omentum.

Examination of the omentum is usually performed transabdominally rather than transvaginally. Bowel gas and adiposity may affect visualization of these subtle findings. Unless you are working in a unit where you scan many women with metastatic spread from ovarian cancer, it is unlikely that you will gain sufficient experience to identify or exclude metastatic spread confidently.

Ultrasound score (U) as for Menstrual status (M)

The ultrasound score (U) is calculated as follows:

- none of the five ultrasound features present = 0
- one of the five ultrasound features present = 1
- between two and all of the five ultrasound features present = 2.

Menstrual status (M)

The menstrual status (M) score is calculated as follows:

- premenopausal status = 1
- postmenopausal status = 3.

Ovarian tumour marker (CA)

Cancer antigen 125 is known as CA125. It is a glycoprotein that may be elevated in women with epithelial ovarian cancer, woman with endometriosis and women with fibroids. The level of CA125 may also rise during pregnancy. It is measured in units per millilitre and the numerical value is used to provide the CA score.

The risk is calculated using the following formula:

RMI SCORE	RISK OF MALIGNANCY
<25	Low risk
25–250	Medium risk
>250	High risk

Table 19.4 Risk of malignancy of an adnexal cyst, categorized according to the risk of malignancy index score

RMI, risk of malignancy index; >, more than; <, less than.

$$RMI = U \times M \times CA125$$

According to the RMI score, a risk of malignancy is categorized as shown in Table 19.4.

The Simple Rules Algorithm

The *simple rules algorithm* describes the subjective assessment of an adnexal cyst using simple ultrasound rules to predict whether an adnexal cyst is likely to be benign or malignant.

There are five ultrasound features of the adnexal cyst which relate to the IOTA classification and which suggest the adnexal cyst is *benign*. They are as follows:

- unilocular
- presence of solid components, the largest of which measures less than 7.0 mm across its largest diameter
- presence of acoustic shadowing
- multilocular with a smooth contour and the largest diameter less than 100.0 mm
- a vascularity colour score of 1, denoting no blood flow.

There are five ultrasound features of the adnexal cyst which relate to the IOTA classification and which suggest the adnexal cyst is *malignant*. They are as follows:

- multilocular solid cyst with an irregular contour and with a largest diameter of at least 100.0 mm
- solid cyst with irregular contour
- at least four papillary projections
- ascites
- a vascularity colour score of 4, denoting high vascularity.

The adnexal cyst is assessed for the presence of any of these features. If one or more of the malignant features are present *and* there are no benign features, the cyst is characterized as malignant. The converse is applied – that is, if one or more of the benign features are present *and* there are no malignant features, the cyst is characterized as benign.

The simple rules are deemed inconclusive if there are both benign and malignant features present *or* if neither benign nor malignant features are present.

Although the simple rules can help determine whether a cyst is likely to be benign or malignant, neither you nor the clinician requesting the ultrasound examination should expect you to be able to diagnose the specific type of cyst on the basis of your ultrasound examination. Depending on the services available in your institution, the more complex adnexal cysts or those which are difficult to determine will be referred for an expert gynaecological ultrasound opinion and/or further imaging, such as magnetic resonance imaging.

The simple rules in practice

Let us now consider how to use the simple rules in practice. We will assume that you as the operator have limited experience of scanning the less common adnexal cysts. You will therefore apply the simple rules in order to try to determine the likelihood of the cyst being benign or malignant.

Case 1 – mucinous cystadenoma (Fig. 19.11)

- multilocular cyst with a smooth contour
- measures 221 × 144 × 158 mm
- anechoic and low-level internal contents, no solid components
- vascularity colour score of 1, denoting no flow.

Case 1 has one benign feature: It has no vascularity demonstrated with colour Doppler. Although it is a multilocular cyst with a smooth contour, its largest diameter is over 100.0 mm therefore this cannot be included as a benign feature. It has no malignant features and therefore would be considered benign based on the simple rules.

Case 2 – fibroma (Fig. 19.3)

- solid cyst with a smooth contour
- measures 118 × 134 × 127 mm
- acoustic shadows
- vascularity colour score of 2, denoting minimal flow.

Case 2 has one benign feature. It has acoustic shadows. It is a solid cyst, but it has a smooth contour, not an irregular one. It has no malignant features and therefore would be considered benign based on the simple rules.

Case 3 – metastatic ovarian carcinoma (Fig. 19.16A and B)

- solid cyst with irregular contour
- measures 102 × 78 × 55 mm
- no acoustic shadows

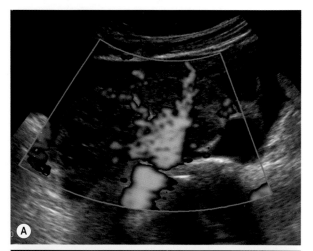

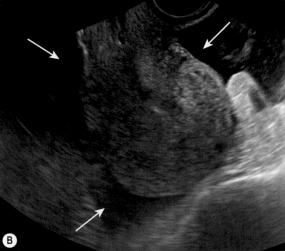

Fig 19.16 • A. A metastatic ovarian carcinoma. The cyst is solid and irregular in outline. It is highly vascular with a vascularity score of 4. B. The same case. Ascites is present, surrounding the uterus (arrows).

- ascites
- vascularity colour score of 4, denoting high vascularity.

Case 3 has no benign features but has three malignant features of a solid cyst with an irregular contour, ascites and vascularity colour score of 4. Therefore, according to the simple rules, this case would be considered likely to be malignant based on its ultrasound features.

WRITING THE REPORT FOR ADNEXAL CYSTS

In addition to the information included in the report template (see Chapter 16), we suggest the following additional information should be included in your reporting of an adnexal cyst.

For each adnexal cyst, include the following:

- the organ from which the adnexal cyst arises; if uncertain, say so
- whether the adnexal cyst is located to the right, left or middle of the pelvis
- measurements of the cyst in three orthogonal planes
- classification (i.e. unilocular, unilocular solid, multilocular, multilocular solid or solid)
- description of the internal contents (i.e. anechoic, low levels, haemorrhagic, etc.)
- whether the contour is smooth or irregular
- subjective assessment of the vascularity
- whether the sliding sign was negative or positive, if employed
- whether the woman experienced any tenderness on scanning
- whether there is any evidence of free fluid or ascites
- conclusion of the scan findings
- whether any other relevant management required after the scan
- recommendations for the purpose and timing of a further scan.

Your role as the operator is to provide in the form of a written or verbal report as accurate a description as possible of the findings identified during your examination. Your aim should be to provide the receiver of the report, who will usually be the referrer, with enough information to enable him or her to make a clinical judgement to assist in the management of the woman. You should be able to differentiate between those adnexal masses which are unlikely to be of clinical relevance and those that are of uncertain significance or have a strong association with clinically significant pathological conditions. You must also remember that an inappropriately written report may be misinterpreted by the reader and result in the woman either being subjected to unnecessary tests and possibly surgery or being denied further investigations which may be necessary to reach the correct diagnosis.

Further reading

Hillaby K, Aslam N, Salim R, Lawrence A, Ruja K S, Jurkovic D 2004 The value of detection of normal ovarian tissue (the 'ovarian crescent' sign) in the differential diagnosis of adnexal masses. Ultrasound Obstet Gynecol 23:63–67

Jacobs I, Oram D, Fairbanks J, Turner J, Frost C, Grudzinskas J G 1990 A risk of malignancy index incorporating CA 125, ultrasound and menopausal status for the accurate preoperative diagnosis of ovarian cancer. BJOG 97: 922–929

Royal College of Obstetrics and Gynaecology 2011 Management of suspected ovarian masses in premenopausal women. Green-top Guideline No. 62. RCOG Press, London

Timmerman D, Valentin L, Bourne T H, Collins W P, Verrelst H, Vergote I 2000 Terms, definitions and measurements to describe the sonographic features of adnexal tumors: a consensus opinion from the International Ovarian Tumor Analysis (IOTA) group. Ultrasound Obstet Gynecol 16:500–505

Timmerman D, Ameye L, Fischerova D, et al 2010 Simple ultrasound rules to distinguish between benign and malignant adnexal masses before surgery; prospective validation by IOTA group. BMJ 341:c6839

Professional issues

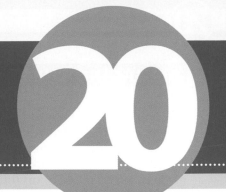

CONTENTS

This chapter discusses professional issues, which are many and varied, ranging from the manner in which the sonographer conducts him- or herself to the responsibility that you as a sonographer have to uphold high-quality and safe delivery of the ultrasound service.

The aims of this chapter are to enable you to do the following:

- understand the sonographer's responsibilities with regard to professional issues
- discuss how to best manage the examination and discuss the findings
- appreciate the manager's responsibilities with regard to professional issues
- appreciate the medicolegal issues relevant to performing and reporting ultrasound scans.

THE REFERRER OF THE ULTRASOUND EXAMINATION

Ultrasound departments should have systems in place which ensure that scan requests are appropriately processed and prioritized in order that women are informed of their appointment in a timely manner. Although the majority of obstetric scans are screening examinations booked at defined gestational ages, others are requested on an ad hoc basis for a clinical indication such as a suspected growth restricted baby. Similarly a gynaecological ultrasound scan may be required as a follow up at a specific timescale or, more acutely, for an indication such as a suspected ovarian torsion.

The referrer should be sufficiently competent to understand when an ultrasound examination is clinically indicated and, perhaps more importantly, when it is not clinically indicated. The correct patient details and a brief relevant clinical history should be included in the ultrasound request. A request for an ultrasound scan should pose a specific question. It is the expectation of the referrer that the ultrasound report will respond to that specific question.

MANAGING THE EXAMINATION

Individual professionalism, together with the requirements of the departmental protocol, should ensure that every examination is performed to an agreed level of competence. Every effort should be made to see the woman on time for her appointment. Unfortunately, ultrasound lists do not always run to time. In the event of any delay, this is best communicated to all those present, and attending in the near future, in the waiting room via the administrative staff at the reception desk on an individual patient basis or by use of a written notice in the waiting area. Informing women of an anticipated delay is a courtesy and also likely to defuse a potentially difficult situation when women, who may well be anxious, express their frustration at being kept waiting beyond their appointment time.

The way in which you approach the ultrasound examination is also influenced by the rapport you develop with the woman and her attenders. You should introduce yourself and any other personnel in the room by name and role. You as the sonographer are much more likely to perform a thorough examination in a relaxed and friendly room than in one with a hostile and suspicious atmosphere. Equally the woman will feel more able to express any concerns she might have if she feels welcomed and informed about the ensuing examination.

The woman should be correctly identified according to the requirements of your departmental protocol. It is imperative that the maternity/hospital notes, ultrasound images and report are correctly identified and all refer to the woman who is having the ultrasound examination. As the sonographer it is your responsibility to perform the ultrasound scan, assimilate the findings and report them. It is therefore your responsibility to ensure that you are able to discharge those functions correctly.

Most women will attend their obstetric ultrasound scan with an accompanying person or persons. If you prefer to scan in silence until you have made a preliminary assessment, then it is important that you should be allowed to do this. However, you should appreciate that the majority of women and their attenders will interpret your silence as suggesting that you have found a problem, unless you explain *before* you start the examination that it is your preferred method of working.

If you find the frequent questioning of an individual (or the activities of accompanying children and attenders) distracting, then you must politely ask that individual to desist in their questioning or the distracting attenders to wait outside so that you can concentrate properly on the examination for which you are responsible. Alternatively, you must develop strategies to cope with these potential distractions while maintaining your concentration.

Invasion of personal space either by an attender or an observer allocated to you by your department might also undermine your ability to concentrate. Again you must politely ask the individual to observe the examination from a different area of the room or develop strategies to cope with such a situation.

DISCUSSING THE FINDINGS

The first issue that you need to consider is where to discuss the findings of your examination. You might consider that the correct procedure is to explain your findings immediately after you have completed the examination. However, this very natural decision could result in the woman receiving information for which she is unprepared, lying on the couch with her abdomen exposed and covered in scanning gel or, if she has had a transvaginal scan, with her legs in stirrups and her underwear removed.

Anyone who has been in such a situation, or a comparable situation, will appreciate the feelings of vulnerability and lack of control that accompany it. These feelings will be accentuated by your relative positions. Thus, although you are sitting beside the woman, you are not communicating with each other at the same height because you are talking down to her and she is talking up to you.

Conversely, inviting the woman to get dressed and taking her to a separate room before telling her your findings (or asking her to wait while you find a colleague to impart them on your behalf) seems, to many, to prolong the agony unnecessarily.

Possibly the best compromise is to ask the woman to dress and sit down on a chair or on the couch in the scanning room. Wait until she is sitting down, and can therefore give you her full attention, before you begin speaking. Do not be tempted to start talking while she is getting dressed. Imagine yourself at your own doctor's surgery. You are getting dressed after a locum, whom you have never met before, has conducted an examination. You are probably embarrassed and anxious. Would you prefer the findings to be given to you while you are struggling to get dressed or would you rather receive them sitting fully clothed on the chair beside the doctor's desk?

Some women will already be anticipating bad news because of findings before the examination. Other women, especially those attending a routine screening examination, will be anticipating normal findings and be unprepared for results that suggest otherwise. Every 'not normal' situation is different, and is made so by the combination of the implications of the ultrasound findings and their interpretation by the woman. Finding the correct words for the first few sentences of the discussion that must follow the completion of such an examination is arguably one of the most difficult tasks that a sonographer faces. Unfortunately, there is no verbal formula that can be applied successfully to all problems in all situations, but there are certain strategies that might be of help.

It is important that bad news is given in a way that the woman is unlikely to misinterpret. If the fetus is dead, then it is preferable to say, 'I'm afraid I have to give you some bad news. Your baby has no heartbeat, so I am very sorry to have to tell you that your baby has died' rather than 'I can't find the fetal heart'. The latter can be interpreted as meaning that the fetus is alive but that you are unable to demonstrate the fetal heart beating because of some technical difficulty.

In a situation where you have identified a serious abnormality, such as spina bifida, a major cardiac defect or severe ventriculomegaly, you may wish to consider using the following opening phrase. 'I am afraid I have to give you some bad news. I have concerns about the appearances of the baby's spine/heart/brain as I am unable to obtain the normal sections'.

The previously described are situations where it might be preferable to break the news to the woman as soon as you are certain of your findings (i.e. while she is still lying on the couch). This position is also easier for all concerned because you might need to seek confirmation of your findings from a colleague who is elsewhere in the department but whom you may wish to ask to scan the woman. Before beginning your discussion, you might want to take a memento type image that can be recorded on hard copy and filed in the notes, to be given to the woman at a later date should she so wish.

Mild ventriculomegaly or echogenic bowel have a higher prevalence at 18–22 weeks than major structural abnormalities, and you will invariably first suspect or detect them early in your scanning career. It is much more likely, therefore, that you will need to explain these findings and their implications to a woman than spina bifida or a cardiac defect. As discussed in previous chapters, such 'not normal' findings need to be considered in the light of the woman's prior screening. Current national recommendations are that ventriculomegaly and echogenic bowel should be referred for a fetal specialist opinion. Any 'not normal' findings should be managed according to local protocol. As discussed in previous chapters, it is these relatively not uncommon findings which are a challenge to the sonographer to impart the correct information without causing the woman anxiety.

The assumption is that these findings, although outside the range of normal appearances, are unlikely to indicate anything other than a normal outcome for the pregnancy. Your body language, the tone of your voice and the eye contact you make with the woman should all emphasize this fact.

Choroid plexus cysts are considered a normal variant and the current recommendation therefore is that they do not need referral for more detailed examination of the fetus. The cysts are often easily identifiable to both the sonographer and woman whilst the brain anatomy is identified. This may prompt a woman to ask such questions as 'What is that you are looking at?' and 'Is it normal?' Describing the choroid plexus cysts as 'cysts on the brain' is unlikely to reassure the woman that the finding is most likely of no significance. It is probably more helpful to explain that adults, children and babies have several glands in the brain that produce fluid in order to 'lubricate' the brain and the spine. Occasionally one of these glands can become temporarily blocked. This can be seen on ultrasound, and this blockage is called a choroid plexus cyst. The vast majority of glands that become blocked become unblocked on their own by 24–26 weeks and the 'cyst' therefore disappears.

It is important to speak slowly and pause frequently to give the woman time to take in what you are saying to her. She must be given the opportunity to ask questions and might need to have the information repeated or explained in a different way. If she becomes upset, do not feel you must comfort her by continuing to talk. In such situations silence can be more supportive than well-meaning chatter.

Irrespective of whether the findings are normal, not normal or abnormal, the information you impart should always be representative of the findings of your examination. It is always better to be honest and truthful.

Your responsibility is to have sufficient, accurate and current knowledge of the range of findings that you are likely to identify in your current role, and their implications. It is unrealistic to assume that you will have the answer to every question a woman might ask you and you should not feel inadequate if you are unable to answer questions that are outside your range of expertise. If you are uncertain or do not know the answer or answers, there are always other people to whom you can refer the woman for information and advice. It is important, however, to develop ways of explaining that you are unable to provide the required information. Using a phrase such as 'that is something that you need to discuss with Dr X or your midwife' is more helpful for the woman, and is a more professional response, than simply saying 'I don't know' or 'I'm not sure, I'll go and ask'.

These skills might not come easily but are an essential component of your role as a sonographer. Providing you learn from every new situation, your communication skills will continue to develop as your expertise and experience grows.

ARRANGING FOLLOW-UP

Your departmental protocol should identify the findings that require ultrasound follow-up and, where indicated, the gestational age at which the follow-up appointments should be made. You must ensure that the necessary appointment is made with the appropriate staff member; it is inappropriate to assume that someone else, or even the woman, will do this on your behalf. It is important that the arrangement of any further appointment is noted on the report and that the woman is aware that a further ultrasound scan appointment has been made for her.

A member of the team of health care professionals involved in the care of the woman should be informed of any clinically significant findings from the examination as soon as possible, preferably before the woman leaves the ultrasound department. This is your responsibility, and you must therefore either make contact yourself or entrust a colleague to do this on your behalf.

THE ULTRASOUND REPORT

The ultrasound report should be clearly written and easy to read. Your name, as the sonographer performing the examination, together with your role and date of the report should always be included. If you have scanned the woman in your capacity as a student, this should be made clear on the report, which *must* be countersigned by whoever has supervised the examination. It is that person who is clinically responsible for the findings as stated in the report.

An ultrasound report should be written in a way that its recipient can understand and, importantly, that the content is relevant. Descriptive terminology such as *anechoic, hypoechoic, hyperechoic* or *acoustic shadowing* can provide useful additional information to your ultrasound colleagues but is unlikely to provide the general practitioner or consultant gynaecologist with useful information on which to base further management decisions. Previous chapters have included a suggested report template according to the ultrasound examination type.

THE SONOGRAPHER'S RESPONSIBILITIES

You have a responsibility to ensure that your professional knowledge and skills are kept up to date. Similarly, accreditation of, for instance, nuchal translucency measurement needs to be current. Furthermore, you must work within your scope of practice and scan safely. If you feel that any of the former are compromised, you must raise your concerns with a senior colleague or your manager. Your department should have a protocol which details the content of each examination and the ensuing pathways where indicated. It is your responsibility to ensure that you understand and comply with your departmental protocols. There should also be local guidance regarding data protection and confidentiality to which you can refer.

DEPARTMENTAL PROTOCOL

Every department should have a protocol that provides the following information:
- the objectives of each type of scan that is undertaken
- the structures that will be sought and evaluated
- a description of what constitutes normal/abnormal findings in those structures
- the measurements that will be taken
- a description of when a measurement or a combination of measurements will be considered abnormal
- the procedures that will be undertaken when a problem is identified
- by what means the findings of normal examinations will be recorded and what images will be recorded
- how examinations will be reported and to whom
- the type of follow up, and its frequency, after the detection of specific findings.

Some consideration needs to be given as to how your ultrasound report informs the reader as to which structures are being examined and measured. If this breakdown is not apparent in the report, it needs to be clearly identified as being a component of a given ultrasound examination in your guidelines.

For example, your local guidelines may include an evaluation of the three vessel and trachea view (3vt) when assessing the fetal heart. Your electronic report may allow a 'drop down' menu, which includes a breakdown of the views which have been assessed; thereby it is possible to record that the 3vt has been assessed as normal or not normal for a given examination. If this breakdown is not possible, your guideline needs to be very clear which views are expected to be assessed when examining the fetal heart.

As an individual you have a responsibility to scan safely. You should be up to date and conversant with your statutory and mandatory training. Ultrasound machines which are poor quality and not fit for purpose and inappropriate appointment times may compromise your ability to scan safely. If you feel any of the former are a concern, you should raise this with your manager in writing.

The departmental protocols should be dated and reviewed on a regular basis. Once a protocol is superseded, it should be kept on file and should not be destroyed. The protocols should reflect the level of service provided by the department. All members of staff, including all new staff members, should be familiar with the contents of the protocols and should ensure that their scanning abilities encompass its requirements. If they do not, this should be addressed urgently by further training followed by assessment. It should be possible for an individual from outside the department to read the protocol and form an accurate description of what each examination includes and the level of expertise being applied.

WORKING WITH A STUDENT

Any student working with a sonographer needs to introduce him- or herself to the woman being scanned. The student should gain the consent of the woman before performing any ultrasound examination. The ultrasound scans should be undertaken under supervision from the qualified sonographer who should be in attendance in the room. The student sonographer should have his or her report countersigned; the ultrasound scan, report and any decisions as a result of the scan are the responsibility of the supervising sonographer.

447

MEDICOLEGAL ISSUES

The increasing reliance that is placed on ultrasound examinations increases the expectations of parents that normal prenatal ultrasound findings equate to a normal baby at delivery. Sadly, this is not always the case, leading to an increasing number of parents seeking litigation. In many instances the problems evident postnatally could not have been detected prenatally and there would therefore be no legal case to answer. In other cases, an abnormal finding is overlooked or its appearance is misinterpreted despite the departmental protocol requiring evaluation of that structure. In such cases it might indeed be the case that the sonographer was negligent and there is therefore a legal case to answer.

For the majority of sonographers, litigation will only be a distant anxiety. However, it is your responsibility as a sonographer to ensure that your actions do not leave you open to litigation. The way to do this is to ensure that every examination you undertake is performed to a standard appropriate to, or above, that required by your department protocol. The range of abnormalities that you should detect and therefore should not overlook will be evident from the contents of your departmental protocol. This information is relevant both to you, the sonographer, and to the woman you are scanning.

In some circumstances it might not be possible to perform an examination to the standard required by your protocol (e.g. in cases of maternal obesity or a persistently difficult fetal position). If this is the case, you should state this fact in your report.

Taking hard copy of a specified number of standard images of a normal examination is good practice because it provides a visual record of the examination. This should be seen as positive evidence of the quality of the examinations you have performed. It can also endorse the technical

difficulties such as maternal obesity mentioned in your report. Should you feel threatened by having to record images, then you should question why this is and ensure that you address the underlying reasons for this appropriately.

The majority of medicolegal cases never reach the courts either because there is no case to answer or because the matter is settled out of court. However, this is likely to be of little comfort when it is first brought to your attention that parents have decided to issue proceedings against your employer and that you were responsible for performing the ultrasound examination of the fetus that subsequently was born with an abnormality. Your departmental protocol should provide the evidence required to support you, assuming it can be demonstrated that you acted within its requirements. You must be aware, however, that if you do not perform an ultrasound examination to the standard required by your departmental protocol and this results in a fetal abnormality being missed, then your actions can be interpreted as negligent because you have breached the duty of care you owe to the woman.

In the event of proceedings being issued for a missed fetal abnormality or an incorrect misinterpretation of an ovarian cyst, the case will be judged by a competent group of similar professionals (i.e. sonographers).

Normally a sonographer's liability is covered vicariously by their employer. However, this is on the proviso that you are working within your scope of practice. If you are working outside your scope of practice or undertaking scans for social reasons, your employer may not guarantee cover and you may need to obtain alternative appropriate indemnity cover.

THE MANAGER'S RESPONSIBILITIES

It goes without saying that the manager of an ultrasound department should ensure that there are systems and resources in place to support all of the previously described scenarios. Guidelines should be drawn up according to the local process. The

recommendations from national bodies, the multidisciplinary team and stakeholders should be considered when reviewing guidelines. Guidelines should be disseminated and sonographers supported and guided in their implementation. It is the manager's responsibility to escalate any problems or issues which may negatively affect the ability of the members of the department for which he or she is responsible to deliver a high quality and safe service.

There needs to be adequate recording and storage of both ultrasound reports and images. Hard copy records are particularly important if a medicolegal issue arises subsequent to the scan being performed. Obviously digital recording is the preferred method of long term storage, but if this is not possible, an adequate alternative needs to be sought. The manager or delegated sonographer should periodically audit the quality of the ultrasound examinations undertaken within the department.

AUDIT OF FINDINGS

Any information that women are given concerning the quality of the ultrasound service that your department provides should be based on the regular audit of your department's results. Such audit might identify the sensitivity of your nuchal translucency programme at 11–14 weeks or your cardiac screening programme at the 18–22 week scan. It might identify the accuracy of estimated fetal weight or the reporting of ovarian cysts. Such results can be used to identify the successful areas of the service and to highlight those areas that produce poor results. Once the reasons for these poor results have been identified, improving this area of service can be addressed.

Further reading

Fetal anomaly screening programme standards: 2015 to 2016. 2015; www.gov.uk/.../fetal-anomalies-screening-programme -standards

Leaflets published by Antenatal Results and Choices (ARC):
a) The Burden of Choice
b) Parents Handbook
info@arc-uk.org

Leaflets published by the Fetal Anomaly Screening Programme (FASP) for the conditions screened for by the NHS FASP screening programme available at www.gov.uk/fetal-anomalies -screening-conditions-diagnosis-treatments

Appendices

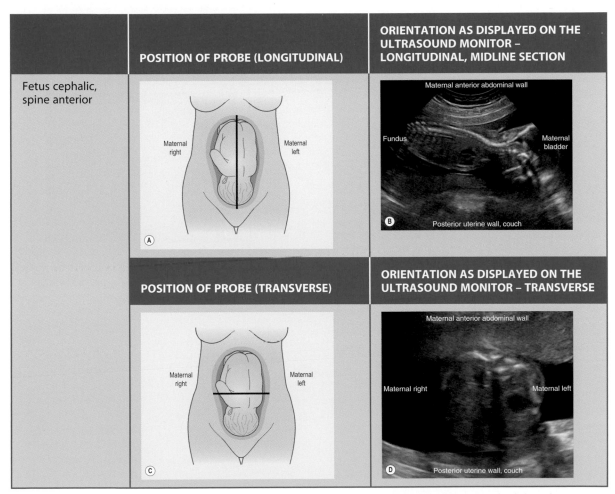

	POSITION OF PROBE (LONGITUDINAL)	ORIENTATION AS DISPLAYED ON THE ULTRASOUND MONITOR – LONGITUDINAL, MIDLINE SECTION
Fetus cephalic, spine anterior	(A) Maternal right / Maternal left	(B) Maternal anterior abdominal wall / Fundus / Maternal bladder / Posterior uterine wall, couch
	POSITION OF PROBE (TRANSVERSE)	ORIENTATION AS DISPLAYED ON THE ULTRASOUND MONITOR – TRANSVERSE
	(C) Maternal right / Maternal left	(D) Maternal anterior abdominal wall / Maternal right / Maternal left / Posterior uterine wall, couch

Probe position on maternal abdomen and corresponding image orientation on ultrasound monitor. Conventional radiological image orientation is used. Anticlockwise rotation of probe is used to move from longitudinal section to transverse section

Continued

Fetus breech, spine anterior

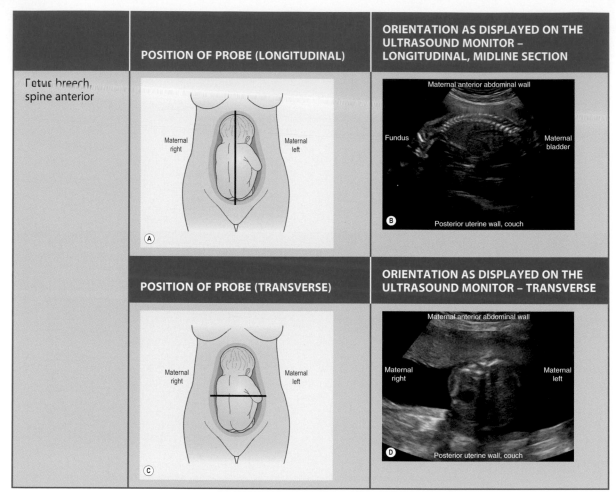

Probe position on maternal abdomen and corresponding image orientation on ultrasound monitor. Conventional radiological image orientation is used. Anticlockwise rotation of probe is used to move from longitudinal section to transverse section

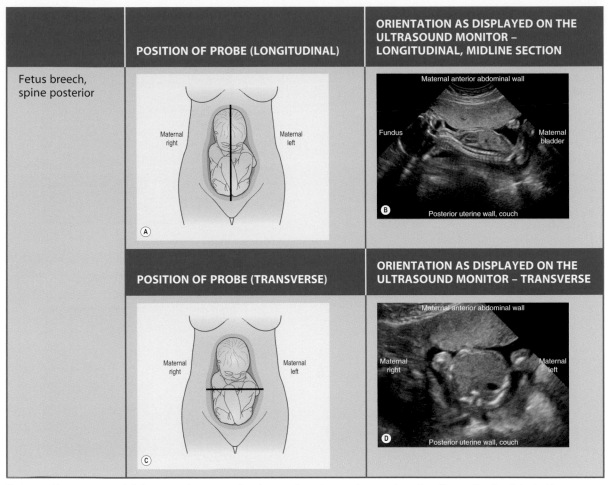

	POSITION OF PROBE (LONGITUDINAL)	ORIENTATION AS DISPLAYED ON THE ULTRASOUND MONITOR – LONGITUDINAL, MIDLINE SECTION
Fetus breech, spine posterior	Maternal right Maternal left (A)	Maternal anterior abdominal wall Fundus Maternal bladder (B) Posterior uterine wall, couch
	POSITION OF PROBE (TRANSVERSE)	ORIENTATION AS DISPLAYED ON THE ULTRASOUND MONITOR – TRANSVERSE
	Maternal right Maternal left (C)	Maternal anterior abdominal wall Maternal right Maternal left (D) Posterior uterine wall, couch

Probe position on maternal abdomen and corresponding image orientation on ultrasound monitor. Conventional radiological image orientation is used. Anticlockwise rotation of probe is used to move from longitudinal section to transverse section

Continued

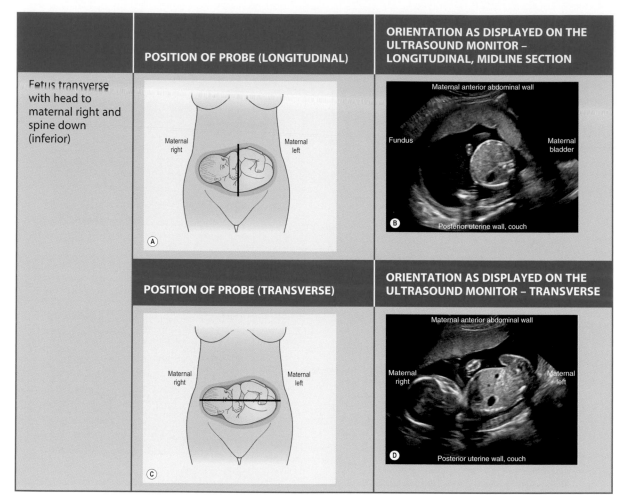

	POSITION OF PROBE (LONGITUDINAL)	ORIENTATION AS DISPLAYED ON THE ULTRASOUND MONITOR – LONGITUDINAL, MIDLINE SECTION
Fetus transverse with head to maternal right and spine down (inferior)	Maternal right — Maternal left (A)	Maternal anterior abdominal wall — Fundus — Maternal bladder — Posterior uterine wall, couch (B)
	POSITION OF PROBE (TRANSVERSE)	ORIENTATION AS DISPLAYED ON THE ULTRASOUND MONITOR – TRANSVERSE
	Maternal right — Maternal left (C)	Maternal anterior abdominal wall — Maternal right — Maternal left — Posterior uterine wall, couch (D)

Probe position on maternal abdomen and corresponding image orientation on ultrasound monitor. Conventional radiological image orientation is used. Anticlockwise rotation of probe is used to move from longitudinal section to transverse section

Equation and look-up table for estimating gestational age (GA) from the crown rump length (CRL) as recommended by current national guidelines

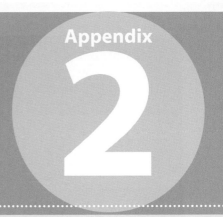

Dating equation using CRL:

$$GA = 8.052 \times (CRL \times 1.037)^{\frac{1}{2}} + 23.73$$

CRL (mm)	GA (WEEKS + DAYS)			CRL (mm)	GA (WEEKS + DAYS)		
	50TH CENTILE	5TH CENTILE	95TH CENTILE		50TH CENTILE	5TH CENTILE	95TH CENTILE
5	6 + 0	5 + 2	6 + 5	21	8 + 5	8 + 1	9 + 3
6	6 + 2	5 + 4	7 + 0	22	8 + 6	8 + 1	9 + 4
7	6 + 3	5 + 6	7 + 1	23	9 + 0	8 + 2	9 + 5
8	6 + 5	6 + 0	7 + 2	24	9 + 1	8 + 3	9 + 6
9	6 + 6	6 + 2	7 + 4	25	9 + 2	8 + 4	9 + 6
10	7 + 1	6 + 3	7 + 5	26	9 + 3	8 + 5	10 + 0
11	7 + 2	6 + 4	8 + 0	27	9 + 3	8 + 6	10 + 1
12	7 + 3	6 + 5	8 + 1	28	9 + 4	8 + 6	10 + 2
13	7 + 4	7 + 0	8 + 2	29	9 + 5	9 + 0	10 + 3
14	7 + 5	7 + 1	8 + 3	30	9 + 6	9 + 1	10 + 3
15	7 + 6	7 + 2	8 + 4	31	9 + 6	9 + 2	10 + 4
16	8 + 1	7 + 3	8 + 5	32	10 + 0	9 + 2	10 + 5
17	8 + 2	7 + 4	8 + 6	33	10 + 1	9 + 3	10 + 6
18	8 + 3	7 + 5	9 + 0	34	10 + 2	9 + 4	10 + 6
19	8 + 3	7 + 6	9 + 1	35	10 + 2	9 + 5	11 + 0
20	8 + 4	8 + 0	9 + 2	36	10 + 3	9 + 5	11 + 1

Continued

Equation and look-up table for estimating gestational age (GA) from the crown rump length (CRL)

CRL (mm)	GA (WEEKS + DAYS)			CRL (mm)	GA (WEEKS + DAYS)		
	50TH CENTILE	5TH CENTILE	95TH CENTILE		50TH CENTILE	5TH CENTILE	95TH CENTILE
37	10 + 4	9 + 6	11 + 1	59	12 + 3	11 + 5	13 + 0
38	10 + 4	10 + 0	11 + 2	60	12 + 3	11 + 6	13 + 1
39	10 + 5	10 + 0	11 + 3	61	12 + 4	11 + 6	13 + 1
40	10 + 6	10 + 1	11 + 3	62	12 + 4	12 + 0	13 + 2
41	10 + 6	10 + 2	11 + 4	63	12 + 5	12 + 0	13 + 3
42	11 + 0	10 + 2	11 + 5	64	12 + 5	12 + 1	13 + 3
43	11 + 0	10 + 3	11 + 5	65	12 + 6	12 + 1	13 + 4
44	11 + 1	10 + 3	11 + 6	66	12 + 6	12 + 2	13 + 4
45	11 + 2	10 + 4	11 + 6	67	13 + 0	12 + 2	13 + 5
46	11 + 2	10 + 5	12 + 0	68	13 + 0	12 + 3	13 + 5
47	11 + 3	10 + 5	12 + 1	69	13 + 1	12 + 3	13 + 6
48	11 + 4	10 + 6	12 + 1	70	13 + 1	12 + 4	13 + 6
49	11 + 4	10 + 6	12 + 2	71	13 + 2	12 + 4	14 + 0
50	11 + 5	11 + 0	12 + 2	72	13 + 2	12 + 5	14 + 0
51	11 + 5	11 + 1	12 + 3	73	13 + 3	12 + 5	14 + 0
52	11 + 6	11 + 1	12 + 4	74	13 + 3	12 + 6	14 + 1
53	11 + 6	11 + 2	12 + 4	75	13 + 4	12 + 6	14 + 1
54	12 + 0	11 + 2	12 + 5	76	13 + 4	13 + 0	14 + 2
55	12 + 1	11 + 3	12 + 5	77	13 + 5	13 + 0	14 + 2
56	12 + 1	11 + 3	12 + 6	78	13 + 5	13 + 0	14 + 3
57	12 + 2	11 + 4	12 + 6	79	13 + 6	13 + 1	14 + 3
58	12 + 2	11 + 4	13 + 0	80	13 + 6	13 + 1	14 + 4

Loughna P, Chitty L, Evans T, Chudleigh T 2009 Fetal size and dating: charts recommended for clinical obstetric practice. Ultrasound 17(3):161–167

Head circumference (HC) dating table and equation

$$\log_e(GA) = 0.010611HC - 0.0000303211HC^2 + 0.43498 \times 10^{-7}HC^3 + 1.848$$

HC (mm)	GA (WEEKS + DAYS)			HC (mm)	GA (WEEKS + DAYS)		
	50TH CENTILE	5TH CENTILE	95TH CENTILE		50TH CENTILE	5TH CENTILE	95TH CENTILE
80	12 + 4	11 + 3	13 + 5	180	20 + 5	19 + 3	22 + 0
85	12 + 6	11 + 6	14 + 1	185	21 + 1	19 + 6	22 + 3
90	13 + 2	12 + 2	14 + 4	190	21 + 4	20 + 2	22 + 6
95	13 + 5	12 + 4	15 + 0	195	22 + 0	20 + 4	23 + 2
100	14 + 1	13 + 0	15 + 3	200	22 + 2	21 + 0	23 + 5
105	14 + 4	13 + 3	15 + 5	205	22 + 5	21 + 3	24 + 2
110	15 + 0	13 + 6	16 + 1	210	23 + 1	21 + 5	24 + 5
115	15 + 3	14 + 2	16 + 4	215	23 + 4	22 + 1	25 + 1
120	15 + 6	14 + 5	17 + 0	220	24 + 0	22 + 4	25 + 5
125	16 + 2	15 + 1	17 + 3	225	24 + 3	22 + 6	26 + 1
130	16 + 4	15 + 4	17 + 6	230	24 + 6	23 + 2	26 + 5
135	17 + 0	15 + 6	18 + 2	235	25 + 3	23 + 5	27 + 1
140	17 + 3	16 + 2	18 + 5	240	25 + 6	24 + 1	27 + 5
145	17 + 6	16 + 5	19 + 1	245	26 + 2	24 + 3	28 + 2
150	18 + 2	17 + 1	19 + 3	250	26 + 5	24 + 6	28 + 6
155	18 + 5	17 + 4	19 + 6	255	27 + 2	25 + 2	29 + 3
160	19 + 1	17 + 6	20 + 2	260	27 + 5	25 + 5	30 + 0
165	19 + 3	18 + 2	20 + 5	265	28 + 2	26 + 1	30 + 4
170	19 + 6	18 + 5	21 + 1	270	28 + 6	26 + 4	31 + 2
175	20 + 2	19 + 1	21 + 4	275	29 + 3	27 + 0	32 + 0

Continued

HC (mm)	GA (WEEKS + DAYS)			HC (mm)	GA (WEEKS + DAYS)		
	50TH CENTILE	5TH CENTILE	95TH CENTILE		50TH CENTILE	5TH CENTILE	95TH CENTILE
280	30 + 0	27 + 3	32 + 4	305	33 + 1	30 + 0	36 + 5
285	30 + 4	27 + 6	33 + 3	310	33 + 6	30 + 3	37 + 4
290	31 + 1	28 + 3	34 + 1	315	34 + 4	31 + 0	38 + 4
295	31 + 5	28 + 6	35 + 0	320	35 + 3	31 + 5	39 + 4
300	32 + 3	29 + 3	35 + 6				

GA, gestational age.
Loughna P, Chitty L, Evans T, Chudleigh T 2009 Fetal size and dating: charts recommended for clinical obstetric practice. Ultrasound 17(3):161–167

Biparietal diameter (BPD) dating table ('outer to inner')

BPD (mm)	ESTIMATED GA (WEEKS + DAYS)	5TH CENTILE (WEEKS + DAYS)	95TH CENTILE (WEEKS + DAYS)	UNCERTAINTY (± DAYS)
21	12 + 5	11 + 6	13 + 5	7
22	13 + 0	12 + 1	14 + 0	7
23	13 + 2	12 + 3	14 + 2	7
24	13 + 4	12 + 4	14 + 4	7
25	13 + 6	12 + 6	14 + 6	7
26	14 + 1	13 + 1	15 + 1	7
27	14 + 3	13 + 3	15 + 3	7
28	14 + 5	13 + 4	15 + 5	7
29	14 + 6	13 + 6	16 + 0	8
30	15 + 1	14 + 1	16 + 2	8
31	15 + 3	14 + 3	16 + 5	9
32	15 + 5	14 + 4	17 + 0	9
33	16 + 0	14 + 6	17 + 2	9
34	16 + 2	15 + 1	17 + 4	9
35	16 + 4	15 + 3	17 + 6	9
36	16 + 6	15 + 5	18 + 2	10
37	17 + 1	15 + 6	18 + 4	10
38	17 + 3	16 + 1	18 + 6	10
39	17 + 6	16 + 3	19 + 2	10
40	18 + 1	16 + 5	19 + 4	10
41	18 + 3	17 + 0	19 + 6	10
42	18 + 5	17 + 2	20 + 2	11

Continued

BPD (mm)	ESTIMATED GA (WEEKS + DAYS)	5TH CENTILE (WEEKS + DAYS)	95TH CENTILE (WEEKS + DAYS)	UNCERTAINTY (± DAYS)
43	19 + 0	17 + 4	20 + 4	11
44	19 + 2	17 + 6	20 + 6	11
45	19 + 4	18 + 1	21 + 2	12
46	19 + 6	18 + 3	21 + 4	12
47	20 + 2	18 + 5	22 + 0	12
48	20 + 4	19 + 0	22 + 2	12
49	20 + 6	19 + 2	22 + 5	13
50	21 + 1	19 + 4	23 + 0	13
51	21 + 4	19 + 6	23 + 3	13
52	21 + 6	20 + 1	23 + 5	13
53	22 + 1	20 + 3	24 + 1	14
54	22 + 4	20 + 5	24 + 4	14
55	22 + 6	21 + 0	24 + 6	14
56	23 + 1	21 + 2	25 + 2	15
57	23 + 4	21 + 4	25 + 4	14
58	23 + 6	21 + 6	26 + 0	15
59	24 + 1	22 + 1	26 + 3	16

GA, gestational age.

Altman D, Chitty L 1997 New charts for ultrasound dating of pregnancy 1997. Ultrasound in Obstetrics and Gynecology (10):174–191

The 11 conditions screened for, together with their current expected detection rates, within the national screening programme

Appendix

5

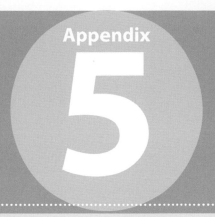

CONDITION	DETECTION RATE (%)
Anencephaly	98
Open spina bifida	90
Cleft lip	75
Diaphragmatic hernia	60
Gastroschisis	98
Exomphalos	80
Serious cardiac abnormalities	50
Bilateral renal agenesis	84
Lethal skeletal dysplasia	60
Edwards' syndrome (trisomy 18)	95
Patau's syndrome (trisomy 13)	95

Equation, head circumference (HC) size chart and HC size table

Equation for estimating HC from gestational age (GA):

$$HC = -109.7 + 15.16(GA) - 0.002388(GA)^3$$

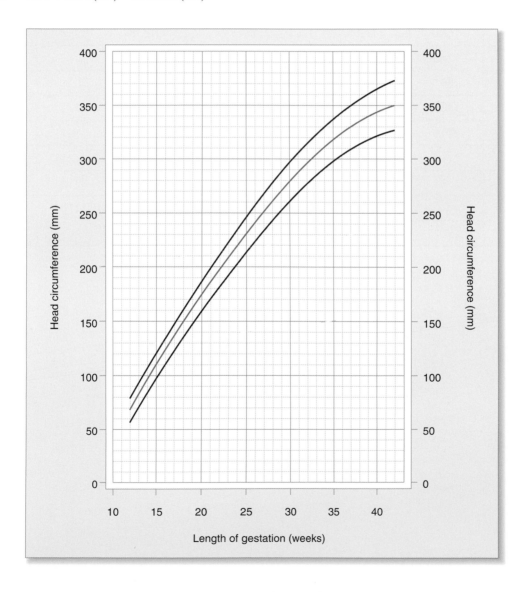

GA (WEEKS)	HC (mm)			GA (WEEKS)	HC (mm)		
	50TH CENTILE	5TH CENTILE	95TH CENTILE		50TH CENTILE	5TH CENTILE	95TH CENTILE
12	68.1	57.1	79.2	28	262.5	245.3	279.6
13	82.2	70.8	93.6	29	271.8	254.3	289.4
14	96.0	84.2	107.8	30	280.7	262.8	298.7
15	109.7	97.5	121.9	31	289.2	270.9	307.6
16	123.1	110.6	135.7	32	297.3	278.6	316.0
17	136.4	123.4	149.3	33	304.9	285.8	324.0
18	149.3	136.0	162.7	34	312.0	292.6	331.5
19	162.0	148.3	175.7	35	318.7	298.8	338.5
20	174.5	160.4	188.6	36	324.8	304.6	345.0
21	186.6	172.1	201.1	37	330.4	309.8	351.0
22	198.5	183.6	213.3	38	335.5	314.5	356.5
23	210.0	194.8	225.3	39	340.0	318.7	361.4
24	221.2	205.6	236.9	40	344.0	322.3	365.8
25	232.1	216.1	248.1	41	347.4	325.3	369.6
26	242.6	226.2	259.0	42	350.3	327.7	372.8
27	252.7	235.9	269.5				

Loughna P, Chitty L, Evans T & Chudleigh T 2009 Fetal size and dating: charts recommended for clinical obstetric practice. Ultrasound 17(3):161–167

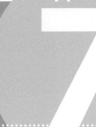
Biparietal diameter (BPD) size chart ('outer to inner')

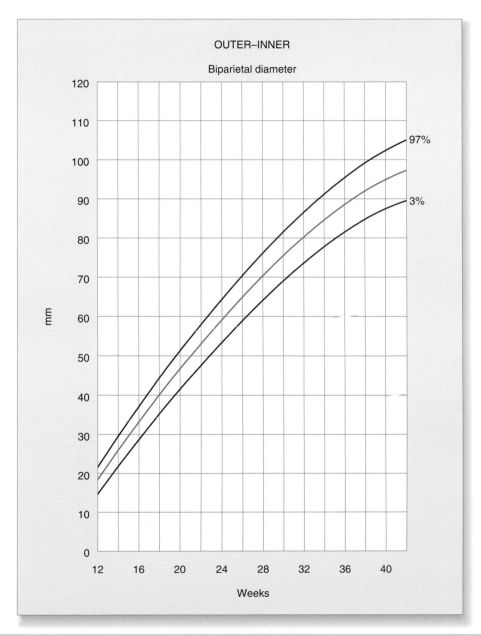

OUTER–INNER

Biparietal diameter

Data from Chitty LS, Henderson A 1994 Charts of fetal size: 2. Head measurements Br J Obstet Gynecol 101:35–43

Equation, abdominal circumference (AC) size chart and AC size table

Equation for estimating AC from gestational age (GA):

$$AC = -85.84 + 11.92\,(GA) - 0.0007902\,(GA)^3$$

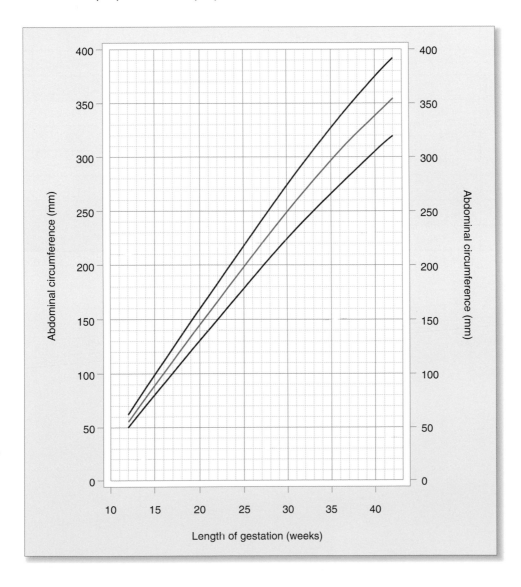

GA (WEEKS)	AC (mm) 50TH CENTILE	AC (mm) 5TH CENTILE	AC (mm) 95TH CENTILE	GA (WEEKS)	AC (mm) 50TH CENTILE	AC (mm) 5TH CENTILE	AC (mm) 95TH CENTILE
12	55.8	49.0	62.6	28	230.6	207.9	253.2
13	67.4	59.6	75.2	29	240.5	216.9	264.2
14	78.9	70.1	87.7	30	250.4	225.8	275.0
15	90.3	80.5	100.1	31	260.1	234.5	285.7
16	101.6	90.9	112.4	32	269.7	243.1	296.3
17	112.9	101.1	124.7	33	279.1	251.5	306.7
18	124.1	111.3	136.9	34	288.4	259.8	317.0
19	135.2	121.5	149.0	35	297.5	267.9	327.0
20	146.2	131.5	161.0	36	306.4	275.8	337.0
21	157.1	141.4	172.9	37	315.1	283.6	346.7
22	168.0	151.3	184.7	38	323.7	291.2	356.3
23	178.7	161.0	196.4	39	332.1	298.6	365.7
24	189.3	170.6	208.0	40	340.4	305.8	374.9
25	199.8	180.1	219.5	41	348.4	312.9	383.9
26	210.2	189.5	230.8	42	356.2	319.7	392.7
27	220.4	198.8	242.1				

Loughna P, Chitty L, Evans T, Chudleigh T 2009 Fetal size and dating: charts recommended for clinical obstetric practice. Ultrasound 17(3):161–167

Equation and dating table for estimating gestational age (GA) from the femur length (FL)

FL dating equation:

$$\text{Log}_e (GA) = 0.034375FL - 0.0037254FL \times \log_e (FL) + 2.306$$

FL (mm)	GA (WEEKS + DAYS)			FL (mm)	GA (WEEKS + DAYS)		
	50TH CENTILE	5TH CENTILE	95TH CENTILE		50TH CENTILE	5TH CENTILE	95TH CENTILE
10	13 + 0	12 + 1	13 + 6	29	18 + 6	17 + 4	20 + 3
11	13 + 2	12 + 3	14 + 1	30	19 + 2	17 + 6	20 + 5
12	13 + 4	12 + 5	14 + 4	31	19 + 4	18 + 1	21 + 1
13	13 + 6	13 + 0	14 + 6	32	20 + 0	18 + 3	21 + 4
14	14 + 1	13 + 1	15 + 1	33	20 + 2	18 + 5	22 + 0
15	14 + 3	13 + 3	15 + 3	34	20 + 5	19 + 1	22 + 2
16	14 + 5	13 + 5	15 + 6	35	21 + 0	19 + 3	22 + 5
17	15 + 0	14 + 0	16 + 1	36	21 + 3	19 + 5	23 + 1
18	15 + 2	14 + 2	16 + 3	37	21 + 5	20 + 1	32 + 4
19	15 + 5	14 + 4	16 + 6	38	22 + 1	20 + 3	24 + 0
20	16 + 0	14 + 6	17 + 1	39	22 + 4	20 + 5	24 + 3
21	16 + 2	15 + 1	17 + 3	40	22 + 6	21 + 1	24 + 6
22	16 + 4	15 + 3	17 + 6	41	23 + 2	21 + 3	25 + 2
23	16 + 6	15 + 5	18 + 1	42	23 + 5	21 + 6	25 + 5
24	17 + 2	16 + 0	18 + 4	43	24 + 1	22 + 1	26 + 1
25	17 + 4	16 + 2	18 + 6	44	24 + 3	22 + 4	26 + 4
26	17 + 6	16 + 4	19 + 2	45	24 + 6	22 + 6	27 + 1
27	18 + 2	16 + 6	19 + 5	46	25 + 2	23 + 2	27 + 4
28	18 + 4	17 + 1	20 + 0	47	25 + 5	23 + 4	28 + 0

Continued

Equation and dating table for estimating gestational age (GA) from the femur length (FL)

FL (mm)	GA (WEEKS + DAYS)			FL (mm)	GA (WEEKS + DAYS)		
	50TH CENTILE	5TH CENTILE	95TH CENTILE		50TH CENTILE	5TH CENTILE	95TH CENTILE
48	26 + 1	24 + 0	20 + 3	58	30 + 4	28 + 0	33 + 4
49	26 + 4	24 + 3	29 + 0	59	31 + 1	28 + 3	34 + 1
50	27 + 0	24 + 5	29 + 3	60	31 + 4	28 + 6	34 + 4
51	27 + 3	25 + 1	30 + 0	61	32 + 1	29 + 2	35 + 1
52	27 + 6	25 + 4	30 + 3	62	32 + 4	29 + 5	35 + 5
53	28 + 2	26 + 0	31 + 0	63	33 + 1	30 + 1	36 + 2
54	28 + 5	26 + 2	31 + 3	64	33 + 4	30 + 4	36 + 6
55	29 + 2	26 + 5	32 + 0	65	34 + 1	31 + 0	37 + 3
56	29 + 5	27 + 1	32 + 3	66	34 + 4	31 + 3	38 + 0
57	30 + 1	27 + 4	33 + 0	67	35 + 1	32 + 0	38 + 5

From Loughna P, Chitty L, Evans T, Chudleigh T 2009 Fetal size and dating: charts recommended for clinical obstetric practice. Ultrasound 17(3):161–167

Equation, femur length (FL) size chart and FL size table

Equation for estimating FL from gestational age (GA):

$$FL = -32.43 + 3.416(GA) - 0.0004791(GA)^3$$

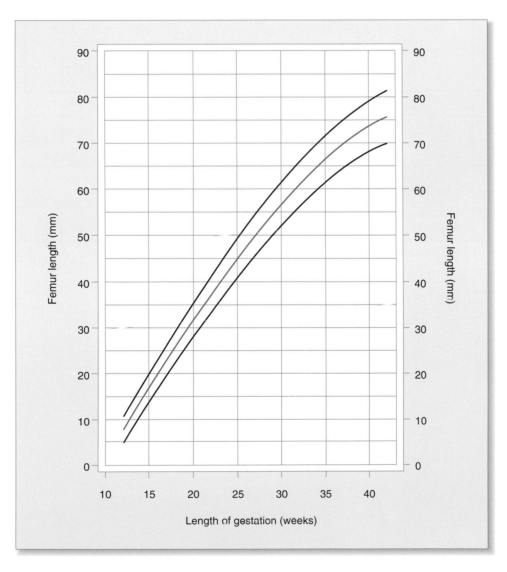

GA (WEEKS)	FL (mm)			GA (WEEKS)	FL (mm)		
	50TH CENTILE	5TH CENTILE	95TH CENTILE		50TH CENTILE	5TH CENTILE	95TH CENTILE
12	7.7	4.8	10.6	28	52.7	48.3	57.1
13	10.9	7.9	13.9	29	55.0	50.4	59.5
14	14.1	11.0	17.2	30	57.1	52.5	61.7
15	17.2	14.0	20.4	31	59.2	54.5	63.9
16	20.3	17.0	23.6	32	61.2	56.4	66.0
17	23.3	19.9	26.7	33	63.1	58.2	68.0
18	26.3	22.8	29.7	34	64.9	59.9	69.9
19	29.2	25.6	32.8	35	66.6	61.5	71.7
20	32.1	28.4	35.7	36	68.2	63.0	73.4
21	34.9	31.1	38.6	37	69.7	64.4	75.0
22	37.6	33.8	41.5	38	71.1	65.7	76.5
23	40.3	36.4	44.3	39	72.4	66.9	77.9
24	42.9	38.9	47.0	40	73.6	68.0	79.1
25	45.5	41.4	49.6	41	74.6	68.9	80.3
26	48.0	43.7	52.2	42	75.6	69.8	81.3
27	50.4	46.0	54.7				

Loughna P, Chitty L, Evans T, Chudleigh T 2009 Fetal size and dating: charts recommended for clinical obstetric practice. Ultrasound 17(3):161–167

Markers of chromosomal abnormality

MARKER	KARYOTYPE	PROBABLE RISK OF ABNORMAL KARYOTYPES LISTED IN COLUMN 2
Agenesis of corpus callosum	Trisomy 13	5%
Cardiac abnormalities	Trisomy 13, 18, 21	15%
Choroid plexus cysts	Trisomy 18	Low
Clasped or overlapping fingers	Trisomy 18	NK
Clinodactyly	Trisomy 21	NK
Cystic hygroma	45 XO, trisomy 13, 18, 21	90%
Diaphragmatic hernia	Trisomy 18	15%
Dilated ureters	Trisomy 18, 21	Low
Duodenal atresia	Trisomy 21	30%
Echogenic focus	Trisomy 21	Low
Echogenic bowel	Trisomy 21	Low
Holoprosencephaly	Trisomy 13, 18	90%
Increased nuchal translucency	Trisomy 21	75%
Increased nuchal fold	Trisomy 21	30%
Severe IUGR	Triploidy, trisomy 18	5%
Ventriculomegaly	Trisomy 21	<1%
Lateral facial cleft	Trisomy 18	<1%
Median facial cleft	Trisomy 13	50%
Multicystic renal dysplasia	Trisomy 18	Low
Non-immune hydrops	45 XO	–
Cystic hygroma	45 XO	99%
Omphalocele	Trisomy 13, 18	30%
Radial aplasia/thumb hypoplasia	Trisomy 13	90%
Rocker bottom feet	Trisomy 18	50%
Sandal gap	Trisomy 21	10%
Short femur or humerus	Trisomy 21	Low
Single umbilical artery	Trisomy 18, 21	5%
Syndactyly/polydactyly	Trisomy 13	–

The figures are the best estimate that can be obtained from the prenatal diagnosis literature.
IUGR, intrauterine growth restriction; low, these markers show a weak association with aneuploidy and on their own do not currently warrant karyotyping; not known; –, risk is not calculable in these markers; <, less than.

Index

Page numbers followed by "*f*" indicate figures, "*t*" indicate tables, and "*b*" indicate boxes.

477

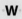
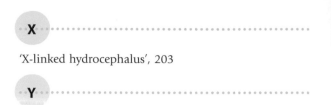